# Cancer Chemotherapy

*A Nursing Process Approach*

## Jones and Bartlett Series in Oncology

*2001 Oncology Nursing Drug Handbook,* Wilkes/Ingwersen/Barton-Burke
*American Cancer Society's Consumers Guide to Cancer Drugs,* Wilkes/Ades/Krakoff
*American Cancer Society's Patient Education Guide to Oncology Drugs,* Wilkes/Ades/Krakoff
*Biotherapy: A Comprehensive Overview, Second Edition,* Rieger
*Blood and Marrow Stem Cell Transplantation, Second Edition,* Whedon
*Cancer and HIV Clinical Nutrition Pocket Guide, Second Edition,* Wilkes
*Cancer Nursing: Principles and Practice, Fifth Edition,* Yarbro, et al.
*Cancer Symptom Management, Second Edition,* Yarbro/Frogge/Goodman
*Cancer Symptom Management, Patient Self-Care Guides, Second Edition,* Yarbro/Frogge/Goodman
*Chemotherapy Care Plans Handbook, Second Edition,* Barton-Burke/Wilkes/Ingwersen
*A Clinical Guide to Cancer Nursing, Fourth Edition,* Groenwald, et al.
*A Clinical Guide to Stem Cell and Bone Marrow Transplantation,* Shapiro, et al.
*Clinical Handbook for Biotherapy,* Rieger
*Comprehensive Cancer Nursing Review, Fourth Edition,* Groenwald, et al.
*Contemporary Issues in Prostate Cancer: A Nursing Perspective,* Held-Warmkessel
*Fatigue in Cancer: A Multidimensional Approach,* Winningham/Barton-Burke
*Handbook of Oncology Nursing, Third Edition,* Johnson/Gross
*HIV Homecare Handbook,* Daigle
*HIV Nursing and Symptom Management,* Ropka/Williams
*Homecare Management of the Bone Marrow Transplant Patient, Third Edition,* Kelley, et al.
*The Love Knot: Ties that Bind Cancer Partners,* Ross
*Medication Errors: Causes, Prevention and Risk Management,* Cohen
*Memory Bank for Chemotherapy, Third Edition,* Preston/Wilfinger
*Oncology Nursing Review,* Yarbro/Frogge/Goodman
*Oncology Nursing Society's Instruments for Clinical Nursing Research, Second Edition,* Frank-Stromborg
*Physicians' Cancer Chemotherapy Drug Manual 2001,* Chu
*Pocket Guide to Breast Cancer,* Hassey Dow
*Pocket Guide to Prostate Cancer,* Held-Warmkessel
*Pocket Guide for Women and Cancer,* Moore, et al.
*Quality of Life: From Nursing and Patient Perspectives,* King/Hinds
*Outcomes in Radiation Therapy: Multidisciplinary Management,* Bruner
*Women and Cancer: A Gynecologic Oncology Nursing Perspective, Second Edition,* Moore-Higgs, et al.

# Cancer Chemotherapy

## A Nursing Process Approach

### THIRD EDITION

**Margaret Barton-Burke, RN, PhD (c), AOCN**
Principal, Oncology Consulting Services
Boston, Massachusetts

**Gail M. Wilkes, RN, MS, AOCN**
Content Manager, CancerSource.com

**Karen C. Ingwersen, RN, MSN, OCN**
Clinical Nurse IV
Beth Israel Hospital
Boston, Massachusetts

**JONES AND BARTLETT PUBLISHERS**
*Sudbury, Massachusetts*

Boston      Toronto      London      Singapore

*World Headquarters*
Jones and Bartlett Publishers
40 Tall Pine Drive
Sudbury, MA 01776
978-443-5000
info@jbpub.com
www.jbpub.com

Jones and Bartlett Publishers Canada
2406 Nikanna Road
Mississauga, ON L5C 2W6
CANADA

Jones and Bartlett Publishers International
Barb House, Barb Mews
London W6 7PA
UK

**Library of Congress Cataloging-in-Publication Data**

Cancer chemotherapy: a nursing process approach/[edited by] Margaret Barton-Burke, Gail Wilkes, Karen Ingwersen.—3rd ed.
     p.; cm.
   Includes bibliographical references and index.
   ISBN 0-7637-1472-0
   1. Cancer—Nursing. 2. Cancer—Chemotherapy. I. Barton-Burke, Margaret. II. Wilkes, Gail M. III. Ingwersen, Karen. IV. Cancer chemotherapy.
   [DNLM: 1. Neoplasms—nursing. 2. Antineoplastic Agents—therapeutic use—Nurses' Instruction. 3. Neoplasms—drug therapy—Nurses' Instruction. WY 156 C213 2001]
RC266 .C34 2001
616.99'4061—dc21

00-062678

*Production Credits*
Acquisitions Editor: Penny M. Glynn
Associate Editor: Christine Tridente
Production Editor: AnnMarie Lemoine
Editorial Assistant: Thomas Prindle
Manufacturing Buyer: Amy Duddridge
Cover Design: Stephanie Torta
Interior Design: Argosy
Composition: Argosy
Printing and Binding: Malloy Lithographing

Printed in the United States of America
05 04 03 02 01    10 9 8 7 6 5 4 3 2 1

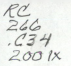
The drug information presented in CANCER CHEMOTHERAPY: A NURSING PROCESS APPROACH has been adapted from manufacturers' current package inserts, standard reference sources, and current research literature on cancer chemotherapy. As such, the information contained in this book has not been tested, verified, or screened by the publisher or authors. The writers and publisher of this book have made every effort to ensure that the dosage regimens set forth in the text are accurate and in accord with current labeling at the time of publication. However, in view of the constant flow of information resulting from ongoing research and clinical experience, as well as changes in government regulations, readers are urged to check the package insert and consult with a pharmacist, if necessary, for each drug that they plan to administer to be certain that changes have not been made in the drug's indications or contraindications or in the recommended dosage for each use. This is particularly important when a drug is new or infrequently employed. While the drugs in this publication were chosen on the basis of frequency of use and appropriate indications, the publisher and authors do not necessarily advocate, and take no responsibility for, the use of the products described herein.

The selection and dosage of drugs presented in this book are in accord with standards accepted at the time of publication. The authors, editors, and publisher have made every effort to provide accurate information. However, research, clinical practice, and government regulations often change the accepted standard in this field. Before administering any drug, the reader is advised to check the manufacturer's product information sheet for the most up-to-date recommendations on dosage, precautions, and contraindications. This is especially important in the case of drugs that are new or seldom used.

# Contents

## PART I    From the Advent of Chemotherapy to Current Research: The Cancer Nurse's Role

### Chapter 1    Oncology Nursing Practice: The Role of the Nurse in Support of Progress in Cancer Treatment    3
*Jean Jenkins, PhD, RN*

### Chapter 2    Cell Cycle Kinetics and Antineoplastic Agents    23
*Karen C. Ingwersen, RN, MSN*

## PART II   Cancer Chemotherapy: Mechanisms and Nursing Care

**Chapter 5    Chemotherapeutic Agents: Standardized Nursing Care Plans
to Minimize Toxicity    187**

**Chapter 6     Drug Interactions in the Cancer Chemotherapy Patient     534**
*Reginald S. King, PharmD*

# PART III  Clinical Application

**Chapter 7     Pediatric Aspects of Cancer Chemotherapy     559**
*Vanessa C. Howard, RN, MSN, FNP*
*Martha May, RN, MSN, FNP*

**Chapter 8     Chemotherapy in the Elderly: Considerations for Clinical Practice     590**
*Constance Engelking, RN, MS*

# Appendices

# Preface to the Third Edition

Ten years ago, I was a member of a group of oncology nurses from the greater Boston area who came together to discuss the idea of a cancer chemotherapy textbook for nurses. Back then there were few books written on the topic, and as a group we asked the question, Who are we to write a book on cancer chemotherapy? We answered that question somewhat naively: "If we don't write it, someone else will. And besides, why shouldn't we write it when we care for patients receiving chemotherapy every day!" That was the beginning of our foray into the world of publishing, where we blended our clinical skills with the expertise of our authors.

The textbook, *Cancer Chemotherapy: A Nursing Process Approach*, was the book that was conceptualized ten years ago. The trifeminate group of authors who developed that book is involved in a trilogy of cancer nursing books, *Cancer Chemotherapy: A Nursing Process Approach*, *Chemotherapy Care Plans Handbook*, and the *2001 Oncology Nursing Drug Handbook*. These works focus on the medications—chemotherapy in particular—used to treat cancer and the nursing care required to care for the person receiving cancer drugs. The nursing process forms the basis for the oncology nurse's scope of practice, and the corresponding nursing diagnoses are integral to appropriate nursing care. Both process and diagnosis become the threads that pull this book together. More than in previous versions, this, the third edition of our text, integrates the nursing process, including nursing diagnosis, with the administration of cancer chemotherapeutic agents. All medication information, care plans, as well as all additional documentation in this book are vital to the safe administration of cancer chemotherapy.

Since publication of the first edition, not only have ten years passed, but a new millennium has begun in cancer care, which has grown in leaps and bounds. In addition to many minor changes in the field of oncology, we have seen major changes as well. These include the biotechnology explosion, an understanding of the human genome, and a partnership between drug companies and regulators whereby more cancer-fighting drugs are produced for human use more rapidly than ever before. Additionally, knowledge about cancer chemotherapeutic agents has grown substantially, and the number and type of available cancer chemotherapeutic agents have more than doubled since this book was first published.

Regardless of the strides that have been made in the field of oncology nursing and regardless of the knowledge that has been gained during the past ten years, the fact remains that people still get cancer. This cancer still needs to be treated, usually with chemotherapy, and the administration of cancer chemotherapy still requires specialized knowledge so that drugs are given safely and patients remain the focus of our care. Therefore, the bulk of this book is Chapter 5, *"Chemotherapeutic Agents,"* along with corresponding care plans. Prior to and following this major chapter, the remainder of the book augments, substantiates, and clarifies the safe administration of cancer chemotherapy. Thus, this volume becomes an enduring product, constantly in need of update but always a foundation for safe nursing care of the cancer chemotherapy patient.

The information provided in this text can be augmented with the detailed information from our other textbooks. Additionally, the second edition of the Oncology Nursing Society's *Cancer Chemotherapy Guidelines and Recommendations for Practice* is a recommended companion text for all nurses who are administering or caring for individuals receiving cancer chemotherapy.

Finally, the information in Cancer Chemotherapy is not meant to replace any hospital formulary or manufacturer's information. The authors and publishers of this book have made every effort to ensure that information and dosage regimens presented in the text are accurate and in accordance with current labeling practices at the time of publication. However, in view of the constant and rapid flow of information resulting from ongoing research and clinical experience, as well as changes in government regulations, nurses are urged to check the package insert and consult with a pharmacist, when necessary, for each drug they plan to administer to be certain that changes have not been made in indications or contraindications or in the recommended dosage for each use. This is particularly important when a drug is new or infrequently used.

# Preface to the Second Edition

Since the first edition of this book was published in 1991, enormous changes have occurred in both the organization and the structure of the health care system. Consequently, these changes have affected the practices of both oncology nursing and medicine. Significantly impacting oncology practice is the shift of cancer care from the inpatient hospital to outpatient clinic, office, and home settings. Additionally, the movement away from the specialist role toward the generalist impacts oncology nursing in particular.

One reason for this impact is that chemotherapy treatments, clinical trials, and other forms of cancer therapy, e.g., bone marrow transplant and colony stimulating factors, are being given in environments no longer under the strict control of either the nurse or the doctor. In fact, symptom management, once the purview of the nurse, is being shared with the clients and their significant other(s). Meanwhile, patient education, nursing's bailiwick, is brief and concise with innovative and creative ways to assess what has been learned about disease and treatment. More important, nurses in many practice settings are being expected to administer chemotherapeutic agents with minimal clinical training and

didactic education. Even more frightening is the move toward medication administration by trained technicians!

This book has as its foundation the Oncology Nursing Society's (ONS) *Cancer Chemotherapy Guidelines and Recommendations for Practice*. In the 1996 guidelines, as in previous editions, ONS recommends that registered nurses—with proper theoretical and clinical training—be the individuals responsible for administering cancer chemotherapeutic agents. The authors of this textbook concur and continue to hold that the nursing process is fundamental to nursing care.

As in the first edition, the nursing process, including nursing diagnosis and care plans, remains the framework for this textbook. The suggested care plans are intended to be individualized and the reader is reminded that not all interventions are appropriate for all clients. The static-appearing care plans, based on the American Nurses Association (ANA)/Oncology Nursing Society (ONS) Standards for Oncology Nursing Practice, are intended to be guidelines adapted to the ever-changing needs of the client.

However, the second edition of this book has intentionally broadened the conceptualizations of chemotherapy, nursing care, and the client. The increased knowledge of the biologic processes that result in cancer combined with the ability to modify these biologic responses permit oncology nurses to rethink the extent of cancer chemotherapy. Because of the ability of chemical agents to alter cellular biology, these agents are now considered biologic response modifiers, along with biological agents. Consequently, a nurse's knowledge of oncology, chemical and biological agents, and the nursing care for the person receiving such therapy must expand as well. The sheer number of new agents makes it increasingly difficult to remember all the particular elements related to specific chemotherapeutic protocols. Thus this textbook attempts to be comprehensive and up-to-date. Finally, nurses have always treated children and adults with chemotherapy. However, the current climate in the health care system suggests that the age of the client receiving chemotherapy will increase from what is currently the norm. The field of geriatric oncology is a rapidly expanding one with oncology nurses becoming experts in this field.

Additionally in the revised edition of this book the authors have painstakingly expanded areas of practice that are at the forefront of chemotherapy usage in the mid-1990s. As in the first edition, the book is organized into three parts.

Part I, **From the Advent of Chemotherapy to Current Research: The Cancer Nurse's Role,** has been expanded to include two new chapters. Chapter 3 on biotherapy, the fourth treatment modality for cancer, is unique in the author's discussion of biotherapy and in her inclusion of the synergy between chemotherapeutic and biological agents. Chapter 4 describes what is on the horizon for chemotherapy, including such topics as bone marrow transplantation, colony

stimulating factors, drug resistance, and chemoprevention.

Part II, **Cancer Chemotherapy: Mechanisms and Nursing Care,** forms the substantive content for the book. In the five years since the first edition, the scientific knowledge about families of chemotherapeutic agents, not only their classification, has burgeoned and relates directly to the number and type of chemotherapeutic agents cited within Chapter 6. Second generations of commonly known agents are becoming the norm. In Chapter 6 drug information has almost doubled to include the number of agents currently in use, as well as those under investigation. Additionally, Chapter 7, on drug interactions, offers a unique perspective concerning clients who receive chemotherapy. In fact, many patients are on other drugs that may cause serious drug interactions or negate the efficacy of chemotherapy. The impact of this area of scientific inquiry is just beginning to be understood.

Finally Part III, **Clinical Application**, has been expanded by adding two chapters, 8 and 9, which include aspects of chemotherapy administration in the pediatric as well as the geriatric population. The former group, pediatric oncology, has been leading chemotherapy science. It is through the use of pediatric clinical trials that amazing cure as well as remission rates have been achieved. However, in the adult population less than 5 percent of all cancer patients are treated on protocol and until recently the geriatric group has been disenfranchised from aggressive chemotherapy treatments and clinical trials. A new focus on both of these specialty areas is explored in this edition.

Appendices present helpful reference material, including Appendix 3, the 1995 Occupational and Safety Health Administration (OSHA) Guidelines in their entirety, and Appendix 9, the Yellow Pages for Cancer Chemotherapy.

The additions to the book serve to illustrate the comprehensive nature of chemotherapy in the 1990s. The book is intended for use by novice as well as advanced practice oncology nurses and the authors are proud to bring this updated edition to you.

# Preface to the First Edition

The original intent of the authors was to develop a quick reference for nurses working with chemotherapeutic agents. The result was a text with an in depth discussion of side effects, administration techniques, and corresponding nursing diagnoses. The care plans suggested by the authors are intended to be individualized for the patient receiving chemotherapy for cancer. While reading this text, keep in mind that not all interventions are appropriate for all patients.

The care plans in this book are presented to the reader with a specific time focus. By this we mean that both patient care and nursing care should be revised constantly. Individualized care should be adapted to the ever changing needs of the patient. Thus, the static care plans in this text are intended to be guidelines from which the practitioner builds an individualized care plan for a patient receiving chemotherapy. The care plans are based on the American Nursing Association (ANA)/Oncology Nursing Society (ONS) Standards for Oncology Nursing Practice.

This book supplements other oncology nursing textbooks and provides "hands on" information to assist the nurse in providing comprehensive care to the patients receiving chemotherapy and to their family. It is designed to be used as a quick reference for more than forty chemotherapeutic agents available in practice settings. The focus of the text is on the chemotherapeutic agents, their side effects, the corresponding nursing diagnoses and care plans, and safe methods of administration and handling of these drugs.

Part I **reviews the history of chemotherapy and the role of the oncology nurse in current chemotherapy research.** In Chapter 1 the authors explore the history of chemotherapy in the treatment of cancer. In addition, the evolution of oncology nursing as a specialty area of practice is discussed. Concluding this chapter is the nursing process theory, which blends the science of chemotherapy administration with the art of nursing care provided for the oncology patient population. Chapter 2 looks at the various professional nursing roles that have evolved since chemotherapy became a standard treatment modality for many persons with cancer.

Part II **provides the core of the whole text—how the drugs work and nursing care plans on major side effects of individual drugs.** Chapter 3 discusses cell cycle kinetics and builds the necessary foundation for the subsequent chapters of the book. Chapter 4 provides an in-depth discussion on the potential side effects of chemotherapy. Standardized nursing care plans are presented that address potential drug toxicities in terms of nursing diagnoses and recommend nursing interventions and outcome criteria based on ANA/ONS practice guidelines. Chapter 5 is the heart of the textbook, where the reader will find the chemotherapeutic agents and abridged version of the care plans from Chapter 4. Standardized nursing care plans are concise and address the potential toxicities specific to each chemotherapeutic agent. The intent is to enable the practitioner to provide safe and effective nursing care to patients receiving chemotherapy.

Part III **reviews technical procedures for administration and safe handling of antineoplastic agents.** Chapters 6 and 7 discuss administration techniques, and include safety checklists and recommendations for management of untoward reactions. Chapter 8 covers the safe handling of antineoplastic agents.

Appendices present helpful reference material, such as acronyms for chemotherapeutic drug regimens, standard doses for accepted drug regimens, and a quick reference chart for common drug side effects.

This text is meant to be used by the advanced practitioner and the novice alike. The theoretical framework is based on nursing diagnosis and standards for nursing practice. Most of the nursing diagnoses included in the text are those approved by the North American Nursing Diagnosis Association (NANDA). The ONS standards of practice and guidelines for care of the person receiving cancer chemotherapy are the theoretical framework for the text.

The beginning practitioner will not only be able to use the nursing diagnoses in the text but will be able to review the basic principles of chemotherapy administration and content on chemotherapeutic agents. The advanced practitioner may use the text as a reference guide.

# Acknowledgements

A book like this does not get written, edited, and produced on its own. There are many people who contribute to the success of the content, as well as the finished product. So we wish to thank the contributing authors, who provided the knowledge upon which this book is founded. We also thank Cathleen Collins Yetman for her copy editing expertise and for helping to make the finished product complete. And we thank Jones and Bartlett Publishers and Argosy.

More importantly, we especially want to acknowledge the people with cancer we have cared for and their family members. They have taught us a great deal about cancer, nursing, and life.

We thank our respective families as well, for without their love, support, and encouragement, projects such as this book would not come to fulfillment. These family members make all the hard work worthwhile.

And finally, I thank my husband. Twenty-six years ago Thom became my mentor and editorial guide, and the knowledge that I (MBB) have gained about writing and life I have learned from this man.

*Margaret Barton-Burke*
*Gail M. Wilkes*
*Karen C. Ingwersen*

# Contributors

**Margaret Barton-Burke**, RN, PhD (c.), AOCN
Principal
Oncology Consulting Services
Boston, Massachusetts

**Constance Engelking**, RN, MS, OCN
Oncology Clinical Nurse Specialist
Westchester County Medical Center
Valhalla, New York

**Vanessa Howard**, RN, MSN, FNP
St. Jude Children's Research Hospital
Memphis, Tennessee

**Karen C. Ingwersen**, RN, MSN, OCN
Clinical Nurse IV
Beth Israel-Deaconess Hospital
Boston, Massachusetts

**Jean F. Jenkins**, RN, PhD, FAAN
Clinical Nurse Specialist
National Cancer Institute
Bethesda, Maryland

**Cynthia R. King**, RN, NP, PhD, FAAN
Nurse Consultant
Special Care Consultants
Rochester, New York

**Reginald S. King**, PharmD, BCOP
Clinical Specialist, Oncology/Bone Marrow
Transplant
Department of Pharmacy
Hahnemann University Hospital
Philadelphia, Pennsylvania

**Martha Langhorne**, MSN, RN, FNP, AOCN
Advanced Practice Nurse
UHS Hospitals & UHS Cancer Care Center
Johnson City, New York

**Martha May**, RN, MSN, FNP
St. Jude Children's Research Hospital
Memphis, Tennessee

**Gail Egan Sansivero**, MS, ANP, AOCN
Nurse Practitioner
The Institute for Vascular Health and Disease
Albany Medical College
Albany, New York

**Gail M. Wilkes**, RN, MS, ANP, AOCN
Content Manager
CancerSource.com
Sudbury, Massachusetts

## Part I

# *From the Advent of Chemotherapy to Current Research*

## *The Cancer Nurse's Role*

# Chapter 1

# Oncology Nursing Practice: The Role of the Nurse in Support of Progress in Cancer Treatment

**Jean Jenkins, PhD, RN**

## EVOLUTION OF ONCOLOGY NURSING

It is a challenging and exciting time for oncology nurses who care for patients receiving chemotherapy. The challenges to nurses are enormous but the professional and personal rewards can be of equal magnitude. Oncology nursing has not always offered these opportunities. Nurses caring for patients with cancer at the turn of the century provided supportive care for patients who felt "isolated and doomed" (Given 1980). As the ability to cure, control, and palliate tumors improved with advances in treatment and supportive measures, the role of nurses became more specialized.

In 1955, the National Cancer Institute (NCI) initiated the Cooperative Clinical Trials Research Program to test new anticancer agents from the NCI's drug development program. The nurse on the clinical research team functioned mainly as a data collector (Henke 1980). As clinical trials became more complex, the research nurse became the liaison with other members of the health care team, coordinating the protocol, answering questions about the research study, and administering the investigational chemotherapy. Perhaps most importantly, the research nurse was the patient's advocate, providing counsel and support. In addition, the expanded role of the nurse included educating the patient and monitoring the patient's response to therapy. The clinical research team with active collaboration in research was seen as a model for cancer care, and the integration of the nurse as a contributing member to research outcomes required expanded knowledge (Hubbard and Gross 1994).

In 1956, the federal government provided educational traineeship grants for cancer nursing education. As the role of chemotherapy as a treatment modality emerged, nurses in large medical centers began administering chemotherapy, sharing the responsibility with physicians (Dangle and Flynn 1987). These nurses became chemotherapy specialists. Chemotherapy in smaller hospitals continued to be the physician's responsibility with the nurse monitoring the patient's response to drug administration.

In 1971, the National Cancer Act provided funds for cancer nursing education and research (Dangle and Flynn 1987), and in 1973 the American Cancer Society sponsored the First National Conference on Cancer Nursing. As the profession of oncology nursing grew, nurses felt a need for collegial support, education, and networking. In 1974, these small interest groups joined together to form a national organization, the Oncology Nursing Society (ONS). Annual ONS Congresses provide cancer nursing education and support and a way for nurses to remain current in this rapidly expanding specialty. Oncology nurses today work to develop the knowledge and skills required in the care of patients receiving chemotherapy in conjunction with other modalities. Currently, oncology nurses enhance the care of patients with cancer through collaborative and independent nursing research that facilitates biomedical research outcomes and improves the patient's ability to live with the chronic illness of cancer.

In this past decade, most oncology nurses became responsible for the administration of chemotherapy. Chemotherapy education programs, providing the theoretical principles for practice, were developed according to ONS and Occupational Safety and Health Administration (OSHA 1993) guidelines. These programs are given in conjunction with a guided clinical practicum, where nurses new to chemotherapy administration can develop skills safely and competently.

The ONS in conjunction with the American Nurses Association (ANA) developed standards of cancer nursing practice that identify specific professional practice and performance standards for the general oncology nurse. These standards identify specific nursing behaviors that permit safe, competent, high-quality patient and family care. A summary of ONS Standards, revised in 1996, appears in Table 1.1. Advanced Practice Standards, developed by the ONS in 1990, expands the concepts of practice roles within the oncology specialty. These roles include clinical nurse specialist, educator, researcher, and administrator.

## THE UNIQUE ROLE OF THE NURSE IN CANCER CHEMOTHERAPY

"Making a nursing diagnosis" is the process of collecting information through assessment and using this information to make judgments about the patient's need for care (Gordon 1987, p.3). "Nursing diagnosis" refers not only to the process of diagnosing but also to the diagnostic judgment reached, which is expressed in a category name (Gordon 1987, p.7).

In the practice of oncology, nurses work intimately with physicians and the drugs they prescribe, specifically chemotherapy. At times, the lines become blurred regarding what are dependent, independent, and collaborative responsibilities when discussing patient care and medical and nursing practice. This text assists the nurse in understanding and translating the specific information about chemotherapy and the nursing care required for safe practice. The care of patients receiving chemotherapy provides fertile ground for innovative clinical nursing practice, and this practice evolves from accurate patient assessment and identification of nursing diagnoses.

The nursing process is the foundation on which nursing care is based. The process includes the following:

- assessment
- diagnosis
- planning
- intervention
- evaluation

### Assessment

Many nurses are uncomfortable using nursing diagnosis. Guzzetta, Bunton, Prinkey, Sherer, and Seifert (1989) believe

**Table 1.1**  Nursing Approaches to Cancer Care: The Oncology Nursing Scope and Standards

**ONS Professional Practice Standards, 1996 (Revised)**

1. The oncology nurse *applies theoretical concepts* as a basis for decisions in practice.

2. The oncology nurse *systematically and continually collects data* regarding the health status of the client, the data are recorded, accessible, and communicated to appropriate members of the multidisciplinary team . . . collects data in the following high-incidence areas:

   a. prevention and early detection
   b. information
   c. coping
   d. comfort
   e. nutrition
   f. protective mechanisms
   g. mobility
   h. elimination
   i. sexuality
   j. ventilation
   k. circulation

3. The oncology nurse *analyzes assessment data* in determining nursing diagnoses.

4. The oncology nurse *identifies expected outcomes* individualized to the client.

5. The oncology nurse *develops an outcome-oriented plan of care* that is individualized and holistic. This plan is based on nursing diagnoses and incorporates preventive, therapeutic, rehabilitative, palliative, and comforting nursing actions to attain expected outcomes.

6. The oncology nurse *implements the nursing plan of care* to achieve the identified outcomes for the client.

7. The oncology nurse *regularly and systematically evaluates the client's responses* to interventions in order to determine the progress toward achievement of expected outcomes and to revise the database, the nursing diagnoses, and the plan of care.

8. The oncology nurse *assumes responsibility for professional development and continuing education and contributes* to the professional growth of others.

9. The oncology nurse *collaborates with the client, the significant others, and the multidisciplinary team* in assessing, planning, implementing, and evaluating care.

10. The oncology nurse *evaluates the quality of care and the effectiveness of oncology practice* in relationship to practice standards, statutes, and regulations.

11. The oncology nurse's *decisions and actions on behalf of clients are determined in an ethical manner.*

12. The oncology nurse *contributes to the scientific base* of nursing practice and the field of oncology *through the review and the application of research.*

*Source:* Adapted from American Nurses' Association. (1996). *ANA and ONS: Statement on the Scope and Standards of Oncology Nursing Practice.* Washington, D.C.: American Nurses' Association. Reprinted with permission.

this discomfort can be traced to a fundamental gap between assessment and formulation of nursing diagnoses. An initial objective nursing assessment is needed for planning care. This assessment should be based on standards of practice. Systematic assessment of the patient is the basic tenet of the nursing process and professional nursing practice. Debate continues within the nursing profession as to whether the tool (structure) or the data gathering (process) is the key to successful nursing process. This text is not meant to endorse either the structure or the process. It does assume that patients must have a comprehensive assessment if a nursing diagnosis is to be made. Guzzetta et al. (1989) assert that if nurses make an incorrect assessment, and collect non-nursing data, they will continue to have problems with nursing perspective, and the appropriate data necessary to assess the patient will not be obtained. The tool used for collecting data does not matter; several assessment tools are available in practice. Many of these tools are institution specific. Some are based on the functional health patterns identified by Gordon (1987).

This text suggests a manageable structure to evaluate the vast amount of information needed to assess a patient prior to administering chemotherapy. The chapters offer assessment criteria in relevant domains:

- biophysical, as in intravenous site selection, degree of bone marrow suppression, and condition of oral mucosa prior to therapy
- cognitive-affective, as in assessing the level of readiness to learn and what information needs to be taught, and
- psychosocial, as in the practitioner's ability to be sensitive to the impact of the diagnosis of cancer and the patient's fear of treatment

## Diagnosis

In 1973, the North American Nursing Diagnosis Association (NANDA), formerly the National Group for the Classification of Nursing Diagnosis, published its first list of nursing diagnoses. Since that time, the interest in nursing diagnosis and its application in clinical settings has grown substantially (Carpenito 1997, 2000).

NANDA continually reviews and updates the approved list of diagnostic categories. The diagnoses previously accepted tend toward descriptions, such as hypothermia, fatigue, and ineffective breast-feeding. NANDA continues the work of renaming the older, more awkward diagnoses, for example, "skin integrity, impaired, actual" (Tribulski 1988). Experience with the cumbersome language of nursing diagnosis has taught the profession a valuable lesson in practicality. This text is one more step toward the practical use of nursing diagnosis in the care of patients with cancer who receive chemotherapy.

Nursing diagnosis is meant to be a shorthand term that helps the nurse make an intellectual jump directly to standards, goals, and interventions. Nursing diagnosis or problem identification in nursing practice is included in revisions of nurse practice acts. Therefore, accountability for nursing interventions, or a nurse's explicit responsibility to a consumer, should be reflected in the nurse's professional practice. The definition of "nursing diagnosis" states that diagnoses are made by professional nurses (Gordon 1987). The revised *ANA and ONS: Statement on the Scope and Standards of Oncology Nursing Practice* (American Nurses' Association 1996) clearly delineates the responsibility of nurses caring for patients with cancer to use nursing diagnoses. Commonly used nursing diagnoses for patients with cancer are listed at the end of the *ONS Scope and Standards*.

Cancer nursing is complex. The complexity of a patient's condition requires that nursing care be comprehensive. Through the language of nursing diagnoses, both the beginning practitioner (novice) and the expert can diagnose clients' conditions using the same terminology.

## Planning

One difference between the novice and the expert is in the repertoire of experiences from which the practitioner develops a plan of care. The care plan serves as a communication tool for the nursing staff. It describes the specific problems or needs of the client and prescribes interventions for directing and evaluating care (Carpenito 1997). Carpenito identifies the following purposes for care planning:

- blueprint to direct charting
- communication tool identifying to the nursing staff what to teach, what to observe, and what to implement
- specific intervention for the individual, the family, and other nursing staff members to implement
- evaluation and review of prescribed care

The plan of care, as prescribed by both the nurse and the physician, is goal directed toward the cure, the stabilization, or the palliation of cancer and the optimization of response to treatment. The authors of this text have attempted to establish priorities of care for the patient receiving specific chemotherapeutic agents. In addition, they have developed nursing care plans based on dependent, independent, and collaborative nursing orders. The plans in Chapter 4 are elaborate in nature but illustrate the maximum care involved with a given diagnosis. They are based on ONS guidelines for the care of patients with cancer. In Chapter 5, an abridged edition of the care plans is included in addition to the fact sheets on chemotherapeutic agents. These plans are meant to be used as a quick reference outlining what the nurse needs to know when administering a specific chemotherapeutic agent.

An additional tool that is now available to facilitate goal setting and measurement of health care quality is the Nursing Outcome Classification (NOC) system (Johnson, Maas, and Moorhead 2000). These patient-focused outcomes provide measures for outcomes that respond to nursing intervention. This standardized nomenclature should be considered in setting expectations and in monitoring direct and indirect caregiving.

## Intervention

Intervention is the actual process of giving care to the patient. The administration of chemotherapy involves knowledge of drug pharmacology and tumor kinetics, patient assessment parameters, and techniques of physical examination. Technical expertise is based on the principles of (1) intravenous therapy and use of venous access devices, (2) drug administration and safe handling of antineoplastic agents, and (3) adult learning.

Most patients receive chemotherapy in an ambulatory setting, so there are time constraints on the nurse-patient interaction. Nurses administering chemotherapy evaluate their patients' tolerance to past chemotherapy and make recommendations for changes in antiemetic therapy to prevent or optimize the control of nausea and vomiting. Nurses take responsibility for educating patients in self-care measures so that patients and their families are able to care for themselves in such a way that tolerance of chemotherapy is optimized.

Nursing interventions core to specialty practice can be used to document and research the effectiveness of nurse-patient interaction (McCloskey, Bulechek, and Donahue 1998). The Nursing Intervention Classification (NIC) system was developed through research at the University of Iowa College of Nursing (McCloskey and Bulechek 2000). These interventions can link to NANDA nursing diagnosis to facilitate selection of nursing interventions appropriate for individuals, families, and communities.

## Evaluation

Evaluation is the final step in the nursing process. When discussing the nursing process, evaluation has different purposes. The first is evaluation of the written plan of care. The second is evaluation of the patient's progress. The third is evaluation of the timeliness of the care plan.

The authors remind the reader that the nursing diagnoses and care plans in this book are a "snapshot" picture in time. These care plans provide a framework by which the nurse can understand the principles and the practice of chemotherapy administration in order to give chemotherapy safely. That is to say, the nurse must know the correct information about the drug in order to administer it safely and to be an informed participant in the treatment; to diagnose and care for the client effectively; and to evaluate the patient's response to nursing care and treatment.

## THE UNIQUE ROLE OF THE NURSE IN CANCER RESEARCH

Through clinical trials, new agents are discovered that enhance the options available to patients with cancer. Nurses continue to expand their contributions to the successful implementation of such clinical trials. The variety of roles assumed by nurses are reviewed after providing an introduction to clinical trials.

## THE DEVELOPMENT OF THE NATIONAL CANCER INSTITUTE AND ANTICANCER DRUG RESEARCH

Clinical chemotherapy research began when the U.S. Public Health Service created the Office of Field Investigations in Cancer at Harvard University in the 1930s. In 1939, the office moved to Bethesda, Maryland, to become part of the newly formed National Cancer Institute (NCI) (Zubrod 1984). A brief history of cancer research support follows:

**1945** NCI satellite units at U.S. Public Health Service Hospital, Baltimore; University of California, San Francisco; George Washington University Medical School, Washington, D.C.

**1953** Establishment of the Clinical Center (hospital) at the National Institutes of Health (NIH); $1 million appropriated by Congress for leukemia research.

**1955** Establishment of the Cancer Chemotherapy National Service Center (CCNSC) at NCI; Clinical Trials Cooperative Groups sponsored at academic institutions and cancer treatment centers.

**1971** National Cancer Act passed by Congress; $100 million approved for cancer research, leading to the development of the National Cancer Program, and the Division of Cancer Treatment, NCI, NIH.

**1990** NCI Designated Comprehensive Cancer Centers guidelines established; NCI Designated Cancer Centers Public Affairs Network formed.

**1992** SPOREs (Specialized Programs of Research Excellence) established to target breast, prostate, and lung cancer basic and clinical research advances.

**1994** NIH Revitalization Act mandates inclusion of women and minorities in NIH funded clinical trials.

**1998** Legislation required the NIH to broaden the public's access to information about clinical trials.

**1999** NCI launched the Cancer Genetics Network, a collaborative infrastructure to facilitate the study of the genetic basis of cancer susceptibility and clinical outcomes.

**2000** Launching of a clinical trials website at http://cancertrials.nci.nih.gov as part of an NCI initiative, the National Clinical Trials Program.

The establishment in 1955 of the CCNSC initiated a significant drug program for cancer research. The CCNSC functioned as a pharmaceutical house run by the NCI that moved agents quickly and safely into clinical trials. In 1965, the program was expanded to review investigational drugs that, upon receiving Investigational New Drug (IND) approval, are moved into clinical trials across the country (Zubrod 1984). Additionally, the NCI's Natural Products Branch (set-up in 1986) coordinates programs directed at the discovery and the development of novel naturally derived agents to treat cancer and AIDS. Through drug-screening mechanisms at the NCI, new agents that appear to have promise in cell line and animal testing are moved into clinical trials with humans.

The Division of Cancer Treatment of the NCI at the NIH plays a major role in cancer research and anticancer drug development. Pharmaceutical companies increasingly are cosponsoring basic and clinical research with the NCI to facilitate and share in the extensive drug testing and approval for commercial use of successful agents (Wittes 1987).

The goal of the NCI and the pharmaceutical industry is to define the activity of new anti-cancer drugs and to make those drugs available to patients with cancer as quickly as possible. The objective of this clinical research is to improve the survival and the quality of life of patients with cancer. Clinical trials provide the methodology to evaluate the toxicity and the effectiveness of new agents. A revitalized system exists for NCI-sponsored clinical trials to facilitate access, development of new ideas, education, and communication. The National Institutes of Health also launched a consumer-friendly database that gives easy access to information about research studies at http://clinicaltrials.gov (Ehrenberger 2000). Hopefully, these websites and other outreach initiatives will reduce barriers and thus enhance access to clinical trial participation by all interested (National Cancer Institute 1999; Wittes and Silva 1999).

The NCI is expanding clinical trials to include studies that are based on molecular targets of prevention and treatment. The pathway to the development of treatments of the future will be based on the cell's signature (National Cancer Institute 1999). Dramatic advances in the understanding of the human genome, the potential influence of genetics for cancer risk, and even drug effectiveness have opened up new opportunities. Nurses should integrate into their repertoire this new knowledge about genetics that ultimately will be the foundation of large-scale clinical trials for patients with or at risk for cancer (Lea, Jenkins, and Francomano 1998).

## CLINICAL TRIALS

A clinical trial is a research study carefully and ethically designed to answer the question of whether a treatment has therapeutic implications (Hubbard and Gross 1994). Also, a clinical trial is a research study that strives to demonstrate a tolerable dose of a drug or drugs, the effects of the drug(s), and the effectiveness of the drug(s) against disease. The hope is to see some evidence of therapeutic improvement that ultimately can be extended to all patients (Livingston and Carter 1982). In cancer clinical trials, the ultimate goals are to help improve the patient's quality of life and to improve survival rates.

The development of anticancer agents has increased greatly due to the success of clinical trials (Carter 1977). Although cell line testing and animal studies can give an idea of what can be expected in terms of toxicity or efficacy, it is only through clinical testing that information regarding the effects of the agents on humans can be obtained (Reich 1982a). Experiments with drug therapies on humans have occurred since ancient times. It was not until the nineteenth century that the need for systematic experiments was stressed in the medical community (Bull 1959). Today, it is extremely unusual for any new therapy to be released for commercial use without undergoing multiple clinical studies to determine therapeutic effectiveness and toxicity (Reich 1982a). The underlying assumption of any good clinical trial is that the agent is worth testing. Other practical considerations include access to the population, numbers of subjects needed, cost considerations, ethical considerations, technical feasibility, competence of the proposed researcher, and scientific merit of the study (Cancer Therapy Evaluation Program 1993).

The facilitation of study implementation and validation of study outcomes rely on the investigator writing a protocol or a proposal that clearly delineates the components of the study. The investigator must define why the study is being done, provide a framework of who is to be included as study participants, and describe how the agent's effects will be evaluated. The protocol also delineates the proposed clinical procedure, including how the agent is administered, and what parameters will be monitored, to ensure that interpretable and generalizable data are available. Table 1.2 lists the essential components of a scientific protocol.

The importance of the introduction and the rationale for the study in the protocol is that it provides the framework of justification for why the agent(s) is being tested. Critical to the protocol are the study objectives because these define the hypothesis that is being tested and the pur-

**Table 1.2  Components of a Scientific Protocol**

1. Objective(s)
2. Introduction and Rationale for the Study
3. Patient Eligibility Criteria
4. Pharmaceutical Information
5. Treatment Plan
6. Procedures for Patient Entry on Study
7. Dose Modification for Toxicity
8. Criteria for Response Assessment
9. Monitoring of Patients
10. Off-Study Criteria
11. Statistical Considerations
12. Record to Be Kept
13. Resources
14. References
15. Informed Consent

*Source:* Cancer Therapy Evaluation Program (CTEP). (1993). *Investigator's Handbook.* Washington, D.C.: National Cancer Institute. http://ctep.info.nih.gov

pose of the study. Patient selection defines the criteria patients must meet in order to be eligible for the study. The study design, the treatment plan, the monitoring parameters, and the pharmaceutical information are all important details for the health care provider interpreting and providing care to patients in clinical trials. Statistical criteria include the number of patients required to answer the questions proposed by the study. Records to be kept, resources for protocol questions, and references about the study also are included in the protocol format or in appendices. Crucial to any clinical trial is informed consent. This description of the study in layperson's terms outlines the study, the expected toxicities, and other resource information for study participants to read and sign prior to study entry. It is essential that the patient willingly enter into a trial with a full understanding of what the study entails. The responsibility to ensure patient understanding is that of the investigator, physician, or nurse.

A clear and descriptive protocol that defines the research question, the scientific data that supports the hypothesis, the planned testing in humans, and the response to treatment results in sound clinical trials (Hubbard and Donehower 1980).

## THE PHASES OF CLINICAL TRIALS

The development of new drugs is a long, complex process. Anticancer agents go through a selection process (drug screen) that was established through NCI (Table 1.3). An article by Gross (1986) contains a diagram that describes the number of compounds that are reviewed initially compared to the actual number of compounds that make it to toxicity studies (clinical trials). As Figure 1.1 shows, only a handful of drugs make it to clinical trials after several years of reviewing and screening.

By the time a drug becomes available to the general medical community, it has gone through extensive testing for toxicity in both animals and humans. Federal law mandates

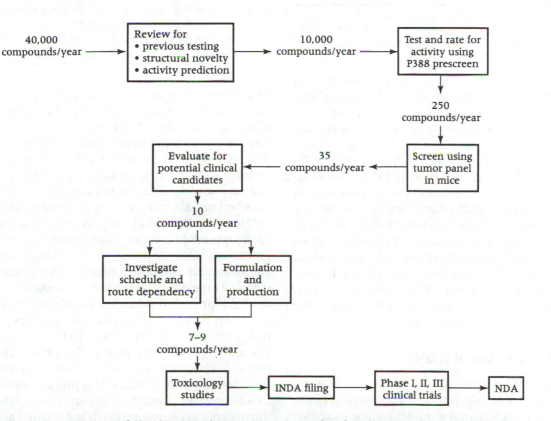

**Figure 1.1**   Phases of the National Cancer Institute (NCI) Drug Development Program
INDA = investigational new drug application; NDA = new drug application

*Source:* Gross, J. (1986). Clinical research in cancer chemotherapy. *Oncology Nursing Forum,* 13(1): 59–65. Reprinted with permission.

**Table 1.3    Steps in Cancer Drug Development**

Define molecular structures

Identify molecular targets

Develop high-throughput screens for high-priority targets

Screen thousands of chemicals and biologicals

Identify the best drug candidates for preclinical development

Laboratory testing and preparing for human trials

Phase I clinical trial

Phase II clinical trial

Phase III clinical trial

Widespread clinical use

*Source:* National Cancer Institute. (1999). *The Nation's Investment in Cancer Research: A Budget Proposal for Fiscal Year 2001.* Bethesda, Md: National Institutes of Health, Publication 99-4373.

**Table 1.4    The Four Phases of Clinical Trials**

Phase I:

    Define toxicities of a new chemotherapeutic agent

    Determine maximum tolerated dose

    Determine new treatment schedule

    Determine new route of administration

Phase II:

    Determine antitumor activity at given dose and schedule

    Further define toxicities

Phase III:

    Compare with conventional treatments

Phase IV:

    Elicit more information about the drug after it is released for commercial use

    Determine the principles for combined modality and the associated problems

that any new drug considered for use in humans must undergo thorough toxicity testing in animals first (Carter 1977). If there is an indication that the drug can be used safely and therapeutically in humans, the drug sponsor applies for Investigational New Drug (IND) approval through the Food and Drug Administration (FDA). Included in the IND application is a careful and ethical description of the planned testing in humans. Before the drug can be tested in humans, the sponsor must submit all the results of the animal studies to the FDA. When the drug has approval, human testing begins (Pines 1981). Human testing is divided into four phases. Table 1.4 defines the four phases of clinical trials.

## Phase I Clinical Trials

A phase I clinical trial is the first clinical phase of testing in humans. The purpose of the phase I clinical trial is to define the *maximum tolerated dose* (MTD). Gross (1986) defines MTD as "the dose at which toxicities are reversible, treatable, and not life threatening."

In addition to establishing the MTD, phase I clinical trials aim at establishing the optimal schedule and safe administration of a given dose. In phase I, the pharmacology of the new drug is looked at as well (Jenkins and Curt 1996). Phase I studies usually are designed to start at a low dose that is not expected to produce serious side effects. Usually, three patients are treated at the initial dose schedule. That initial dose is based on toxicology reports from the animal studies (Simon 1997). There are approximately five dose escalations in a phase I study. Three or more patients usually are enrolled for each dose escalation (Gross 1986).

Careful monitoring and recording of toxicities is essential to this phase of clinical trials. The nurse plays a key role in this phase. The nurse is often the one who administers the treatment and, therefore, is in a prime position to observe for toxicities (Gross 1986). The nurse's role in clinical research is discussed at a later point in this chapter. The completion of phase I studies is marked by the description of toxicities observed, the severity of the toxicities, and an establishment of doses for further studies.

Patients who are involved in phase I studies usually have exhausted conventional therapy. The purpose of phase I is not to find antitumor activity, but to establish a safe dose in humans. A drug is not considered inactive because it does not show any antitumor activity in phase I. It should always be considered for phase II studies unless it produces unacceptable toxicities (Reich 1982b).

## Phase II Clinical Trials

After a starting dose is established through phase I studies, the new drug moves into phase II testing. The purpose of phase II trials is to determine antitumor toxicity of the agent in a variety of cancers (Hubbard and Gross 1994). Carter (1977) describes a twofold approach to phase II studies: drug oriented and disease oriented. In the *drug-oriented approach*, a drug is evaluated when used in a variety of cancers. Although this has been the commonly used approach in the past, it has certain limitations (Simon 1997). There can be misleading results because of patient selection. Response rates can be affected for many reasons. Although the number of patients might be large, there might be relatively few patients with a particular disease who have the potential to respond to the drug, and prior extensive therapy can alter the drug response (Carter 1977). Carter notes that perhaps the greater danger is not in overestimating the responsiveness of a new drug, but in underestimating a drug and failing to study it effectively.

The second approach to phase II studies as outlined by Carter (1977) is the *disease-oriented approach*. This approach evaluates a drug in the treatment of a specific type of cancer. Usually, these studies fall into two categories: controlled randomized studies or nonrandomized

sequential studies. The *nonrandomized* phase II study looks at patients with a specific disease of a subcategory (pancreatic versus all gastrointestinal cancers or squamous cell cancer of lung versus all lung cancer). In a *randomized* study, a patient is randomly assigned to two or more therapeutic regimens. One of the reasons for randomizing patients is to eliminate any conscious or unconscious bias on the part of the researcher.

The requirement of phase I as well as phase II studies is that the benefits must outweigh the risks. Patients must be evaluated carefully for eligibility for phase II trials. Aside from detecting the antitumor activity of a new drug, phase II trials also build on the knowledge obtained through phase I studies. Carter (1977) points out that drug toxicity, administration, and scheduling may be more clearly defined. At the end of the phase II study, there should be adequate information on the efficacy and the nature of toxicities to justify further study. This justification for further study should be based on the concept of risk-benefit ratio, which is discussed in the next section of this chapter.

## Phase III Clinical Trials

The goal of phase III clinical trials is to establish the new drug as an effective treatment by comparing it with conventional treatments (Lake and Jenkins 1993). Patients are randomized in a phase III study in an effort to eliminate any conscious or unconscious bias of the investigator. The purpose of evaluating the new treatment is to determine absolute efficacy and safety. The drug can be administered in a variety of ways: alone, combined with standard therapy, or substituted for drugs in standard therapy. The new agent also can be compared with single or combined drugs already known to be effective (Gross 1986). The goal of phase

III trials is to determine whether the new drug demonstrates (1) greater usefulness than conventional therapy, (2) equivalent or less toxicity, (3) greater potential in combination, or (4) an improvement in survival and quality of life of cancer patients (Fischer, Knobf, and Durivage 1997).

## Phase IV Clinical Trials

Phase IV clinical trials study the new treatments combined with other modalities. Patients who are eligible are those who have localized disease with significant incidence of recurrence after surgery or radiation (Hubbard and Gross 1994). This phase evaluates adjuvant therapy and the potential for producing long-term survival or cure.

## ETHICAL ISSUES IN CLINICAL RESEARCH

Clinical trials have become an integral part of the advancement of quality care for persons with cancer. Clinical trials may involve any disease or treatment, but they must include the protocol components described earlier. One of the most important components is a section that carefully outlines how the patients' rights are protected (Gross 1986).

Basic ethical principles should form the cornerstone of any sound clinical trial. The primary principle of a clinical trial should be that the patient will benefit from the drug (Carter 1977). The benefits of the clinical trial must outweigh the potential harm or risk to the patient. Ethical principles are based on respect for human dignity, autonomy (self-determination), and veracity. Individuals are believed to have dignity and worth and are not just a means of accomplishing some objective (Lynch 1988).

The basic ethical principles and guidelines involving research subjects evolved from the Nuremberg War Trials in 1945. Social outcry at the abuses of medical experiments performed on prisoners in the Nazi concentration camps prompted the Nuremberg Code. The purpose of the Nuremberg Code of 1947 was to establish ethical guidelines for research involving human subjects (Belmont Report 1979). Subsequent codes followed the guidelines of the Nuremberg Code. Among these were the Helsinki Declaration of 1964 and the 1971 U.S. Department of Health, Education, and Welfare Guidelines (Belmont Report 1979). These formal doctrines outlined the basic laws and regulations for individuals participating in medical research (Lynch 1988).

The development of federal guidelines for clinical research resulted from the evidence of several abuses of research studies. In 1932, the Tuskegee Syphilis Study looked at the untreated course of syphilis. The subjects were not offered the available treatment of arsenic and mercury. Later, in 1953, when penicillin became the acceptable treatment, the subjects again were not offered the available drug (Bandman 1985). In 1963, in a study of the immune system, unsuspecting patients at the Jewish Chronic Disease Hospital in New York were injected with live cancer cells (Belmont Report 1979). In 1964, in order to secure placement in an otherwise over-crowded facility, the parents of mentally retarded children allowed experiments in hepatitis transmission and immunization to be performed on their children (Bandman 1985). These instances highlighted the fact that violations of human rights existed even after the acceptance of the Nuremberg Code. The need to regulate research and to protect research subjects was met with the establishment of the National Research Act of 1974. This act established the National Commission for the Protection of Human Subjects of Biomedical and Behavioral

Research. The purpose of this commission was to advise the Secretary of the Department of Health, Education, and Welfare (HEW) of the impact of research on ethical, legal, and social issues. Through this commission, the basic guidelines for informed consent were developed. The Research Act helped establish the Institutional Review Boards (IRBs), which protect research subjects through monitoring and documenting adherence to federal guidelines.

In 1979, the National Commission for the Protection of Human Subjects of Biomedical and Behavioral Research published *The Belmont Report: The Ethical Principles and Guidelines for the Protection of Human Subjects of Research*. This report came to be known as the "Belmont Report" and has been adopted universally as policy on the conduct of human research.

From the Belmont Report (1979) evolved three general principles that are particularly relevant to ethical research involving human subjects:

1. *Respect for Persons*

   This principle addresses two ethical issues. The first is that *individuals are autonomous;* capable of self-determination. They make judgments about personal goals. No one should obstruct the autonomous actions by denying the individual the freedom to act on those judgments or by withholding information needed to make those judgments. The second issue addresses the fact that there are *some individuals,* who, due to illness, mental disability, or restricted liberty, have diminished autonomy and *are entitled to protection.* The degree of protection depends on the risk of harm versus the likelihood of benefit to the individual and should be reevaluated on an ongoing basis.

2. *Beneficence*

   The principle of beneficence is defined as "acts of kindness or charity that go beyond street obligation" (Belmont Report 1979). Two expressions of beneficent action are (1) do no harm and (2) maximize benefits and minimize risks. The principle of beneficence is an integral component in clinical research involving patients.

3. *Justice*

   The principle of justice states that *equals should be treated as equals.* This principle addresses the issue of equal distribution of a treatment. Sometimes different treatments might be given based on age, experiments, competence, deprivation, and position. Justice demands that treatment be provided to individuals who are likely to benefit from the treatment.

The Belmont Report (1979) also recommends that (1) informed consent, (2) risk/benefit assessment, and (3) selection of subjects involved in research be considered when applying the three basic principles to clinical research.

1. *Informed Consent*

   Informed consent is mandatory in clinical trials (Simon 1997). Informed consent contains three major elements: information, comprehension, and voluntariness. *Information* ensures that individuals are given sufficient information regarding the research procedure, the objectives, the risks versus benefits, the alternative treatments, and the statement outlining the opportunity for the individual to ask questions or to withdraw from the study without being penalized. *Comprehension* refers to the ability of the individual to understand the information. Provisions must be made to adapt the presentation of the information so that the individual can understand. *Voluntariness* refers to the fact that the individual has given consent without coercion or inducement.

2. *Risk/Benefit Assessment*

The justification for research is based on the ratio of risk to benefit. The guidelines established in the Nuremberg Code and subsequent federal regulations require that the benefits to the individual subject and the benefit to society at large from the research must outweigh the risks to the subjects involved in the research. The risks and benefits must be discussed thoroughly and included in the informed consent.

3. *Selection of Subjects*

The ethical principle of justice guides the selection of subjects for clinical trials. The researcher needs to exhibit fairness in the selection of subjects. Subjects should not be offered treatment that would not benefit them. There should be no preference in selection of groups of subjects (e.g., adults before children). There should be no implied benefit for being involved in a given study (e.g., prisoners would not receive any special treatment for agreeing to be a part of study). Unfair advantage should not be taken of potential subjects (prisoners and other institutionalized people should not be considered a potential study group because they are confined).

Historically, it has been determined that women have not always been represented adequately in clinical trials. The NIH Revitalization Act of 1990 requires the inclusion of minorities and women in study populations so that research findings can be of benefit to all persons. If there is to be any exclusion of study subjects, a clear compelling rationale must be provided for NIH-supported or NIH-conducted studies (Harden and McFarland 2000). Compliance with this requirement was monitored to ensure greater applicability of study outcomes (Tejeda et al. 1996).

Ethical principles are essential components of research involving human subjects. Every clinical trial must address both scientific and humanistic questions. By maintaining ethical standards in clinical trials, we ensure that individual rights are protected (Office of Science and Technology Policy 1991).

## THE ROLES OF NURSES IN CLINICAL ONCOLOGY

In 1950, the American Nurses' Association adopted the Code for Nurses (American Nurses' Association 1994). It defines a code of ethical conduct and principles that help guide and evaluate nursing practice. These ethical guidelines are similar to the ethical principles discussed in the previous section. The Code for Nurses is based on the most fundamental principle: respect for persons. The other principles, which are offshoots of the basic principle, are autonomy (self-determination), beneficence (doing good), nonmalficence (avoiding harm), veracity (truth telling), confidentiality (respecting privileged information), fidelity (keeping promises), and justice (treating fairly).

The Code for Nurses provides a framework within which ethical decision making can take place. This code plays an important role in the field of cancer research. The nurse involved in research plays a vital role in ensuring the protection of the integrity, the privacy, and the rights of patients involved in research. The nurse who is involved in research should be fully knowledgeable about the intent and the nature of the research in order to be able to protect patients' rights (American Nurses' Association 1994).

Nurses have cared for cancer patients for many years, often on specialized units for the care of cancer patients (Henke 1980). Many of these units may be involved in clinical research. As the treatments for cancer became more complex, the role of nurses in cancer research evolved. Today, the nurse involved in clinical research is an integral part of the research team. As the needs of cancer patients increase, the nurse provides more complex nursing care. Responsibilities of nurses involved in cancer research are data collection, education, emotional support, and identification and prevention of serious toxicities (Klimaszewski et al. 2000).

There are different nursing roles in a cancer research setting. These roles have different foci, but some job responsibilities can overlap in some cancer research settings. The roles of nurses in cancer research include clinical nurse specialist, clinical research nurse, and oncology nurse. The two focus areas are (1) involvement in the conduction of clinical trials and (2) care for patients undergoing cancer research trials (Jenkins and Curt 1996). Another key role for nurses in clinical oncology is that of chemotherapy administration in a variety of settings. As the health care system changes, more of these chemotherapeutic agents are being administered in both the outpatient and home settings.

## Clinical Nurse Specialist

Specialization in nursing is a concept that has been evolving since 1943, when Frances Ruter envisioned the role of the "nurse clinician." This nurse clinician was a nurse who had an advanced degree and remained actively involved in clinical practice (Yasko 1983). During the 1950s and the 1960s, the term "clinical specialist" was applied to the nurse with a master's degree in nursing and a specialization in a particular field of nursing (e.g., oncology, cardiology, or neurology) (Crabtree 1979). This role of clinical nurse specialist (CNS) grew out of the increasing patient populations requiring specialized care and the increasing new and complex technology and treatment methods (Hart, Lekander, Bartels, and Tebbitt 1987). It generally is agreed that the purpose of the CNS is to improve patient care (Crabtree 1979) and to improve the standards of nursing practice (Yasko 1983).

During the first half of the century, there was no formalized education for nurses who worked with cancer patients. Their education was gained through clinical experience. During the 1950s and the 1960s, efforts to promote graduate education for clinical specialization in cancer nursing were spearheaded by the American Cancer Society and the National Cancer Institute, both of which were early voices for cancer nursing (Spross 1983). These educational programs allowed cancer nurses to develop proficiency in caring for cancer patients. Few entry-level nursing programs included any content on caring for clients with cancer (Yasko 1983). Since the early 1970s, the Oncology Nursing Society (ONS) has helped to develop the role of the oncology clinical nurse specialist (OCNS). Cancer nursing emerged as a specialty through the activities and rapid growth of the ONS.

The roles of the OCNS parallel the traditional roles of the CNS. These roles include clinician, consultant, educator, change agent, and researcher (Spross 1983). They are of the utmost importance when the OCNS is involved with clinical trials. To improve the care of the research patient, the OCNS may become the consultant and educator. As an expert in cancer nursing, the OCNS becomes a resource to patients and their families, providing them with the appropriate education. These educational interventions evolve throughout the course of the disease and treatment. The OCNS develops an expertise for assessing the learning needs of patients and families involved in research. The assessment of needs also extends to the nursing staff. Guiding nurses who care for patients undergoing research is another aspect of the role of the OCNS as an educator (Welch-McCaffrey 1986). As a clinician working with research patients, the OCNS helps to monitor the research treatment and to minimize any untoward side effects. As a researcher, the OCNS actively takes part in the design of protocols. Through this collaborative work relationship with the investigator, the OCNS can have an opportunity to review the impact that the proposed study might have on resources. Preparing for a new population, assessing the impact on staffing or bed capabilities, ensuring that adequate supplies and equipment are obtained, and preparing staff for protocol implementation are only a few of the issues the OCNS needs to address for study implementation (Engelking 1992). The OCNS involved in research can provide important assistance in ensuring that research is conducted safely.

## Clinical Research Nurse

The role of the clinical research nurse evolved during the 1970s, a time when clinical trials were being evaluated for their therapeutic potential in treating advanced cancer (Hubbard and Gross 1994). One of the first roles that brought out the need for collaboration in clinical research, the clinical research nurse, changed the focus of nursing from being task oriented to sharing the responsibility for the safe administration of investigational therapies.

Hubbard and Donehower (1980) point out that as an integral member of the research team, the nurse develops fundamental knowledge of clinical research and an understanding of the complex needs of the patient involved in clinical research. The authors also report that the research nurse has the opportunity to participate in patient care rounds and conferences that help researchers learn more about the biology of cancer, as well as the natural history of a particular cancer.

Recently, through the involvement of clinical research nurses, nursing considerations have been included in research protocols. The research nurse plays a major role in data collection and analysis, and in the publication of research data. In some settings, this nurse also develops a role as investigator in the clinical trials (Tokarsky 2000). As the role of the clinical research nurse in clinical trials evolved, oncologists became aware of the value of nursing in improving the quality of clinical trials (Hubbard and Gross 1994).

Throughout the phases of clinical trials, the research nurse plays a vital role as caregiver and treatment administrator, observer of toxic side effects, monitor and recorder of these side effects, resource for patient, patient advocate, data manager, and coordinator of patient care (Gross 1986). Direct patient care is not the primary focus of the research nurse; rather the focus is the improvement of patient care through the conduct of safe and ethical clinical trials.

## Oncology Nurse

The role of the oncology nurse has changed over the last decade and now takes various forms. For example, some oncology nurses provide direct patient care, and others focus on the improvement of care as a result of the safe conduct of research trials. Although these roles have different foci, they both attempt to meet the needs of cancer patients. This section focuses on the role of the oncology staff nurse who concentrates on the delivery of *direct patient care*.

In some research settings, the role of the oncology nurse overlaps with the responsibilities of the research nurse. Although the oncology staff nurse might not be involved in the design of the protocol or the analysis of data and might not become a co-investigator, the nurse remains a vital member of the research team. As the acuity of patients and the complexity of clinical trials increase, the oncology nurse provides sophisticated care to the cancer patient. The oncology nurse might be the administrator of investigational therapies. As such, the nurse is often the one to observe and monitor reactions or side effects to treatments (Engelking 1991). The accuracy of these observations and documentation of toxicities are of the utmost importance, especially in phase I trials, where toxicities are defined. As well as being the backbone of clinical research, documentation serves as legal proof of patient care—medical and nursing. Assessments, judgments, and interventions must be documented. According to Shine (1989), the nurse must chart in an objective, accurate, thorough, and timely manner, using institutionally approved abbreviations. Regardless of the quality of care given or the toxicity noted, if it is not documented in the medical record, technically it did not happen (Shine 1989).

Additionally, such forces as managed care and capitation are changing the face of oncology nursing care, particularly in the field of chemotherapy administration. These factors, as well as the increasing knowledge about the safety and efficacy of chemotherapeutic agents, are influencing the settings in which chemotherapy is given. The outpatient clinic, the oncologist's office, and the home environment quickly are becoming the setting for chemotherapy administration even when clinical trials are being implemented. Consequently, oncology nurses in these settings are challenged to work with chemotherapeutic agents in the same way as the research nurses and their inpatient clinical counterparts.

The oncology nurse becomes a resource for the patient undergoing cancer research. Education of both the patient and his or her family may be provided by the nurse. The nurse becomes both educator and advocate for the patient involved in research. The nurse must constantly assess the patient's understanding of the proposed treatment. Evaluating patient needs, the oncology nurse gives consistent and accurate information to the patient and family. This information needs to be simple and concise. It might contain the nature of the proposed research, the methods of administration of treatment, and the potential risks from side effects. Often this information already is addressed by the physician but the nurse is responsible for constantly reinforcing it (Lynch 1988).

As patient advocate, the oncology nurse helps the patient make clear decisions based on individual goals and values. The nurse helps the patient to communicate these goals clearly to the health team. Ensuring that the patient receives and understands the essential information and that there is adequate time for questions and answers, is a vital aspect of patient advocacy. Listening to a patient's fears and anxieties surrounding the unknown is an essential role for the nurse. Often patients feel more comfortable discussing particular fears and anxieties with oncology nurses because of their availability and frequent contact (Lynch 1988). The nurse might become the liaison between the health care team and the patient. As patient advocate, the nurse is crucial in facilitating communication and collaboration and ensuring informed consent.

The role of the oncology nurse as patient advocate and educator is very important in the research setting. The oncology nurse helps the patient understand the purpose, the procedure, the risks, the benefits, and the potential side effects of the research protocol, as well as the interventions to reduce the impact it has on his or her lifestyle.

## CONCLUSION

The Oncology Nursing Society (ONS) Scope and Standards of Practice form the framework on which the practice of oncology nursing is built. Reference is made throughout this text to tools published by the ONS, the American Cancer Society, and the National Cancer Institute. The suggestion of these tools is to make the reader aware of the fact that standards of practice are available, as are similar publications to operationalize these standards and implement them in a practical manner. It is up to the reader to use what is available to provide optimal care to the patient receiving cancer chemotherapy.

Several roles have evolved in cancer nursing in a research setting. Many of the responsibilities overlap. Of importance is the fact that nurses involved in cancer research have demonstrated, through their respective roles, that they have made a significant contribution to the conduct of safe and ethical clinical trials and have established themselves as invaluable resources in supporting or conducting cancer research. Finally, nurses caring for cancer patients who require chemotherapy are in the frontlines of cancer care. These nurses make all the difference to the patient's quality of life throughout his or her cancer experience.

## BIBLIOGRAPHY

American Nurses' Association. (1994). *Code for Nurses with Interpretive Statements*. Washington, D.C.: American Nurses' Association.

———. (1996). *ANA and ONS: Statement on the Scope and Standards of Oncology Nursing Practice*. Washington, D.C.: American Nurses' Association.

Bandman, E.L. (1985). Protection of human subjects. *Topics in Clinical Nursing* 7(2): 15–23.

Belmont Report. (1979). See National Commission for the Protection of Human Subjects of Biomedical and Behavioral Research.

Bull, J.P. (1959). Historical development of clinical therapeutic trials. *Journal of Chronic Disease* 10(3): 218–248.

Cancer Therapy Evaluation Program (CTEP). (1993). *Investigator's Handbook*. Washington, D.C.: National Cancer Institute.

Carpenito, L.J. (1997). *Handbook of Nursing Diagnosis*. 7th ed. Philadelphia: Lippincott.

———. (2000). *Nursing Diagnosis Application to Clinical Practice*. 8th ed. Philadelphia: Lippincott.

Carter, S.K. (1977). Clinical trials in cancer chemotherapy. *Cancer* 40(1): 544–557.

Crabtree, M.S. (1979). Effective utilization of clinical specialists within the organizational structure of hospital nursing service. *Nursing Administration Quarterly* 4(1): 1–11.

Dangle, R.B., and Flynn, K. (1987). Historical perspective. In C.R. Ziegfeld (ed.): *Core Curriculum for Oncology Nursing*. Philadelphia: W.B. Saunders, 375–390.

Ehrenberger, H. (2000). Clinical trials are just a click away. *ONS News* 15(4): 7.

Engelking, C. (1991). Facilitating clinical trials. *Cancer* 67(6): 1793–1797.

———. (1992). Clinical trials: impact evaluation and implementation considerations. *Seminars in Oncology Nursing* 8(2): 148–155.

Fischer, D.S., Knobf, M.K., and Durivage, H. (1997). *The Cancer Chemotherapy Handbook*. 5th ed. St. Louis: Mosby.

Gordon, M. (1987). *Nursing Diagnosis Process and Application*. 2nd ed. New York: McGraw-Hill.

Gross, J. (1986). Clinical research in cancer chemotherapy. *Oncology Nursing Forum* 13(1): 59–65.

Guzzetta, C., Bunton, S., Prinkey, L., Shever, A., and Seifert, P. (1989). *Clinical Assessment Tools for Use with Nursing Diagnoses*. St. Louis: Mosby.

Harden, J.T., and McFarland, G. (2000). Avoiding gender and minority barriers to NIH funding. *Journal of Nursing Scholarship* 32(1): 83–86.

Hart, C.N., Lekander, G., Bartels, D., and Tebbitt, B.V. (1987). Clinical nurse specialists: An institutional process for determining priorities. *Journal of Nursing Administration* 17(6): 31–35.

Henke, C. (1980). Emerging roles of the nurse in oncology. *Seminars in Oncology* 7(1): 4–8.

Hubbard, S.M., and Donehower, M.G. (1980). The nurse in a cancer research setting. *Seminars in Oncology* 7(1): 9–17.

Hubbard, S., and Gross, J. (1994). Principles of clinical research. In J. Gross and B. Johnson (eds.): *Handbook of Oncology Nursing.* 2nd ed. Boston: Jones & Bartlett, 195–218.

Jenkins, J., and Curt, G. (1996). Implementation of clinical trials. In S. Baird, R. McCorkle, and M. Grant (eds.): *Cancer Nursing.* 2nd ed. Philadelphia: W.B. Saunders, 470–484.

Johnson, M., Maas, M., and Moorhead, S. (eds.). (2000). *Nursing Outcomes Classification (NOC).* 2nd ed. St. Louis: Mosby.

Klimaszewski, A., Aikin, J.L., Bacon, M.A., DiStasio, S.A., Ehrenberg, H.E., and Ford, B.A. (2000). *Manual for Clinical Trials Nursing.* Pittsburgh: Oncology Nursing Press.

Lake, P., and Jenkins, J. (1993). Cancer chemotherapy: Clinical trials. *Cancer Nursing* 16(6): 486.

Lea, D., Jenkins, J., and Francomano, C. (1998). *Genetics in Clinical Practice: New Directions for Nursing and Health Care.* Boston: Jones & Bartlett.

Livingston, R.B., and Carter, S.K. (1982). Experimental design and clinical trials: Clinical perspectives. In R.B. Livingston, S.K. Carter, and E. Glatstein (eds.): *Principles of Cancer Treatment.* New York: McGraw-Hill, 34–45.

Lynch, M. (1988). The nurse's role in the biotherapy of cancer: Clinical trials and informed consent. *Oncology Nursing Forum* 15(6) (suppl): 23–27.

McCloskey, J.C., and Bulechek, G.M. (eds.). (2000). *Nursing Interventions Classification (NIC).* 3rd ed. St. Louis: Mosby-Year Book.

McCloskey, J.C., Bulechek, G.M., and Donahue, W. (1998). Nursing interventions core to specialty practice. *Nursing Outlook* 46(2): 67–76.

National Cancer Institute. (1999). *The Nation's Investment in Cancer Research: A Budget Proposal for Fiscal Year 2001.* Bethesda, Md.: National Institutes of Health, Publication 99-4373.

National Commission for the Protection of Human Subjects of Biomedical and Behavioral Research. (1979). *The Belmont Report: Ethical Principles and Guidelines for the Protection of Human Subjects of Research.* Washington, D.C.: U.S. Department of Health and Human Services, Publication (OS) 78-0012.

NIH guidelines on the inclusion of women and minorities as subjects in clinical research. (1994). *Federal Register* 59 (Separate Part IV): 11146–11151.

Occupational Safety & Health Administration (OSHA). (1993). Hazardous drug handling (OSHA Instruction CPL 2-2.20B CH4). Washington, D.C.: OSHA, Draft: 24-1 to 24-33.

Office of Science and Technology Policy. (1991). Federal policy for the protection of human subjects, notices and rules. In *Federal Register 56* (117): 28002–28032.

Pines, W.L. (1981). *A Primer on New Drug Development.* FDA Consumer. U.S. Dept. of Health and Human Resources. Public Health Service. Washington, D.C.: Food and Drug Administration, Office of Public Affairs, Publication (FDA) 81-3021.

Reich, S.D. (1982a). Clinical trials—A review of terms and principles: Part I. *Cancer Nursing* June 5(3): 232–233.

———. (1982b). Clinical trials—A review of terms and principles—statistical considerations: Part II. *Cancer Nursing* October 5(5): 399–402.

Shine, K.N. (1989). Areas of liability for nurse defendants. *Forum: Risk Management Foundation of the Harvard Medial Institutions,* 10(1).

Simon, R.M. (1997). Design and analysis of clinical trials. In V.T. DeVita Jr., S. Hellman, and S.A. Rosenberg (eds.): *Cancer: Principles and Practice of Oncology.* Philadelphia: Lippincott, 513–528.

Spross, J. (1983). An overview of the oncology clinical nurse specialist's role. *Oncology Nursing Forum* 10(3): 54–58.

Tejeda, H.A., Green, S.B., Trimble, E.L., Ford, L., High, J.L., Ungerleider, R.S., Friedman, M.A., and Brawley, O.W. (1996). Representation of African-Americans, Hispanics, and Whites in National Cancer Institute cancer treatment trials. *Journal of the National Cancer Institute* 88(5): 812–816.

Tokarsky, J. (2000). Nursing companion studies. In A.D. Klimaszewski, J.L. Aikin, M.A. Baron, S.A. DiStasio, H.E. Ehrenberger, and B.A. Ford (eds.): *Manual for Clinical Trials Nursing.* Pittsburgh: Oncology Nursing Press, 157–159.

Tribulski, J.A. (1988). Nursing diagnosis: Waste of time or valued tool? *RN* 51(1): 30–34.

Welch-McCaffrey, D. (1985). Rationale, development and evaluation of a chemotherapy certification course for nurses. *Cancer Nursing* 8(5): 255–262.

———. (1986). Role performance issues for oncology clinical nurse specialists. *Cancer Nursing* 9(6): 287–294.

Wittes, R.E. (1987). Current emphasis in the Clinical Drug Development Program of the National Cancer Institute. *NCI Updates,* 1(12):1–15.

Wittes, R.E., and Silva, J. (1999). Role of clinical trials informatics in the NCI's cancer informatics infrastructure. *Proc AMIA Symposium,* 950–954.

Yasko, J. (1983). A survey of oncology clinical nursing specialists. *Oncology Nursing Forum* 10(1): 25–30.

Zubrod, C.G. (1984). Origins and development of chemotherapy research at NCI. *Cancer Treatment Reports* 68(1): 9–19.

# Chapter 2

# Cell Cycle Kinetics and Antineoplastic Agents

## Karen C. Ingwersen, RN, MSN

Cancer has existed as a disease for many centuries, although it often is thought that cancer is a disease of the modern world. The earliest evidence of cancer comes from Egyptian remains, revealing that such cancers as osteogenic sarcoma and nasopharyngeal carcinomas existed in the year 2500 B.C. (Shimkin 1977). In order to understand the development of chemotherapy, the theory undergirding its use and the role of the oncology nurse in administering chemotherapy agents, it is helpful to review the history of cancer therapy.

## HISTORY OF CANCER THERAPY

The disease of cancer dates back as far as prehistoric times. There is evidence that cancer affected animals long before humans were on earth. The studies of the remains of a Cretaceous dinosaur and a Pleistocene cave bear indicate the existence of tumors of the vertebrae (Brothwell 1967). Evidence of malignant neoplasms was documented in Egyptian mummies some 5000 years ago (Wells 1963). The number of cases of these prehistoric and ancient tumors are small, but they support the assumption that cancer is a very old disease,

afflicting animals and man long before written history.

As cancer dates back to antiquity, so too is there evidence in the earliest Egyptian writing of medical treatment for benign tumors (such as lipomas and polyps) and for malignant cancers of the stomach and uterus (Breasted 1930). Early treatment of these tumors by the Egyptians consisted of surgical removal of benign lipomas and polyps with a knife or a red-hot iron. Cancer of the stomach was treated with boiled barley mixed with nuts, and cancer of the uterus was treated with a mix of fresh dates and pig's brain, which was then introduced into the vagina (Ebbell 1937).

As early as the Greco-Roman period (500 B.C.–A.D. 500), cancer was recognized and given a grave prognosis. Evidence of cancer was documented in the writings of Hippocrates (the "father of medicine") and other medical authorities of the period, such as Celsus, Artaesus, and Galen (Shimkin 1977). Shimkin's book describes the predominant theory regarding cancer during this period. At this time in history, the body of man was defined by the four Humors: blood, phlegm, yellow bile, and black bile. When in proper proportions in regard to mixture, quantity, and force, man remained healthy. If any Humor was out of proportion (diminished or increased), man became ill. The four Humors were the biological counterparts for air, fire, water, and earth, which in certain proportions produced heat, cold, wet, and dry. Cancer was believed to be the result of an excess of black bile (also called *melanchole* or *atrabilis*). Cancer was and still is, in many respects, a melancholy disease.

The Medieval period (A.D. 500–1500) saw little progress in science and medicine. These years were dominated by political and religious struggles. Cancer was still believed to be caused by an excess of black bile. Superficial tumors and ulcers were treated by wide excision and cauterization. Caution was used if tumors could not be treated by excision. The more extensive tumors and ulcers were treated with caustic pastes, and treatment included a combination of phlebotomy, herbal potions, diet, powder of crab, and other symbolic charms. Medicine during this time remained a combination of astrology, herbal potions, caustic pastes, excisions and cauterizations, and bloodletting. None of the pastes, potions, or symbolic charms had any benefit systemically, but some did have escharotic effects on local tumors. In particular, arsenic paste might have had an antitumor effect. The use of arsenic compositions continued throughout the centuries up to 1865, when marked improvements were observed by Lissauer after a solution of potassium arsenite (Fowler's Solution) was given to a patient with chronic leukemia. A few years later, Billroth demonstrated a dramatic response of lymphosarcoma to Fowler's Solution (Haddow 1970). The Renaissance and Reformation periods (1500–1600) saw a continuation of the treatment of cancer through the use of excisions and caustic powders and pastes. Cancer was beginning to be studied more as the field of anatomy began to develop (Shimkin 1977).

Shimkin (1977) describes the evolution of cancer treatments through the centuries. The seventeenth century saw a change in the theory of cancer. Cancer was no longer thought to be a result of an excess of black bile, but was now seen as a result of stasis and abnormalities of lymph. Surgery continued to be used for local tumors. In breast tumors, the technique of mastectomy was used. Without anesthesia or antiseptic techniques, the breast was removed by a total slice removal followed by cauterization. In addition, the opinion that cancer was contagious began to develop during this century.

Up to this time in history, the chemotherapy of cancer remained a treatment using caustic pastes and potions, which showed little concrete value. An important development occurred in the 1600s that would later encourage the investigation of the chemotherapy of cancer. The success of the use of chemotherapy for cancers is linked directly to the successful discovery of the use of chemotherapy for infections. Beginning in 1630, the first real chemotherapeutic *drug* (chemical used to treat disease) was used by the Jesuits who used a tea made from the bark of the chinchona tree to treat malaria. In addition, dysentery was treated by using a drug from the bark of a tree in Brazil. From these crude and simple extracts came quinine and emetine (ipecac), which have become well established in the treatment of malaria and amoebic dysentery, respectively (Burchenal 1977). These drugs can be considered the first successful curative chemotherapeutic agents. They were used without knowledge of the etiology of disease, the identity of chemicals, or the action of the drugs (DeVita 1982). These successes provided the support that drugs could cure diseases. However, further advances in both the chemotherapies of infectious diseases and cancer would have to wait until the early twentieth century, when Paul Ehrlich, the "father of chemotherapy," made important discoveries that affected both the course of infectious diseases and the course of cancer treatment.

During the eighteenth century, surgery remained the primary means for treating localized tumors. The theory that cancer was originally a localized, resectable disease caused by inflammation was developed during this time. Attention was being given to the disease known as cancer, and the first hospitals specifically for cancer opened in France (1740) and England (1792). The treatment of cancer was emerging but was still in an embryonic state. Toward the end of the century, it was discovered that environmental carcinogens could be epidemiologically linked to cancer. The use of snuff and the exposure to chimney soot was related causally to nasal cancers and scrotal cancers, respectively.

The nineteenth century was an age of inventions. The field of oncology was ushered into a new era. A better understanding of tumor histology resulted from the invention of the achromatic microscope. The use of anesthesia as well as the introduction of antisepsis allowed for the surgical removal of deeper cancers of internal organs. As mentioned before, the first chemical agent to be used against a malignant disease was arsenic, in the form of potassium arsenite. Another mixture was used against a malignant disease in 1893 by Coley. This was a mixture of streptococci and bacilli (Coley's toxins), which demonstrated an objective response in sarcoma. The treatment was dangerous, and its results were unpredictable. Still, a few people were cured of cancer in the nineteenth century.

Three discoveries that occurred at the turn of the twentieth century had a great impact on the treatment of cancer. The first event was the development of the radical "en bloc" mastectomy by Halsted, whereby the primary tumor and the draining lymph nodes were removed surgically. Second, the discovery of X-rays by Roentgen opened a new modality besides surgery, to treat tumors that could now be visualized. Radiation therapy was introduced following the discovery of the radioactivity of uranium in 1896 by Becquerel and of radium in 1898 by Marie and Pierre Curie. The use of radiation therapy in the treatment of cancer first occurred in 1896; by 1905, the first patient with carcinoma of the uterus was treated with radium. During this time, cancer was seen as an incurable disease (Dangle and Flynn 1987). In 1913, the American Cancer Society (ACS) was established as a voluntary organization dedicated to the control and the elimination of cancer in the United States.

## ADVENT OF CANCER CHEMOTHERAPY

A third event was to form the backbone for programs that would help develop cancer chemotherapeutic agents. The idea that drugs could be used in the treatment of malignant disease was supported by the great successes seen with the synthetic chemicals and the natural products used to cure parasitic and common bacterial infections and tuberculosis in rodent models and humans. At the turn of the twentieth century, Paul Ehrlich, who coined the term *chemotherapy* and was named the "father of chemotherapy," made tremendous advances in the discovery of chemicals used to control infections (Burchenal 1977). Ehrlich tested these drugs on rodent models, the model most likely to predict the effectiveness of these drugs in humans. It was the theory of using rodent models that led George Clowes of Rosewell Park Memorial Institute in the early 1900s to develop inbred rodent lines that could carry transplanted rodent tumors. These rodent models provided the testing ground for the early cancer chemotherapeutic agents (DeVita 1982). Later potential cancer chemotherapeutic drugs were investigated and tested for their effect against tumors in humans. Cancer chemotherapy had come a long way from the ineffective use of metallic salts, such as arsenic, copper, and lead by the early Egyptian and Greek civilizations.

The modern era of chemotherapy was initiated by the discovery of the effective use of estrogens in prostate and breast cancer (Shimkin 1977). The alkylating agents were discovered under the cloak of wartime secrecy, when a group of investigators connected to the Chemical Warfare Service looked at the toxic effects of poison gases. In an accident in Naples Harbor, sailors were exposed to poisonous mustard gas. As a result, many developed marrow and lymphoid hypoplasia (Knobf, Fischer, and Welch-McCaffrey 1984). Looking at these results, it was thought that a derivative of this gas could be useful in treating cancers. Given a code designation of HN2 (and subsequently known as *nitrogen mustard*), this agent was used to treat lymphomas. It was given first to patients with Hodgkin's disease at Yale University in 1943. The patients' tumors responded to the treatment (i.e., tumors became smaller). The results of these investigations were not made public until 1946 because of the secret nature of the Chemical Warfare Program (DeVita et al. 1979). The clinical effect of nitrogen mustard caused great excitement among researchers interested in treating cancers but was short-lived, as all the patients relapsed. From these studies came other such derivatives as Myleran and melphalan (Burchenal 1977).

In 1947, a significant discovery by Dr. Sydney Farber was made in the treatment of childhood acute leukemia (Farber, Diamond, and Mercer 1948). He demonstrated the activity of the antifols as effective cancer agents. A related drug, methotrexate, would later be developed as an effective agent in treating choriocarcinomas (DeVita et al. 1979). The use of chemotherapy agents against solid tumors was disappointing until 1956, when methotrexate was used successfully against advanced choriocarcinoma, leading to more than 50% of patients being cured of their disease. Also that year, the first patient with Wilm's tumor was cured using chemotherapy, and the first bone marrow transplant was performed (Dangle and Flynn 1987). As a result of these important discoveries, the development of cancer chemotherapeutic agents began in earnest. It was these dramatic results in the treatment of leukemia and choriocarcinoma that led the U.S. Congress to appropriate $5 million for the development of the Cancer Drug Development Program, established through the National Cancer Institute (NCI). Through this program, many of our known chemotherapeutic agents have been developed (Saunders and Carter 1977).

The appropriations of such funds opened up the more reliable testing and development of cancer chemotherapeutic agents. In the past 40 years, 30 or more agents were developed that have efficacy against a variety of malignant diseases. Over the years, changes have occurred in treatment regimens that have brought dramatic results against certain cancers. Single-agent drug therapy was the accepted treatment regimen in the earlier days of chemotherapy development. Today combination chemotherapy has resulted in long-term remissions (Krakoff 1977), more effective prevention of resistance, and tolerable side effects with maximal dose (Murinson 1981). A cure is possible now in patients with gestational choriocarcinoma, advanced Hodgkin's disease, non-Hodgkin's lymphomas, Burkitt's lymphoma, childhood leukemias, and testicular cancers. Increased survival has been reported in many other lymphomas and leukemias (Stonehill 1978).

Another approach that has shown evidence of increased survival rates and longer disease-free intervals is the use of adjuvant chemotherapy (Groenwald 1987). It is known that, despite surgery and radiation, many cancers recur. This recurrence is believed to be a result of undetectable micrometastases. The modern use of chemotherapy primarily evolved from a need to treat metastatic, disseminated disease. Adjuvant chemotherapy has proved effective in Wilm's tumor, osteosarcoma, Ewing's sarcoma, embryonal rhabdomyosarcomas in children, nonseminomatous testicular cancer, and both premenopausal and postmenopausal breast cancer (Cline and Haskell 1980).

Forty years ago, it was believed that chemotherapy was ineffective against cancer. Fifteen years ago, only hematologic and embryonic tumors were thought to be treatable by cancer chemotherapy. Today combination chemotherapy and adjuvant chemotherapy have achieved great success in the treatment of malignant disease. However, there is still a long way to go. The prospects for the future lie in several areas that are just now being explored.

## THE CELL CYCLE AND ITS IMPORTANCE

The cell cycle describes a sequence of steps through which both normal and neoplastic cells grow and replicate. This process of cell growth and replication involves five steps, or phases, which are designated by the letters and subscripts $G_0$, $G_1$, S, $G_2$, and M. The phases of the cell cycle are shown in Figure 2.1.

The letter G denotes gap phases: time periods in which cells are either preparing for the more active phases of DNA (deoxyribonucleic acid) synthesis and mitosis, or resting. $G_1$ is referred to as the *first gap* or *first growth phase*. During this phase, the cell prepares for DNA synthesis by producing RNA (ribonucleic acid) and protein. $G_1$ includes a *resting phase* called $G_0$. Cells in $G_0$ are considered to be out of the cell cycle, that is, cellular activity does not include replication when the cell is in $G_0$. Cells can remain in $G_0$ for varying lengths of time, and can be recruited back into $G_1$ according to the organism's needs. In this way, cells in $G_0$ are in a "cellular reservoir": resting cells can be drawn from $G_0$ to add to the supply of dividing cells in the cell cycle (Bingham 1978).

The *synthesis* of DNA is the major event occurring during the S phase. DNA is the genetic code of information necessary for the growth, repair, and reproduction of the cell. Normal and neoplastic cells differ in the amount of time they spend in the S phase. Many antineoplastic drugs work by causing irreparable disruption in the organization of the DNA code during DNA synthesis. The disruption ultimately results in cell death. The S phase lasts between 10 and 30 hours (Brown 1987).

$G_2$ is the *second growth period* or *second gap*. The synthesis of RNA and proteins continues as the cell prepares itself for mitosis. The production of the mitotic spindle apparatus (where chromosomes are condensed in preparation for division) also occurs during this phase. $G_2$ lasts between 1 and 12 hours.

Actual cell division, or *mitosis*, occurs during the M phase. The mitotic process consists of four phases: prophase, metaphase, anaphase, and telophase. The major events occurring during the M phase are pictured in Figure 2.2.

During the M phase, the cell divides into two daughter cells, each one containing the same number and kind of chromosomes as the parent cell. At the completion of the M phase, the cells either reenter the cell cycle at $G_1$ to undergo further maturation and replication or await activation by resting in $G_0$. Normally, cells spend about an hour in M.

The amount of time required to complete the cell cycle (called the *generation time*) varies depending upon the type of cell. Although the time from the beginning of S to the end of M seems to be fairly constant, the time the cell spends in $G_1$ can vary greatly (from 12 to 48 hours). The temporal length of $G_1$ determines the rate of cell proliferation (Baserga 1981).

Current research into cyclins might tell us more about the growth and regulation of the cell. Cyclins are proteins that cause the cell to enter mitosis and begin division. It is the absence of cyclin that enables the cell to change from metaphase to anaphase.

Cyclin research also has helped to elucidate cell cycle activity for malignant cells. It has been found that in some cancer cell lines, a genetic protein that interacts with cyclin and inhibits cell division is missing. Malignant cells from a variety of tumors bear abnormalities in a four-protein molecular structure responsible for cell cycle control (cyclin is one of the four proteins).

Another active area of research is the study of a cellular process called *apoptosis*. Apoptosis occurs when proteins in the nucleus of the cell fragment the cell's nuclear DNA, resulting in cell death. The absence of growth factors or hormones in some malignant cells can lead to apoptosis, whereas various other genetic events have been found to lead to a resistance to apoptosis. Treatment with some chemotherapeutic agents, monoclonal antibodies, oncolytic viruses, and other agents has resulted in a breakdown of resistance to apoptosis in some cancer cells (Sinkovics 1991).

Further elucidation of the molecular mechanisms underlying apoptosis might shed light on the question of why some tumor cells survive chemotherapy and others do not (Sen and D'Incalci 1992).

Antineoplastic drugs affect both normal and malignant cells by altering cellular activity during one or more phases of the cell cycle. Although both types of cells die as a result of irreparable damage caused by chemotherapy, normal cells have a greater ability to repair minor damage and to continue living than do neoplastic cells. The increased vulnerability of malignant cells is exploited to achieve the therapeutic effects seen with the administration of antineoplastic drugs.

Most antineoplastic agents are classified according to their structure or cell cycle activity. Two major classes of chemotherapeutic agents have been established: cell cycle phase-specific and cell cycle phase-nonspecific.

**Figure 2.1   Stages in the Cell Replication Cycle**
S = DNA synthesis; $G_2$ = the gap between DNA synthesis and mitosis; M = mitosis; and $G_1$ = the gap between the end of mitosis and the start of DNA synthesis ($G_0$ = resting phase, no replication)

*Source:* Groenwald, S. (1987). *Cancer Nursing: Principles and Practice.* Boston: Jones & Bartlett. Reprinted with permission.

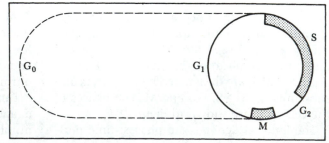

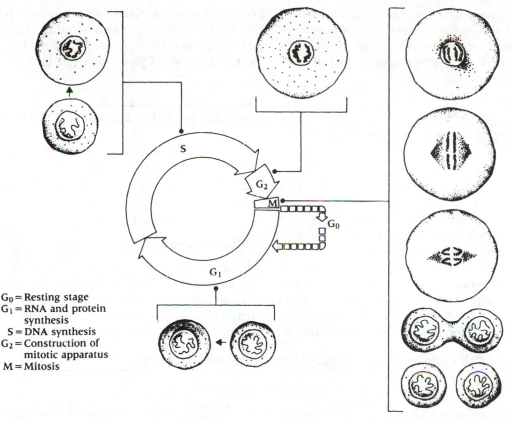

**Figure 2.2**   The Cell Cycle

*Source:* Goodman, M.S. (1987). *Cancer: Chemotherapy and Care.* Bristol Myers Oncology Division. Reprinted with permission.

## CELL CYCLE PHASE-SPECIFIC AGENTS

*Cell cycle phase-specific agents* kill proliferating cells only in a specific phase of the cell cycle (phases $G_1$ through M) (Brown 1987). For example, the vinca alkaloids, vincristine and vinblastine, are lethal only to cells in the M phase, whereas hydroxyurea and cytosine arabinoside (cytarabine) inhibit DNA synthesis and therefore are specific to the S phase. Because phase-specific agents depend on cells being in a specific phase to work, they are most effective against cells that are rapidly cycling.

Rapid cycling ensures that the cell passes through the phase in which it is vulnerable to the effects of the drugs. The antimetabolites and bleomycin are examples of phase-specific agents (see Table 2.1).

Some authors (Knobf et al. 1984) classify phase-specific agents under a broad class of agents called *cell cycle-specific agents.* These drugs damage both proliferating and resting cells, although they tend to be more effective against actively dividing cells than those in $G_0$ (Knobf et al. 1984). Therefore, cells that spend most of their time in $G_0$ are not affected significantly by cycle-specific agents. For purposes of simplicity and clarity, and because the distinctions between the classes of antineoplastic drugs often are relative, the drugs are classified as either cell cycle phase-specific or cell cycle phase-nonspecific.

## CELL CYCLE PHASE-NONSPECIFIC AGENTS

*Cell cycle phase-nonspecific agents* do not depend on the phase of the cell cycle to be active. Rather, these agents affect cells in all phases of the cell cycle: resting cells are as vulnerable as dividing cells to the cytotoxic effects of these agents. Consequently, phase-nonspecific agents have been found to be some of the most effective drugs against slow-growing tumors (Knobf et al. 1984). However, because DNA is the target site for these drugs, maximum cell

kill is not possible when cells are in the S phase at the time of drug administration. Nitrogen mustard, dacarbazine, and mitomycin are some examples of phase-nonspecific agents.

## CHEMOTHERAPY AND CELL KINETICS

A basic understanding of tumor cell kinetics is helpful in comprehending the rationales behind various chemotherapy schedules and regimens.

### Tumor Growth

Tumors grow by a progressive, steady expansion. According to Brown (1987), three characteristics of cells should be considered when assessing tumor growth: cell cycle time, growth fraction, and rate of cell loss. *Cell cycle*

**Table 2.1  Cell Cycle Activity of Selected Chemotherapeutic Agents**

| *Cell Cycle Phase-Specific Agents* | | | |
| --- | --- | --- | --- |
| **G$_1$ Phase** | **G$_2$ Phase** | **S Phase** | **M Phase** |
| L-asparaginase | bleomycin | cytarabine | docetaxel |
| prednisone | etoposide | 5-fluorouracil | paclitaxel |
| | irinotecan | gemcitabine | vinblastine |
| | topotecan | hydroxyurea | vincristine |
| | | methotrexate | vindesine |
| | | thioguanine | |

| *Cell Cycle Phase-Nonspecific Agents* | | | |
| --- | --- | --- | --- |
| **Alkylating Agents** | **Nitrosoureas** | **Antibiotics** | **Miscellaneous** |
| busulfan | carmustine (BCNU) | dactinomycin | dacarbazine |
| chlorambucil | lomustine (CCNU) | daunorubicin | procarbazine |
| cisplatin | semustine (MeCCNU) | doxorubicin | |
| cyclophosphamide | streptozocin | mitomycin | |
| ifosfamide | | | |
| mechlorethamine | | | |
| melphalan | | | |

*Source:* Adapted from Goodman, M.S. (1987). *Cancer: Chemotherapy and Care.* Bristol-Myers Oncology Division. Reprinted with permission.

*time* is defined as the amount of time needed for the cell to complete an entire cycle from mitosis to mitosis. Cycle times for cancer cells vary from 24 to 120 hours, with most ranging from 48 to 72 hours. It is interesting to note that some of the more rapidly dividing normal cells (e.g., colon and rectum crypt cells at 39–48 hours and bone marrow precursor cells at 19–40 hours) have similar, if not faster, cell cycle times than cancer cells. It originally was thought that cancer cells cycled and grew faster than normal cells (Brown 1987). It is easily understandable, then, how toxicities to normal cells occur, as chemotherapy acts on *all* rapidly dividing cells, not just those that are malignant. The *growth fraction* is the fraction of cells in the tumor that are cycling at a given time. In the early stages of tumor development (i.e., when tumor volume is low), the growth fraction is high, and the tumor doubles its volume relatively rapidly. As the tumor grows, however, space becomes restricted, and it outgrows its blood and nutrient supply so that the *tumor doubling time* decreases. Common tumor doubling times range from 5 days to 2 years.

The last factor influencing net tumor growth is the *rate of cell loss*, which is the fraction of cells that die or leave the tumor mass. Tumor growth is the net effect of the three factors mentioned above and follows a *Gompertzian growth curve* (see Figure 2.3).

The growth curve is a visual depiction of the idea that, as the tumor mass increases in size, tumor doubling time slows. The earliest point at which a solid tumor can be detected clinically is when it contains $5 \times 10^8$ cells (at this point, it measures 1 cm in diameter) (Gussack, Brantley, and Farmer 1984).

Tumor growth characteristics at least partially determine the choice of chemotherapeutic agents used against a tumor. For example, when tumor volume is low, a relatively large percentage of cells are dividing and thus are

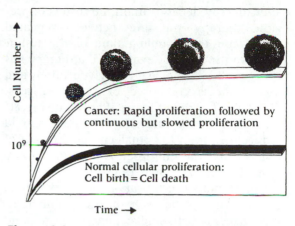

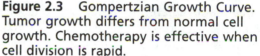

**Figure 2.3  Gompertzian Growth Curve. Tumor growth differs from normal cell growth. Chemotherapy is effective when cell division is rapid.**

*Source:* Goodman, M.S. (1987). *Cancer: Chemotherapy and Care.* Bristol-Myers Oncology Division. Reprinted with permission.

vulnerable to chemotherapeutic agents that affect dividing cells (cell cycle phase-specific agents). Likewise, when tumor volume is high, fewer cells divide and agents effective regardless of cell division characteristics (phase-nonspecific agents) are used (Goodman 1987).

## Cell Kill Hypothesis

The *cell kill hypothesis* is the theoretical ability of chemotherapeutic agents to kill cancer cells. According to the hypothesis, which was first described in studies by Skipper and Shabel and their colleagues (Skipper, Shabel, and Wilcox 1964; Skipper, Shabel, and Wilcox 1965; Skipper 1968), drugs kill cancer cells on the basis of *first order kinetics*: a certain drug dosage kills a constant percentage of cells rather than a constant number of cells. Repeated doses of therapy thus are needed to reduce the total number of cells, and the number of cells left after therapy depends upon the results of previous therapy, the time between repeated doses, and the doubling time of the tumor (Belinson 1980). For example, if a therapy has a 90% cell kill rate against a given tumor and the tumor is composed of a million cells, 100,000 cells are left living after the first treatment. Repeated treatments eventually should reduce the tumor to a small enough number of cells so that the immune system can kill any remaining cells (Brown 1987).

Unfortunately, cells can mutate over time, causing them to be resistant to chemotherapy. Also, patients with similar tumors can respond to treatment differently, sometimes making therapeutic decisions difficult (Goodman 1987). Consequently, the cell kill hypothesis cannot serve as the only predictor of a host's response to chemotherapy. For further discussion of tumor resistance to chemotherapy, the reader is referred to the end of this chapter and to Chapter 3.

### Relevance of Cytostatic versus Cytotoxic Agents in Designing Chemotherapeutic Regimens

One way in which chemotherapeutic regimens are planned uses the principles of synchronization and recruitment. *Synchronization* refers to the process of increasing the percentage of tumor cells that are in a specific phase of the cell cycle (Hill 1978). This can be done by administering *cytostatic* agents (those that block or retard cell development in a specific phase of the cell cycle) or by administering *cytotoxic* agents (which kill cells in a specific sensitive phase and lead to a relative increased percentage of cells in the insensitive phases). Also, low doses of antineoplastic agents tend to cause cells to arrest or "block" in certain phases,

whereas high doses tend to cause cell death, particularly in certain phases (Gussack et al. 1984). According to Hill (1978), the chemotherapeutic purpose of synchronization is to gather cells in a specific phase of the cell cycle so that they are rendered vulnerable to agents that are cytotoxically specific for that phase. For example, cytosine arabinoside's cytostatic properties cause cells to arrest at the boundary of phases $G_1$ and S (the $G_1$/S boundary) (Hill 1978). In causing this $G_1$/S arrest, an increased percentage of cells are "caught" in late $G_1$–early S, rendering them vulnerable to agents specific for the S phase.

*Recruitment* is another theoretical construct used to design chemotherapeutic regimens. The term refers to the transformation of resting cells into dividing (or cycling) cells. It can occur as an indirect consequence of cell killing when cell population depletion leads to the recruitment of resting cells back into the cell cycle. Cells that are recruited in this way are more vulnerable to the effects of drugs that work when cells are dividing (i.e., cycle phase-specific drugs) (Gussack et al. 1984). The principles of synchronization and recruitment are depicted in Figure 2.4.

## CLASSIFICATION OF ANTINEOPLASTIC AGENTS

Antineoplastic agents are drugs that are used specifically for the purpose of killing cancer cells. The terms *cancer chemotherapeutic drugs* and *cytotoxic compounds* are interchangeable. Cancer chemotherapeutic drugs generally are grouped into seven major classes: alkylating agents, antimetabolites, antibiotics, plant alkaloids, hormones, miscellaneous agents, and investigational agents.

## Alkylating Agents

The alkylating agents are members of one of the two primary classes of cytotoxic compounds useful in the treatment of cancer. They are highly reactive compounds that work by interacting chemically with the cellular DNA to prevent replication of the cell. More specifically, by substituting an alkyl group for the hydrogen atoms in cellular molecules, alkylating agents cause single- and double-strand breaks in DNA to cross-link and bond covalently (Chabner and Myers 1985). The DNA strands are thus unable to separate, an action necessary for the replication of cellular genetic material. Alkylating agents also prevent replication by causing a misreading of the DNA code and by inhibiting RNA, DNA, and protein synthesis in rapidly dividing tissues (Chabner and Myers 1985). The nucleic acid base most often involved in the process is guanine, but adenine and cytosine also have undergone alkylation as a result of drug administration. A schematic diagram showing sites and mechanisms of action of all the major chemotherapeutic agents is shown in Figure 2.5.

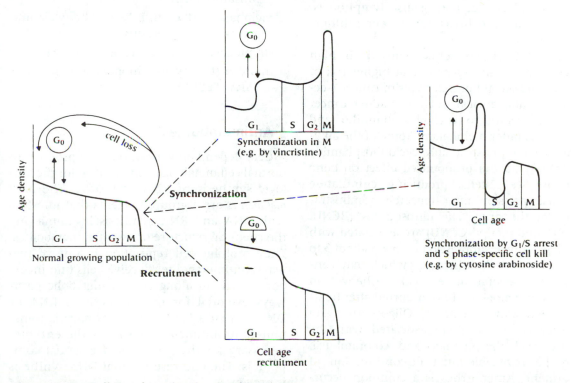

**Figure 2.4   Cell Synchronization and Recruitment**

*Source:* van Putten, L.N. (1976). *European Journal of Cancer* 12: 79. Reprinted with kind permission from Elsevier Science Ltd, The Boulevard, Langford Lane, Kidlington OX5 1GB, UK.

As a class, alkylating agents are considered cycle nonspecific. They exert their lethal effects on cells throughout the cell cycle, but tend to be more effective against rapidly dividing cells. One author postulates that this may be because rapidly dividing cells have less time to repair damage caused in $G_1$ before they enter the sensitive S phase of the cycle (Chabner and Myers 1985). Because alkylating agents are active against cells in $G_0$, they can be used to "debulk" (reduce the size of) tumors, causing resting cells to be recruited into active division. At this point, those cells are vulnerable to the cell cycle specific agents.

The alkylating agents have been proven to be cytotoxically active against lymphomas, Hodgkin's disease, breast cancer, and multiple myeloma.

Unfortunately, patients exposed to high doses of alkylating agents are at higher risk of developing second primary sites of cancer (secondary malignancies), such as bladder cancer (after exposure to cyclophosphamide) and leukemias (after melphalan). Some of the alkylating agents (most notably, cyclophosphamide and AZQ) have a pronounced effect on bone marrow stem cells, producing cumulative myelosuppression after repeated administrations of the drug. The nitrosoureas (BCNU, CCNU, and methyl-CCNU) are associated with a delayed myelosuppression with a nadir at 3 to 5 weeks after administration, which may continue for several more weeks. Changes in gonadal function also have occurred after treatment with alkylating agents. Oligospermia and azospermia, most often associated with the agents cyclophosphamide and chlorambucil, may be reversible after discontinuation of treatment. Amenorrhea is a common occurrence, but it too may be reversible in some patients.

*Common Alkylating Agents*

busulfan (Myleran)

carboplatin (Paraplatin)

carmustine (BiCNU, BCNU)

chlorambucil (Leukeran)

cisplatin (*Cis*-Platinum, CDDP, Platinum, Platinol)

cyclophosphamide (Cytoxan, Endoxan, Neosar)

dacarbazine (DTIC-Dome, Imidazole Carboximide)

estramustine phosphate (Estracyte, Emcyt)

ifosfamide (Ifex, IFX, Isophosphamide)

lomustine (CCNU, CeeNU)

mechlorethamine (Nitrogen Mustard, Mustargen, $HN_2$)

melphalan (Alkeran, L-PAM, Phenylalanine Mustard, L-Sarcolysin)

streptozocin (Streptozotocin, Zanosar)

thiotepa (triethylene thiophosphoramide, TSPA, TESPA)

## Antimetabolites

Cells depend on various nutrient products of normal cell metabolism, *metabolites*, for the biologic synthesis of RNA and DNA. The *antimetabolites* are a group of agents that interfere with DNA and RNA synthesis by mimicking the chemical structure of essential metabolites. They prohibit cell replication in one of two ways: antimetabolites deceive cells into incorporating them along certain metabolic pathways essential for the synthesis of RNA or DNA so that a false genetic message is transmitted; or antimetabolites block the enzymes necessary for the synthesis of essential compounds. The end result is that DNA synthesis is prevented.

Most antimetabolite cytotoxic activity occurs during the synthetic phase (S) of the cell cycle. It logically follows, then, that these agents would be most effective when used against rapidly cycling cell populations. This explains

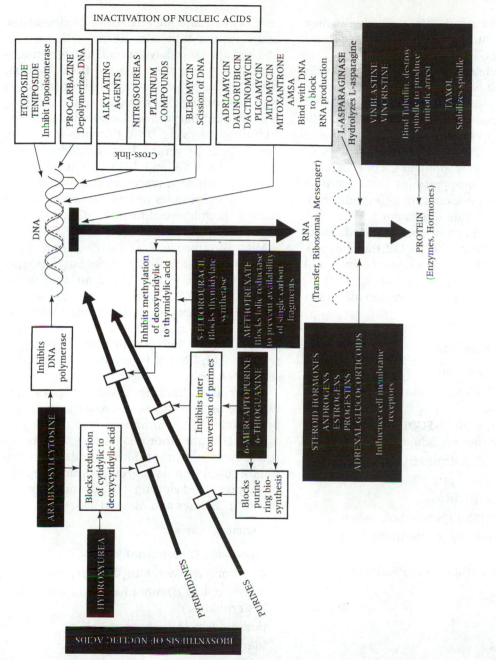

**Figure 2.5**  Mechanism of Action of Chemotherapeutic Agents

*Source:* Krakoff, I. (September/October 1991). Cancer chemotherapeutic and biologic agents. *CA—A Cancer Journal for Clinicians* 41(5): 266. Reprinted with permission.

why antimetabolites are more effective against fast-growing tumors than against slow-growing tumors.

The most common toxicities to normal cells occur as a result of the agent's attack on rapidly dividing cell populations. For example, oral mucosal cells, bone marrow stem cells, and cells lining the GI tract are affected by antimetabolite administration. Toxicities that follow such cytotoxic activity include stomatitis, bone marrow depression (myelosuppression), and diarrhea (and other GI sequelae resulting from death of normal cells and tissue sloughing).

Commonly used antimetabolites include folate antagonists (methotrexate, DDMP, trimetrexate), purine antagonists (6-mercaptopurine and 6-thioguanine), fluoropyrimidines (5-fluorouracil, FUDR) and cytosine arabinoside (ARA-C, cytarabine).

*Common Antimetabolites*

capecitabine (Xeloda)

cytarabine (ARA-C, Cytosar-U, cytosine arabinoside)

floxuridine (FUDR, 5-FUDR, 5-fluoro-2'-deoxyuridine)

5-fluorouracil (fluorouracil, Adrucil, 5-FU)

gemcitabine (Gemzar)

hydroxyurea (Hydrea)

6-mercaptopurine (purinethol, 6-MP)

methotrexate (Amethopterin, Mexate, Folex)

6-thioguanine (thioguanine, tabloid)

## Antibiotics

The antitumor antibiotics are agents that are isolated from microorganisms (Knobf et al. 1984). They have both antimicrobial and cyto-

toxic activity, although the latter predominates. As a class, the antibiotics are cell cycle nonspecific and appear to have several different mechanisms by which they produce their cytotoxic effects. For example, bleomycin's primary action is to produce single- and double-strand breaks in DNA. The anthracyclines (daunomycin and doxorubicin) intercalate DNA (forming a bond so that DNA is prevented from functioning as a template for RNA and DNA synthesis), cause oxidation-reduction reactions, and react directly with cell membranes at low concentrations to change membrane function (Chabner and Myers 1985).

Mitomycin produces cellular reactions similar to those of the anthracyclines but also functions as an alkylator. Mithramycin inhibits DNA-directed RNA synthesis, whereas actinomycin-D's primary action is the intercalation of DNA (Chabner and Myers 1985). To summarize, antibiotics function by either binding or reacting with DNA or by inhibiting the synthesis of RNA or both.

Major dose-limiting toxicities associated with the antibiotics are myelosuppression (all but bleomycin); skin and GI toxicity (actinomycin D); pneumonitis leading to fibrosis (bleomycin); cardiotoxicity and mucositis (doxorubicin and daunorubicin); and hepatic, renal, and blood clotting dysfunctions (mithramycin) (Chabner and Myers 1985).

*Common Antibiotics*

bleomycin (Blenoxane)

dactinomycin (actinomycin D, Cosmegan)

daunorubicin (Daunomycin, Rubidomycin, Cerubidine)

doxorubicin (Adriamycin)

idarubicin (Idamycin)

mithramycin (Mithracin, plicamycin)

mitomycin (Mutamycin)

mitoxantrone (Novantrone)

## Plant Alkaloids (Mitotic Inhibitors)

The search for new cytotoxic compounds led to the screening of many plant extracts. Four compounds of note (vincristine, vinblastine, etoposide, and teniposide) have survived clinical trials to become recognized as worthwhile antineoplastic agents. Vincristine and vinblastine are called vinca alkaloids and are derived from the shrub *Vinca rosea*. Teniposide and etoposide are derived from products of the mandrake plant.

Plant alkaloids work by crystallizing the microtubular mitotic spindle proteins during metaphase, which arrests mitosis and causes cell death. At high concentrations of drug, an inhibition of nucleic acid synthesis and protein synthesis has also been noted. The action of plant alkaloids is considered cell cycle phase-specific, occurring during the M phase. Teniposide and etoposide are premitotic in their cytotoxic activity, exerting most of their effect in $G_2$ (Knobf et al. 1984).

Major dose-limiting toxicities of plant alkaloids include myelosuppression (with vinblastine, etoposide, and teniposide) and neurotoxicity (with vincristine and, to a lesser extent, vinblastine).

*Common Plant Alkaloids*

etoposide (VP 16-213, Vepesid, epipodophyllotoxin)

teniposide (VM-26)

vinblastine (Velban, vinblastine sulfate)

vincristine (Oncovin, vincristine sulfate)

vinorelbine (Navelbine)

## Hormones

The growth and development of certain tumors depend to some extent on their existing in a specific hormonal environment (Brown 1987; Goodman 1988). When that environment is changed, tumor growth is impaired or arrested. Breast, thyroid, prostate, and uterine cancers are examples of solid tumors that are sensitive to hormonal manipulation. With these diseases, the action of hormones or hormone antagonists depends upon the presence of hormone receptors in the tumors themselves (e.g., estrogen receptors in breast cancers). Normally, proteins in the cytoplasm of a cell act as receptors that bind to hormones and transfer them to the nucleus of the cell. Once there, the hormone receptors facilitate the binding of chromatin to the nucleus—a process necessary for the synthesis of messenger RNA, which transmits the genetic information necessary for the synthesis of new proteins. The blocking of this process occurs when hormones or their antagonists are administered. Commonly used gonadal or sex hormones are estrogens—diethyl-stilbestrol (DES), ethinyl estradiol (Estinyl); progestins—medroxyprogesterone acetate (Provera), megestrol acetate (Megace); antiestrogens—tamoxifen citrate (Nolvadex); androgens—fluoxymesterone (Halotestin, Utadren), testosterone propionate (Oreton); and antitesterones—leuprolide acetate (Lupron), bicalutamide (Casodex), flutamide (Eulexin).

Corticosteroids, such as prednisone and prednisolone, comprise another class of agents useful in the treatment of certain neoplasms. The discovery of their lympholytic action led to their use against lymphatic leukemias, myeloma, and malignant lymphoma. Some evidence exists to suggest that corticosteroids also can recruit malignant cells out of the $G_0$ phase of the cell cycle and into active division, making them vulnerable to damage caused by cell cycle-specific chemotherapeutic agents (Bingham 1978).

Side effects from hormonal therapy occur as a result of the administering of higher than physiological doses of a drug to achieve the desired antineoplastic effects (Brown 1987). For the sex hormones, they include changes in secondary sexual characteristics (e.g., deepening of voice and hirsutism), changes in libido, and fluid retention. For the corticosteroids, side effects include hypertension, fluid retention, hyperglycemia, ulcers, osteoporosis, emotional instability, muscle wasting, increased appetite, Cushingoid features, increased susceptibility to infection, and masking of fevers.

*Common Hormonal Agents*

Adrenocorticoid Agents
   cortisone
   dexamethasone
   hydrocortisone
   methylprednisone
   methylprednisolone
   prednisone
   prednisolone

Androgens
   fluoxymesterone (Halotestin, Ora-Testryl)
   testolactone (Teslac)
   testosterone propionate (Neo-hombreol, Oreton)

Estrogens
   conjugated equine estrogen (Premarin)
   diethylstilbestrol (DES)
   diethylstilbestrol diphosphate (Stilphostrol, Stilbestrol diphosphate)
   ethinyl estradiol (Estinyl)

Antiestrogens
   tamoxifen citrate (Nolvadex)

Antitesterones
   bicalatamide (Casodex)

   flutamide (Eulexin)
   leuprolide acetate (Lupron)

Progesterones
   medroxyprogesterone acetate (Provera, Depo-Provera)
   megestrol acetate (Megace, Pallace)

## Miscellaneous Agents

Miscellaneous agents are those agents whose mechanisms of action differ from the major classes mentioned above. One of the most commonly used of these agents is L-asparaginase.

Asparagine is a nonessential amino acid required by some tumor cells for normal growth and development. The enzymes needed to synthesize asparagine are present in many normal tissues but are lacking in certain tumors, especially those arising from T-lymphocytes (Chabner and Myers 1985). Cells that lack these enzymes derive asparagine from circulating pools of amino acids. L-asparaginase depletes these pools rapidly and completely. Because normal tissues can synthesize their own asparagine, L-asparaginase has very little toxicity to normal tissues. However, it is a foreign protein, and can cause serious anaphylactic reactions.

*Common Miscellaneous Agents*

L-asparaginase (Elspar)
mitotane (Lysodren)
mitoxantrone (Novantrone)
procarbazine (Matulane)

## *Camptothecins*

The camptothecins are drugs that inhibit the enzyme topoisomerase I. Topoisomerase I is one of the enzymes responsible for relaxing the tension in the DNA helix by causing single-strand breaks in the helix, and eventually reattaching them in the religation step of the process. Topotecan and irinotecan work by binding to topoisomerase I, thereby arresting the cell in the $G_2$ phase.

Dose-limiting toxicities include diarrhea (with irinotecan) and myelosuppression (with both irinotecan and topotecan).

### Common Camptothecins

irinotecan (Camptosar, Camptothecan-11, CPT-11)

topotecan (Hycamptin)

## Taxanes

Like the plant alkaloids, paclitaxel (Taxol) and docetaxel (Taxotere) are plant derivatives, originally from the needles of the Pacific yew tree. The taxanes promote microtubule assembly and stability, thereby blocking the cell cycle in mitosis. Docetaxel is more potent in enhancing microtubule assembly, and induces apoptosis.

Hypersensitivity reactions/anaphylaxis are not uncommon during administration of taxanes. Patients should be monitored closely, especially in the initial phase of the infusion. Dose-limiting toxicities include myelosuppression and neurotoxicity (peripheral neuropathy).

### Common Taxanes

docetaxel (Taxotere)

paclitaxel (Taxol)

## Investigational Chemotherapeutic Agents

Investigational agents are those agents that currently are undergoing clinical trials and thus are not yet approved by the U.S. Food and Drug Administration (FDA). Such agents include not only new drugs but also approved drugs that are being administered in a manner different from that for which approval was obtained previously.

In clinical trials, drugs are procured directly from the National Cancer Institute (NCI) or indirectly through cooperative group protocols (the Cancer and Leukemia Group B, the Pediatric Oncology Group, etc.) and cancer centers. Although patients generally need to be treated on an NCI-approved protocol to receive investigational drugs, such agents may be obtained in certain circumstances directly from the pharmaceutical company for "compassionate use." This term refers to the use of an investigational agent off protocol in a patient for whom no other clinically established treatment options exist. For a thorough discussion of clinical trials, the reader is referred to Chapter 1.

## RATIONALE OF SINGLE-AGENT THERAPY VERSUS COMBINATION THERAPY

Single-agent therapy was used often in the early history of cancer chemotherapy. Starting in the 1960s, however, combinations of chemotherapeutic agents were found to produce superior clinical responses with less overall toxicity than single-agent therapy (Knobf et al. 1984). With a few exceptions, combination chemotherapy has replaced single-agent therapy in the medical management of cancer.

The major disadvantage of single-agent therapy led to clinical trials with combinations of drugs. Some of the disadvantages noted were: single agents were unsuccessful at achieving long-term remissions; they produced cell lines that were resistant to further drug therapy; and they produced severe or lethal toxicities when given in doses adequate to irradicate the tumor (Hubbard 1981). The most significant of these disadvantages is tumor drug resistance, as this was found to be the most common reason for treatment failure.

The improved therapeutic effects of combination chemotherapy resulted from both the additive and synergistic effects of the drugs used. According to Carter and Livingston (1982), three conceptual approaches have been used in designing drug combinations. The *biochemical approach* asserts that by using drugs that individually produce different biochemical damage, one can attack different sites in the biosynthetic pathways or inhibit processes that are necessary for the normal function of essential macromolecules. The goal of the biochemical approach is to decrease the production and the availability of the end products needed by the tumor for normal growth and development.

The *cytokinetic approach* is based on principles of cell cycle kinetics. This approach suggests that drugs should produce changes in cells that render them more vulnerable to cycle-specific agents. For example, it is known that "debulking" a tumor by surgery or chemotherapy causes an increase in the growth fraction (the number of cells undergoing active division) of the remaining cells. Activating cells in this way would make them vulnerable to cycle-specific agents.

The third approach is the *empirical approach*. Numerous effective combinations of agents have evolved through the use of individual agents that alone have demonstrated antineoplastic activity against a particular tumor. When combined, the mechanisms of action of the different drugs often complement each other to produce maximal cell kill. A distinct advantage of combination chemotherapy is that the toxicities of the individual drugs often differ, allowing the administration of nearly full tolerated doses without severe toxicity. One example of an empirically derived drug combination is MOPP (mechlorethamine, vincristine, prednisone, procarbazine) for the treatment of Hodgkin's disease. The effect on

the bone marrow of the drug combination MOPP plus ABVD (adriamycin, bleomycin, vinblastine, dacarbazine) used against Hodgkin's disease is shown in Figure 2.6.

A closer look at this drug combination illustrates some of the principles used in the empirical approach:

PRINCIPLE *Each drug in the combination should be active against the tumor when used alone.*
Mechlorethamine, vincristine, procarbazine, prednisone, doxorubicin, bleomycin, vinblastine, and dacarbazine all have been shown to be active against Hodgkin's disease.

PRINCIPLE *The mechanisms of action of the different drugs should complement each other to produce maximal cell kill.*
The drugs listed above are both cell cycle phase-specific and cell cycle phase-nonspecific. For example, dacarbazine and mechlorethamine are alkylating agents and are cell cycle phase-nonspecific, whereas vincristine and vinblastine are both specific for the S and M phases. Using these drugs in combination theoretically ensures that cells will be affected regardless of their cycling characteristics at the time of drug administration.

PRINCIPLE *Drugs that produce toxicities in different organ systems should be combined so that maximal doses of each can be administered without excessive morbidity.*
In the MOPP combination, mechlorethamine is a potent myelosuppressant, whereas vincristine's dose-limiting toxicity is often neurotoxicity. Prednisone does not affect bone marrow, but sometimes causes imbalances in glucose metabolism and protein breakdown (Knobf et al. 1984).

Procarbazine's dose-limiting toxicities are nausea and vomiting and myelosuppression, although the myelosuppression occurs much later than that of mechlorethamine (Goodman 1987).

**PRINCIPLE**  *Drugs should be combined that have toxicities occurring at different times.*

As mentioned, mechlorethamine's myelosuppressive nadir occurs at 10–14 days,

whereas procarbazine's is 2–3 weeks after cessation of therapy (Knobf et al. 1984). This phenomenon is illustrated in Figure 2.6.

Some of the advantages of combination chemotherapy are: it allows for maximal cell kill within the range of toxicity tolerated by

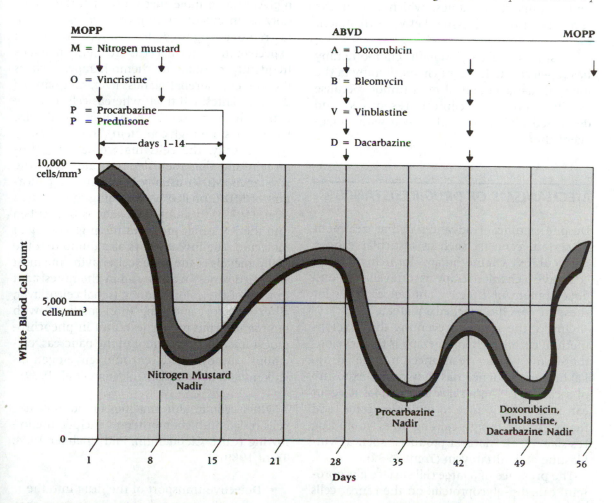

**Figure 2.6**  The Effect of MOPP Combined with ABVD on the White Blood Cell Count

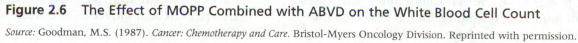

*Source:* Goodman, M.S. (1987). *Cancer: Chemotherapy and Care.* Bristol-Myers Oncology Division. Reprinted with permission.

the patient for each drug; it provides for a broader range of coverage of new resistant tumor cell lines (this seems to be the major reason for the success of combination chemotherapy over single-agent therapy); and it prevents or slows the development of new resistant cell lines (DeVita 1982). An important advance made with the institution of combination of chemotherapy was the use of intermittent treatment schedules, which permit the recovery of normal tissues between treatment cycles.

In summary, combination chemotherapy has replaced single-agent chemotherapy in the medical management of most tumors because of its improved clinical responses and decreased toxicity over that seen with single-agent therapy.

## MECHANISMS OF DRUG RESISTANCE

Despite significant advances in the treatment of certain cancers, such as testicular cancer, with curative chemotherapy, for many cancers "curative" chemotherapy is unavailable, and development of effective anticancer drugs for these tumors has reached a plateau.

One of the factors preventing the development of curative chemotherapy is the development of tumor resistance to the drug. Laboratory evidence has shown that exposure of a cancer cell to a *single* antineoplastic agent can lead to resistance to multiple agents, and many of the drugs causing this "multidrug resistance" are natural products, such as vinblastine and adriamycin (Trent 1989).

The presence of a large cell surface glycoprotein, called p-glycoprotein, on the cancer cells appears to be one of the most important causes of multidrug resistance. Cancer cells with multidrug resistance have a very high number of these cell surface glycoproteins, whereas cells sensitive to chemotherapy agents have very few if any (Trent 1989).

According to Kartner and Ling (1989), the p-glycoprotein molecule works like a pump so that chemotherapeutic drugs enter the cell but then are pumped quickly back out of the cancer cells, leaving cells undamaged by the chemotherapy. Certain normal body cells have p-glycoprotein molecules on their surface, possibly as an evolutionary protective mechanism to remove ingested toxins. As might be expected, these normal cells are found in organs frequently resistant to chemotherapy, such as the kidneys, adrenal glands, liver, and parts of the gastrointestinal tract, whereas cells that are extremely chemosensitive, such as blood cells, have almost no p-glycoprotein (Trent 1989).

Genetically, the cells that contain p-glycoprotein and that then demonstrate multidrug resistance (MDR) usually have gene amplification of MDR, or PGY1. According to Goldstein et al. (1989), this amplified gene is transcribed into the RNA that produces the p-glycoprotein molecule. The investigators also found that the highest levels of the gene (cells having the most amplified genes) were found in chemoresistant cancers of the colon, kidney (renal cells), liver, adrenal cortex, and lung (non-small cell with neuroendocrine properties), and in pheochromocytoma, islet cell tumor of the pancreas, carcinoid tumor, and chronic myelogenous leukemia in blast crisis (Goldstein et al. 1989).

Other cellular abnormalities found in cancer cells resistant to chemotherapy include the following (Curt, Clendeninn, and Chabner 1984; Trent 1989):

- Defective transport of the drug into the cell with increased drug excretion so that there are decreased intracellular concentrations of the drug

- Defective drug metabolism
- Increased drug inactivation
- Altered DNA repair with increased cell efficiency to excise or repair DNA damage caused by the drug
- Altered drug target, so drug cannot recognize intracellular target (i.e., enzyme, nucleotide)

Current research efforts include the following:

- Identifying agents that inactivate the p-glycoprotein molecule in cells (Kartner and Ling 1989)
- Screening agents that overcome resistance to known drugs
- Identifying drugs that effect cellular pathways leading toward cell division or apoptosis
- Identifying chemomodifiers that may be combined with chemotherapy agents to increase their effectiveness, such as the calcium channel agents and VX170
- Finding drugs that interact with unique chromosomal abnormalities of tumors

As more is learned about the mechanisms of drug resistance, models can be developed and tested that target these mechanisms and attempt to make the cancer cells sensitive to chemotherapeutic agents. For a more in-depth discussion of multidrug resistance and of current prospects in cancer treatment the reader is referred to Chapter 3.

## CONCLUSION

Drug therapy, supportive therapy, bone marrow transplantation, and biological response modifiers are in the forefront of cancer treatment methodology. All of these therapies are used in combination to enhance drug effective-

ness. New drugs are being tested and developed in a variety of programs through the National Cancer Institute, as well as in programs in pharmaceutical companies. The development of new drugs has been the cornerstone of cancer chemotherapy. Newer theories of chemotherapy administration, such as neoadjuvant or induction chemotherapy, confers a definite survival advantage in several sarcomas and improves surgical results in other solid tumors. Although chemoprevention has been shown to prevent the development of second primary cancers in patients with head and neck cancers, it is being explored in other tumors. Newer strategies related to a more effective use of chemotherapy, hormones, and biological agents are underway.

*Supportive therapy* has improved the survival of cancer patients. With the availability of platelets, hemorrhage is no longer a leading cause of death. Infections still remain a problem for many patients, but the development of antibiotic agents and growth factors has improved survival rates.

Both allogeneic (matched-donor) and autologous (self-donor) *bone marrow transplantations* have shown success in a variety of cancers. This area is just being explored and holds a great deal of promise. Also, the use of growth factors to hasten bone marrow recovery permits more consistent, and higher, drug dosing.

The field of cancer treatments has grown over the years. More than 40 chemotherapeutic agents have proven useful in treating malignant diseases. The development of new drugs is slow, and prospects for the future lie not only in trying to prevent disease but also in more effective use of established drugs, more intensive supportive therapy, and exploring the field of immunology.

Cancer chemotherapy, hormones, and biotherapy are here to stay. The science is constantly changing in an attempt to improve the survival of persons with cancer as well as their quality of life. The new millennium will see continuing changes in therapeutics, such as the technology of bone marrow transplantation, genetic re-engineering, and drug development; oncology nursing will be in the forefront of these scientific and practice advancements.

## BIBLIOGRAPHY

### Chemotherapy

Baserga, R. (1981). The cell cycle. *New England Journal of Medicine* 304(8): 453–459.

Belinson, J.L. (1980). Understanding how chemotherapy works. *Contemporary Obstetrics and Gynecology* 21: 2–17.

Bingham, C.A. (1978). The cell cycle and cancer chemotherapy. *American Journal of Nursing* July 78(7): 1201–1205.

Breasted, J.H. (1930). *The Edwin Smith Surgical Papyrus*. Chicago, Ill.: University of Chicago Press.

Brothwell, D. (1967). The evidence of neoplasms. In D. Brothwell and A.T. Sanderson (eds.): *Disease of Antiquity*. Springfield, Ill.: C.C. Thomas, 320–345.

Brown, J. (1987). Chemotherapy. In S. Groenwald (ed.): *Cancer Nursing: Principles and Practice.* Boston: Jones & Bartlett, 348–384.

Burchenal, J.H. (1977). The historical development of cancer chemotherapy. *Seminars in Oncology*, 4(2): 135–146.

Carter, S., and Livingston, R. (1982). Principles of cancer chemotherapy. In S. Carter, E. Glatstein, and R. Livingston (eds.): *Principles of Cancer Treatment*. New York: McGraw-Hill, 95–110.

Chabner, B.A., and Myers, C.E. (1985). Clinical pharmacology of cancer chemotherapy. In V.T. DeVita, Jr., S. Hellman, and S.A. Rosenberg (eds.): *Cancer: Principles and Practice of Oncology*. Philadelphia: Lippincott, 287–327.

Cline, M.J., and Haskell, C.H. (1980). *Cancer Chemotherapy*. 3rd ed. Philadelphia: Saunders.

Dangle, R.B., and Flynn, K. (1987). Historical perspective. In C.R. Ziegfeld (ed.): *Core Curriculum for Oncology Nursing*. Philadelphia: Saunders, 375–390.

DeVita, V.T., Jr. (1982). Principles of chemotherapy. In V.T. DeVita, Jr., S. Hellman, and S.A. Rosenberg (eds.): *Cancer: Principles and Practice of Oncology*. Philadelphia: Lippincott, 276–292.

DeVita, V.T., Jr., Oliverio, V., Jr., Muggia, F., et al. (1979). The drug development and clinical trials programs of the division of cancer treatment. National Cancer Institute. *Cancer Clinical Trials* 2(3): 195–216.

Ebbell, B. (1937). *The Papyrus Ebers: The Greatest Egyptian Medical Document*. Copenhagen: Levin and Munksgaard.

Farber, S., Diamond, L., Mercer, R., et al. (1948). Temporary remissions in acute leukemia in children produced by folic acid antagonists, 4-aminopteroyglutamic acid (aminopterin). *New England Journal of Medicine* 238: 787–793.

Goodman, M.S. (1988). Concepts of hormonal manipulation in the treatment of cancer. *Oncology Nursing Forum* 15(5): 639–647.

———. (1987). *Cancer: Chemotherapy and Care*. Bristol-Myers Oncology Division.

Groenwald, S. (1987). *Cancer Nursing: Principles and Practice*. Boston: Jones & Bartlett.

Gussack, G.S., Brantley, B.A., and Farmer, J.C. (1984). Biology of tumors and head and neck cancer chemotherapy. *Laryngoscope* 94(9): 1181–1187.

Haddow, A. (1970). David A. Karnofsky memorial lecture: Thoughts on chemical therapy. *Cancer* 26(4): 737–754.

Hill, B.T. (1978). Cancer chemotherapy: the relevance of certain concepts of cell cycle kinetics. *Biochimica and Biophysica Acta* 516: 389–417.

Hubbard, S.M. (1981). Chemotherapy and the nurse. In L.B. Marino (ed.): *Cancer Nursing*. St. Louis: Mosby.

Knobf, M.K.T., Fischer, D.S., and Welch-McCaffrey, D. (1984). *Cancer Chemotherapy: Treatment and Care*. 2nd ed. Boston: G.K. Hall Medical Publishers.

Krakoff, I. (September/October 1991). Cancer chemotherapeutic and biologic agents. *CA—A Cancer Journal for Clinicians* 41(5): 266.

Krakoff, I.H. (1977). Systemic cancer treatment: cancer chemotherapy. In J. Horton and G.J. Hill (eds.): *Clinical Oncology*. Philadelphia: Saunders.

Murinson, D.S. (1981). Clinical pharmacology. In S.N. Rosenthal and J.M. Bennett (eds.): *Practical Cancer Chemotherapy*. Garden City, N.Y.: Medical Examination.

Saunders, J.F., and Carter, S.K. (eds.) (1977). USA-USSR Monograph: Methods of Development of New Anticancer Drugs. *National Cancer Institute Monograph*, 45. Washington D.C.: U.S. Department of Health, Education, and Welfare, Public Health Service, Publication 76-1037.

Sen, S., and D'Incalci, M. (1992). Apoptosis: Biochemical events and relevance to cancer chemotherapy (review). *FEBS Letters* 307(1): 122–127.

Shimkin, M.S. (1977). *Contrary to Nature*. Washington D.C.: U.S. Department of Health, Education, and Welfare, Public Health Service, Publication 76-720.

Sinkovics, J.G. (1991). Programmed cell death (apoptosis): Its virological and immunological connections (review). *Acta Microbiologica Hungarica* 38(3–4): 321–324.

Skipper, H.E. (1968). In *The Proliferation and Spread of Neoplastic Cells*, 21st Annual Symposium on Fundamental Cancer Research at M.D. Anderson Hospital and Tumor Institute, Houston, Texas. Baltimore: Williams and Wilkins, 213–233.

Skipper, H.E., Shabel, F.M. Jr, and Wilcox, W.S. (1964). *Cancer Chemotherapy Reports* 35: 1–111.

———. (1965). *Cancer Chemotherapy Reports* 45: 5–28.

Stonehill, E.H. (1978). Impact of cancer therapy on survival. *Cancer* 42(2 Suppl): 1008–1014.

van Putten, L.N. (1976). Cell synchronization and recruitment (figure). *European Journal of Cancer* 12: 79.

Wells, C. (1963). Ancient Egyptian Pathology. *Journal of Laryngology and Otology* 77: 261–265.

## Mechanisms of Drug Resistance

Curt, G.A., Clendeninn, N.H., and Chabner, B.A. (1984). Drug resistance in cancer. *Cancer Treatment Reports* 68(1): 87–99.

Gerlach, J.H., Kartner, N., Bell, D.R., and Ling, V. (1986). Multidrug resistance. *Cancer Surveys* 5(1): 25–46.

Goldstein, L.J., Galaski, A., Fojo, M., Willingham, M., Lai, S.L., Gazdar, A., and Pirker, R. (1989). Expression of a multidrug resistance gene in human cancers. *Journal of the National Cancer Institute* 81(2): 116–124.

Kartner, N., and Ling, V. (1989). Multidrug resistance in cancer. *Scientific American* 260(3): 44–51.

Trent, J.M. (1989). Mechanisms of drug resistance. In *Proceedings, Advances in Clinical Oncology*. Snowbird, Utah: March 1989, 33–35.

# Chapter 3

# New Frontiers of Chemotherapy

**Cynthia R. King, PhD, NP, RN**

## INTRODUCTION

Over the years, the use of chemotherapeutic agents has resulted in the successful treatment of many malignant diseases. Today, several exciting innovative uses of chemotherapy and other agents exist that hold promise as cancer therapies. These include hematopoietic stem cell transplantation (HSCT) which includes bone marrow transplantation and peripheral stem cell transplantation, biological response modifiers (BRMs), and modulators, or multidrug resistance (MDR). The purpose of this chapter is to provide information on HSCT, colony stimulating factors (CSFs), BRMs, MDR, and chemoprevention. Oncology nurses in all settings eventually will be responsible for the care of patients with cancer who are receiving or have received these new treatment modalities. This information will help prepare oncology nurses to provide high-quality nursing care to these patients.

## HEMATOPOIETIC STEM CELL TRANSPLANTATION

### History

The first bone marrow transplant (BMT) was performed in 1891 by Brown-Sequard. This marrow was given by mouth and unfortunately it was not successful. In 1937, Schretzanmayr administered bone marrow intramuscularly (Santos 1983). Intravenous (IV) marrow was given to a woman with gold-induced aplastic anemia in 1939. The donor was her brother. This was the first true transplant attempt (Deeg, Klingemann, Phillips, and van Zant 1999). In 1957, French and Yugoslav physicians treated radiation-exposed laboratory workers with allogeneic BMT. There was temporary engraftment, but it is not clear whether the benefit was long-term (Bekkum and deVries 1967).

In the 1960s, attention was directed to animal studies and to better understanding the genetic factors involved in marrow grafting and hematopoiesis. At that time, knowledge also was increasing regarding histocompatibility, tissue typing, blood component therapy, conditioning regimens, and supportive measures (Buchsel 1993b; Deeg, Klingemann, Phillips, and van Zant 1999; Thomas and Storb 1970).

Between 1969 and 1975, BMT was used to treat severe aplastic anemia or acute leukemia when other therapies failed (Thomas et al. 1975). Six-month survival rates increased from 20–70% as more effective conditioning regimens were developed and supportive care of patients was refined further (Whedon

1991a). In 1979, the first peripheral stem cell transplants (PSCTs) were performed. The cells were infused over 8–14 days; consequently, these transplants were not successful because engraftment did not occur. Finally, from 1984–1986, successful PSCTs were performed in which stem cells were infused over 1–2 days (Kessinger, Armitage, Landmark, and Weisenburger 1986; Reiffers et al. 1986).

Bone marrow transplantation and peripheral blood stem cell transplantation (now termed PBCT) are treatments that are included in the overall term hematopoietic stem cell transplantation (HSCT). The number of these transplants performed each year has increased significantly since the 1970s. Bortin and colleagues (Bortin, Horowitz, and Gale 1988; Bortin, Horowitz, and Rimm 1992) reported that there were 200 transplant centers by 1990. These centers were performing 5,000 transplants annually. As many as 20–25 new transplant teams join the International Bone Marrow Transplant Registry (IBMTR) each year. Horowitz and Rowlings (1997) reported that in 1995 at least 18,000 autologous transplants and 12,000 allogeneic transplants were performed. Over the past 40 years, HSCT has developed into a successful treatment modality because of advances in the biological sciences, development of new drugs and protocols, improvements in transfusion technologies, and supportive care provided by health care professionals.

## Types of Transplant

There are three types of HSCT. They are described below and are named according to the source from which the healthy cells are obtained. In each case, the cells could be obtained from the bone marrow or the peripheral blood. Thus, transplants can be bone marrow transplants (BMTs) or peripheral blood stem cell transplants (PBCTs).

### Autologous

The cells are obtained directly from the patient, and then are reinfused back into the patient after the chemotherapy and/or radiation. The use of autologous bone marrow transplantation (ABMT) is limited significantly by the need for the marrow to be healthy and free from disease. With ABMT, the marrow is harvested when the patient is in remission and is cryopreserved until needed for transplant. With autologous PBCT (APBCT), the cells are collected by pheresis just prior to the transplantation and are cryopreserved.

### Syngeneic

The cells are obtained from an identical twin and thus are matched perfectly to the patient. Because it is uncommon for a patient to have an identical twin, these transplants are performed infrequently. A higher incidence of leukemic relapse has been reported in syngeneic transplants than in allogeneic transplants. This may be due to the antileukemic effect of graft-versus-host-disease (GVHD).

### Allogeneic

The cells are obtained from a donor (related or unrelated) and are given to the patient. Matching the donor and the patient is important. Some recipients receive cells from an "HLA matched" relative. Other individuals do not have a phenotypically identical sibling or family member and must receive matched cells from an unrelated donor (e.g., the National Marrow Donor Program Registry) or from a partially matched related or unrelated donor. The ultimate success of an allogeneic transplant depends on how well the donor and the patient are matched. Matched unrelated transplants are generally more successful than partially matched transplants. There are higher complications and lower survival rates for partially matched transplants.

## Umbilical Cord Blood Cells

It is now known that umbilical cord blood is rich in hematopoietic stem cells and can be used successfully for engraftment. Cord blood cells now can be used as a source of cells for HSCT for HLA-matched unrelated individuals. Unfortunately, there is little cord blood available. Thus, this method is practical only as a source of stem cells for transplanting infants and small children. Several advantages of this method include the following: these cells are a potential resource that usually is discarded, there might be qualitative features of these cells that make them superior to bone marrow or peripheral blood stem cells in terms of proliferative potential, and because the cord blood cells are of fetal origin they have reduced immuno-competence so they may be less likely to cause GVHD. However, disadvantages exist to the use of cord blood. Specifically, the small size of the number of cells collected and the longer time for engraftment (O'Connell and Schmit-Pokorny 1997; van Zant 1999). Despite the disadvantages, the optimal cryo-preservation of umbilical cord blood has been discovered (Donaldson et al. 1996) and individuals have been transplanted successfully with cord blood (Zix-Kieffer et al. 1999). Newer sources of stem cells in the future might include cadaveric and fetal liver cells).

## Indications

Transplants may be performed for malignant and/or some nonmalignant disorders. Tables 3.1 and 3.2 provide overviews of the indications for HSCTs. Transplants can be used for both hematologic malignancies (e.g., acute and chronic leukemias and preleukemias) and nonhematologic malignancies (e.g., lymphomas, multiple myeloma, neuroblastoma, and selected solid tumors). Severe aplastic ane-mia (SAA) and thalassemia, and severe combined immune deficiencies (SCIDs), are examples of nonmalignant disorders that are treated successfully with transplantation. Most of the HSCTs done for nonmalignant diseases are done in children. Overall, HSCTs are used to 1) replace marrow or stem cells in patients whose marrow is diseased or deficient, and 2) as a rescue after high-dose chemotherapy is given (Billett 1992; Deeg et al. 1999; Gale and Butturini 1992; Goldstone 1992; Gorin 1992; Jagannath, Vesole, and Bartogie 1992; King 1993; O'Connell and Schmit-Pokorny 1997; Vose, Phillips, and Armitage 1992).

### Table 3.1   Malignant Disorders Treated with HSCT

Acute myelogenous leukemia

Acute lymphocytic leukemia

Chronic myelogenous leukemia

Chronic lymphocytic leukemia

Hairy cell leukemia

Non-Hodgkin's lymphoma

Burkitt's lymphoma

Hodgkin's lymphoma

Multiple myeloma

Neuroblastoma

Myelodysplastic syndromes

Gliomas

Lung cancer

Ovarian cancer

Brain cancer

Sarcomas

Breast cancer

Testicular cancer

Melanoma

*Source:* Adapted from Whedon, M.B. (1991b). Autologous bone marrow transplantation. In M.B. Whedon, *Bone Marrow Transplantation: Principles, Practice, and Nursing Implications.* Boston: Jones & Bartlett, 20–48.

**Table 3.2** Nonmalignant Disorders Treated with HSCT

| Hematologic Disorders | Congenital Disorders | Mucopolysaccharidoses |
|---|---|---|
| Aplastic anemia | Severe combined immuno-deficiency (SCID) | Hurler's disease |
| Diamond-Blackfan anemia | Wiskott-Aldrich syndrome | |
| Fanconi's anemia | Functional T-cell deficiency | |
| Sickle cell anemia | | |
| Thalassemia | | |
| Chediak-Higashi syndrome | | |
| Chronic granulomatous disease | | |
| Congenital neutropenia | | |
| Paroxysmal nocturnal hemoglobinuria | | |

*Source:* Adapted from Whedon, M.B. (1991b). Autologous bone marrow transplantation. In M.B. Whedon, *Bone Marrow Transplantation: Principles, Practice, and Nursing Implications.* Boston: Jones & Bartlett, 20–48.

## Treatment Process

Even though different types of HSCT and a variety of clinical indications exist, the treatment process is similar for all. This treatment process has several stages or phases. The sequence includes evaluation of the patient for eligibility, admission to the unit, administration of the conditioning regimen, infusion of the marrow/stem cells, recovery of the patient as cells engraft, discharge, and post-transplant rehabilitation.

### Evaluation Phase

During the evaluation phase, the patient is screened for eligibility and is educated about the procedure and the potential complications. Other factors that may determine eligibility include whether the disease is responsive to chemotherapy and/or radiation, the disease is in an early stage, and the source of the stem cells is free of disease. Type of disease, stage of disease, and age are among several factors that further determine eligibility. The patient also must have an appropriate source of marrow/stem cells, be free of other serious health conditions, have adequate venous access, have

adequate financial resources, and provide informed consent. Additionally, a thorough physical exam is performed, as well as baseline tests and studies (Table 3.3). The comprehensive pretreatment evaluation is conducted by physicians, nurses, and other disciplines. Nurses often coordinate these activities (Buchsel 1993b; King 1993; O'Connell and Schmit-Pokorny 1997; Whedon 1991a).

*Donor Search.*

Not all patients who require an allogeneic transplant have an HLA-matched sibling. The figure varies based on ethnicity, but about 1 in 3 patients has a matched sibling. If the patient does not have a sibling, then a search begins for the matched unrelated donor (MUD). The searches are done through donor registries throughout the world. Between 1988 and 1990, the number of unrelated donor transplants doubled from 5% to 10% (O'Connell and Schmit-Pokorny 1997).

*HLA Tissue Typing.*

An important component to the success of an allogeneic HSCT is the compatibility of the

**Table 3.3  Tests Performed During Evaluation of an HSCT Patient**

**Laboratory Tests**

Complete blood count (CBC)

Hepatitis screen (A, B, C)

Human immunodeficiency virus (HIV)

Cytomegalovirus (CMV)

Herpes simplex virus (HSV)

PT/PTT

Liver profile

Renal profile

Endocrine profile

Blood group typing

**Other Tests**

Pulmonary function tests

Chest X-ray

Echocardiogram

MUGA scan

**Evaluations**

Nutritional evaluation

Psychologic assessment

Social work evaluation

Dental exam

**Staging Tests**

Bone marrow aspirate and biopsy

Radiological tests (CT, MRI, bone scans)

Tumor markers

donor and the recipient. This is determined by a tissue typing system called the Human Leukocytic Antigen (HLA system). This system includes at least six antigen groups located on chromosome 6. They are HLA-A, -B, -C; -DR, -DQ, and -DP (Welte 1994). This HLA system allows the body's immune system to differentiate self from nonself (or foreign cells) and mount an attack against foreign cells (Weinberg 1991). The search for a matched donor involves comparing HLA-A, -B, -C, and -DR antigens. When an appropriate HLA match is found, that individual is educated and evaluated for eligibility. He or she undergoes a physical exam and laboratory testing. Additionally, the donor requires counseling. He or she is never pressured into volunteering. The identity of the donor remains unknown to the patient and the transplant center.

*Harvest/Pheresis.*

If the patient is to receive autologous marrow or stem cells, these are harvested/pheresed during the evaluation phase or upon admission to the transplant unit. Bone marrow cells are obtained through a procedure called a bone marrow harvest. The procedure for "harvesting" bone marrow is the same for autologous and allogeneic BMT. This procedure is performed in the operating room. The donor is given either spinal or general anesthesia and is placed in the prone position. After both posterior iliac crests are cleansed, multiple aspirations are performed bilaterally. The cells are obtained in 2–5 ml aspirates. As many as 100–200 aspirates may be necessary to obtain the appropriate number of marrow cells. Generally, the equivalent of 10–15 ml/kg of body weight is collected. Only 6–10 punctures are required in the skin because the needles are redirected several times in each site. Throughout the procedure, marrow cell counts are performed to determine the appropriate number of cells for engraftment. Often $1–8 \times 10^8$ cells/kg body weight (500–1000cc) are collected from the donor (Buchsel 1993b; King 1993; Whedon 1991a). It is easier to aspirate cells from a healthy allogeneic donor than from a previously treated patient. The entire process takes 1–2 hours.

After the cells are collected, they are placed in a heparinized tissue culture medium and are filtered through a series of fine mesh screens to remove fat and bone particles. Then the cells are placed in blood administration bags and either are taken to the patient (allogeneic) or are frozen (autologous) (Buchsel 1993b; King 1993; Whedon 1991a).

For autologous BMT, the cells are either frozen either intact or after purging the malignant cells from the sample by one of several methods. This freezing process involves adding a preservative, such as dimethyl sulfoxide (DMSO), to the cells, placing the bag between two flat aluminum plates, and storing the cells at the lowest possible temperature. Then the cells are stored in liquid nitrogen at approximately −196°C or in vapor phase at −80°C in order to block all enzymatic pathways of cell metabolism to maintain cell viability. The rate of freezing is slow to decrease the shock to the cells (Buchsel 1993b; King 1993; Whedon 1991b). Some viability of cells is lost during the freezing and thawing processes. It has been shown, however, that significant viability can be maintained after storing cells for many years (Deeg et al. 1999).

If there is concern that the autologous cells contain malignant cells, then removal of the malignant cells is attempted by purging. This may result in the loss of some normal cells, thus additional BM or PBCs may be collected. There are pharmacological and physical methods for purging cells. The pharmacological techniques include 4-hydroperoxycylophosphamide (4-HC), mafosfamide, cisplatin, VP-16, vincristine, methylprednisolone, mero-cyanine 540, immunologic methods, monoclonal antibodies and complement, immunotoxins, monoclonal antibodies and magnetic microspheres, and toxins. The physical methods for purging cells include lectin agglutination, counterflow elutriation, photoactive agents, long-term bone marrow culture, and positive selection for normal early progenitors. It still remains controversial whether to purge cells.

Peripheral blood stem cells (PBCs) are obtained by a process called pheresis. PBCs are 10–100 times less concentrated than bone marrow cells, and thus more volume is collected with pheresis. A cell separator machine is used for pheresis. The donor/patient is connected to the machine, blood is withdrawn and separated, and unneeded components are returned to the donor/patients. Each pheresis session is generally 2–4 hours long. A donor/patient may need as few as 3 sessions or as many as 10 sessions over a span of days to weeks. After each session, the cells are frozen with DMSO.

Some transplant centers "mobilize" stem cells prior to collection. Mobilized stem cells are PBCs whose numbers have been increased deliberately prior to pheresis. It has been shown that mobilized stem cells can accelerate (by 1 week) the rate of marrow recovery following transplant. PBCs are mobilized or stimulated by the use of chemotherapeutic agents, colony-stimulating factors (CSFs), or both. When mobilization is effective, it decreases the number of pheresis sessions required to collect an adequate number of cells for durable engraftment. Unfortunately, the method of mobilization is unpredictable and does not always produce significant increases in circulating cells. After the chemotherapy has been administered, it is difficult to determine the best time to begin collections. The optimum time of mobilization occurs in approximately 10–14 days but lasts only 3–4 days. It would be helpful if the optimum time of mobilization could be determined by culture assays, but it takes 14 days to quantify stem cells from culture assays.

Different methods exist to determine the appropriate number of blood cells to collect via pheresis, including the number of mononuclear cells (MNCs), colony-forming units-granulocyte and monocyte (CFU-GM), and CD34-positive cells. The pheresis procedure generally is tolerated well by patients, although they may experience citrate toxicity, hypovolemia, thrombocytopenia, headache, and chilling.

It is still not standard to collect umbilical cord blood at most institutions. Usually, an obstetrician or nurse midwife collects the cells after the delivery of the placenta. The amount collected ranges from 42–282 ml.

## Admission

The second phase involves admission and orientation to the transplant unit. The admission is often overwhelming for the patient and his or her family. After the patient is admitted to the unit, the primary nurse performs a thorough physical assessment, as well as an evaluation of psychological and social background and coping strategies. At this time, the nurse initiates an individualized comprehensive care plan or care map for the patient.

During the admission phase, the physicians and nurses make sure patients are thoroughly informed and consent to the transplant. This is important because after the conditioning regimen has been administered, patients cannot discontinue treatment. Furthermore, a fully informed patient is more likely than an uninformed patient to adhere to his or her treatment regimen. There should be adequate opportunity for questions throughout the process (King 1993).

### Alternative Care Models.

Some transplants (mostly PBCTs) are offered in settings other than hospitals. These alternative settings include a combination of inpatient, outpatient, and home care. These programs are designed to provide safe, quality, cost-effective care that decreases the need for hospitalization. An important part of these models is adequate supportive care and qualified personnel and support systems. There also are specific patient criteria including the following:

- Remain afebrile
- Maintain a platelet count of $> 20,000$ m$^3$, without any active bleeding
- Make daily clinic visits for assessments and procedures
- Take adequate nutrition and fluids daily as well as oral medications
- Understand how to access emergency care
- Maintain written schedule of medications

There are also several criteria that a caregiver should meet, including:

- Be responsible for home care
- Transport patient to and from clinic visits
- Assist with care as needed
- Monitor patient's compliance with medications and self-care
- Understand how to access emergency care

Some of the different models of care for transplantation are traditional HSCT, early discharge HSCT, and outpatient HSCT. The traditional model involves the evaluation occurring as an outpatient. Then admission for the conditioning regimen, supportive care, and recovery until adequate engraftment. Then the patient receives follow-up care as an outpatient. Early discharge also involves evaluation, placement of a central venous catheter, harvest, or apheresis all on an outpatient basis. The patient then is admitted only for the conditioning regimen. When the conditioning regimen is complete, the patient is cared for as an outpatient unless they develop serious infections or complications. Outpatient HSCT involves the patient having the entire procedure from evaluation to recovery as an outpatient unless they develop serious infections or complications.

## Conditioning Regimen

The third phase involves the administration of the conditioning or preparative regimen. This usually begins within 24–48 hours of admission. The regimen physiologically prepares the patient for the new healthy stem cells. The conditioning regimen has two main purposes: (1) to immuno-suppress the patient (host), which decreases the risk of graft rejection and allows for engraftment, and (2) to eradicate residual malignant cells while having tolerable morbidity and mortality (Phillips 1999, Wiebe, Smith, and DeGregorio 1992). This process is described by a variety of terms, including ablation, preparative regimens, and condition-ing regimen.

The conditioning regimen plays a significant role in the ability to achieve and sustain success-ful engraftment following transplantation. It con-sists of high-dose chemotherapy and/or radiation. No one specific conditioning protocol is adminis-tered to all patients. The regimen is selected based on a variety of factors: (a) patient's disease, (b) chemosensitivity of the tumor, (c) type of trans-plant, (d) past treatment protocols, and (e) cur-rent medical condition. Obtaining adequate antihematopoietic and immunosuppressive activ-ity may require the administration of multiple chemotherapeutic agents and radiation. New dosage schedules medications and combinations of drugs are continually developed. In part, the choice of the chemotherapeutic agents depends on such pharmacologic factors as cell cycle speci-ficity, pharmacodynamics, pharmacokinetics, drug interactions, and overlapping toxicities of agents (Phillips 1999; Wiebe et al. 1992). Specifi-cally, the choice of agents for high-dose chemotherapy is based on the following consider-ations:

Effectiveness of the agent against the
    specific tumor
Steepness of the dose-response curve for

the agent in experimental and clinical
    trials
Difference between the transplant dose and
    the standard dose
Nonadditive toxicity when given in
    combination with other agents
Non–cross-resistance with other agents
    used in the conditioning regimen
    (Frei 1992)

Chemotherapy drugs usually are adminis-tered by central venous catheter (CVC) or by mouth over 2–6 days. These agents affect both diseases and healthy cells. Predominately, they affect the most rapidly dividing cells (e.g., mouth, throat, and gastrointestinal tract).

Some of the chemotherapeutic agents used in transplantation are presented in Table 3.4. It is important to remember that different transplant centers use different protocols; therefore, other agents may be used at particular centers.

When radiation is administered as part of the conditioning regimen, it usually is given as total body irradiation (TBI), total lymphoid irradiation (TLI), or total abdominal irradiation (TAI) for immunosuppression or to eradicate disease. TBI also is used for its antileukemic effect. It provides effective tumor kill because of its ability to penetrate the central nervous system (CNS). The addition of TBI does reduce the risk of graft rejection to less than 50%. The dose given ranges from 500–1600 Cgy.

In preparation for TBI, the patient has a spe-cial consultation session in which he or she is placed in various positions on the treatment table while measurements are taken and recorded. Purple marks are drawn on the skin to ensure appropriate margins for the radia-tion. TBI may be given in one dose or in mul-tiple doses ("fractionated") over several days. Each session takes approximately 30–60 min-utes and is painless. Giving multiple doses over several days appears to minimize the risk of

**Table 3.4**  Chemotherapeutic Agents Used in Transplantation

| Agent | Dose | Toxicity | Agent | Dose | Toxicity |
|---|---|---|---|---|---|
| ATG (anti-thymocyte globulin) | 15 mg/kg | Tachycardia<br>Azotemia<br>Serum sickness<br>Anaphylaxis<br>Edema | dacarbazine | 1250 mg/m$^2$ | Myelosuppression<br>Nausea/vomiting<br>Anorexia<br>Veno-occlusive disease<br>Neurological toxicities<br>Paresthesias |
| busulfan | 1–4 mg/kg | Myelosuppression<br>Stomatitis<br>Hyperuricemia<br>Hyperuricosaria<br>Amenorrhea<br>Gynecomastia<br>Cataracts<br>Interstitial pulmonary fibrosis | | | Facial flushing<br>Photosensitivity<br>Teratogenicity |
| | | | etoposide | 30–60 mg/kg | Myelosuppression<br>Nausea/vomiting/diarrhea<br>Cardiac dysfunction<br>Anaphylaxis<br>Bronchospasm<br>Pancreatitis |
| carboplatin | 400 mg/m$^2$ | Myelosuppression<br>Nausea/vomiting<br>Stomatitis<br>Renal toxicities<br>Hepatic toxicities<br>Peripheral neuropathies | | | Stomatitis<br>Paresthesias<br>Peripheral neuropathies |
| | | | ifosfamide | 7500 mg/m$^2$ | Hemorrhagic cystitis<br>Nausea/vomiting<br>Anorexia<br>Stomatitis<br>Renal toxicity<br>Neurological toxicities<br>Hepatic toxicities<br>Hallucinations/confusion<br>Teratogenicity |
| carmustine | 15 mg/kg | Myelosuppression<br>Severe hypotension<br>Tachypnea<br>Dyspnea<br>Increased BUN<br>Headache<br>Subacute hepatitis | | | |
| cyclophos-phamide | 50–200 mg/kg | Hemorrhagic cystitis<br>Myelosuppression<br>Tachycardia<br>Cardiomyopathy<br>Congestive heart failure<br>Shortness of breath<br>Hypotension<br>Stomatitis<br>Nausea/vomiting<br>Anorexia<br>Amenorrhea<br>Azoospermia<br>Teratogenicity | melphalan | 30–180 mg/m$^2$ | Myelosuppression<br>Stomatitis<br>Anaphylaxis<br>Skin rash<br>Headache<br>Teratogenicity |
| | | | mitomycin C | 20 mg/m$^2$ | Myelosuppression<br>Nausea/vomiting/diarrhea<br>Anorexia<br>Stomatitis<br>Renal toxicities<br>Phlebitis<br>Blurred vision |
| cytarabine | 1–3 g/m$^2$ | Myelosuppression<br>Nausea/vomiting/diarrhea<br>Stomatitis<br>Cardiomegaly<br>Abdominal pain<br>Skin rash<br>Anorexia<br>Ataxia<br>Thrombophlebitis<br>Cerebellar toxicity<br>Staggered gait<br>Slurred speech | thiotepa | 30–400 mg/m$^2$ | Myelosuppression<br>Nausea/vomiting/diarrhea<br>Stomatitis<br>Amenorrhea<br>Hyperuricemia<br>Skin rash<br>Headache/dizziness |

*Source:* Adapted from Franey, R.J., and Yee. G.J. (1994). Regimen-related toxicity after bone marrow transplantation. *Highlights on Antineoplastic Drugs* 10: 60–75; King C.R. (1993). *Bone Marrow Transplantation Clinical Background Manual.* Paramus, N.J.: Roche Professional Service Centers; Phillips, G.L. (1999). Conditioning Regimens. In H.J. Deeg, H.G. Klingemann, G.L. Phillips, and G. van Zant (eds.): *A Guide To Blood and Marrow Transplantation* (pp. 67–88). 3rd ed. Berlin: Springer; Wiebe, V.J., Smith, B.R., and DeGregorio, M.W. (1992). Pharmacology of agents used in bone marrow transplant conditioning regimens. *Critical Reviews in Oncology-Hematology* 13(13): 241–270. Reprinted with permission.

side effects. Blocking techniques can be used to protect certain organs, such as lungs and kidneys (Labar et al. 1989; Lawton 1989; Vitale et al. 1989). In recent years, some protocols have substituted newer chemotherapeutic agents and removed TBI from the conditioning protocol (Kanfer and McCarthy 1989; Tutschka, Copelan, and Kapoor 1989).

In the past, the conditioning regimens were always given in the hospital after the patient was admitted to the transplant unit. Now these regimens may be given as an inpatient or outpatient. At some institutions, the chemotherapy might be given daily on an outpatient basis. In this case, the patient is admitted to the hospital only as their physical condition necessitates. Other transplant centers are administering chemotherapy daily on an inpatient basis, and then discharging the patient prior to or just after the infusion of the cells. Additionally, different isolation techniques are used. These include reverse isolation, reverse isolation with special air handling systems, high efficiency particulate air (HEPA) filters, or laminar airflow (LAF). Despite the type of isolation and whether the patient receives the conditioning regimen as an inpatient or an outpatient, the patient and family should be taught many important self-care activities, such as mouth care, use of incentive spirometer, skin care, personal hygiene, specific diet, neutropenic precautions, exposure to other individuals, and amount and type of activity.

## Infusion of Cells

Over the years, various routes have been used for infusing marrow/stem cells, including the following: intraperitoneal, intrasplenic, and oral. Currently, the route of choice is intravenous (IV). Cells may be infused via IV piggyback or pushed via a syringe. Nurses are generally the health care professionals responsi-

ble for preparing the patient and the family and for infusing the cells: however, policies do vary at different transplant centers. Standing orders, premedications, and emergency medications are prescribed by the physician and are available at the time of the infusion (King 1993).

This day of infusing the cells generally is referred to as day 0. The cells represent "new life" to the patient and family. Even though this is a very important day for the patient and family it may be anticlimactic because the actual administration is similar to the infusion of any other blood product.

When autologous marrow or stem cells are used, the frozen cells are brought to the patient's room or nursing unit and are thawed in a warm (37°–38°C) water bath prior to infusion. To maintain maximum viability of the cells, only one bag is thawed at a time. As the cells are administered and pass through the patient's system, the patient excretes DMSO (the preservative) through his or her lungs. This may produce an odd smell that is often described as "garlic" or "creamed corn." The odor may remain for 24–36 hours and the patient may experience nausea and vomiting. In addition to the DMSO, the thawing process causes red blood cell (RBC) lysis. After the marrow/stem cells are infused, the patient develops hemoglobinuria, or dark red urine, for 2 hours secondary to the lysis of the RBCs (King 1993).

When allogeneic marrow cells are used, the cells are brought to the patient care area after they have been collected from the donor and processed in the blood bank. Recipients of allogeneic cells do not have to contend with the pungent odor produced by DMSO.

Patients may experience several potential reactions to the infusion. Side effects most commonly reported include chills, fever, shortness of breath (SOB), hypotension, chest pain, rash, nausea, vomiting, decreased urine output, and malaise. Additional side effects include respiratory distress syndrome, renal failure, fluid overload, abdominal cramping, and diarrhea. Most centers premedicate patients with diphenhydramine. Additionally, they may administer acetaminophen or hydrocortisone to prevent hypersensitivity reactions (Roy, Veys, and Jackson 1989; Smith et al. 1987). Because of the number of potential side effects, nurses must monitor the following frequently: vital signs, intake and output, and signs of sensitivity reaction. The rate of infusion may be decreased slightly to alleviate side effects.

When the cells are infused, they travel to the bone marrow spaces. This is called homing. In 7–14 days, these new, healthy cells begin to establish normal function.

## Recovery

The recovery period begins the day after the infusion of the marrow/stem cells. This is called Day +1. During this period, the patient waits for engraftment of the cells and a normal blood count. This may take 14–21 days or longer. Recovery occurs at variable speeds based on the nature and the status of the primary disease; previously administered chemotherapy and radiation; the type of conditioning regimen; any medications for the prevention of GVHD; and the use of antiviral agents.

Recovery may be difficult if one or more potentially life-threatening complications develop. Except for GVHD, which occurs only with allogeneic transplants, the complications

**Table 3.5    Acute Complications Associated with HSCT**

| Complication | Nursing Interventions |
|---|---|
| Myelosuppression | |
|    Anemia | Provide rest, blood products |
|    Granulocytopenia | Prevent infections, give CSFs |
|    Thrombocytopenia | Prevent bleeding, give platelets |
| Infections | |
|    Bacterial, viral, fungal | Give antimicrobials and CSFs, isolation |
| Cardiac | Cardiac monitoring, auscultation |
| Pulmonary | |
|    Interstitial pneumonitis | Lung assessment, give antimicrobials |
|    Pulmonary edema | Diuretics, I & O, weight |
|    Pulmonary infections | Assess for fever and changes in pulmonary status, give antimicrobials |
| Gastrointestinal | |
|    Stomatitis | Oral assessment, oral care |
|    Parotitis | Ice packs |
|    Xerostomia | Oral care, artificial saliva |
|    Nausea/vomiting | Give antiemetics on schedule |
|    Diarrhea | Assess I & O, F & E status, give antidiarrheal agent |
| Hepatic | |
|    Veno-occlusive disease | Maintain F & E balance, decrease effects of ascites, assess weight |
| Renal insufficiency | Assess F & E status, weight, I & O, blood urea nitrogen/creatinine |
| Graft-versus-host disease | Assess skin, liver, GI tract, I & O, maintain F & E balance |
|    Psychosocial | Provide support to patient/family, encourage patient to express emotions, listen to concerns |

CSFs = colony-stimulating factors; I = intake; O = output; F = fluid; E = electrolyte; GI = gastrointestinal from autologous and allogeneic BMT and PBCT are very similar.

The acute complications associated with transplantation can occur simultaneously. One may exacerbate another. The treatment of one complication may place the patient at risk for another complication, and the complications may be subtle or obvious. Some of the acute complications and nursing interventions are shown in Table 3.5.

Nurses play a vital role in preventing complications and providing supportive care. Every nurse involved in caring for transplant patients must understand how to recognize and treat infections, because infections in neutropenic patients often result in sepsis and death. Nurses are instrumental in encouraging patients to comply with daily exercise, mouth care, and incentive spirometry.

## Discharge and Rehabilitation

The goal of HSCT is to cure the patient and to return him or her to a productive life. It is important that there be a smooth transition for the patient and the family from the protected environment of the transplant center to the daily routine at home. The average length of hospitalization (if the HSCT is performed completely inpatient) varies from patient to patient. The length of stay depends on the patient's condition, the type of transplant, and the conditioning regimen used. Many new advances in supportive care (including colony-stimulating factors) have decreased the length of stay significantly.

Some centers have a professional discharge planner, whereas others use staff nurses or HSCT coordinators to anticipate discharge needs. It is essential that someone act as the liaison between the inpatient and outpatient units in order to provide continuity of care as patients leave the transplant center.

Education is a significant part of the discharge process. Nurses play a key role in educating patients and families on granulocytopenic precautions, preparation of the home environment, care

of the central venous catheter, good hygiene, hand-washing techniques, oral care, when to contact health care professionals, appropriate activities, and appropriate nutrition.

Each transplant center has established specific discharge criteria. There are some generally accepted guidelines for discharge (Table 3.6). Patients may leave the transplant unit when they meet the discharge criteria and are medically stable. Many centers discharge patients directly home. Some centers discharge patients to an outpatient setting, such as hospital-owned apartments. This may be an option, for example, if a patient meets only some of the discharge criteria and no longer requires the intensive care provided in the transplant unit (Buchsel 1993a; Buchsel 1993b; King 1993).

**Table 3.6   Discharge Criteria**

Absolute neutrophil count (ANC) > 500–1000

Platelets > 15,000–20,000

Hematocrit > 25–30% for adults and children

Able to take in > 50% of baseline nutrient requirement

Able to take oral medications

Nausea and vomiting controlled with oral medications

Diarrhea controlled at < 500 ml/day

Afebrile for at least 48 hours

Adequate home environment

Adequate support and resources at home

*Source:* Adapted from Buchsel, P.C. (1991). Ambulatory care: Before and after BMT. In M.B. Whedon, (ed.): *Bone Marrow Transplantation: Principles, Practice, and Nursing Implications.* Boston: Jones & Bartlett.

It is essential that all HSCT patients and families receive verbal and written instructions prior to discharge. Critical information to cover includes signs and symptoms to report to the transplant team, bleeding precautions, infection control practices, central venous catheter care, dietary restrictions, medication instructions, follow-up appointments, and what to do in an emergency. Phone numbers should be provided for how to reach the transplant team 24 hours a day, 7 days a week.

During the early post-transplant period, the patient may need daily to weekly examinations at the outpatient clinic. These visits will include blood tests, chest X-rays, bone marrow aspirations, lumbar punctures, and blood products. Some transplant patients receive immunosuppressive agents, immunoglobulin therapy, colony stimulating factors (CSFs), or total parenteral nutrition (TPN) as outpatients. During the first few months, post-transplant emphasis is placed on the prevention of infection because infection is a leading cause of readmission to the hospital (Buchsel 1993a; Buchsel 1993b).

Long-term complications are those that occur 100 or more days after transplant. As more transplants are performed each year, it becomes more important for nurses in all settings to be knowledgeable regarding these complications. Most of these late effects of transplantation result from the chemotherapeutic agents and/or radiation given as the conditioning regimen. Table 3.7 displays various long-term complications observed post-transplant (Buchsel 1986; Buchsel 1993b).

## Care of the Transplant Patient

The success of HSCT is dependent in part on the supportive care provided by nurses and the ability to prevent or manage the potential acute and long-term complications associated with therapy. Caring for HSCT patients is complex, intensive, and challenging. Yet many of the nursing interventions used with transplant patients are the same as those used with oncology patients receiving standard or intensive chemotherapy (see Table 3.5). The nursing interventions provided in chapter 4 concerning potential toxicities are applicable to transplant patients. Additionally, transplant nurses may need to prevent menses by administering

**Table 3.7**  Long-Term Complications Associated with Transplantation

| Complication | Time Posttransplant |
|---|---|
| Chronic graft-versus-host disease | ≥100 days |
|   Skin | |
|   Gastrointestinal tract | |
|   Liver | |
|   Oral | |
|   Ocular | |
|   Vaginal | |
| Infectious complications | 100–365 days |
|   Bacterial | |
|   Viral | |
|   Fungal | |
| Pulmonary complications | 100–400 days |
|   Interstitial pneumonitis | |
|   Cytomegalovirus | |
|   *Pneumocystis carinii* | |
|   Obstructive disease | |
| Genitourinary effects | 4–26 months |
|   Bladder shrinkage | |
|   Radiation nephritis | |
| Dental decay | 3 months–1 year |
| Cataracts | 1.5–5 years |
| Neurological complications | 1 month–5 years |
|   Leukoencephalopathy | |
| Psychosocial complications | Weeks to years |
|   Emotional | |
|   Body image changes | |
|   Financial/employment | |
| Retarded growth and development | Months to years |
| Gonadal dysfunction | Months to years |
| Secondary malignancies | 1–15 years |

*Source:* Adapted from Buchsel, P.C. (1986). Long-term complications of allogeneic bone marrow transplantation: Nursing implications. *Oncology Nursing Forum* 13: 61–70; Buchsel, P.C. (1993b). Bone marrow transplantation. In S.L. Groenwald, M.H. Frogge, M. Goodman, and C.H. Yarbro (eds.): *Cancer Nursing: Principles and Practice* 3rd ed. (pp. 393–434). Boston: Jones & Bartlett.

oral contraceptives or prevent infection by requiring the patient to abstain from fresh fruits and vegetables or to adhere to a low-bacteria diet. Depending on the institution, the specific neutropenic precautions also may

include following particular isolation procedures (wearing gowns, gloves, or masks),
teaching visitors HSCT precautions, observing
strict personal hygiene, using surveillance cultures, or administering prophylactic antibiotics.

To be sure all HSCT patients receive quality
supportive care throughout the transplant
process, many centers are developing extensive care plans; critical pathways; standing
orders for medications (e.g., chemotherapy,
antibiotics, and colony stimulating factors), lab
work, hydration, and infusion of cells; and
patient-teaching books and documentation
tools in order to provide quality care in the
most cost-effective manner. Generally, the
documentation tools and standing orders complement the care plans or critical pathways.
What is important in pathways or maps are
timelines for implementation and expected
outcomes. Table 3.8 outlines some of the key
elements to be included in a critical pathway
or care map. Most transplant centers maintain
the copyright of their critical pathways or care
maps, but they share with individuals or other
centers that request a copy. With the increased
use of care plans, critical pathways, and other
tools, some transplant centers have been able
to decrease the cost of care, decrease the
length of hospitalization, and enhance communication between departments and team
members (Burns, Tierney, Long, Lambert, and
Carr 1995). One type of algorithm that is used
commonly with HSCT patients to help improve
the quality of care and to decrease the cost of
care and the length of stay is one used for prophylactic and empiric antibiotic therapy in the
febrile neutropenic HSCT patient. An example
of a portion of a typical algorithm appears in
Figure 3.1. In some centers, this is accompanied by standing orders or guidelines for the
HSCT team to follow.

**Table 3.8** Elements of Critical Pathways or Care Maps

Disease Status Staging
Co-morbidities
Type of transplant
Study/protocol
Allergies
ABO type
CMV status
HSV status
Clinical consultants (e.g., renal, dietary, pulmonary, psychiatry)
Blood component therapy
Tests procedures
Conditioning regimen (chemotherapy/radiation)
Physical assessment
  Neurological
  Pulmonary
  Cardiovascular
  Nutritional/hydration
  Mobility
  Skin integrity
  Pain
Prophylaxis of infection
Management of acute complications
Discharge criteria
Date critical pathway or care map reviewed
Signature of health care professional who reviewed critical pathway or care map

## BIOLOGICAL RESPONSE MODIFIERS

The field of biotechnology has emerged over
the past decade. Biotechnology uses organisms
and their cellular, subcellular, and molecular
components to produce proteins and antibodies targeted at specific cancers producing a new
modality for treating cancer patients. Biological response modifiers (BRMs), biotherapy, are

**On Day 0 (day of infusion of cells) prophylactically start ciprofloxacin 500 mg po q 12 hrs and fluconazole 200mg q 24 hrs and acyclovir 800mg po q 12 hrs if patient is herpes simplex virus positive or has a history of genital or oral herpes.**

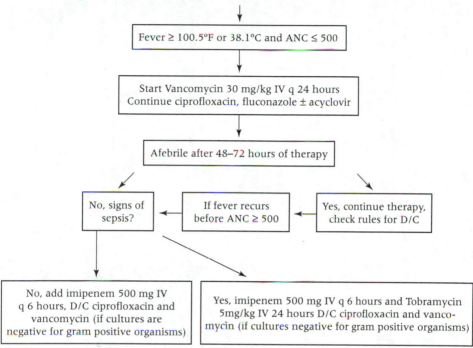

Fever ≥ 100.5°F or 38.1°C and ANC ≤ 500

Start Vancomycin 30 mg/kg IV q 24 hours
Continue ciprofloxacin, fluconazole ± acyclovir

Afebrile after 48–72 hours of therapy

No, signs of sepsis?

If fever recurs before ANC ≥ 500

Yes, continue therapy, check rules for D/C

No, add imipenem 500 mg IV q 6 hours, D/C ciprofloxacin and vancomycin (if cultures are negative for gram positive organisms)

Yes, imipenem 500 mg IV q 6 hours and Tobramycin 5mg/kg IV 24 hours D/C ciprofloxacin and vancomycin (if cultures negative for gram positive organisms)

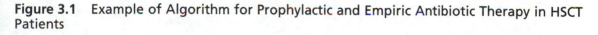

**This algorithm continues based on the patient's febrile status and ANC count. Each HSCT center uses a different combination of antibiotics based on what antibiotics are on formulary, the organisms most commonly cultured, and physician preference.**

**Figure 3.1** Example of Algorithm for Prophylactic and Empiric Antibiotic Therapy in HSCT Patients

agents derived from biological sources that affect biological responses.

These biological agents are capable of the following: producing direct antitumor activity; restoring, augmenting, or modulating the host's immune system; and interfering with tumor cell differentiation, transformation, or metastasis. Most agents are proteins or glycoproteins that exert biological effects by binding to cell-surface receptors specific for them. Cytokines are sub-

stances released from activated lymphocytes and include interferons (INFs), interleukins (ILs), tumor necrosis factor (TNF), and hematopoietic growth factors or colony stimulating factors (CSFs). Other BRMs are the monoclonal antibodies (MoAbs) and immunomodulators. Although many BRMs are still investigational, many are being approved for use. The following is a brief overview of BRM. Table 3.9 highlights the side effects seen in patients treated with BRMs and

**Table 3.9 Side Effects of Biological Response Modifiers**

| System | Interferons | Interleukin-2 | Hematopoietic Growth Factors | Monoclonal Antibodies | Tumor Necrosis Factor |
|---|---|---|---|---|---|
| Central nervous System | Impaired concentration, headache, lethargy, confusion | Impaired concentration, headache, lethargy, confusion, anxiety psychoses | Rare | Rare | Confusion, rare seizures |
| General | Constitutional symptoms,* fatigue* | Constitutional symptoms,* fatigue,* weight gain during therapy followed by weight loss* | Mild constitutional symptoms, fatigue (mostly with GM-CSF) | Constitutional symptoms, allergic reactions rare anaphylaxis | Constitutional symptoms,* rigors,* fatigue* |
| Cardiovascular | Hypotension, tachycardia, arrhythmias, rare myocardial ischemia | Hypotension,* edema,* ascites, arrhythmias, decreased systemic vascular resistance* | Rare hypertension with epoetin alfa | Hypotension, chest pain | Hypotension,* arrhythmias |
| Pulmonary | Rare | Dyspnea, pulmonary edema | Rare occurrence of dyspnea with first dose of GM-CSF | Dyspnea, wheezing | Dyspnea |
| Renal/hepatic | Proteinuria, elevated liver enzymes* | Oliguria,* increased BUN and creatinine,* proteinuria, azotemia, increased bilirubin, SGOT, SGPT, LDH | Rare elevation of LDH, alkaline phosphatase with G-CSF | Rare | Increased bilirubin, liver enzymes |
| Gastrointestinal | Nausea/vomiting, diarrhea, anorexia* | Nausea/vomiting,* diarrhea,* anorexia,* mucositis | Rare | Nausea/vomiting | Nausea/vomiting, anorexia, diarrhea |
| Genitourinary | Impotence, decreased libido | Decreased libido | Rare | Rare | Decreased libido |
| Integument | Alopecia, rash | Rash* dry desquamation,* erythema,* pruritis,* inflammatory reaction at injection sites* | GM-CSF,/G-CSF: inflammation at injection site, rare occurrence of rash | Urticaria, rash, pruritis | Inflammatory reaction at injection sites |
| Hematologic | Leukopenia,* anemia, thrombocytopenia | Anemia,* thrombocytopenia, lymphopenia,* eosinophilia* | Leukocytosis,* eosinophilia (GM-CSF) | In hematologic malignancies, leukopenia | Thrombocytopenia, granulocytopenia |
| Musculoskeletal | Myalgias,* arthralgias* | Myalgias, arthralgias | Bone pain* with GM-CSF/G-CSF | Rare arthralgias | Myalgias, arthralgias |

*Common side effects

*Source:* Rieger, P.T. (1996). Biotherapy—The Fourth Modality. In M. Barton-Burke, G. Wilkes, and K. Ingwersen, *Cancer Chemotherapy: A Nursing Process Approach.* 2nd ed. pp. 43–73. Sudbury, Mass: Jones & Bartlett.
Adapted with permission from Rumsey, K.A.. and Rieger, P.T. (1992). *Biological Response Modifiers.* Chicago: Precept Press.

**Table 3.10** Plan of Care for Patients Receiving Biological Response Modifier Therapy

| Nursing Diagnosis (Potential/Actual) | Expected Outcomes | Assessment | Nursing Interventions |
|---|---|---|---|
| I. *Altered comfort related to:* | | | |
| A. Chills | I. A. 1. Pt/significant other demonstrates self-care behaviors for management of chills<br>2. Pt reports acceptable control of chills | I. A. 1. Assess severity and duration of chills and document<br>2. Monitor vital signs frequently and report changes to physician | I. A. 1. Keep pt warm<br>2. Avoid icy fluids<br>3. Medicate with meperidine 25–50 mg IVPB, as ordered<br>4. Instruct pt/significant other in self-management of chills |
| B. Fever 101°–104°F (38.4°–40.0°C) | B. 1. Pt/significant other demonstrates self-care behaviors for management of fever<br>2. Pt reports acceptable control of temperature<br>3. Pt reports temperatures uncontrolled with medication of unrelated to normal pattern | B. 1. Monitor temperature every 1–4 hrs<br>2. Report to physician fevers > 104°F despite antipyretics or other control measures | B. 1. Encourage po fluids<br>2. Medicate with antipyretic as ordered<br>3. For temps > 103°F despite antipyretic, consider tepid sponge bath or shower; ice packs to temperature-control areas; hypothermia blanket, if indicated<br>4. Instruct pt/significant other to monitor temperature<br>5. As therapy continues, teach family to monitor temperature pattern in response to medication; report unusual spikes to health care team<br>6. Instruct pt/significant other in self-management of fever<br>7. Instruct pt/significant other to report to physician if fever does not resolve after therapeutic measures |
| C. Pruritus | C. 1. Pt/significant other identifies/demonstrates measures to control pruritus<br>2. Pt reports acceptable control of pruritus | C. 1. Assess pruritus onset/duration and characteristics, factors that relieve/aggravate the condition, treatment used previously | C. 1. Water-based lotion and/or cream to affected area prn<br>2. Use colloidal oatmeal baths in bathwater (tepid water instead of hot)<br>3. Consider use of room humidifier<br>4. Administer medications as ordered; may need aggressive, around-the-clock administration<br>5. Encourage use of distraction (relaxation techniques, reading, needlework, etc.)<br>6. Teach signs/symptoms of skin changes to report<br>7. Discuss measures to promote skin hydration<br>8. Teach measures to prevent further skin irritation<br>9. Teach relaxation techniques as necessary<br>10. Teach pt to substitute rub, pressure, or vibration for scratching (e.g., rub arms with lotion) |

*(continued)*

**Table 3.10** Plan of Care for Patients Receiving Biological Response Modifier Therapy *(continued)*

| Nursing Diagnosis (Potential/Actual) | Expected Outcomes | Assessment | Nursing Interventions |
|---|---|---|---|
| II. *Pain related to myalgias, arthralgias, headaches* | II. A. Pt/significant other demonstrates self-care behaviors for the management of myalgias and headaches<br>B. Pt reports acceptable control of pain | II. A. Assess need for analgesia<br>B. Assess characteristics of pain<br>C. Assess adequacy of pain control | II. A. Acetaminophen 650 mg po q 3–4 hs as ordered<br>B. Apply moist heat to aching areas<br>C. Instruct pt/significant other in self-management of myalgias and headaches |
| III. *Diarrhea related to treatment with biologic agents* | III. A. Pt/significant other identifies measures to correct or control diarrhea<br>B. Pt reports acceptable control of diarrhea | III. A. Abdominal assessment every 8 hs and prn<br>B. Monitor intake and output every 8 hs<br>C. Monitor stools for frequency, volume, and consistency and document<br>D. Assess for complications of diarrhea (e.g., dehydration)<br>E. Assess perineal/perianal region for skin status | III. A. Administer IV fluid as ordered<br>B. Encourage adequate po fluid intake<br>C. Administer medications that control diarrhea as ordered<br>D. Encourage hygiene measures. May consider use of sitz bath and/or barrier creams<br>E. Teach complications of diarrhea (e.g., fluid electrolyte imbalance, skin breakdown) and prevention measures<br>F. Teach signs and symptoms to report |
| IV. *Altered nutritional status (less than body requirements) related to anorexia, mucositis, nausea, vomiting* | IV. A. Pt maintains adequate nutritional status<br>B. Pt/significant other verbalizes understanding of nutritional needs<br>C. Pt/significant other demonstrates measures to increase nutritional uptake | IV. A. Weigh pt regularly and record<br>B. Initiate a calorie count if indicated to assess intake | IV. A. Provide appetizing foods consistent with pt preference<br>B. Provide high-calorie, low-bulk foods<br>C. Use nutritional supplements<br>D. Refer to dietitian for consultation<br>E. Try small, frequent meals<br>F. Try cool foods if pt is sensitive to food odors<br>G. Give antiemetics as ordered; in some cases, around-the-clock administration might be necessary<br>H. Discuss with health care team the need for tube feedings, or hyperalimentation (IVH), if nutritional status becomes severely compromised<br>I. Instruct pt/significant other in measures to provide adequate nutrition |

| Nursing Diagnosis | Expected Outcomes | Assessment | Interventions |
|---|---|---|---|
| V. Altered oral mucous membranes related to treatment with biological agents | A. Pt recognizes and report changes in mucous membranes<br>B. Pt demonstrates oral hygiene protocol | V. A. Perform oral exam to include palate, gingiva, dorsum of tongue, undersurface of tongue, floor of mouth, buccal mucosa, oral pharynx inner surface of lips<br>B. Assess normal oral hygiene routine | V. A. Encourage pt to perform oral hygiene after meals and at bedtime<br>B. Begin use of salt and soda mouth rinses every 2 hs and prn<br>C. Provide lubricant for lips<br>D. Encourage use of soft toothbrush<br>E. Consider oral irrigations prn to hydrate mouth and for comfort<br>F. Avoid use of agents that further dry the oral mucosa<br>G. Explain rationale for prophylactic oral hygiene protocol<br>H. Teach proper oral hygiene protocol<br>I. Teach signs/symptoms to report to nurse/physician |
| VI. Fatigue related to treatment with biological agents | A. Pt maintains independence in activities of daily living and/or uses measures to prevent further immobility<br>B. Pt verbalizes understanding of cause of fatigue | VI. A. Assess effect of fatigue on activities of daily living<br>B. Assess usual pattern of sleep and rest<br>C. Assess for signs and symptoms associated with fatigue<br>D. Assess for cofactors that may influence fatigue (e.g., anemia, poor nutritional intake, pain) | VI. A. Encourage pt to arrange most strenuous activities according to peak energy level<br>B. Encourage pt to seek assistance with activities of daily living as necessary<br>C. Encourage pt to maintain mobility<br>  1. Ambulatory pt: mild exercise (e.g., walking as tolerated)<br>  2. Bedridden pt: turn every 2 hs; active/passive range of motion<br>D. Encourage pt to take short naps as required to increase energy level<br>E. Treat cofactors that may contribute to fatigue as appropriate<br>F. Teach pt/significant other about fatigue as an expected side effect of biotherapy and self-management strategies to prevent sequelae |
| VII. Altered skin integrity related to treatment with biological agents | A. Pt/significant other verbalizes understanding of factors that may cause alteration in skin integrity<br>B. Skin integrity is maintained<br>C. Pt/significant other demonstrates behaviors to maintain skin integrity | VII. A. Observe skin daily for any breaks, discoloration, redness<br>B. Observe injection sites for changes (e.g., inflammatory reactions)<br>C. Observe IV sites for phlebitis | VII. A. Turn bedfast pt every 2 hs<br>B. Rotate injection sites for IM/SQ agents<br>C. Apply moist heat to any inflamed areas<br>D. Apply water-based lotion and/or cream to entire body 2–3 times a day for dry desquamation<br>E. Consider use of room humidifier for dryness<br>F. Instruct pt/significant other in individual measures for maintenance of skin integrity<br>G. Instruct pt/significant other in causative factors |

*(continued)*

**Table 3.10**  Plan of Care for Patients Receiving Biological Response Modifier Therapy (*continued*)

| Nursing Diagnosis (Potential/Actual) | Expected Outcomes | Assessment | Nursing Interventions |
|---|---|---|---|
| VIII. *Altered tissue perfusion related to treatment with biologic agents* | VIII. A. Pt maintains adequate blood pressure | VIII. A. Assess orthostatic vital signs every 1–4 hs, daily weights, intake and output every 8 hs<br>B. Assess respiratory and cardiovascular system every 8 hs or clinic visit for increased heart rate, decreased blood pressure, complaints of dizziness, complaints of shortness of breath, rales<br>C. Assess for fluid shifts as evidenced by peripheral edema, ascites rales, weight gain, decreased urine output | VIII. A. Administer IV fluids, colloids, and vasopressors as ordered<br>B. Institute comfort measures as necessary<br>C. Institute safety concerns: ambulate with assistance, rise from lying to sitting position slowly<br>D. Encourage po fluid intake<br>E. Teach pt/significant other about expected side effects of biotherapy and temporary nature of side effects<br>F. Teach pt/significant other to monitor for side effects while at home (daily weight, temperature tid, etc.) and notify physician of any changes or problems<br>G. Teach pt/significant other to recognize these signs and symptoms: peripheral edema, shortness of breath, decreased urinary output, weight gain ≥ 5 pounds<br>H. Teach pt to rise from lying position slowly |
| IX. *Potential for injury related to allergic reaction* | IX. A. Pt immediately reports signs and symptoms of anaphylaxis | IX. A. Prior to administration, review prior allergic episodes to include agent thought to be responsible, description of the episode (reaction to agent)<br>B. During administration, assess for shortness of breath/ wheezing, sneezing/coughing, local or generalized urticaria and/or erythema/itching, hypotension, tachycardia cyanosis unconsciousness, emesis and/or diarrhea | IX. A. Administer test dose if ordered<br>B. Ensure that emergency equipment is available<br>C. Ensure that emergency drugs (epinephrine, diphenhydramine, hydrocortisone) are available when administering MABs<br>D. Teach pt to report pain or tightness in chest dyspnea; inability to speak; generalized itching; symptoms of uneasiness, agitation, warmth, dizziness; desire to urinate or defecate |

| Nursing Diagnosis | Expected Outcomes | Assessment | Interventions |
|---|---|---|---|
| X. *Altered thought processes related to treatment with biological agents (e.g., confusion slowed mentation, somnolence)* | X. A. Pt/significant other verbalizes understanding of factors that may cause alteration in thought processes  B. Pt/significant other recognizes changes in thinking or behavior  C. Pt maintains reality orientation | X. A. Assess mental status prior to therapy  B. Assess mental status on each shift or clinic visit and when indicated  C. Assess amount of premedication and/or analgesics pt is receiving | X. A. Orient to time and place if necessary  B. Allow verbalization of feelings  C. Refer to mental health professional if indicated  D. Report changes in mental status to physician  E. Initiate safety measures if indicated  F. Provide memory prompts for orientation (e.g., clocks, calendar, family photos)  G. Instruct pt/significant other how biological therapy may cause alteration in thought process  H. Inform pt/significant other that this side effect is temporary |
| XI. *Altered coping related to changes in disease status and/or new therapy* | XI. A. Pt recognizes potential/actual stressors and facilitates own coping strategies | XI. A. Assess pt's perception of stressors and beliefs about the causes  B. Assess pt's past use of coping strategies  C. Evaluate pt's ability to solve problems | XI. A. Encourage pts to verbalize thoughts and feelings about changes in disease status and new therapy  B. Identify available resources for support and encourage participation (e.g., American Cancer Society, support groups, chaplain)  C. Teach relaxation techniques  D. Teach problem-solving techniques |
| XII. *Knowledge deficit related to medication self-administration* | XII. A. Pt/significant other demonstrates self-administration of agent if indicated | XII. A. Assess ability of pt/significant other to be responsible for self-administration | XII. A. Utilize teaching aids (e.g., written materials, videotape, injection models)  B. Instruct pt/significant other in reconstitution of agent  C. Instruct pt/significant other in IM/SQ injection technique |
| XIII. *Knowledge deficit related to treatment with biological therapy* | XIII. A. Pt/significant other verbalizes expected side effects of agent, reportable signs and symptoms, and treatment plan | XIII. A. Assess knowledge of side effects  B. Assess understanding of therapeutic plan | XIII. A. Instruct pt/significant other of expected side effects and reportable signs and symptoms  B. Instruct pt/significant other regarding required laboratory and diagnostic tests  C. Instruct pt/significant other on therapeutic plan |

*Source:* Adapted with permission from Rumsey, K.A., and Rieger, P.T. (1992). *Biological Response Modifiers.* Chicago: Precept Press. Rieger, P.T. (1996). Biotherapy—The Fourth Modality. In M. Barton-Burke, G. Wilkes, and K. Ingwersen: *Cancer Chemotherapy: A Nursing Process Approach.* 2nd ed. pp. 43–73. Sudbury, Mass: Jones & Bartlett. Reprinted with permission.

Table 3.10 offers a standardized care plan for the patient receiving biotherapy.

## Interferons

The interferons are a family of glycoproteins that are produced by a variety of immune cells. There are three major types of interferon: alpha, beta, and gamma. Interferon-alpha (INF-α) is produced primarily by leukocytes, interferon-beta (INF-β) by fibroblasts, and interferon-gamma (INF-γ) by T lymphocytes. The biological effects of interferon are mediated by its binding to receptors on cell-surface membranes. INF-α and INF-β share a receptor, whereas INF-γ has its own receptor. After binding to the receptor, interferon is internalized, degraded, and ultimately causes the production of other intracellular proteins.

## Interleukins

Interleukins (ILs) are proteins that exist as natural components of the human immune system. Most interleukins are capable of inducing multiple biological activities in a variety of target cells. Interleukin-1 (IL-1) is produced by a variety of cells and has multiple effects, including acting as an endogenous pyrogen, inducing the release of lymphokines, enhancing antibody responsiveness, mediating the inflammatory response, and serving as a hematopoietic growth factor. Common side effects include chills, fever, constitutional symptoms, hypotension at higher doses, tachycardia, and inflammation at the injection sites.

Interleukin-2 (IL-2) (Aldesleuken, Proleukin) is a lymphokine that was first termed T-cell growth factor because it is produced by helper T-cells following antibody-antigen reaction (processed antigen is mounted on macrophage) and IL-1. IL-2 amplifies the immune response to an antigen by immunomodulation and immunorestoration. IL-2 stimulates T-lymphocyte proliferation, enhances killer T-cell activity, increases antibody production (secondary to increased B-cell proliferation), helps to increase synthesis of other cytokines (IFNs, IL-1, -3, -4, -5, -6, CSFs), and stimulates production and activation of natural killer (NK) cells and other cytotoxic cells (LAK and TIL) (Wilkes, Ingwersen, and Barton-Burke 2000). IL-2 has proven to be a potent stimulator of immune response and pivotal to the body's immune response. The biological effects of IL-2 include supporting the growth of T-lymphocytes, stimulating cytotoxic T-cells, stimulating the activity of natural killer cells and other interleukins, as well as enhancing humoral immunity through the production of antibodies.

Interleukin-3 (IL-3) is a multilineage factor that is closely linked to the GM-CSF gene on chromosome 5q. The primary source of IL-3 is the activated T lymphocyte. It acts at an earlier stage than GM-CSF by binding to early progenitor cells, stimulating the growth of early progenitor cells (CFU-blast and CFU-GEMM) as well as more committed cells (e.g., CFU-GM, CFU-Eo, and CFU-MEGG) (Figure 3.2), species-specific stimulation of bone marrow progenitor cells (CFU-GEMM [colony-forming unit-granulocyte, erythocyte, megakaryocyte, and macrophage]). Production of immature neutrophils is enhanced when the drug is administered after GM-CSF. IL-3 acts at a specific stage of the cell cycle prior to the S (synthesis) phase and produces changes in macrophages. IL-3 may affect more cell types than either GM-CSF or G-CSF. It also has been shown to synergize with other HGFs in stimulating hematopoiesis. When used alone in HSCT patients, IL-3 has accelerated the recovery of neutrophils and platelets. However, the results appear to be similar to those

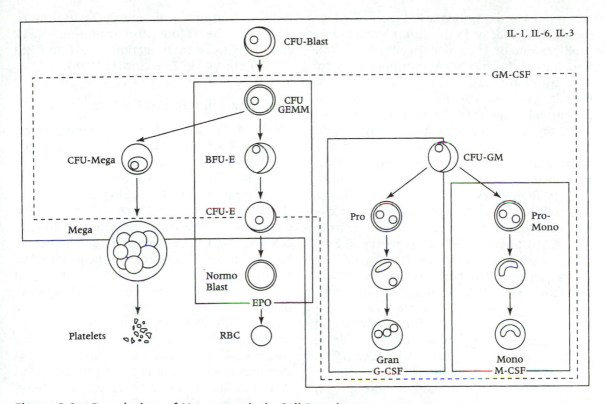

**Figure 3.2**   Regulation of Hematopoietic Cell Development

CFU = colony-forming unit; CFU-Gemm = CFU-granulocyte erythroid macrophage-megakaryocyte; Mega = megakaryocytes; CFU-GM = CFU-granulocyte macrophage; Pro = promyelocyte; Mono = monocyte; Gran = granulocyte; BFU-E = burst-forming unit

*Source:* Gabrilove, J. (1988). Introduction and overview of hematopoietic growth factors. *Seminars in Hematology* 26(2) (Suppl 2): 1–4. Reprinted with permission.

of GM-CSF and some trials have noted high rates of dose reduction or drug discontinuation with IL-3 (Dix and Yee 1997; Weinthal 1996). The recommended dose of IL-3 is 250 $\mu g/m^2/day$ IV. Potential toxicities include fever, headache, flushing, bone pain, lethargy, nausea, vomiting, and local erythema at the injection site (Dix and Yee 1997; Jassak 1993; Mazanet and Griffin 1992; Weinthal 1996).

Interleukin-4 (IL-4) is produced primarily by activated T-cells and stimulates the growth of resting B-cells, acting like a B-cell growth factor. It also acts as a growth factor by stimulat-ing the B-cell to replicate its own deoxyribose nucleic acid (DNA), inducing T-cell growth, enhancing the production of IL-2, and activating granulocytes, macrophages, megakaryocytes, thymocytes, and mast cells. IL-4 also serves as a costimulant with selected colony-stimulating factors for the production of progenitor cells (Rieger, 1996). Side effects of IL-4 include nasal congestion, diarrhea, nausea, vomiting, fatigue, anorexia, headache, elevated liver enzymes, gastroduodenal ulceration (rare), dyspnea, and capillary leak syndrome.

Interleukin 6 (IL-6) is a CSF that acts primarily as a cofactor in the differentiation and proliferation of cytotoxic T-cells (Dorr and Von Hoff 1994) has been antitumor activity. IL-6 also stimulates the differentiation of megakaryocytes, resulting in increased peripheral platelets (thrombopoiesis). IL-6 mediates increased osteoclast activity and bone absorption and probably augments IL-3 activity. IL-6 is produced by T-lymphocytes, monocytes, and endothelial cells, and fibroblasts (Wilkes, Ingwersen, and Barton-Burke 2000). It has little effect on neutrophil recovery. IL-6 also is being tested in clinical trials with GM-CSF or G-CSF following HSCT. Side effects associated with IL-6 have been flu-like symptoms, transient, mild elevations in transaminases, alkaline phosphatase, creatinine, and fasting blood glucose levels. There also have been dose-limiting toxicities of atrial fibrillation and hepatotoxicity at doses of 30 µg/kg per day. (Dix and Yee 1997; Lazarus 1997; Weinthal 1996).

Interleukin-11 Opreleukin (Neumega) (IL-11) is a CSF that seems to be similar in function to IL-6. IL-11 is a thrombopoietin growth factor that stimulates directly the bone marrow stem cells and megakaryocyte progenitor cells so that the production of platelets is increased. IL-11 is produced by recombinant DNA technology. It results in higher platelet nadir and accelerates time to platelet recovery postchemotherapy (Wilkes, Ingwersen, and Barton-Burke 2000). It is an early acting HGF. When used alone and with other HGFs, IL-11 stimulates megakaryocytes, erythroid, and myeloid colony growth and stimulates the number of immunoglobulin-secreting B lymphocytes in vitro. IL-11 appears to be synergistic with G-CSF, IL-3, IL-6, and SCF to produce multilineage colonies. Dose-limiting toxicities have been fluid retention and atrial arrhythmias. Although the results are promising, IL-11 continues to be investigational (Dix and Yee 1997; Lazarus 1997; Weinthal 1996).

## Colony Stimulating Factors

One of the most significant advances during the past decade has been the development and the increasing availability of hematopoietic colony stimulating factors (CSFs) or hemato-poietic growth factors (HGFs). CSFs are a class of glycoprotein hormones that stimulate the production and the differentiation of blood cells, accelerate bone marrow recovery, and bolster the immune system. In essence, they help to regulate hematopoiesis. CSFs play a significant role in high-dose chemotherapy and HSCTs. They stimulate early hematopoietic reconstitution. The reason to use CSFs despite the infusion of large numbers of allogeneic or autologous cells is that patients still suffer profound neutropenia and thrombocytopenia. This puts the patient at great danger for life-threatening infections and hemorrhage. Without CSFs, absolute neutrophil count (ANC) recovery takes 21 days or longer and platelet recovery takes 60 days or more. HGFs also play an important role if the new cells fail to engraft. Causes for engraftment failure include the following: (a) disease relapse, (b) post-transplant infections, (c) low numbers of infused hematopoietic stem cells, (d) extensive chemotherapy prior to marrow collection, (e) graft-versus-host-disease, (f) drug toxicity, (g) use of matched unrelated or mismatched related allogeneic donor marrow, or (h) T-cell depletion of donor cells (Glaspy and Ambersley 1990; Koloc and Schannweber 1993; Lazarus 1997).

There are a variety of CSFs (Table 3.11), which are produced by several cell types in response to numerous stimuli. The first HGF to be described was erythropoietin (EPO) in 1906. It was dis-

**Table 3.11    Selected Colony Stimulating Factors (CSFs)**

| CSF | Target Cell | Activity |
|-----|-------------|----------|
| EPO | Erythrocyte (RBC) | Increases proliferation and differentiation of erythrocytes |
| G-CSF | Neutrophils | Acts synergistically with GM-CSF and IL-3 |
| GM-CSF | Neutrophils, monocytes/macrophages, eosinophils | Increases proliferation and differentiation of progenitor cells |
| M-CSF | Macrophages | Increases differentiation of monocytes/macrophages and works against antifungal infections |
| IL-3 | Neutrophils, eosinophils, macrophages, basophils, megakaryocytes, erythrocytes, stem cells | Increases growth of stem and progenitor cells |
| Pixy321 (IL-3 + GM-CSF) | Early, intermediate, and late progenitor cells | Increases growth of stem and progenitor cells and platelets |
| TBO | Megakaryocytes | Increases proliferation and differentiation of megakaryocytes |
| IL-6 | Megakaryocytes | Increases proliferation and differentiation of megakaryocytes |
| IL-11 | Megakaryocytes, Erythroid, and Myeloid colony growth and Immunoglobulin-secreting B lymphocytes | Increases proliferation and differentiation of megakaryocytes |
| SCF | One of the earliest acting HGFs in development | Alone little activity. In combination may increase progenitor cells and increase platelet recovery |

EPO = erythropoietin, G-CSF = granulocyte CSF; GM-CSF = granulocyte-macrophage CSF; M-CSF = macrophage CSF; IL-3 = Interleukin 3; Pixy321 = Interleukin-3 plus GM-CSF; TBO = thrombopoietin; IL-6 = Interleukin 6; IL-11 = Interleukin 11; SCF = Stem cell factor
*Source:* Adapted from Maxwell, M.B., and Maher, K.E. (1992). Chemotherapy induced myelosuppression. *Seminars in Oncology Nursing* 8(2): 113–133.

covered during experiments in which plasma from anemic animals was transfused into normal animals. From these experiments, it was determined that hormonal factors present in the body regulate the production of RBCs (Mazanet and Griffin 1992).

## PRODUCTION AND FUNCTION

It was not until the 1960s that the other CSFs were defined and isolated. These agents were produced finally in large quantities in the 1980s. Certain CSFs are single lineage (EPO, G-CSF, M-CSF, and TBO), whereas others are multilineage (GM-CSF, IL-3). Four major human HGFs (G-CSF, GM-CSF, M-CSF, and IL-3) are produced in the hematopoietic micro-environment of the bone marrow. They are produced primarily by T-lymphocytes, monocytes, macrophages, endothelial cells, and fibroblasts (Haeuber 1991).

When CSFs bind to receptors, they signal the target cell to initiate intracellular processes. This results in the proliferation and the maturation of hematopoietic cells. HGFs also can be classified by their activity on specific hematopoietic cells—early, intermediate, or late acting. Early acting CSFs target the pluripotent stem cells, whereas the late acting CSFs target committed progenitor cells. Intermediate acting HGFs have the ability to act on uncommitted and committed progenitor cells. Each HGF specifically affects hematopoiesis, but it requires a combination of early, intermediate, and late acting CSFs to reproduce the normal process of hematopoiesis.

## Erythropoietin

In 1989, erythropoietin (EPO) became the first CSF to be approved by the Food and Drug Administration (FDA). Erythropoietin regulates and is essential for the growth and development of erythrocytes (RBCs). The primary stimulus for the production and the release of EPO is hypoxia. It is produced by interstitial cells of the liver and/or kidney. Once produced, the hormone travels to the hematopoietic tissue and activates the proliferation and the differentiation of erythroid progenitor cells. These progenitor cells then differentiate into mature erythrocytes. Thus, EPO is a late acting HGF. Erythropoietin can be used in combination with multilineage CSFs to enhance the differentiation of megakaryocyte progenitors. Erythropoietin is approved for anemias in patients with chronic renal failure, zidovudine-treated HIV infected patients, and chemotherapy patients with nonmyeloid malignancies (Dix and Yee 1997; Jassak 1993; Mazanet and Griffin 1992). However, EPO also has been evaluated in HSCT patients. The use of EPO in HSCT patients remains controversial. Overall, it appears that autologous HSCT patients experienced no difference in transfusion requirements whether or not they received EPO. Allogeneic patients with GVHD

and those receiving cyclosporin and methotrexate have shown an advantage in receiving EPO compared to control patients because they required fewer transfusions and had shorter hospitalizations (Biggs et al. 1995; Klaesson et al. 1994; Steegmann et al. 1992).

For oncology patients suffering from anemia, EPO is administered at a dose of 150 U/kg subcutaneously (SQ) three times per week. An increase in the hematocrit is observed usually within 14–21 days. Generally, EPO is well tolerated. Some patients experience worsening or development of hypertension, thrombocytosis, hyperkalemia, increased blood urea nitrogen concentrations, iron deficiency, and flu-like symptoms (Dix and Yee 1997).

## Granulocyte Factors

The two major granulocyte stimulating (GSFs) factors are granulocyte CSF (G-CSF) and granulocyte-macrophage CSF (GM-CSF). Both G-CSF and GM-CSF have been used in the care of oncology and HSCT patients. Overall, they have been shown to (1) decrease the number of neutropenic days, (2) provide more rapid recovery of neutrophils, (3) increase the number of progenitor cells, (4) decrease the amount of antibiotics used, (5) assist patients to continue chemotherapy, and (6) decrease the number of hospitalizations. Thus, they have the capacity to minimize the degree and the duration of myelosuppression and allow for dose intensification of chemotherapy and radiation, as well as to reduce the number of infections (Dix and Yee 1997; Mazwell and Maher 1992; Ogawa 1994).

Activated monocytes, macrophages, activated neutrophils, fibroblasts, endothelial cells, interleukin-1 (IL-1), tumor necrosis factor (TNF), and bacterial endotoxins produce G-CSF9 (filgrastim [Neupogen]). G-CSF is a recombinant DNA protein that regulates the production of neutrophils in the bone marrow (proliferation, differentiation, activation of mature neutophils). The drug is produced by the insertion of the human G-CSF gene into *Escherichia coli* bacteria (Wilkes, Ingwersen, and Barton-Burke 2000). It predominately enhances the growth of granulocyte colonies by affecting the proliferation and the differentiation of late neutrophil progenitor and precursor cells. Unlike GM-CSF, which stimulates neutrophils and eosinophils, G-CSF activates only neutrophils. G-CSF also can act as a chemotactic signal for phagocytes (Dix and Yee 1997; Mazanet and Griffin 1992).

The recommended dose for G-CSF for the treatment of chemotherapy-induced neutropenia is 5–10 µg/kg/day SQ for up to 14 days. The higher doses are used in HSCT patients (Dix and Yee 1997; Jassak 1993). The most common side effect is mild to moderate bone pain. This most frequently occurs at high doses and is well controlled with nonnarcotic analgesics. Less frequently observed toxicities include thrombocytopenia, epistaxis, gastrointestinal distress, anemia, osteoporosis, and palpable splenomegaly (Dix and Yee 1997; Haeuber and DiJulio 1989; Koloc and Schannweber 1993; Mazwell and Maher 1992; Ogawa 1994).

GM-CSF is a multilineage human growth factor (HGF) with a broader spectrum of activity that affects all levels of granulocytes and stimulates the production of monocytes and macrophages. It exerts its effects by interacting with specific receptors on the plasma membrane of granulocytes and macrophages. GM-CSF induces synthesis of other cytokines and enhances cytotoxic action (Wilkes et al. 2000). It is made by endothelial cells, fibroblasts, marrow stromal cells, and T-lymphocytes. This HGF stimulates the growth of committed bone marrow progenitor cells, such as CFU-GEMM, CFU-E, and CFU-GM (Mazanet and Griffin 1992). GM-CSF is given subcutaneously (SQ) or intravenously and is administered in doses of 250 µg/m$^2$/day for about 21 days or when the absolute neutrophil count is above 1500 for 1–3 days. The toxicities associated with GM-CSF include fever, fatigue, myalgias, loss of appetite, rash, bone pain, phlebitis, and thrombosis at the site of the IV infusion (Dix and Yee 1997; Haeuber and DiJulio 1989; Jassak 1993; Neumanaitis 1993).

## Macrophage Colony Stimulating Factor

Macrophage CSF (M-CSF) is a single-lineage factor that was purified in 1975. It is different from the other HGFs in terms of structure and biologic activity. It is produced by monocytes, granulocytes, fibroblasts, marrow stromal cells, and endothelial cells. M-CSF has been shown to increase monocyte and macrophage numbers, increase macrophage antitumor and antimicrobial activity, and promote the release of other CSFs (G-CSF, GM-CSF, IL-1, TNF, and interferon). M-CSF acts predominately on the growth of macrophage colony formation and stimulates the release of IL-1, TNF, interferon, and plasminogen activator (Mazanet and Griffin 1992). M-CSF has been studied as an antifungal agent in HSCT patients with invasive fungal infection. Some studies have shown longer survival with M-CSF than with antifungals (Lazarus 1997).

## Pixy321

Pixy321 is an investigational recombinant protein that combines both IL-3 and GM-CSF using an amino acid linker protein. This was developed to combine the early, rapid-onset action of GM-CSF on committed late neutrophil progenitors with the slower, sustained, late onset effect of IL-3 on earlier and intermediate progenitors of many lineages. Pixy321 appears to accelerate both neutrophil and platelet recovery. It generally has been given in a dose of 125 µg/m$^2$ SQ or IV per day. It generally is well tolerated but can produce local erythema, tenderness, and pruritis after SQ injection. Some patients also experience flu-like symptoms and bone pain. Clinical trials continue with Pixy321 after HSCT and to mobilize PBCs (Dix and Yee 1997; Lazarus 1997; Weinthal, 1996).

## Thrombopoietin

Thrombopoietin (TBO) is a hormone thought to be responsible for the production and the maturation of megakaryocytes (which produce platelets) in both animals and humans. It is required for the day-to-day maintenance of platelet counts. Thrombopoietin has been shown to (1) increase platelet counts, (2) increase platelet size, and (3) increase the percentage of precursor cells. Thrombopoietin recently has been purified and cloned (Schick 1994; McDonald 1992). Thrombocytopenia has been a serious complication after chemotherapy, radiation, and HSCT as well as for patients with aplastic anemia or acquired immune deficiency syndrome (AIDS). Other CSFs (e.g., G-CSF, GM-CSF, and erythropoietin) have not been shown to increase platelet counts. Some researchers have suggested that combinations of IL-1,IL-3, IL-6, IL-11, Pixy321 (IL-3 plus GM-CSF), or stem cell factor may increase platelet counts on a limited basis; however, none of these hormones acts specifically on the megakaryocytes. Thrombopoietin can cause a fourfold increase when given to normal mice. The optimal dose and side effects of this new hormone are still being evaluated, but thrombopoietin is an important advance in the treatment of thrombocytopenia (Lazarus 1997; McDonald 1992; Schick 1994).

## Stem Cell Factor

Stem cell factor (SCF) is a potent CSF that acts on the earliest and most immature hematopoietic progenitors, but appears to have little effect on hematopoiesis when administered alone. It has been shown to be synergistic with many of the other HGFs. Stem cell factor has many potential clinical uses, including treatment of bone marrow failure states, ex vivo expansion of hematopoietic progenitor and stem cells for marrow transplantation, gene transfer therapy, and mobilization of peripheral blood progenitor and hematopoietic stem cells. It generally is well tolerated with some mild to moderate injection reactions as well as systemic symptoms of angioedema, dyspepsia, and hypotension. It continues to be investigated alone and in combination with many other HGFs (Dix and Yee 1997; Lazarus 1997)

## Monoclonal Antibodies

Monoclonal antibodies (MoAbs) are highly specific in their ability to recognize proteins on the surface of cells. A large number of MoAbs that recognize specific cancer-associated antigens are under investigation for treatment of specific cancers. OncoScint CR/OV is a MoAb that recognizes both colorectal and ovarian adenocarcinomas and has been approved for the detection of both primary and metastatic tumors. The recently approved trastuzumab (Humanized anti-HER-2-antibody, rhuMAb-HER2, Herceptin) is a recombinant humanized monoclonal antibody targeted against the Human Epidermal Growth Factor receptor (HER2). HER2 is overexpressed in a number of cancers, including 25–30% of breast cancers. This monoclonal antibody is believed to act through three different mechanisms: (1) antagonizing function of growth-signaling

(2) signaling immune cells to attack and kill malignant cells with this receptor, and (3) add to the cytotoxicity induced by traditional chemotherapy (Wilkes et al. 2000). Rituximab is a MoAb directed against the $CD_{20}$ antigen receptor on B-cell lymphocytes and is indicated for the treatment of refractory or relapsed low-grade or follicular $CD_{20}$ positive B-cell non-Hodgkin's lymphoma. This anti-$CD_{20}$ antibody is genetically engineered (chimeric monoclonal antibody) and directed against the $CD_{20}$ antigen found on the surface of normal and malignant B-cell lymphocytes. The $CD_{20}$ antigen is also present (expressed) on more than 90% of B-cell non-Hodgkin's lymphoma (NHL) cells, but fortunately is not found on normal bone marrow stem cells, pre–B-cells, or other normal tissues. A section of the rituximab (Fab domain) $CD_{20}$ binds to the $CD_{20}$ antigen on B-lymphocytes; another section of the rituximab (Fc domain) calls together other immune effectors, resulting in lysis of the B-lymphocyte (Wilkes et al. 2000). Other MoAbs are in development and are expected to be approved soon. One example is tositumomab, $I^{131}$ tositumomab an investigational iodine-131–labeled anti-B1 murine monoclonal antibody directed against the $CD_{20}$ B-lymphocyte antigen found on the surface of some normal lymphocytes, and lymphocytes in non-Hodgkin's lym-phoma (NHL). The agent contains two parts: an IgG2 murine monoclonal antibody directed against the $CD_{20}$ surface antigen, and antibody labelled with iodine-131. The antibody attaches to the $CD_{20}$ surface antigen on the lymphocytes, directly killing the cells by inducing apoptosis, and mediating antibody-dependent cell killing, plus delivering ionizing radiation directly to the cell. Radiation is delivered directly to the tumor cells, as well as some normal cells with $CD_{20}$ antigens (Wilkes et al. 2000).

## Immunomodulators

Immunomodulators are substances that have the ability to stimulate immune responses. Bacillus Calmette-Guérin (BCG) and *Corynebacterium parvum (C. parvum)* are examples of early immunomodulators that were used against a variety of tumors but seemed effective only when used in a patient with minimal tumor burden. Another immunomodulator, levamisole, has received regulatory approval recently for the treatment of Dukes' C (stage III) colon cancer.

## Tumor Necrosis Factor

Tumor necrosis factor (TNF) is pivotal in the pathogenesis of infection, inflammation, and injury, and it is part of the beneficial processes of host defenses and tissue homeostasis. It is a cytokine produced primarily by activated macrophages that is capable of directly killing cells by halting cell growth in $G_2$ phase of the cell cycle, by cytotoxicity, and by inducing hemorrhagic necrosis. It also activates the immune system by increasing the production and activity of natural killer (NK) cells, as well as the production and activity of B-cells, and neutrophils. TNF (cachectin) binds to target cell membranes and appears to halt cell growth in the $G_2$ phase of cell cycle (cytostatic), is cytotoxic, and may cause vascular endothelial injury in tumor capillaries, leading to hemorrhage and necrosis of tumor cells. Numerous clinical trials have evaluated the efficacy of TNF both alone and in combination in a variety of cancers, however, therapeutic responses have remained unimpressive (Wilkes et al. 2000).

## APPLICATIONS

The therapeutic uses of CSFs are being studied in clinical trials throughout the United States and abroad. CSFs may be used alone or in combination. Many HGFs are used to prevent myelosuppression associated with AIDS, antineoplastic chemotherapy, HSCT, myelodysplasticsyndromes, and aplastic anemia. Additionally, several factors have been used to mobilize peripheral stem cells. It is known that IL-3, G-CSF, and GM-CSF all stimulate neutrophil production, but GM-CSF and G-CSF also enhance their function. Thus, combining IL-3 with G-CSF or GM-CSF can be more potent in stimulating granulocyte recovery than when any of these are used alone. Other current or investigational uses of CSFs include as antimicrobial agents (M-CSF) and to facilitate gene insertion (Il-1, Il-3, IL-6, and SCF) (Glaspy and Ambersley 1990; Jassak 1993; Lazarus 1997; Mazanet and Griffin 1992; Neumanaitis 1993; Ogawa 1994).

## NURSING CARE RELATED TO CSFs

Nursing care provided to patients receiving growth factors is similar to care for patients receiving any type of biological agent. Care should include a thorough pretreatment assessment, education, monitoring of adverse effects and toxicities, laboratory monitoring, and individualized nursing interventions (Haeuber 1991; King 1995).

A comprehensive nursing assessment of the patient should be obtained prior to initiating CSF therapy. This assessment should include physical factors as well as psychological and social factors and the need for support services. If the patient is to self-administer G-CSF subcutaneously at home, support services can be required (King 1995). It is essential that patients and families have a thorough understanding of the types of human blood cells and their roles in the body, the need for an HGF, the method of administration, the potential side effects, the importance of monitoring side effects, and whom and when to call if problems develop (Haeuber 1991; Maxwell and Maher 1992). Nurses generally provide this education to patients and families. Formal teaching tools are often helpful (e.g., pamphlets and videos) for instruction and reinforcement of information. Some institutions have developed standard checklists for teaching purposes. Standard teaching sheets may ensure that no information is missed and serve as documentation of information that has been taught over several days (Haeuber 1991; King 1995).

In addition to assessment and education, oncology nurses are involved actively in symptom management when adverse effects develop from the administration of CSFs. Generally, side effects are mild; however, some patients might experience discomfort secondary to these effects (see Table 3.9).

Therapy with BRMs has advanced immensely in the past few years. These factors have allowed health care providers to improve supportive care provided to patients with cancer. CSFs have greatly affected the quality of life of oncology patients by decreasing the length of stay for neutropenic patients, decreasing the number of neutropenic episodes, decreasing the number of transfusions required, and decreasing antibiotic use.

## MULTIDRUG RESISTANCE

Despite significant advances in the development and the use of antineoplastics to cure cancer, there remains the perplexing biologic problem of resistance to chemotherapy. This represents a major problem in oncology. Exposure of cancer cells to one single antineoplastic agent can lead to resistance to multiple agents. This is called multidrug resistance (MDR) (DeVita 1990; Leyland-Jones et al. 1993).

**Table 3.12**  Antineoplastics Associated with Multidrug Resistance

dactinomycin
daunorubicin hydrochloride
doxorubicin hydrochloride
etoposide
mitomycin
mitoxantrone
taxol
trimetrexate
vincristine
vinblastine

*Source:* Adapted from Leyland-Jones, B., Dalton, W., Fisher, G.A., and Sikic, B. (1993). Reversal of multidrug resistance to cancer chemotherapy. *Cancer* 72(Suppl. 11): 3483–3488.

**Table 3.13**  Mechanisms of Drug Resistance

Altered membrane transport
Altered target enzyme
Defective drug metabolism
Decreased drug activation
Enhanced DNA repair
Increased drug degradation
Subcellular redistribution

*Source:* Adapted from Leyland-Jones, B., Dalton, W., Fisher, G.A., and Sikic, B. (1993). Reversal of multidrug resistance to cancer chemotherapy. *Cancer* 72(Suppl 11): 3483–3488.

Biedler and Riehm made the first report of MDR in 1970. In 1976, Juliano and Ling reported the association of MDR with a surface glycoprotein called p-glycoprotein. The *p* stands for permeability. The glycoprotein has been identified on the surface of cells of a number of tumors in normal tissue, and it is one of the most important causes of MDR. For example, generally high levels are found in colon, renal cell, and islet cell cancer, as well as in CML in blast crisis. It has been found that this protein is more likely to be present in patients with any tumor type if they have relapsed after exposure to chemotherapy. The normal cells that have high levels of p-glycoprotein are located in organs that are frequently resistant to chemotherapy (e.g., kidneys, liver, and adrenal glands) (DeVita 1990; Moscow and Cowan 1988).

P-glycoprotein has been described as working as an efflux pump, such that antineoplastic agents enter the cell but are then immediately pumped back out. Thus, the cancer cells are left undamaged by the chemotherapy (De Vita 1990).

A number of antineoplastic agents have been associated with MDR (Table 3.12). The majority of these are large and are natural products. All of these agents are hydrophobic. Currently, it is hypothesized that these agents compete with p-glycoprotein as transport substrates (Leyland-Jones et al. 1993).

Additional mechanisms of drug resistance may coexist with MDR (Table 3.13). These mechanisms may render cancer cells refractory to modulation by MDR inhibitors (Leyland-Jones et al. 1993). In 1981, Tsuruo discovered the possibility of modulating MDR when verapamil inhibited the drug efflux characteristic of MDR P-388 leukemia cells, increased the accumulation of vincristine in parenteral leukemia cells, and improved the survival of mice bearing resistance P-388 leukemia. It is most likely that verapamil modulates drug resistance by competitive inhibition of p-glycoprotein. Since 1981, a variety of other agents have been found to modulate MDR activity (Table 3.14). These compounds have been found to have chemosensitizing capabilities similar to those of verapamil. The mechanism in overcoming drug resistance appears to be related to the blocking of enhanced drug efflux from cells, leading to increased intracellular drug accumulation (Leyland-Jones et al. 1993).

As more is learned about MDR and its causes, and modulation, oncology nurses are taking a more active role in this new frontier.

Specifically, inpatient and outpatient nurses are involved in research, education, and clinical care related to MDR. Few patients and families understand MDR. Thus, knowledge deficit is a major problem in which oncology nurses can effectively intervene (Table 3.15).

The resistance of many cancers to drugs has been a major stumbling block to the successful elimination of malignant cells. The field of MDR modulation is young but holds significant promise. Clinical trials are being conducted with a variety of modulating agents that would inactivate the p-glycoprotein in cells. Additionally, there are clinical trials in which chemotherapeutic agents are being combined with chemomodifiers to increase their effectiveness. Researchers are working on the identification and the development of more MDR reversal agents. In the future, improvements in the effectiveness of chemotherapy may result from understanding and preventing mechanisms of MDR.

Research is underway to identify and characterize new natural products that circumvent MDR. There are two categories of agents being evaluated based on their interactions with p-glycoprotein: (1) they potentiate cytotoxicity of classical anticancer drugs by inhibiting the function of p-glycoprotein or (2) they act as direct cytotoxins to both drug sensitive to MDR cells. Some new agents that act as antagonists to p-glycoprotein include a novel porphyrin (e.g., tolyporphin), new alkaloids and

**Table 3.14    Modulators of Multidrug Resistance**

| |
|---|
| Calcium channel blockers |
|   AHC-52 |
|   Diltiazem |
|   Nicardipine |
|   Nimodipine |
|   Verapamil |
| Calmodulin inhibitors |
| Cyclosporine A |
| Inactive anthracyclines and vinca alkaloids |
| Megestrol acetate |
| Local anesthetics |
| Quinine |
| Quinidine |
| Reserpine |
| Tamoxifen citrate |

*Source:* Adapted from Leyland-Jones, B., Dalton, W., Fisher, G.A., and Sikic, B. (1993). Reversal of multidrug resistance to cancer chemotherapy. *Cancer* 72(Suppl 11): 3483–3488.

depsipeptide called hapalosin. These can all bind directly to p-glycoprotein and allow for greater cytotoxicity by such agents as taxol, vinblastine, and actinomycin. In the second category, there are several cyanobacterial extracts that show equal cytotoxicity toward drug-sensitive and MDR cells suggesting their toxins are not transported by p-glycoprotein. One group of cytotoxic macrolides called scytophcins has this property (especially cryptophycin) (Smith, Prinsep et al. 1994; Smith, Zhang et al. 1994; Stratmann et al. 1994).

**Table 3.15    Nursing Care Plan for Multidrug Resistance (MDR)**

| Nursing Diagnosis (Potential/Actual) | Expected Outcome | Nursing Interventions |
|---|---|---|
| *Knowledge deficit related to MDR* | Pt/significant other verbalizes understanding of MDR causes and treatment | Instruct pt/significant other on what MDR is, the causes, and the current treatment |
| | | Administer modulator as ordered |
| | | Instruct pt/significant other on potential side effects of modulator |

# CHEMOPREVENTION

Chemoprevention is a new treatment modality involving intervention with specific agents to inhibit neoplastic development prior to or during the premalignant process. This is done to suppress carcinogenesis before invasive cancer develops (Lippmann, Benner, and Hong 1994; Ren and Lien 1997). This new approach has been created to be used in addition to established therapies rather than to replace accepted modalities. Animal models have demonstrated that specific agents can prevent premalignant lesions from progressing to invasive cancer. Additionally, epidemiologic studies have suggested that certain dietary items can inhibit carcinogenesis in humans (Lippman, Benner, and Hong 1993).

Two main theories are involved in chemoprevention. The first is the theory of multistep epithelial carcinogenesis and the fact that carcinogenesis in epithelial tissues develops in sequential steps. The first step involves premalignant changes, and the process ultimately progresses to invasive cancer. The second concept is field carcinogenesis. This theory describes carcinogen exposure as damaging the epithelium and predisposing the entire carcinogen-exposed field to the development of multiple independent cancers. Exposure of the aerodigestive tract to cigarette smoke and exposure of the skin to sunlight are examples (Lippman et al. 1993; Lippman et al. 1994).

The National Cancer Institute has established a Cancer Prevention Research Program, which currently is sponsoring many chemoprevention trials. To hunt for chemoprevention agents, hundreds of compounds have been isolated from the human body, foods, and plants. Many of these involve retinoids (including beta-carotene), calcium, hormone antagonists (tamoxifen and finasteride), plant phenolics (green tea, flavinoids, and curcumin), soybeans, aspirin, and ibuprofen. The clinical trials are directed at 12 major cancer targets (breast, prostate, colon, head, neck, esophagus, lung, bladder, cervix, skin, liver, and multiple myeloma) (Table 3.16).

The most commonly studied retinoid is 13, cis-retinoic acid (13cRA). In high doses, it

**Table 3.16   Chemoprevention Clinical Trials**

| Disease | Agents Used in Clinical Trials |
|---|---|
| Breast | Fenretinide alone or with tamoxifen |
| | Exemestane (selective estrogen receptor modulator) |
| Prostate | Antiandrogens |
| | Antiestrogens |
| | Soy proteins |
| | Fenretidine |
| Colon | Ursodiol |
| | Calcium alone or with vitamin D |
| | NSAIDs (piroxicam, COX-2 inhibitors) |
| Head and Neck | 13-cis-retinoic acid and interferon and vitamin E |
| | Fenretinide |
| | 13-cis-retinoic acid and curcumin |
| Esophagus | COX-2 inhibitors |
| Lung | Fenretidine |
| | Oltipraz |
| Bladder | Fenretidine |
| | COX-2 inhibitors |
| Cervix | Fenretidine |
| | 9-cis-retinoic acid |
| Skin | Fenretidine |
| | COX-2 inhibitors |
| | Topical tea polyphenols |
| Liver | Oltipraz |
| Multiple myeloma | DHEA Biaxin |

has been found to reverse oral leukoplakia and to prevent second tumors of the head, the neck, and the skin. Beta-carotene has been included in some chemoprevention studies based on its antioxidant properties and its in vivo conversion to retinol (the natural form of Vitamin A). Calcium appears to be promising for the prevention of colon cancer. Tamoxifen is a synthetic, nonsteroidal antiestrogen that has been used in primary and adjuvant treatment of breast cancer. It has also been shown to reversibly suppress primary and second primary breast carcinogenesis in rodents. A new retinoid, fenretinide, is the most promising chemoprevention agent. It appears to be effective in preventing chemically induced breast and bladder cancer in rodents. Research has just begun to evaluate the effectiveness of fenretinide and tamoxifen together. The combination may be even more active in primary and second primary breast disease prevention than is either agent alone (Lippman, Benner, and Hong 1993).

## RETINOIDS

Retinoids are a class of more than 3,000 natural derivatives and synthetic analogues of Vitamin A. They are effective modulators of epithelial differentiation and carcinogenesis. It appears that the biological activities of retinoids are mediated by nuclear receptors that are part of the steroid-thyroid hormone family of receptors. Research to date indicates that certain retinoids can inhibit the development of invasive cancer at many epithelial sites, including the head and neck and the lung (Lippman, Benner, and Hong 1993).

Beta-carotene is a plant carotenoid with pro-vitamin A activity that is hypothesized to decrease cancer risk by trapping organic free radicals and/or deactivating excited oxygen molecules (a byproduct of some metabolic functions) and thus preventing tissue damage (Hennekens 1994). Research has shown an inverse relationship between the risk of cancer and the consumption of fruits and vegetables rich in beta-carotene. Beta-carotene is found in abundant quantities in yellow fruits and vegetables (including carrots, yellow squash, tomatoes, and dark green leafy vegetables). Additionally, this pro-vitamin A is beneficial because it is natural, readily available, and inexpensive. Unfortunately, yellowing of the skin can occur if the blood concentration reaches more than 5.6 micromoles/liter. This yellowing, however, is reversible. Some researchers believe that beta-carotene's antioxidant properties, not its retinol (pro-vitamin A) activity, cause the cancer prevention effects. Beta-carotene is one of the most important substances for inactivating singlet oxygen and free radicals that damage RNA and DNA and promote tumors (McClinton-Adams 1994; Michels and Willett 1994).

## ANTIOXIDANTS AND OTHER NATURAL PRODUCTS FROM THE HUMAN BODY

Antioxidant vitamins (e.g., beta-carotene, Vitamin E, and Vitamin C) are hypothesized to have chemopreventive effects. It currently is thought that these vitamins decrease cancer risk by inhibiting oxidation processes that may occur from exogenous sources or as the product of normal metabolism. More specifically, they decrease the risk of cancer by trapping organic free radicals and/or by deactivating excited oxygen molecules and thus preventing tissue damage. Beta-carotene, Vitamin C, and Vitamin E are important because the body cannot synthesize these compounds (Hennekens 1994; Michels and Willett 1994).

Beta-carotene has relatively good antioxidant properties, whereas retinol does not. Beta-carotene has been found to be protective for lung cancer in most studies. Although not proven, an association between total beta-carotene and a modest reduction in breast cancer risk has been demonstrated through research (Michels and Willett 1994).

Vitamin C (ascorbic acid) is a water-soluble antioxidant. It circulates in the extracellular fluid, but it is also an intracellular antioxidant. It is quickly and effectively absorbed from the diet. Vitamin C is found in fruits and vegetables, specifically in citrus fruits and potatoes. Associations have been noted between a high intake of Vitamin C and a reduced risk of stomach, esophageal, oral, pharyngeal, and laryngeal cancers (Michels and Willett 1994).

Vitamin E is a fat-soluble antioxidant and one of the body's primary defenses against oxidation. It is available in many foods. As much as 30% of Vitamin E comes from vegetable oils or products created from these oils (e.g. margarine and salad dressings). Another 20% comes from fruits and vegetables, and 15% comes from fortified cereals and grain products. Meat, poultry, fish, eggs, and nuts supply only a small amount of Vitamin E. To date, the only association of Vitamin E and reduced risk of cancer has been with pharyngeal and lung cancer (Michels and Willett 1994).

There are no definitive data on the role of antioxidants and cancer because it has been difficult to control for all factors associated with vitamin intake that might independently affect cancer risk (Hennekens 1994).

Other natural products from the human body that are being studied include Vitamin D, calcium, dehydroepidandrosterone (DHEA), and coenzyme $Q_{10}$. It has been suggested that a deficiency in Vitamin D may increase the risk of prostate cancer and colorectal cancer. The main studies with calcium have been conducted with colon cancer. An increase in Vitamin D and dietary calcium has been shown to decrease the risk of colon cancer, especially in men. DHEA has inhibited tumor development in the thyroid and the small intestine in animals, but has had side such effects as weight loss and hepatomegaly. Coenzyme $Q_{10}$ has shown some possibility of assisting tumor regression in breast cancer if given in high doses (Ren and Lien 1997).

## NATURAL PRODUCTS FROM FOODS AND VEGETABLES AND OTHER HIGHER PLANTS

Many natural products from foods, vegetables, and other higher plants are being studied as chemopreventive agents. These include celery seed oil, parsley leaf oil, sulforaphane, isoflavonoids, lignans, protease inhibitors, tea polyphenols, and curcumin. There is considerable interest in tea polyphenols because tea is one of the most widely consumed beverages in the world. Individuals who drink green tea tend to have a lower risk for gastric cancer (Ren and Lien 1997).

Despite the many clinical trials in progress there is currently no definitive data to prevent a clear identification of the type and the concentration of agents to use to prevent cancer in humans. Nonetheless, nurses should continue to advocate a balanced diet for all patients. More clinical trials are required to learn about effective chemopreventative and therapeutic agents.

## TOXINS

Immunotoxins and recombinant toxins are a new class of cytotoxic agents. These toxins are made up of monoclonal antibodies (MoAbs) or growth factors that are coupled with bacterial or plant toxins. Toxins can selectively target and kill cells that either express particular antigens or have growth factor receptors on their surfaces. The effectiveness of toxins in the treatment of cancer currently is being studied (Pai and Pastan 1994).

Ricin, pseudomonas exotoxin A (PE), and diptheria toxin (DT) have been the most commonly used immunotoxins. Recently, these three have been cloned and expressed in *Escherichia coli*. Consequently, recombinant toxin molecules that produce less toxiciy to the host can now be selected and produced. Recombinant toxins with PE and DT can be produced in large quantities for clinical applications. In addition to exploring the use of immunotoxins as cytotoxic agents in cancer patients, some researchers are exploring the use of immunotoxins in bone marrow purging prior to transplantation (Pai and Pastan 1994).

Successful clinical trials with toxins have involved patients with lymphomas and leukemias. This might be due in part to the fact that these cancers are more responsive to chemotherapy than solid tumors. Some clinical trials have compared intravenous bolus administration with continuous infusion, but no improvement in antitumor activity was noted in these trials. A major challenge for researchers involves the inability to deliver repeated doses of toxins to patients because of antibody formation against the toxin. Despite obstacles, research continues to define the role of toxins in cancer therapy (Pai and Pastan 1994).

## CONCLUSION

In the past decade, fewer new antineoplastic agents have been developed, but well-accepted chemotherapeutic agents and other agents are being used in new ways. These innovative treatments—HSCT, colony stimulating factors, biological response modifiers, modulators of multidrug resistance, chemopreventive agents, and toxins—hold significant promise and new frontiers as cancer therapies. As these therapies become more widely used, they offer new challenges for oncology nurses.

## BIBLIOGRAPHY

Bekkum, D.W., and deVries, M.J. (1967). *Radiation Chimeras*. London: Logos Press.

Biggs, J., Atkinson, K., Booker, V., CorCannon, A., Dart, G.V., Dodds, A., Downs, K., Szer, J., Turner, J., and Washington, R. (1995). Prospective randomized double blind trial of the invivo use of recombinant human erythropoietin in bone marrow transplantation from HLA identical sibling donors. *Bone Marrow Transplantation* 15(1): 129–134.

Biedler, J.L., and Riehm, H. (1970). Cellular resistance to actinomycin D in Chinese hamster cells in vitro: Cross-resistance, radioautographic, and cytogenetic studies. *Cancer Research*, 30(4), 1174–1184.

Billett, A.L. (1992). High-dose therapy in acute lymphoblastic leukemia. In J.O. Armitage and K.A. Antman (eds.): *High-Dose Cancer Therapy*. Baltimore: Williams and Wilkins, 607–618.

Bortin, M.M., Horowitz, M.M., and Gale, R.P. (1988). Current status of bone marrow transplantation humans. *National Immunology and Cell Regulation* 7(5–6): 334–350.

Bortin, M.M., Horowitz, M.M., and Rimm, A.A. (1992). Progress report from the International Bone Marrow Transplant Registry. *Bone Marrow Transplantation* 10(2): 113–122.

Buchsel, P.C. (1993a). Ambulatory care for the bone marrow transplant patient. In P.C. Buchsel and C.H. Yarbro (eds.): *Oncology Nursing in the Ambulatory Setting: Issues and Models of Care*. Boston: Jones & Bartlett, 185–216.

Buchsel, P.C. (1993b). Bone marrow transplantation. In S.L. Groenwald, M.H. Frogge, M. Goodman, and C.H. Yarbro (eds.): *Cancer Nursing: Principles and Practice* 3rd ed. Boston: Jones & Bartlett, 393–434.

Buchsel, P.C. (1991). Ambulatory care: Before and after BMT. In M.B. Whedon (ed.): *Bone Marrow Transplantation: Principles, Practice and Nursing Implications*. Boston: Jones & Bartlett.

Buchsel, P.C. (1986). Long-term complications of allogeneic bone marrow transplantation: Nursing implications. *Oncology Nursing Forum* 13: 61–70.

Burns, J.M., Tierney, K.D., Long, G.D., Lambert, S.C., and Carr, B.E. (1995). Critical pathway for administering high-dose chemotherapy followed by peripheral blood stem cell rescue in the outpatient setting. *Oncology Nursing Forum* 22(8): 1219–1224.

Deeg, H.J., Klingemann, H.G., Phillips, G.L., and van Zant, G. (1999). *A Guide To Blood and Marrow Transplantation*. 3rd ed. Berlin: Springer.

DeVita, V.T., Jr. (1990). The problem of resistance. *Principles and Practice of Oncology Updates* 4: 1–12.

Dix, S.P., and Yee, G.C. (1997). Pharmacologic and Biologic Agents. In M.B. Whedon and D. Wujcik (eds.): *Blood and Marrow Stem Cell Transplantation: Principles, Practice, and Nursing Insights*. 2nd ed. Boston: Jones & Bartlett.

Donaldson, C., Armitage, W.J., Denning-Kendall, P.A., Nicol, A.J., Bradley, B.A., and Hows, J.M. (1996). Optimal cryopreservation of human umbilical cord blood. *Bone Marrow Transplantation* 18(4): 725–731.

Dorr, R.T., and von Hoff, D.D. (1994). *Cancer Chemotherapy Handbook*. 2nd ed. Norwalk, Conn: Appleton & Lange.

Franey, R.J., and Yee, G.J. (1994). Regimen-related toxicity after bone marrow transplantation. *Highlights on Antineoplastic Drugs* 10: 60–75.

Frei, E. (1992). Pharmacologic strategies for high-dose chemotherapy. In J.O. Armitage and K.A. Antman (eds.): *High-dose Cancer Therapy*. Baltimore: Williams and Wilkins, 3–13.

Gabrilove, J. (1988). Introduction and overview of hematopoietic growth factors. *Seminars in Hematology* 26(2)(suppl 2): 1–4.

Gale, R.P., and Butturini, A. (1992). Intensive therapy of chronic myelogenous leukemia. In J.O. Armitage and K.A. Antman (eds.): *High-dose Cancer Therapy*. Baltimore: Williams and Wilkins, 619–625.

Glaspy, J.A., and Ambersley, J.M. (1990). The promise of colony stimulating factors in clinical practice. *Oncology Nursing Forum* 17(supp 1): 20–24.

Goldstone, A.H. (1992). High dose therapy for the treatment of non-Hodgkin's lymphoma. In J.O. Armitage and K.A. Antman (eds.): *High Dose Cancer Therapy*. Baltimore: Williams & Wilkins.

Gorin, N.C. (1992). High-dose therapy for acute myelocytic leukemia. In J.O. Armitage and K.A. Antman (eds.): *High-dose Cancer Therapy*. Baltimore: Williams and Wilkins.

Haeuber, D. (1991). Future strategies in the control of myelosuppression. The use of colony stimulating factors. *Oncology Nursing Forum* 18(Suppl 2): 6–12.

Haeuber, D., and Di Julio, J.E. (1989). Hemopoietic colony stimulating factors: An overview. *Oncology Nursing Forum* 16: 247–255.

Hennekens, C.H. (1994). Antioxidant vitamins and cancer. *American Journal of Medicine* 97(Suppl 3A): 2S–4S; discussion, 22S–28S.

Horowitz, M.M., and Rowlings, P.A. (1997). An update from the international bone marrow transplant registry and the autologous blood and marrow transplant registry on current activity in hematopoietic stem cell transplantation. *Current Opinion in Hematology* 4(6): 395–400.

Jagannath, S., Vesole, D., and Barlogie, B. (1992). High-dose therapy, autologous stem cells, and hematopoietic growth factors for the management of multiple myeloma. In J.O. Armitage and K.A. Antman (eds.): *High-dose Cancer Therapy*. Baltimore: Williams and Wilkins, 638–650.

Jassak, P.J. (1993). Biotherapy. In S.L. Groenwald, M.H. Frogge, M. Goodman, and C.H. Yarbro (eds.): *Cancer Nursing: Principles and Practice*. Boston: Jones & Bartlett, 366–392.

Kanfer, E.J., and McCarthy, D.M. (1989). Cytoreductive preparation for bone marrow transplantation in leukemia: To irradiate or not? *British Journal of Haematology* 71(4): 447–450.

Kessinger, A., Armitage, J.O., Landmark, J.D., and Weisenburger, D.D. (1986). Reconstitution of human hematopoietic function with autologous cryopreserved circulating stem cells. *Experimental Hematology* 14(3): 192–196.

King, C.R. (1995). The outpatient management of myelosuppression. *Clinical Perspectives in Oncology Nursing* 1(4): 1–12.

King, C.R. (1993). *Bone Marrow Transplantation Clinical Background Manual*. Paramus, N.J.: Roche Professional Service Centers.

Klaesson, S., Ringden, O., Ljungman, P., et al. (1994). Reduced blood transfusion requirements after allogeneic bone marrow transplantation: Results of a randomized double-blind study with high-dose erythropoietin. *Bone Marrow Transplantation* 13(4): 397–402.

Koloc, G., and Schannweber, K. (1993). Recombinant granulocyte colony-stimulating factor. *Journal of Intravenous Nursing* 16(4): 234–238.

Labar, B., Bogdanic, V., and Nemet, D. (1989). Total body irradiation with or without lung shielding for allogeneic bone marrow transplantation. *Bone Marrow Transplantation* 4(Suppl 3): 108.

Lawton, C.A. (1989). Technique modifications in hyperfractionated total body irradiation for T lymphocyte depleted bone marrow transplants. *International Journal of Radiation Oncology, Biology and Physiology* 17(2): 319–322.

Lazarus, H.M. (1997). Recombinant cytokines and hematopoietic growth factors in allogeneic and autologous bone marrow transplantation. In J. Winter (ed.): *Blood Stem Cell Transplantation*. Boston: Kluwer Academic Publishers.

Leyland-Jones, B., Dalton, W., Fisher, G.A., and Sikic, B. (1993). Reversal of multidrug resistance to cancer chemotherapy. *Cancer* 72(Suppl 11): 3483–3488.

Lippman, S.M., Benner, S.E., and Hong, W.K. (1994). Retinoid chemoprevention studies in upper aerodigestive tract and lung carcinogenesis. *Cancer Research* 54(Suppl 7): 2025S–2028S.

Lippman, S.M., Benner, S.E., and Hong, W.K. (1993). Chemoprevention: Strategies for the control of cancer. *Cancer* 72(Suppl 3):984–990.

Maxwell, M.B., and Maher, K.E. (1992). Chemotherapy induced myelosuppression. *Seminars in Oncology Nursing* 8(2): 113–133.

Mazanet, R., and Griffin, J.D. (1992). Hematopoietic growth factors. In J.O. Armitage and K.A. Antman (eds.): *High-dose Cancer Therapy*. Baltimore: Williams and Wilkins, 289–313.

McClinton-Adams, J.L. (1994). Cancer prevention with beta-carotene. *Annals of Pharmacotherapy* 28(4): 470–471.

McDonald, T.P. (1992). Thrombopoietin: Its biology, clinical aspects, and possibilities. *American Journal of Pediatric Hematology/Oncology* 14(1): 8–21.

Michels, K.B., and Willett, W.C. (1994). Vitamins and cancer. A practical means of prevention? In V.T. DeVita, Jr., S. Hellman, and S.A. Rosenberg, (eds.): *Important Advances in Oncology 1994*. Philadelphia: Lippincott.

Moscow, J.A., and Cowan, K.H. (1988). Multidrug resistance. *Journal of National Cancer Institute* 80(1): 14–20.

Neumanaitis, J. (1993). Granulocyte-macrophage-colony-stimulating factor: A review from preclinical development to clinical application. *Transfusion* 33(1): 70–83.

O'Connell, A.S., and Schmit-Pokorny, K. (1997). Blood and marrow stem cell transplantation: Indications, procedure, process. In M.B. Whedon and D. Wujcik (eds.): *Blood and Marrow Stem Cell Transplantation: Principles, Practice, and Nursing Insights*. 2nd ed. Boston: Jones & Bartlett.

Ogawa, M. (1994). The role of granulocyte colony stimulating factor with dose-intensive chemotherapy. *Seminars in Oncology* 21(Suppl 1): 7–9.

Pai, L.H., and Pastan, I. (1994). Immunotoxins and recombinant toxins for cancer treatment. In V.T. DeVita, Jr., S. Hellman, and S. Rosenberg (eds.): *Important Advances in Oncology 1994*. Philadelphia: Lippincott.

Phillips, G.L. (1999). Conditioning Regimens. In H.J. Deeg, H.G. Klingemann, G.L. Phillips, and G. van Zant (eds.): *A Guide To Blood and Marrow Transplantation*. 3rd ed. Berlin: Springer, 67–88.

Reiffers, J., Bernard, P., David, B., Vezon, G., Sarrat, A., Marit, G., Moulinier, J., and Broustet, A., (1986). Successful autologous transplantation with peripheral blood hemopoietic cells in a patient with acute leukemia. *Experimental Hematology* 14(4): 312–315.

Ren, S., and Lien, E.J. (1997). Natural products and their derivatives as chemoprevention agents. *Progress in Drug Research* 48, 147–171.

Rieger, P.T. (1996). Biotherapy – The Fourth Modality. In M. Barton-Burke, G. Wilkes, and K. Ingwersen: *Cancer Chemotherapy: A Nursing Process Approach*. 2nd ed. Sudbury, Mass: Jones & Bartlett, 43–73.

Roy, V., Veys, P., and Jackson, F. (1989). Adult respiratory syndrome following autologous bone marrow transfusion. *Bone Marrow Transplantation*, 4(6), 711-712.

Rumsey, K.A. and Rieger, P.T. (1992). *Biological Response Modifiers*. Chicago: Precept Press.

Santos, G.W. (1983). History of bone marrow transplantation. *Clinical Haematology* 12(3): 611–639

Schick, B.P. (1994). Clinical implications of basic research: Hope for treatment of thrombocytopenia. *New England Journal of Medicine* 331(13): 875–876.

Smith, C.D., Prinsep, M.R., Caplan, F.R., Moore, R.E., and Patterson, G.M.L. (1994). Reversal of multiple drug resistance by tolyporphin, a novel cyanobacterial natural product. *Oncology Research* 6(4–5): 211–218.

Smith, C.D., Zhang, S., Mooberry, S.L., Patterson, G.M.L., and Moore, R.E. (1994). Cryptophycin: A new microtubule depolymerizing agent active against drug-resistant cells. *Cancer Research* 54(14): 3779–3784.

Smith, D.M., Weisenburger, D.D., Bierman, P.M., Kessinger, Vaughan, and Armitage (1987). Acute renal failure associated with autologous bone marrow transplantation. *Bone Marrow Transplantation* 2(2): 195–201.

Steegmann, J., Lopez, J., Otero, M., et al. (1992). Erythropoietin treatment in allogeneic BMT accelerates erythroid reconstitution: Results of a prospective controlled randomized trial. *Bone Marrow Transplantation* 10(6): 541–546.

Stratmann, K., Burgoyne, D.L., Moore, R.E., Patterson, G.M.L., and Smith, C.D. (1994). Hapalosin, a cyanobacterial cyclic depsipeptide with multidrug-resistance reversing activity. *Journal of Organic Chemistry* 59(24): 7219–7226.

Thomas, E.D., and Storb, R. (1970). Techniques for human marrow grafting. *Blood* 36(4): 507–515.

Thomas, E.D., Storb, R., Cliff, R.A., Fefer, A., Johnson, L., Neiman, P.E., Lerner, K.G., Glucksberg, H., Buckner, C.D. (1975). Bone marrow transplantation. *New England Journal of Medicine* 292(17): 895–902.

Tutschka, J., Copelan, E.A., and Kapoor, N. (1989). Replacing total body irradiation with busulfan as conditioning of patients with leukemia for allogeneic marrow transplantation. *Transplant Proceedings* 21(Pt3), 2952–2954.

van Zant, G. (1999). Stem cell sources. In H.J. Deeg, H.G. Klingemann, G.L. Phillips, and G. van Zant (eds.): *A Guide to Blood and Marrow Transplantation*. 3rd ed. Berlin: Springer.

Vitale, V., Scarpati, D., Frassoni, P. et al. (1989). Total body irradiation: Single dose, fractions, dose, rate. *Bone Marrow Transplantation* 4(Suppl 1): 233–235.

Vose, J.M., Phillips, G.L., and Armitage, J.O. (1992). Autologous bone marrow transplantation for Hodgkin's disease. In J.O. Armitage and K.A. Antman (eds.): *High-dose Cancer Therapy*. Baltimore: Williams and Wilkins, 651–661.

Weinthal, J.A. (1996). The role of cytokines following bone marrow transplantation: Indications and controversies. *Bone Marrow Transplantation* 18 (Suppl 3): S10–S14.

Whedon, M.B. (1991a). Allogeneic bone marrow transplantation: Clinical indications, treatment, process and outcomes. In M.B. Whedon, *Bone Marrow Transplantation: Principles, Practice and Nursing Implications*. Boston: Jones & Bartlett, 3–19.

———. (1991b). Autologous bone marrow transplantation. In M.B. Whedon, *Bone Marrow Transplantation: Principles, Practice and Nursing Implications*. Boston: Jones & Bartlett, 20–48.

Wiebe, V.J., Smith, B.R., and DeGregorio, M.W. (1992). Pharmacology of agents used in bone marrow transplant conditioning regimens. *Critical Reviews in Oncology-Hematology* 13(13): 241–270.

Wilkes, G., Ingwersen, K., and Barton-Burke, M. (2000). *2001 Oncology Nursing Drug Handbook*. Sudbury, Mass: Jones & Bartlett.

Zix-Kieffer, I., Langer, B., Eyer, D., Acar, G., Racadot, E., Schlaeder, G., Oberlin, F., and Lutz, P. (1996). Successful cord blood stem cell transplantation for congenital erythropoietic porphyria (Gunther's disease). *Bone Marrow Transplantation* 18: 217–220.

# Part II

# Cancer Chemotherapy

## Mechanisms and Nursing Care

# Chapter 4

# Potential Toxicities and Nursing Management

## Gail M. Wilkes, RN, MS, AOCN

## INTRODUCTION

Cancer is a disease of the cell. Cancer chemotherapeutic agents, or antineoplastic agents, interfere with cell replication to bring about either tumor cell kill (cytotoxic drugs) or cessation of growth (cytostatic drugs). Although studies have been made using monoclonal antibodies to target tumor cells, we are largely unable to target chemotherapy agents directly against malignant cells exclusively, thus sparing normal, rapidly dividing cells. As a result, we see temporary damage in normal frequently dividing, or proliferating, cell populations, such as bone marrow, gastrointestinal mucosa, gonads, and hair follicles. Damage to normal cells usually is temporary because normal cells have more efficient repair mechanisms than malignant cells.

In addition, certain drugs may have an affinity for specific organ(s) in the body and cause organ toxicity over time. For example, doxorubicin, an anthracycline drug, may cause myofibril damage in the heart, leading to increased risk of cardiomyopathy with cumulative drug doses over 450–550 mg/m$^2$.

As nurses, we are taught to monitor patient tolerance of drugs and to discuss drug discon-tinuance with the physician when signs or symptoms of drug toxicity are observed. As oncology nurses caring for patients receiving chemotherapy, we expect certain toxicities, such as neutropenia, that would otherwise not be tolerated with other medications. Our role as patient educators is to teach patients and families self-care, and our competent assessment and intervention to minimize complications and optimize patient tolerance of therapy are crucial for patient safety and quality of life. We work closely with other members of an interdisciplinary team to accomplish this. In order to better understand chemotherapy-related toxicities, it is important to understand the timing and the mechanism of occurrence.

Perry and Yarbro (1984) have classified common toxicities by time of occurrence, whether onset is immediate, early, or late. These include the following:

1. *Immediate onset, hours to days after administration*: nausea/vomiting, phlebitis, hyperuricemia, renal failure, anaphylaxis, skin rash, teratogenicity. Specific drugs may cause hemorrhagic cystitis (Cytoxan), radiation recall (actinomycin D), fever/chills (bleomycin), hypertension (procarbazine), and hypotension (etoposide).

2. *Early onset, days to weeks*: leukopenia, thrombocytopenia, alopecia, stomatitis, diarrhea, megaloblastosis. Specific drugs may cause paralytic ileus (vincristine), hypercalcemia (estrogens, antiestrogens), hypomagnesemia (cisplatin), pancreatitis (L-asparaginase), fluid retention (estrogen, steroids), pulmonary infiltrates (metho-trexate, bleomycin), and ototoxicity (cisplatin).

3. *Delayed onset, weeks to months*: anemia, aspermia, hepatocellular damage, hyperpigmentation, pulmonary fibrosis. Specific drugs may cause peripheral neuropathy (paclitaxel, vincristine, cisplatin), cardiac necrosis (Adriamycin, cyclophosphamide), SIADH (cyclophosphamide, vincristine), and hemolytic-uremic syndrome (mitomycin C).

4. *Late onset, months to years*: sterility, hypogonadism, premature menopause, second malignancy. Specific drugs may cause hepatic fibrosis/cirrhosis (methotrexate), encephalopathy (methotrexate, CNS radiation), and cancer of the bladder (cyclophosphamide).

This chapter focuses on common toxicities and examines pathophysiologic mechanisms, nursing management, and patient teaching strategies to minimize complications and to optimize patient tolerance of treatment.

The first section addresses chemotherapy-induced damage to rapidly proliferating normal cell populations: the bone marrow, the gastrointestinal tract epithelium, the hair follicles of the scalp, and the gonads.

The next section deals with specific organ toxicities, drugs implicated, and specific principles the interdisciplinary team uses to monitor for or prevent toxicity. Appendix I presents the National Cancer Institute (NCI) schema for grading common toxicities and provides a mechanism to define, compare, and evaluate toxicity in chemotherapy regimens. The NCI updates its criteria, and the reader is urged to visit the NCI Website (http:// ctep.info.nih.gov/CTC3/CTC.html).

---

## Section A. *Toxicity to Rapidly Proliferating Normal Cell Populations*

---

## I. BONE MARROW DEPRESSION (BMD)

### Introduction

The bone marrow is an organ that is constantly active, responding to the human body's need for white blood cells to protect against infection, red blood cells to carry oxygen to the body's cells, and platelets to prevent bleeding. Chemotherapy works by interfering with cell division of frequently dividing cells, so the bone marrow stem cells, which divide frequently to provide the formed blood cell elements as needed by the body, are often temporarily injured by chemotherapy. In fact, bone marrow depression may become the dose-limiting toxicity for many drugs. In order to understand the potential damage of chemotherapy on the bone marrow, it is helpful to review the normal development of blood cells in the bone marrow. It is believed that all cells develop from a pluripotent stem cell, which has the ability to differentiate and mature into the formed blood cell elements seen in the peripheral blood (see Figure 4.1). Figure 4.2 illustrates the scientific developments in understanding the influence of growth factors in the maturation of formed blood cell elements.

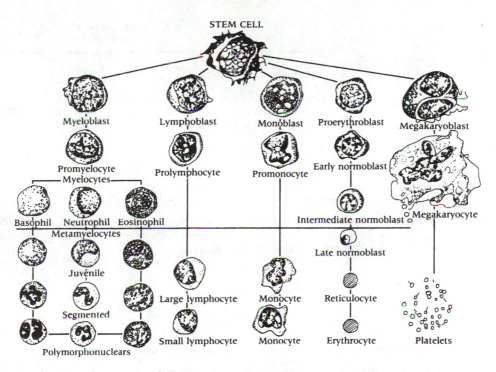

**Figure 4.1** The Development of the Various Formed Elements of the Blood from Bone Marrow Cells

*Leukocytes*, or white blood cells, are composed of five different cell types, which can be separated into two groups: those with granules in their cytoplasm (*granulocytes*) and those without. Most important of the granulocytes are the *neutrophils*, which are the body's first line of internal defense against infection or invading microorganisms. These cells represent the largest number of white blood cells and converge at the site of infection. Thus, when the infection is severe, so many neutrophils are needed to halt the infection that the bone marrow releases immature neutrophils, called *bands* or *stabs*, or perhaps even more immature cells, into the peripheral bloodstream. This is called a *shift to the left*. There is an increased percentage of neutrophils and usually an increased number of white blood cells overall (leukocytosis) in a left shift. Bacterial infections in general cause a rise in the percentage of neutrophils, whereas viral infections may decrease the neutrophil count (McConnell 1986). Other granulocytes are the *eosinophils*, which are active against allergens and parasites, and *basophils*, which have a role in histamine production and fibrinolysis and are released during chronic inflammation. The white blood cells without granules are the *lymphocytes*, which provide cell-mediated immunity (T-cells) and antibody production (B-cells), and the *monocytes*, which represent the body's second line of defense, destroying remaining microorganisms and removing debris from the site of infection. Monocytes are helpful in phagocytosing both mycobacteria and fungi. Monocytes that migrate into the surrounding tissue are called *macrophages*.

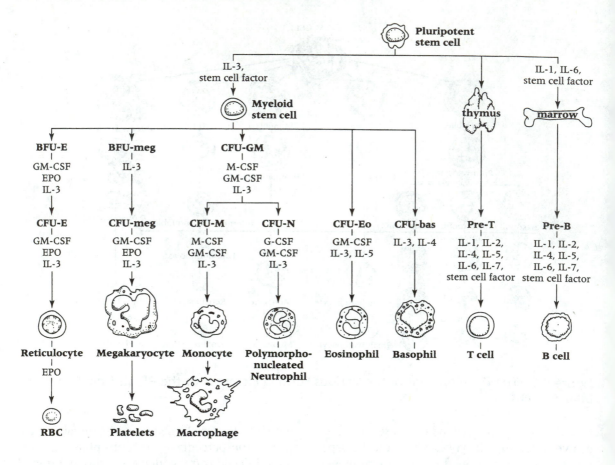

**Figure 4.2**   Role of Growth Factors in the Maturation of Formed Blood Cell Elements

Chemotherapy does not affect circulating, mature blood cells because they are no longer dividing. Rather, chemotherapy damages stem cells that have a cell generation time of 6–24 hours (Brager and Yasko 1984), decreasing the bone marrow's ability to replace the body's used blood cell elements, in particular the neutrophils and platelets. Because all blood cells have a fixed life span (white blood cells 6 hours, platelets about 10 days, and red blood cells about 120 days), the effect in lowering the blood counts occurs at a predictable time after the chemotherapy is administered, usually 7–14 days depending on the specific drug. The *lowest* point reached in the peripheral blood count after chemotherapy is administered is called the *nadir* (see Table 4.1).

Certain alkylating agents, such as mechlorethamine (nitrogen mustard) and the nitrosoureas (e.g., lomustine [CCNU]) cause direct stem cell suppression (Dorr and Fritz 1980; Dorr and von Hoff 1994). Fortunately, many cells in the bone marrow are not actively dividing, with as many as 15–50% of stem cells in the $G_0$ or resting stage, so the stem cells can escape from cell cycle phase-specific agents. As

**Table 4.1  Bone Marrow Depression: Expected Time of Drug Nadirs**

| Drug Class | Nadir | Recovery |
|---|---|---|
| **I. Alkylating Agents** | | |
| a. mechlorethamine (nitrogen mustard) | 7–15 days | 28 days |
| b. melphalan (Alkeran) | 10–12 days | 42–50 days |
| c. busulfan (Myleran) | 11–30 days | 24–54 days |
| d. chlorambucil (Leukeran) | 14–28 days | 28–42 days |
| e. cyclophosphamide (Cytoxan) | 8–14 days | 18–25 days |
| f. ifosfamide | mild | After 2 weeks |
| g. cisplatin (Platinol) | 14 days | 21 days |
| h. carboplatin | 18–24 days | 4–6 weeks |
| i. dacarbazine (DTIC) | 21–28 days | 28–35 days |
| j. nitrosoureas | | |
|     carmustine (BCNU) | 26–30 days | 35–49 days |
|     lomustine (CCNU) | 40–50 days | 60 days |
|     semustine (MeCCNU) | 28–63 days | 82–89 days |
|     streptozocin (Zanosar) | As single agent, nonmyelosuppressive | |
| k. thiotepa (TESPA) | 5–30 days | 40–50 days |
| **II. Antimetabolites** | | |
| a. cytosine arabinoside (Ara-C) | 12–14 days | 22–24 days |
| b. fluorouracil (5-FU) | 7–14 days | 16–24 days |
| c. methotrexate (MTX) | 7–14 days | 14–21 days |
| d. mercaptopurine (6MP) | 7–14 days | 14–21 days |
| e. hydroxyurea (Hydrea) | 18–30 days | 21–35 days |
| f. 5-Azacytadine | 14–17 days | 28–31 days |
| g. gematabine (Gemzar) | 5–6 days | ≤7 days |
| h. fludarabine (Fludara) | 13 days | 3–25 days |
| i. capecitabine (Xeloda) | 14 days | 21 days |
| **III. Plant Alkaloids** | | |
| a. paclitaxel (Taxol) | 8–11 days | 21 days |
| b. vincristine (VCR) | 4–5 days but relatively nonmyelosuppressive | 7 days |
| c. Velban (Vlb) | 5–9 days | 14–21 days |
| d. vindesine | 5–10 days | 10 days |
| e. vinorelbine (Navelbine) | 7–8 days | 15–17 days |
| **IV. Podophyllotoxins** | | |
| a. etoposide (VP-16) | 9–14 days | 20–22 days |
| b. VM-26 | 3–14 days | 28 days |
| c. irinotecan (Camptosar) | 21 days | 28 days |
| d. topotecan (Hycamptin) | 11–15 days | 21 days |
| **V. Antibiotics** | | |
| a. bleomycin (Blenoxane) | Nonmyelosuppressive | |
| b. daunorubicin (Daunomycin, Cerubidine) | 10–14 days | 21 days |
| c. doxorubicin (Adriamycin) | 10–14 days | 21–24 days |
| d. dactinomycin (Actinomycin D) | 14–21 days | 22–25 days |
| e. mitomycin C (Mutamycin) | 28–42 days | 42–56 days |
| f. mithramycin (Mithracin) | 14 days | 21–28 days |
| g. epirubicin (Ellence) | 10–14 days | 21 days |
| **VI. Steroids (do not cause myelosuppression)** | | |
| **VII. Miscellaneous** | | |
| a. mitoxantrone (Novantrone) | 8–10 days | After 2 weeks |
| b. procarbazine (Matulane) | 25–36 days | 36–50 days |
| c. asparaginase (Elspar) | Nonmyelosuppressive | |

*Source:* Modified from Dorr, R.T., and Fritz, W. (1980). *Cancer Chemotherapy Handbook:* 103–104. Reprinted by permission of Elsevier Science Publishing Company, Inc.

shown in Table 4.1, phase-specific agents, such as the antimetabolites, cause fairly rapid nadirs (7–30 days) with brisk recovery, followed by cell cycle nonphase-specific agents such as doxorubicin, with nadirs occurring in 10–14 days and recovery in 21–24 days. Finally, cell cycle nonspecific agents, such as the nitrosoureas, produce delayed and prolonged bone marrow depression, with nadirs occurring in 26–63 days and recovery in 35–89 days (Bergsagel 1971) (see Figure 4.3). Thus, in combination chemotherapy, a drug with an early nadir and recovery in 21–28 days can be administered every 3–4 weeks, in contrast to those with delayed bone marrow depression,

which can be administered only every 6–8 weeks. In addition, agents such as the nitrosoureas, may have a cumulative effect, causing severe and less reversible damage to the bone marrow, decreasing bone marrow reserve, and resulting in protracted bone marrow depression (leukopenia and thrombocytopenia). Certain chemotherapeutic agents do not cause significant bone marrow depression. These are vincristine, bleomycin, cisplatin in moderate doses, L-asparaginase, and steroid hormones.

The degree of bone marrow depression is also influenced by other host factors, as seen in Table 4.2

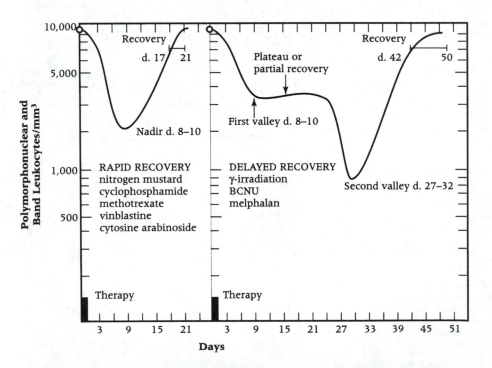

**Figure 4.3** Times to Recovery of Peripheral Granulocyte Counts Following Administration of Antitumor Drugs

*Source:* From Bergsagel, D.E. (1971). Assessment of massive-dose chemotherapy of malignant disease. *Canadian Medical Association Journal* 104: 31–36. Reprinted with permission.

**Table 4.2**  Factors Affecting the Degree of Bone Marrow Depression

| Factor | Influence |
| --- | --- |
| 1. Age | Advancing age often is associated with reduced functional bone marrow reserves so recovery may be delayed. Studies have shown that many elderly patients are able to tolerate full doses (Blesch 1988). |
| 2. Drug dose | The higher the dose of a myelosuppressive drug, the greater the degree of bone marrow suppression. Of greatest importance is the depression of the granulocytes (see Figure 4.4). |
| 3. Nutritional state | Protein-calorie malnutrition may reduce the ability to repair normal cells damaged by chemotherapy. |
| 4. Bone marrow reserve | When reserve is limited, bone marrow recovery is delayed with prolonged neutropenia or thrombocytopenia, and a subsequent need to delay treatment or reduce drug dosage. Reserves may be reduced in individuals who have histories of significant alcohol abuse (fatty marrow) and those with tumor invasion of the bone marrow (myelophthisic), with bone marrow failure. |
| 5. Ability to metabolize drug | Renal or hepatic dysfunction can decrease drug metabolism and elimination, resulting in prolonged, elevated circulating blood levels of drug with consequent increased toxicity. |
| 6. Prior treatment | Radiation to sites of bone marrow production (ends of long bones, skull, sternum, ribs, vertebrae, sacrum, upper and lower limb girdles) or prior chemotherapy may cause bone marrow atrophy or fibrosis and decreased bone marrow reserves (hypocellularity). |
| 7. Sequestration of drug | Such drugs as methotrexate are sequestered in physiologic effusions and then slowly released into the systemic circulation with prolonged toxicity. |

## Nursing Management of the Patient with Bone Marrow Depression

Infection occurs frequently in the course of cancer illness and treatment. It is a very serious complication and is the most common cause of cancer deaths (Brandt 1984). Thus, nursing care is directed toward the prevention of infection if possible, or early identification and intervention to prevent further injury. *The single most important risk factor for bacterial infection is a decreased number of neutrophils* (Fox 1981), so it is essential to be familiar with the calculation of the absolute neutrophil count in caring for patients receiving chemotherapy. Normal values for the elements in a white blood cell differential are shown in Table 4.3. In determining the numbers of cell elements, 100 cells are examined, and the differential shows how many of the 100 cells are each type of white blood cell. Because the immature neutrophil, called the *band*, is effective in fighting against infection, the number of bands is added to the number of neutrophils first. This figure is easily converted to a percentage by dividing by 100. Thus, to calculate the absolute number of neutrophils in the total white blood count, the number of neutrophils and bands in 100 white blood cells examined is converted to a percentage, then this index is multiplied times the total number of white blood cells because it is known that this percentage of them should be neutrophils. The formula looks like this:

$$\frac{Number\ of\ neutrophils\ mm^3}{(absolute\ neutrophil\ count)} =$$

$$\frac{white\ blood\ cell\ count}{(number\ of\ cells/mm^3)} \times \frac{\%\ of\ neutrophils}{(including\ band\ forms)}$$

For example, your patient has a total white blood count of 10,000/mm³. He has no clinical signs of infection, and the differential shows that there are 65 neutrophils, 2 bands, 1 eos, 3 monos, and 29 lymphs. This number should total 100. Because you are interested in the number of neutrophils that fight against infection, you add the neutrophils (65) and the bands (2), arriving at 67. Thus, 67 of the 100 cells are able to fight against bacterial infection. This number is converted to a percentage: $67 \div 100 = 0.67$, and then multiplied by the total white blood count to approximate the total or absolute number of neutrophils in the body. This equals 6700/mm³, which falls within the normal range of Table 4.3

**Table 4.3** Normal Values of the White Blood Count Differential

| Cell Element | Percentage of Total | Absolute Count |
|---|---|---|
| Total WBC Leukocytes | 100 | 5000–10,000/mm³ |
| Neutrophils | 50–70 | 2500–7000/mm³ |
| Lymphocytes | 20–40 | 1000–4000/mm³ |
| Monocytes | 2–6 | 100–600/mm³ |
| Eosinophils | 1–4 | 50–400/mm³ |
| Basophils | 0.5–1 | 25–50/mm³ |

*Source:* Modified from McConnell, E.A. (1986). Leukocyte studies: What the counts can tell you. *Nursing* 86 (March): 42–43. All rights reserved. Reprinted with permission.

Normally, leukocytes number 5000–10,000/mm³ cells, and of these, neutrophils represent roughly 50–70%. A normal neutrophil count is 3150–6200/mm³, with polymorphonuclear cells (*segs*) accounting for 3000–5800/mm³ and bands for 150–400/mm³. *Neutropenia* is defined as a neutrophil count less than 2500/mm³. It is easy to understand why *neutropenia is the single most important risk factor in bacterial infection:* there are inadequate numbers of these protective cells to phagocytose and wall off invading microorganisms, and if immature cells are released, they are limited in their effectiveness. The relative risk of bacterial infection *increases* as the absolute neutrophil count *decreases*: there is no significant risk when the absolute neutrophil count is 1500–2000/mm³; there is minimal risk at 1000–1500/mm³, moderate risk at 500–1000/mm³, and severe risk when the absolute neutrophil count is less than 500/mm³ (Fox 1981).

In the past, (1960–1970), bacterial infections were most often related to gram-negative microorganisms; however, within the past decade gram-positive infections are more prevalent (Wilkes, Ingwersen, and Barton-Burke 1999, 464). The longer the duration of neutropenia, the greater the risk for infection.

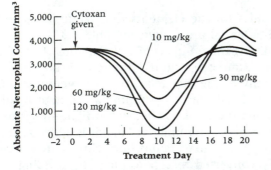

**Figure 4.4** Effect of Increasing Doses of Cyclophosphamide on Peripheral Blood Granulocyte Counts

*Source:* From Braine, H.G. (1980). Infectious complications of granulocytopenia after cancer chemotherapy. In M.D. Abeloff (ed.): *Complications of Cancer: Diagnosis and Management.* Baltimore/London: Johns Hopkins University Press: 152. Reprinted with permission of the Johns Hopkins University Press.

In a study by Bodey et al. (1966), the risk was 60% if neutropenia lasted 3 weeks; if the absolute neutrophil count (ANC) was $<100/mm^3$ during this time, the risk was 100%. Further compromise may occur with lymphopenia occurring 1–2 days after chemotherapy, with recovery in 2–3 days, and if steroids are used in treatment, corticosteroid-induced T-cell lymphocyte and macrophage dysfunction can occur (Brager and Yasko 1984). Invasion by microorganisms and infection can be reduced in the neutropenic patient by maintaining intact skin and mucous membrane barriers, eliminating exposure to infecting organisms, such as those on the hands of health care workers, and maintaining a well-nourished state, which promotes immunocompetence with functioning lymphocytes and antibody formation.

In addition, restoration of an adequate neutrophil count to prevent febrile neutropenia can be induced by granulocyte colony-stimulating factors: G-CSF (filgrastim, Neupogen) and GM-CSF (sargramostim, Leukine, Prokine).

Studies have shown that it is the patient's own normal flora that cause approximately 85% of infections in the neutropenic patient. Fever is usually the first sign of infection, and because of the absence of significant numbers of neutrophils, other signs are absent, such as pus formation or consolidation on a chest X-ray. Fever (101°F, or 38.3°C) in a neutropenic patient, if untreated, can result in death within 48 hours in up to 50% of patients, because sepsis can develop so quickly (Carlson 1985). Thus, infection becomes a medical emergency. Although 40–60% of patients with fever never show a culture-proven infection (Pizzo 1993), cultures of potential sites of infection are done, a chest X-ray is taken, and empiric broad-spectrum antibiotic coverage is started to suppress colonizing organisms. If fever persists, then antifungal therapy usually is instituted. In addition, herpes virus infections are common, especially in patients with hematologic malignancies or undergoing bone marrow transplantation (Zaia 1990).

The most common infective organisms are the gram-negative bacilli, such as *Pseudomonas aeruginosa*, *Enterobacteriaceae*, *Klebsiella pneumoniae*, and *Escherichia coli*; next common are fungi, such as *Candida albicans* and *C. aspergillus* (Pizzo 1993), and the increasing incidence of fungi appears related to the widespread use of prophylactic antibiotics. Also, gram-positive organisms are becoming more common, such as *Staphylococcus aureus*, *Staphylococcus epidermidis*, *Corynebacteria* and *Clostridia spp*, due to increased use of implanted venous access devices and the development of effective antibiotics against gram negative bacteria. (Wilkes, et al. 1999, 464). The most common sites of infection are the upper and lower respiratory tract (i.e., pneumonia) and the blood (bacteremias); other less commonly occurring sites are pharynx (pharyngitis or stomatitis), esophagus (esophagitis), perianal region, skin, urinary tract, and central nervous system (Rodriguez and Ketchel 1981).

It is important to look at the potential routes of exposure that may lead to the colonization of organisms in the neutropenic patient. These are shown in Figure 4.5, and include health care providers who do not wash their hands and carry microorganisms from one patient to another; fresh fruits or leafy vegetables, which may contain *klebsiella* or *pseudomonas*; standing water, which may contain *pseudomonas*; fresh flowers or plants; and the air. In order to reduce the acquisition of new potential pathogens, patients with an ANC of 500 or less are placed on neutropenic precautions. Scrupulous hand washing with soap, water, and friction prior to entering the patient's room and between contact with different parts of the patient's body is the most effective method to

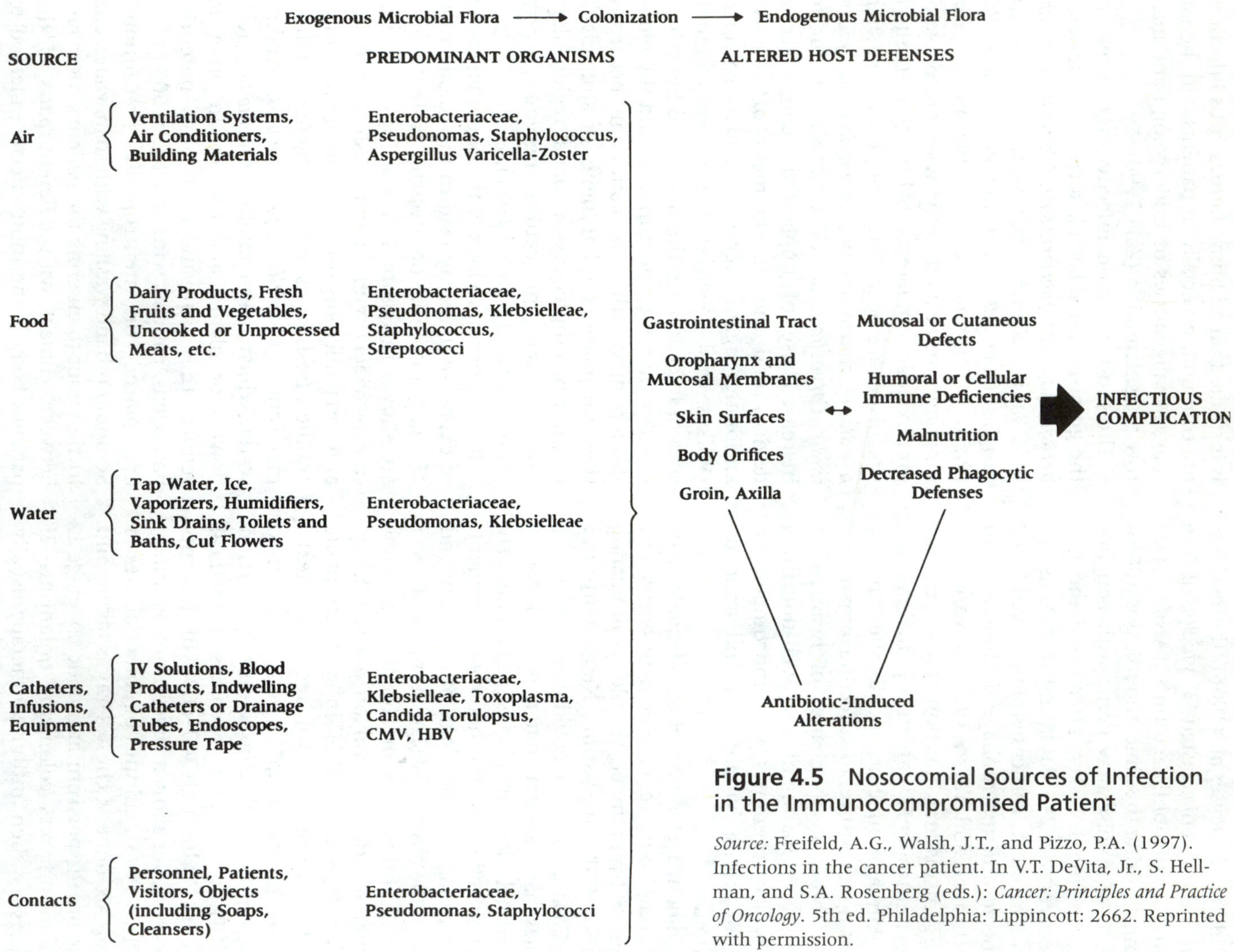

Exogenous Microbial Flora ⟶ Colonization ⟶ Endogenous Microbial Flora

| SOURCE | PREDOMINANT ORGANISMS | ALTERED HOST DEFENSES |
|---|---|---|
| **Air** | Ventilation Systems, Air Conditioners, Building Materials | Enterobacteriaceae, Pseudonomas, Staphylococcus, Aspergillus Varicella-Zoster |
| **Food** | Dairy Products, Fresh Fruits and Vegetables, Uncooked or Unprocessed Meats, etc. | Enterobacteriaceae, Pseudonomas, Klebsiellleae, Staphylococcus, Streptococci |
| **Water** | Tap Water, Ice, Vaporizers, Humidifiers, Sink Drains, Toilets and Baths, Cut Flowers | Enterobacteriaceae, Pseudomonas, Klebsiellleae |
| **Catheters, Infusions, Equipment** | IV Solutions, Blood Products, Indwelling Catheters or Drainage Tubes, Endoscopes, Pressure Tape | Enterobacteriaceae, Klebsiellleae, Toxoplasma, Candida Torulopsus, CMV, HBV |
| **Contacts** | Personnel, Patients, Visitors, Objects (including Soaps, Cleansers) | Enterobacteriaceae, Pseudomonas, Staphylococci |

Gastrointestinal Tract
- Oropharynx and Mucosal Membranes
- Skin Surfaces
- Body Orifices
- Groin, Axilla

→ Antibiotic-Induced Alterations

Mucosal or Cutaneous Defects

Humoral or Cellular Immune Deficiencies

Malnutrition

Decreased Phagocytic Defenses

**INFECTIOUS COMPLICATION**

**Figure 4.5**  Nosocomial Sources of Infection in the Immunocompromised Patient

*Source:* Freifeld, A.G., Walsh, J.T., and Pizzo, P.A. (1997). Infections in the cancer patient. In V.T. DeVita, Jr., S. Hellman, and S.A. Rosenberg (eds.): *Cancer: Principles and Practice of Oncology.* 5th ed. Philadelphia: Lippincott: 2662. Reprinted with permission.

prevent the spread of microorganisms (Pizzo 1989). If possible the patient should be placed in a private room but research has shown that there is no significant difference in infection rates between neutropenic patients receiving standard hospital care and those on simple protective isolation as long as scrupulous hand washing is used (Golden 1971; Neuseff and Maki 1981). Total protected environments using laminar flow rooms and gastrointestinal (GI) decontamination have reduced significantly the incidence of infection in neutropenic patients; because of the cost and the availability of these environments, they are used primarily for patients undergoing bone marrow transplants (Bodey 1984).

The standardized nursing care plan for the patient experiencing bone marrow depression, with the potential for neutropenia and injury related to infection, is shown at the end of this section. Nursing interventions are aimed at the prevention of infection by maintaining intact skin and mucous membranes and minimizing exposure to environmental sources of infection, as well as early diagnosis and intervention if infection occurs. Because most chemotherapy is administered to ambulatory patients in outpatient settings, patient and family education to prepare the patient for self-care, and specifically for protection from infection and self-assessment if infection occurs, should begin before chemotherapy is initiated.

While the routine use of granulocyte colony-stimulating factor (G-CSF, Neupogen) in conjunction with bone marrow suppressive chemotherapy has largely prevented febrile neutropenia, it is still critical to teach patients and families how to prevent, monitor for, and seek medical care for infections.

Bone marrow depression, and neutropenia specifically, often represent the dose-limiting toxicity of chemotherapy.

Chapter 3 describes in greater detail the role of granulocyte-macrophage colony-stimulating factor (GM-CSF), a glycoprotein that controls the production, the differentiation, and the function of the granulocytes and the monocyte macrophages.

## Bone Marrow Depression: Thrombocytopenia

Platelets are formed in the bone marrow and, as shown in Figure 4.6, arise from megakaryocytes. As they are released from the bone marrow, the megakaryocytes break into tiny fragments called *platelets*. Platelets are important in blood coagulation and represent a key element in hemostasis. Platelets are important in maintaining capillary (vascular) integrity: platelets adhere to sites of injury in the blood vessel wall creating a plug that stops blood loss; also, platelets release Factor 3, which initiates clot formation and participates in clot retraction (Wroblewski and Wroblewski 1981).

As has been discussed previously, chemotherapy does not damage mature, circulating formed blood cell elements. Rather, the damage to the rapidly dividing progenitor stem cells prevents the platelets from being replaced once they have completed their usefulness in the body. This decrease in platelets is gradual because the life span of a platelet is about 10 days, with a nadir that often occurs after that of the white blood cell. Recovery of the white blood cell count usually occurs first, followed by the platelets, and lastly the red blood cell count. Bone marrow depression of the platelet stem cells may result in *thrombocytopenia*, a decrease in platelet count of less than $100,000/mm^3$, and increased risk of bleeding. The normal platelet count is $150,000-350,000/ mm^3$. Risk of serious bleeding increases as the platelet count decreases: it is mild when the platelet count is $50,000-100,000/mm^3$; moderate when

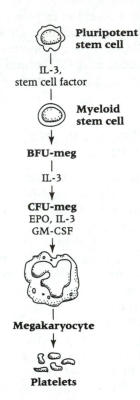

**Figure 4.6**  Normal Maturation of Platelets

20,000–50,000/mm³; and severe when less than 20,000/mm³, with increased risk of spontaneous bleeding. This risk further increases as platelets fall below 10,000/mm³, especially for GI or central nervous system (CNS) hemorrhage, and usually requires platelet transfusion.

Drugs that inhibit prostaglandin synthesis or that interfere with platelet function or production increase the risk of bleeding. These medications should be avoided if possible and include all aspirin-containing drugs and nonsteroidal anti-inflammatory drugs (NSAIDs) (see Table 4.4). Other factors that increase the risk of bleeding are bone marrow infiltration by tumor (such as leukemia and metastatic cancer, which crowd out the normal cell elements in the bone marrow and decrease the number of precursor

megakaryocytes) and radiation-induced depression of bone marrow stem cells when the radiation port includes active marrow sites of skull, ribs, sternum, vertebrae, pelvis, and ends of long bones. Oprelvekin (Neumega® IL-II) is indicated for the prevention of severe thrombocytopenia and to decrease the need for platelet transfusions in patients with nonhematological malignancies receiving myelosuppressive chemotherapy. Nursing care is directed at the prevention of bleeding or, if this is not possible, the early identification and intervention to minimize bleeding. This is described in the standardized nursing care plan for care of the patient with bone marrow depression at the end of this section.

Bone marrow depression causes several changes in a patient's physiological and psychosocial functioning. Figure 4.7 illustrates the potential patient problems associated with bone marrow depression and their interrelatedness. These changes are discussed in the care plan for bone marrow depression.

Initial patient education prior to chemotherapy administration includes avoidance of medications that increase the risk of bleeding, self-assessment for signs of bleeding, and avoidance of injury (Table 4.5). Assessment by the nurse of injury potential (bleeding) includes laboratory platelet count and its relationship to the expected nadir for specific chemotherapy drugs received, past nadir counts, and medications that may interfere with platelet function. Patient assessment is directed to the systems where most frequent bleeding due to thrombocytopenia occurs (Heyman and Schiffer 1990):

*gastrointestinal:* guaiac emesis, feces; monitor orthostatic vital signs if bleeding is suspected and patient can tolerate it;

*skin and mucous membranes:* inspect for petechiae (pinpoint capillary hemorrhages on distal extremities); presence of ecchymoses or

**Table 4.4  Medications That May Interfere with Platelet Function**

### Nonprescription Products Containing Aspirin

| Product | (Manufacturer) | Product | (Manufacturer) |
|---|---|---|---|
| Alka-Seltzer Effervescent Tablets | (Miles Laboratories) | Ecotrin Tablets | (Smith Kline Consumer) |
| Alka-Seltzer Plus Cold Medicine | | Empirin Tablets | (Burroughs Wellcome) |
| Tablets | (Miles Laboratories) | Excedrin Tablets & Capsules | (Bristol-Myers Products) |
| Anacin Tablets and Capsules, | | | |
| Maximum Strength | (Whitehall) | 4-Way Cold Tablets | (Bristol-Myers Products) |
| Arthritis Pain Formula Tablets | (Whitehall) | | |
| Arthritis Strength Bufferin Tablets | (Bristol-Myers Products) | Goody's Headache Powder | (Goody's) |
| Arthropan Liquid | (Purdue Frederick) | | |
| A.S.A. Tablets/Aspirin Tablets | | Maximum Bayer Aspirin | (Glenbrook) |
| A.S.A. Enseals | (Lilly) | Measurin Caplets | (Winthrop Pharmaceuticals) |
| Ascriptin Tablets | (Rorer Consumer) | Midol Caplets | (Glenbrook) |
| Ascriptin Tablets, Extra Strength | (Rorer Consumer) | Mobigesic Tablets | (Ascher) |
| Aspergum | | Momentum Muscular | |
| | | Backache Formula Tablets | (Whitehall) |
| Bayer Aspirin Tablets | (Glenbrook) | | |
| Bayer Children's Aspirin Tablets | (Glenbrook) | Os-Cal-Gesic Tablets | |
| Bayer Children's Cold Tablets | (Glenbrook) | | |
| Bayer Timed-Release Aspirin Tablets | (Glenbrook) | Pabalate | (Robins) |
| Bufferin Tablets | (Bristol-Myers Products) | Pepto-Bismol Tablets & Suspension | (Proctor & Gamble) |
| Bufferin, Arthritis Strength Tablets | (Bristol-Myers Products) | | |
| Bufferin, Extra Strength Tablets | (Bristol-Myers Products) | St. Joseph Aspirin for Children | (Plough) |
| | | St. Joseph Cold Tablets for Children | (Plough) |
| Cama Arthritis Pain Reliever | (Sandoz Consumer) | Sine-Off Sinus Medicine Tablets— | |
| Congesprin Chewable Tablets | (Bristol-Myers Products) | Aspirin Formula | (Smith Kline Consumer) |
| Cope Tablets | | Supac Tablets | (Mission) |
| Coricidin "D" Decongestant Tablets | (Schering) | Synalgos Capsules | (Wyeth-Ayerst) |
| Coricidin Tablets | (Schering) | | |
| Cosprin 325 Tablets | (Glenbrook) | Triaminicin Tablets | (Sandoz Consumer) |
| Cosprin 650 Tablets | (Glenbrook) | Trigesic | (Squibb) |
| Dasin Capsules | (Beechum Labs) | Vanquish Caplets | (Glenbrook) |
| Doan's Pills | (CIBA Consumer) | | |
| Duradyne Tablets | | | |

### Prescription Products Containing Aspirin

| Product | (Manufacturer) | Product | (Manufacturer) |
|---|---|---|---|
| Axotal Tablets | (Adria) | Methocarbamol with Aspirin Tablets | (Par) |
| | | Micrainin Tablets | (Wallace) |
| B-A C Tablets and Capsules | (Mayrand) | Mobidin Tablets | (Ascher) |
| Bufferin with Codeine No. 3 Tablets | | | |
| | | Norgesic & Norgesic Forte Tablets | (3M Riker) |
| Darvon with A.S.A. Pulvules | (Lilly) | | |
| Darvon Compound Pulvules | (Lilly) | Pabalate-SF Tablets | (Robins) |
| Darvon Compound-65 | (Lilly) | Percodan & Percodan-Demi | |
| Darvon-N with A.S.A. | (Lilly) | Tablets | (DuPont Pharmaceuticals) |
| Disalcid Capsules | (3M Riker) | Propoxyphene Compound 65 | (Lemmon) |
| Easprin | (Parke-Davis) | Robaxisal Tablets | (Robins) |
| Empirin with Codeine Tablets | (Burroughs Wellcome) | | |
| Equagesic Tablets | (Wyeth-Ayerst) | Synalgos-DC Capsules | (Wyeth-Ayerst) |
| Fiorinal Tablets | (Sandoz Pharmaceuticals) | Talwin Compound Tablets | (Winthrop Pharmaceuticals) |
| Fiorinal with Codeine | (Sandoz Pharmaceuticals) | Trilisate Tablets and Liquid | (Purdue Frederick) |
| Magan Tablets | (Adria) | Zorprin Tablets | (Boots-Flint) |
| Magsal Tablets | (U.S. Pharmaceuticals) | | |

*Important note:* Not a complete list. Other products may also contain aspirin or similar ingredients. Always ask the doctor or pharmacist before taking any medication.

*Source:* Adapted from Medical Economics Company. (1998). *Physicians' Desk Reference.* Oradell, N.J.: Medical Economics Company.

oozing of blood from gums, nose; prolonged oozing from venipuncture sites;

*genitourinary:* hemestick urine, assess for heavy or prolonged menses;

*respiratory:* assess for blood in sputum;

*central nervous system (intracranial):* monitor for any changes in neurological vital signs—blurred vision, spots in visual fields, headaches, disorientation, loss of coordination, changes in mental status, irritability, changes in pupil size, reactivity to light.

If the platelet count is less than 50,000/ mm$^3$, then platelet precautions should be instituted. Intervention is aimed at preventing injury by maintaining intact skin and mucosal membrane barriers. Intramuscular injections, rectal manipulation, deep endotracheal suctioning, and urinary catheterization should

**Table 4.5   Patient Instructions to Avoid Injury Related to Thrombocytopenia**

1. Use soft toothbrush or sponge-tipped applicator.
2. Use electric razor rather than blade razor.
3. Have regular bowel movements (prevent constipation).
4. Avoid vaginal douches, rectal suppositories, and enemas.
5. Avoid aspirin, aspirin-containing drugs, and other medications that interfere with platelet function. Avoid alcohol.
6. Blow nose gently; don't bend over so that head is below shoulders.
7. Use water-based lubricant prior to sexual intercourse; avoid anal intercourse.
8. Avoid use of dental floss and toothpicks.
9. Avoid cutting toenails and fingernails; use nail file.
10. Avoid bumps or falls.
11. If taking corticosteroid medication, make certain you take medication with food and eat in-between meal snacks.
12. Avoid tight-fitting or constrictive clothing.
13. Report any signs of bleeding or changes in neurologic status.

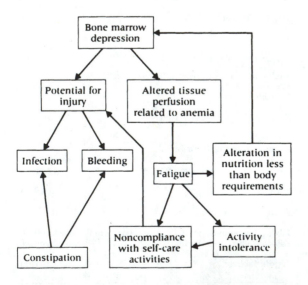

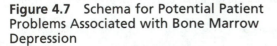

**Figure 4.7** Schema for Potential Patient Problems Associated with Bone Marrow Depression

be avoided because bleeding may occur secondary to damage to mucosal surfaces or injury to the skin. Pressure should be applied to venipuncture sites for at least 5 minutes so that an effective platelet plug can form, and venipunctures should be minimized. If the female patient has prolonged menses or menses occur during thrombocytopenia, discuss with the physician the use of medroxy-progesterone or other hormones to delay menses (Haeuber and Spross 1994) or to induce amenorrhea. A safe environment should be maintained for the patient at all times.

Hemorrhage is a life-threatening complication of thrombocytopenia. Early GI bleeding may be detected by testing emesis and stool for occult blood. In order to reduce the risk of intracranial hemorrhage, discourage the patient from heavy lifting and using the Valsalva maneuver (Wroblewski and Wroblewski 1981).

Platelet transfusion usually is administered if there are signs or symptoms of bleeding, or in some cases if the platelet count is less than 20,000/mm³. A transfusion of 10 units usually increases the platelet count 70,000–90,000/ mm³, unless the patient is sensitized or febrile or there is HLA incompatibility. The most common allergic reactions to platelet transfusion are fever and chills resulting from sensitization to previously transfused platelets, and these are treated with diphenhydramine (Benadryl) and acetominophen (Tylenol). However, because fever and chills destroy circulating platelets, future platelet transfusions should be preceded by prophylactic diphenhydramine and acetominophen or Solucortef (Brager and Yasko 1984). Fortunately, most platelets transfused in patients with cancer are irradiated, filtered, or washed to remove leukocytes that can trigger an allergic response.

## Anemia

Red blood cells (RBCs), or *erythrocytes*, by virtue of hemoglobin, carry molecules of oxygen to the tissues to meet their metabolic needs and to remove carbon dioxide to the lungs for elimination. Red blood cells also help in acid-base buffering of the blood. When the number of circulating red blood cells declines, decreased amounts of oxygen are delivered to the cells, with consequent signs and symptoms of impaired tissue oxygenation. The severity of symptoms is a function of the severity of the anemia.

Anemia resulting from bone marrow depression (see Table 4.6) related to chemotherapy occurs rarely, or considerably later than the nadirs for white blood cells and platelets because the life span of the red blood cell is approximately 120 days. Certain chemotherapeutic agents can cause anemia over time, and these include cisplatin. Other factors influencing the development of anemia include decreased red blood cell precursors by tumor infiltration of the bone marrow; concomitant or previous radiation to active bone marrow with resulting fibrosis; and active bleeding, such as menses with severe thrombocytopenia. The red blood cell development is shown in Figure 4.8. The red blood cells are released from the bone marrow as *reticulocytes*, and the

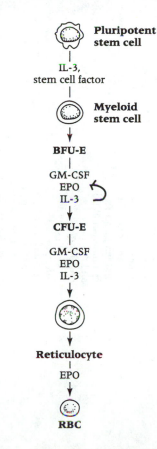

**Figure 4.8** Maturation of Red Blood Cells

**Table 4.6  Standardized Nursing Care Plan for the Patient Experiencing Bone Marrow Depression**

| Nursing Diagnosis | Expected Outcomes | Nursing Interventions |
|---|---|---|
| I. A. *Potential for altered health maintenance* | A. Pt will manage self-care as evidenced by verbal recall or return demonstration of instructions for self-assessment of oral temperature; examination of skin and mucous membranes; signs and symptoms of infection and bleeding; measures to avoid exposure to infection; measures to avoid injury and bleeding; and when and how to notify the health care provider | I. A. 1. Assess baseline knowledge, learning style, level of anxiety of pt and significant other<br>2. Develop and implement teaching plan<br>  a. Purpose and goal of chemotherapy<br>  b. Specific drugs<br>    1) mechanism of action<br>    2) potential side effects, including bone marrow suppression as appropriate<br>  c. Self-care measures<br>    1) assessment and care of skin, oral mucosa to prevent infection, trauma<br>    2) assessment of temperature BID, or if feels as if fever, and instructions to call health care provider if temperature is over 101°F (38.5°C)<br>    3) signs and symptoms of infection (fever, sore throat, cough, painful urination)<br>    4) signs and symptoms of bleeding (nose or gum bleeding, capillary or large "black and blues")<br>    5) measures to minimize exposure to infection and trauma as described in NCI booklet *Chemotherapy and You: A Guide to Self-Help*<br>  d. Provide written information to reinforce teaching, such as the booklet above, free from the NCI |
| B. *Potential for noncompliance with self-care activities* | B. Pt and significant other will comply with prescribed measures 90% of the time | B. 1. Reinforce teaching prior to treatment as nurse does prechemo assessment and prior to pt leaving clinic or hospital after treatment administration<br>2. Evaluate compliance through telephone call to pt following treatment or discharge or visiting nurse home visit<br>3. If pt or significant other is having difficulty with managing self-care activities, consider visiting nurse referral or hospitalization if pt is neutropenic or thrombocytopenic and unable to safely care for self |
| C. *Knowledge deficit related to purpose and self-administration techniques of cytokine growth factors, which may be given to prevent complications of febrile neutropenia, anemia, or bleeding* | C. Pt and significant other will verbally describe and demonstrates technique for administration of growth factors if ordered | C. 1. Provide teaching regarding side effects and administration techniques using video, pt education booklets, and demonstration/return demonstration<br>2. If unable to manage administration, contact community nursing agencies<br>3. Pt/family teaching materials available through the pharmaceutical companies that make cytokine growth factors |

II. *Potential for altered nutrition: less than body requirements*

II. A. Pt will maintain within 5% of pretreatment weight

B. Recovery from nadir approximates expected time based on specific chemotherapy agents

II. A. Assess food preferences

B. Encourage foods high in proteins, calories, iron, and folic acid

C. Discourage excessive alcohol intake

D. Review dietary instructions with pt and person responsible for preparing food

E. Review teaching material with pt and family from NCI booklet *Eating Hints* for pts receiving chemotherapy, a free publication

III. *Potential for injury: infection and bleeding related to bone marrow depression*

III. A. Pt will remain free of infection, bleeding, and tissue hypoxia

B. Pt will experience minimal complications of bone marrow suppression as evidenced by return to normal temperature and neutrophil count and absence of major bleeding

III. A. Assessment of potential for injury related to bone marrow depression

1. Expected nadir from specific agents administered, nadir from prior treatment cycle if appropriate
2. Major life stressors and coping ability
3. Sexual history and self-care habits re: hygiene
4. Sleep pattern
5. Elimination pattern
6. Nutritional pattern
7. History and physical exam
   a. Symptoms of infection: fever, pain (swallowing, with elimination, etc.), erythema, presence of exudate
   b. Symptoms of bleeding: dizziness, presence of blood in excretia
   c. Symptoms of anemia: fatigue, dyspnea on exertion, angina
   d. Skin, mucous membranes: are they intact, color, evidence of petechiae or ecchymoses, exudate
   e. Breath sounds, pulmonary exam
   f. CNS exam
   g. Laboratory data: complete blood count, WBC differential, absolute neutrophil count

B. Institute neutropenic precautions for absolute neutrophil count < 500/mm³
   1. Protect pt from exposure to microorganisms
      a. Provide private room if possible
      b. Place sign on door requiring *all* persons who enter to wash their hands meticulously prior to entering the room, that persons with colds or infections should not enter, and that no flowers, fresh fruits, or vegetables should be brought into the room
      c. Place card in nursing cardex instructing that *no* intramuscular injections, rectal temperatures, or medications should be administered PR

*(continued)*

**Table 4.6** Standardized Nursing Care Plan for the Patient Experiencing Bone Marrow Depression (*continued*)

| Nursing Diagnosis | Expected Outcomes | Nursing Interventions |
| --- | --- | --- |
| | | d. Plan scrupulous hygiene with pt for oral care, daily bath, and meticulous perineal hygiene |
| | | e. Inspect all intravenous sites and change dressings using aseptic technique; sites should be changed every 48 hours or earlier if there is any indication of phlebitis |
| | | f. Avoid invasive procedures, such as urinary catheterization if possible |
| | | g. Wash hands meticulously prior to entering room and between each physical contact with the pt; monitor that all other persons wash their hands prior to entering; ensure that the nurse caring for the pt does not care for any other pt who is infected |
| | | 2. Continually assess for presence of infection |
| | | a. Monitor vital signs every 4 hours or more frequently if temperature is elevated |
| | | b. Monitor absolute neutrophil count |
| | | c. Inspect potential sites of infection: mouth, pharynx, rectum, wounds, intravenous sites, and others, remembering that usual signs of infection, such as pus and erythema, may be absent |
| | | d. Monitor for changes in character, color, and amount of excretia (sputum, urine, stool) |
| | | e. Report signs and symptoms of infection to physician and obtain cultures, administer antipyretics and antibiotics as ordered |
| | | 3. Instruct pt in stress-reducing activities to promote relaxation and satisfactory sleep/rest patterns |
| | | C. Institute platelet precautions for pt with platelet count less than 50,000/mm$^3$ |
| | | 1. Protect pt from trauma and potential bleeding |
| | | a. Place sign in nursing cardex that no IM or rectal medications should be administered, no aspirin or prostaglandin inhibiting medications should be administered, and no rectal temperatures should be taken |
| | | b. Minimize number of venipunctures and apply pressure to site at least 5 minutes until bleeding stops |
| | | c. Avoid invasive procedures, such as deep endotracheal suctioning, enemas, douches |
| | | d. Teach pt to brush teeth with soft brush or sponge applicator to prevent trauma to gums; avoid flossing |
| | | e. Provide safe environment, padding side rails when in use and removing clutter and obstructing furniture from room |
| | | f. Prevent constipation by administering stool softeners as ordered, and encourage fluid intake of 3 liters per day |

|  |  |  |
|---|---|---|
|  |  | 2. Continually monitor for signs and symptoms of bleeding<br>  a. Minor bleeding, such as petechiae, ecchymoses, epistaxis; occult blood in stool, urine, emesis<br>  b. Major bleeding, such as hematemesis, melena, heavy vaginal bleeding; changes in orthostatic vital signs > 10 mmHg in blood pressure or increase in heart rate > 100 beats per minute; changes in neuro vital signs<br>  c. Monitor platelet count, hematocrit daily<br>  d. Notify MD re: signs and symptoms of bleeding, and transfuse platelets as ordered |
| IV. *Potential for altered tissue perfusion related to anemia* | IV. A. Pt will be without signs and symptoms of severe anemia | IV. A. Assess signs and symptoms of anemia<br>  1. Hematocrit: mild (31–37%), moderate (25–30%), or severe (<25%)<br>  2. Presence of symptoms of mild anemia (paleness, fatigue, slight dyspnea, palpitation, sweating on exertion); moderate anemia (increased severity of symptoms of mild anemia); and severe anemia (headache, dizziness, irritability, angina, dyspnea at rest, compensatory tachycardia, and tachypnea)<br>B. Encourage pt to change positions gradually, slowly moving from lying to sitting position and sitting to standing position. Encourage slow, deep breathing during position changes<br>C. Reassure pt that fatigue is related to anemia and hopefully will improve with transfusion<br>D. Replace red blood cells as ordered, expecting that the 1 unit of RBCs will increase the hematocrit; washed or leukocyte-poor red blood cells are used to prevent antibody formation if the pt is planning to go for a bone marrow transplant<br>E. Assess activity tolerance and need for oxygen for activity or at rest<br>F. Review foods that are high in iron and folic acid and encourage pt to include these in the diet |
| V. *Potential for constipation* | V. A. Pt will move bowels at least once every day | V. A. Provide pt education about the goal and means of preventing constipation, such as stool softeners, oral fluids to 3 quarts per day, high-fiber diet, adequate exercise<br>B. Discuss a bowel regime with physician to promote soft, regular bowel movements, especially if the pt is receiving narcotic analgesia |

*(continued)*

**Table 4.6** Standardized Nursing Care Plan for the Patient Experiencing Bone Marrow Depression *(continued)*

| Nursing Diagnosis | Expected Outcomes | Nursing Interventions |
|---|---|---|
| VI. *Potential for activity intolerance related to fatigue of anemia, malaise* | VI. A. Pt will maintain minimal activity | VI. A. Teach pt to increase rest and sleep periods and to alternate rest and activity periods<br>B. Encourage pt to incorporate foods high in iron in diet, such as liver, eggs, lean meat, green leafy vegetables, carrots, and raisins<br>C. Assess need for homemaker, home health aide, and visiting nurse at home<br>D. Assess for psychological manifestations of fatigue:<br>  1) depression<br>  2) anxiety<br>  3) loss of independence<br>  4) decreased level of concentration<br>  5) difficulty making decisions<br>E. Teach pt to prioritize activities deciding what pt must do and those that can be delegated<br>F. Teach pt to eat several small meals a day, and select high energy foods, such as potatoes, rice, pasta<br>G. If pt able, teach pt to start and maintain an exercise program, starting slowly<br>  1) gradually increase activity<br>  2) low-impact exercises, such as stretching, muscle strengthening<br>  3) cardiovascular exercises |

cells mature in the blood with the help of vitamin $B_{12}$. Erythropoietin, an endogenous hormone produced by the kidneys, stimulates production of red blood cells. Recombinant erythropoietin (epoetin alfa, ProCrit) stimulates the division and differentiation of erythrocyte stem cells in the bone marrow. The drug may be useful in preventing aplasia-induced anemia and is given subcutaneously three times per week. It is contraindicated in patients with uncontrolled hypertension. For this drug therapy to be effective, for example, in the treatment of patients receiving chemotherapy, the patient's endogenous erythropoietin level should be ≤ 200 μ/ml. Recombintant erythropoietin often is used to prevent the development of anemia or to prevent the need for red blood cell transfusion in patients receiving cisplatin chemotherapy. Recently, studies have indicated that a weekly dose of 40,000 μ SQ is equally effective (Cheung et al. 1998).

Classifications of anemia are shown in Table 4.7.

Physical assessment of the patient with anemia may show compensatory changes in vital signs, with increased heart rate and depth of respiration in an effort to try to increase the oxygenation of the tissues. Skin may be blanched, nail beds pallid, and mucous membranes pale, especially the conjunctiva. Nursing interventions are directed at replacing red blood cells through transfusions when the hematocrit is 25 or less and patient teaching to minimize fatigue and facilitate early identification of symptoms.

## II. MUCOSITIS

Mucositis refers to an inflammation of the mucous membranes and occurs as a sequela of chemotherapy administration because of damage to the frequently dividing cells in the mucosal epithelium that lines the GI tract. Mucositis is further specified as to its anatomic location: when it occurs in the oral cavity, it is called *stomatitis*; in the esophagus, *esophagitis*; in the intestines, *mucositis* usually is manifested by diarrhea; and in the rectum, *proctitis*.

The epithelial cells lining the GI mucosa are subjected to "wear and tear" by chemical, mechanical, and thermal factors as the ingested food is chewed, swallowed, digested, and expelled. Thus, there is demand for frequent replacement of the mucosal epithelium cells so that the millions of epithelial cells normally shed during digestion are replaced (cell birth = cell death).

**Table 4.7** Degrees of Anemia

|  | Hemoglobin (G/100 ml) | Hematocrit (%) | Symptoms |
|---|---|---|---|
| Normal male | 14–18 | 42–52 |  |
| Normal female | 12–16 | 37–47 |  |
| Mild anemia |  | 31–37 | Pale, fatigue, slight dyspnea on exertion; palpitation and sweating with exertion |
| Moderate anemia |  | 25–30 | Increased severity of symptoms of mild anemia |
| Severe anemia |  | < 25 | Headache, dizziness, irritability; dyspnea on exertion and at rest; angina, compensatory tachycardia, tachypnea |

*Source:* Modified from Brager, B.L., and Yasko, Y.M. (1984). *Care of the Client Receiving Chemotherapy*. Reston, Vir.: Reston Publishing Co., 96, 106, 178, 180.

## Stomatitis

The stem cells of the oral mucous membranes are found in the deep squamous epithelium, which lies above the basement membrane. These cells have a life span of 3–5 days, with the outer epithelial layer being replaced entirely every 7–14 days (Beck and Yasko 1984). Stem cell replication is rapid, taking about 32 hours, with estimated phases of the cell cycle as follows: mitosis (8 hours), $G_1$ (14 hours), S (10–11 hours), $G_2$ (10–19 minutes) (Lavalle and Proctor 1978). Unfortunately, chemotherapy agents cannot distinguish between malignant and normal frequently dividing cells, so the mucosal stem cells are injured directly. No longer can these stem cells replace oral mucosal cells lost through normal sloughing, and the decreased renewal of epithelial cells results in thinning of the mucosa (Frattore, Larson, and Mostofi 1986). There is evidence of beginning tissue damage in 5–7 days after chemotherapy administration: pale, dry mucous membranes, burning sensation, dry tongue with raised papillae, and ridging of buccal mucosa. This damage may progress to severe inflammation and ulceration with pain, as shown in Figure 4.9, and then recovery occurs within 2–3 weeks without scarring (Engelking 1988).

Figure 4.9 illustrates the development of stomatitis utilizing a stress response model. The phases of Alarm, Resistance, Exhaustion, and Recovery are represented over a span of 21 days.

An objective evaluation of the degrees of stomatitis was developed by Capizzi et al. (1970) and used in the Oncology Nursing Society's *Guidelines for Cancer Nursing Practice* (Goodman and Stoner 1991). This assessment includes the physical assessment of the mucous membranes for color, intactness, evidence of ulceration, bleeding, or infection, as well as the functional assessment of the patient's ability to eat and drink. The degrees of stomatitis were labeled Grades I–IV:

Grade I    Erythema of oral mucosa

Grade II   Isolated small ulcerations or white patches. Patient able to eat and drink.

Grade III  Confluent ulceration or white patches covering > 25% of oral mucosa. Patient able to drink only fluids.

Grade IV   Hemorrhagic ulceration, ulceration covering > 50% of oral mucosa. Patient unable to drink fluids or to eat.

According to Frattore et al. (1986), the nonkeratinized surfaces of the buccal and labial mucosa, ventral and lateral tongue surfaces, soft palate, and floor of the mouth are the areas most commonly affected.

Factors that aggravate the degree of stomatitis are drug dose, nutritional deficits, poor oral hygiene, and concurrent radiotherapy to the head and neck (Yasko 1983). The incidence of stomatitis is approximately 40% and is associated with the antimetabolites (especially methotrexate and 5-fluorouracil), antibiotics (especially bleomycin and doxorubicin), and plant alkaloids (Dreizen, Boday, and Rodriguez 1975). More recent estimates on the incidence of oral complications in adult patients are 23%–80% with leukemia, 12% with sarcoma or carcinoma, and 33% with lymphoma (Nieweg, Van Tinteren, Poelhuis, and Abraham-Inpijn 1992).

Taste alterations are another effect of direct cell injury. There are about 10,000 taste buds located on the papillae that cover the tongue. The taste cells that comprise each taste bud are renewed every 5–7 days and often are damaged by chemotherapy. Thus, mild or more severe stomatitis may be accompanied by taste alterations, and this can be a very distressing

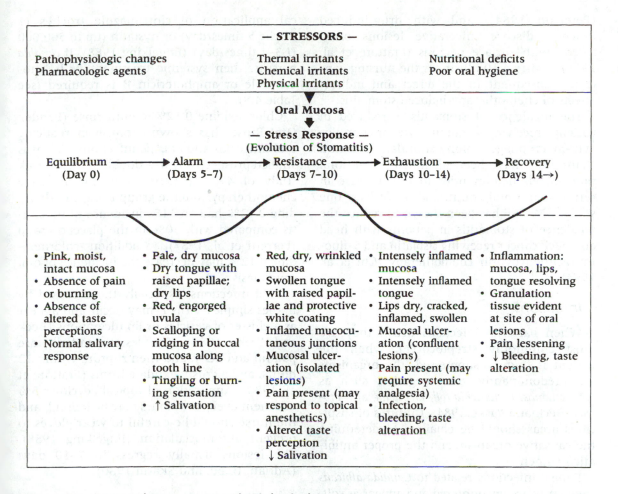

**Figure 4.9** Mucosal Response to Physiological Stressors

*Source:* Adapted from Engelking, C. (1988). Managing stomatitis: A nursing process approach. In *Supportive Care for the Patient with Cancer.* Richmond, Vir.: A.H. Robins, 20–28.

side effect. Pain resulting from erythema and ulceration often lead to dysphagia and difficulty speaking. Nutritional deficits are intensified and further aggravate the damaged mucosa and delay healing.

Indirect injury to the oral mucosa is related to bone marrow suppression, as there is increased risk of infection and bleeding. Severe stomatitis usually precedes the drug-induced

nadir by 2–3 days. As the nadir occurs, neutropenia increases the risk of superinfection by normal oral flora. After injury to the mucosa has occurred, infection by bacterial, fungal, or viral organisms can occur. Also, the mucosal barrier is no longer intact, so a portal of entry for microorganisms into the systemic circulation now exists. Adult patients often have periodontal disease with chronic oral infection

(Peterson 1984), and with drug-induced mucosal disease, ulcerative lesions often spread with surface necrosis (Frattore et al. 1986). Figure 4.10 illustrates the nursing concerns subsequent to the direct and indirect effects of chemotherapy-induced stomatitis.

The incidence of stomatitis is reduced in patients receiving a granulocyte or granulocyte-macrophage colony-stimulating factor. Neutrophils have been identified on the oral mucosal epithelium prior to the increase in serum neutrophil count, and, in at least one study, GM-CSF has been shown to reduce the incidence of stomatitis in patients with head and neck cancer receiving cisplatin and 5-fluorouracil/leucovorin chemotherapy (Chi et al. 1994).

### Infections

When bacterial infections occur, they are most commonly streptococcal; when the patient is immunosuppressed, the organisms are predominantly gram negative, such as *pseudomonas*, *Escherichia coli*, *klebsiella*, and *proteus* (Beck and Yasko 1984). Cultures of suspicious areas should be obtained to determine the causative organism and the proper antibiotic regimen.

Fungal infections related to *Candida albicans* frequently are encountered and appear as soft, white, cottage cheese-like patches containing candida and epithelial cells, often overlying red, raw, or bleeding mucosa (Beck and Yasko 1984). This fungus is responsible for one-half of all oral infections during antileukemic therapy and for almost two-thirds of oral infections in patients receiving chemotherapy for solid tumors (Frattore, et al. 1986). Risk for fungal infection increases for patients on corticosteroid therapy or prolonged antibiotic therapy with broad-spectrum agents (Frattore et al. 1986). Antifungal treatment begins with topical application of clotrimazole troches (1 troche 5 times/day) or nystatin (up to 500,000 U 3–4 times/day) (Engelking 1988). If *candida* persists, then systemic treatment with ketoconazole or amphotericin B is required (see Table 4.8).

Chlorhexidine 0.12% mouth rinse (Peridex Oral Rinse) has shown promise in reducing oral mucositis and *candida* infections. This was studied prospectively in a double-blind 5-week study of 49 in-patients receiving intensive chemotherapy, and the group using chlorhexidine 0.12% had an 11% incidence of mucositis compared with 50% in the placebo group (Ferretti et al. 1987). In addition, chlorhexidine 0.12% may decrease the incidence of oral candidiasis.

Viral infections, especially those caused by herpes simplex virus I, may occur and appear as a cluster of vesicles or lip ulcerations (Beck and Yasko 1984). The lesions initially are painful and itchy, and then rupture within 12 hours, and a crusty exudate forms (Frattore et al. 1986). Application of topical acyclovir 5% ointment every 3–6 hours may be helpful, and the nurse should be careful to wear gloves to prevent autoinocculation (Engelking 1988). The lesions usually regress in 7–10 days (Adrian, Hood, and Skarin 1980).

### Nursing Interventions

Nursing interventions begin prior to chemotherapy administration with a thorough patient assessment of the oral cavity and risk factors, such as cigarette smoking, alcohol use, periodontal disease, poor oral hygiene, poor nutritional status, and concurrent radiotherapy to head or neck. Dental work may need to be performed prior to chemotherapy. In order to effectively examine the oral cavity, a flashlight, a tongue blade, a gauze pad, and gloves are needed. Inspect the upper inner lip

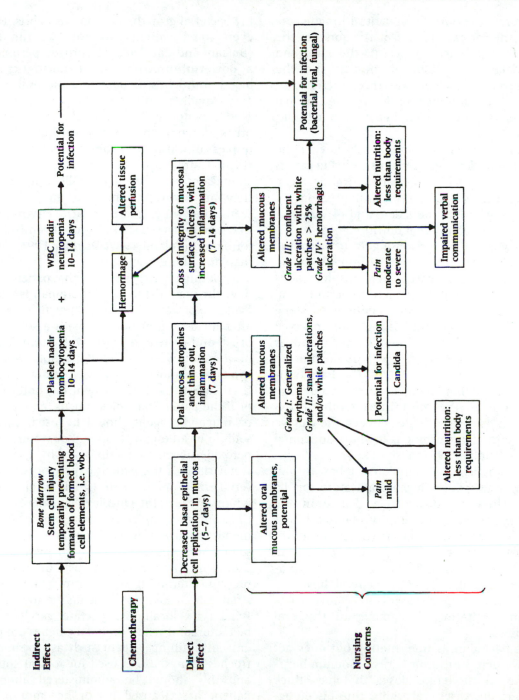

**Figure 4.10** Sequelae of Mucositis

and gums; the dorsal and ventral tongue surfaces; the lateral borders of the tongue; the inner cheek (buccal mucosa); the hard and soft palate; the floor of mouth; and the oropharynx for color, moisture, presence of debris, and presence of lesions. A normal mucosa is pink, moist, intact, and without debris.

After a patient is identified as having the potential to develop stomatitis, nursing care is aimed at (1) teaching the patient oral cleansing and self-care, (2) preventing oral infection, (3) identifying early dysfunction, and (4) promoting comfort and optimal nutrition.

The goal of oral cleansing is to keep the mucosa moist, clean, and without debris so that the mucosal barrier remains infection-free. Patients should be taught to perform oral cleansing after meals and at bedtime, brushing with a soft toothbrush, flossing with unwaxed dental floss, and using a mouthwash that does not contain alcohol, as this will dry the mucosa (Goodman and Stoner 1985). The Bass technique of toothbrushing is recommended by many nurses: the soft-bristled toothbrush is held at a 45-degree angle between the gingiva and teeth, and brushing is in short horizontal strokes (Dudjak 1987; Yasko 1983).

If the patient is edentulous or has an oral lesion, soft sponge-tipped applicators can be used. There is considerable debate in the oncology nursing community about the best oral cleanser, and it appears that it is the frequency and the consistent practice of oral care rather than the agent that minimizes oral complications (Dudjak 1987). In general, however, the purpose of the cleanser is to remove debris without irritation or damage to the oral mucosa.

Normal saline is nonirritating but does not remove debris or formed crusts. Sodium bicarbonate in moderate doses dissolves thick mucous; decreases oral acidity, thus discouraging bacterial growth; and loosens debris. However, some patients do not like the taste (Bersani and Carl 1983). Hydrogen peroxide is a powerful mucosolvent, oxidizing crusted blood and debris, deodorizing the oral cavity, and providing antimicrobial action (Engelking 1988). Unfortunately, though, peroxide can break down granulation tissue, and has an unpleasant taste for some patients, despite rinsing after use. Lemon glycerine swabs should not be used for the following reasons: they are drying to mucosa, may decalcify teeth, and they create an acid environment that encourages bacterial growth and plaque formation (Poland 1987; Daeffler 1994; Goodman and Stoner 1991).

Most nursing experts agree that patients who have the potential to develop stomatitis, but no evidence of stomatitis, should practice oral care after meals and at bedtime with a soft toothbrush and paste and gargle with normal saline or a mouthwash without alcohol. Dentures should be removed to cleanse the oral mucosa. If saliva is thick, if the patient has oral cancer, or if the patient has thick mucus, an oxidizing or mucolytic agent should be used, such as sodium bicarbonate (1 tsp in 8 oz water) or 1:4 peroxide/normal saline followed by a saline or water rinse. If the patient experiences Grade I (erythema) or Grade II (small ulceration or white patches), the Oncology Nursing Society's *Guidelines for Cancer Nursing Practice* recommends cleansing every 2 hours with normal saline, or cleansing every 4 hours with an oxidizing/mucolytic agent if crusts or debris are present, alternating with warm saline gargles. Analgesics, such as viscous xylocaine or Benadryl/xylocaine/Kaopectate gargles, may be required. If white candidal patches are present, an antifungal agent such as clotrimazole troches or nystatin is used for topical control, and this should be administered after the patient has cleansed his or her mouth. For

**Table 4.8** Potential Oral Infections Seen in Patients with Stomatitis

| Infectious Organism | Appearance | Management | | |
| --- | --- | --- | --- | --- |
| | | Drug | Dose | Comments |
| *Fungi* *Candida albicans* (moniliasis; thrush) | Soft, whitish, or cream-colored strands or patches covering all or part of tongue, lips, or buccal mucosa; patches adhere to underlying mucosa; when removed, mucosa is bright red and moist underneath (Daeffler 1994) | clotrimazole 10 mg (Mycelex) troche | Dissolve slowly in mouth 5 troches/day for 2 weeks | All topical drugs are applied to clean mucosa, and then NPO for 15–30 mins; do not use if xerostomia is present |
| Aspergillosis | Lesions often on palate: painful, yellowish ulcers surrounded by black border (Frattore et al. 1986) | nystatin (Mycostatin) suspension | Swish 500,000 U q 4–6 hrs, keep in mouth for 2 min, and then discard/ swallow | Topical drug |
| | | ketoconazole 200 mg/day (Nizoral) | 1 tablet daily for 1–2 weeks | Systemic therapy if topical treatment ineffective |
| *Bacteria* *Staphylococcus aureus* | Exudative, purulent, and encrusted erosions; less commonly encountered; in the neutropenic patient, lesion is smaller with less pus and appears as dry, raised, yellow-brown plaque (Frattore et al. 1986) | Antibiotic therapy/ chlorhexidine digliconate 0.12% (Peridex Oral Rinse) | Swish and spit 15 cc for 30 seconds BID | Antibiotics based on organism sensitivity Prophylaxis in patients receiving intensive chemotherapy, radiation therapy, or BMT |
| Gram negative bacteria | Raised, creamy, moist, glistening site of infection; nonpurulent; smooth edges; seated on painful, red, superficial ulcers | | | |
| *Pseudomonas aeruginosa* | Raised lesions enclosed by a red halo; initially dry, yellowish center turning purple-to-black with necrosis; necrotic core sloughs off, disclosing bright red granulation tissue (Frattore et al. 1986) | | | |

*(continued)*

**Table 4.8**   Potential Oral Infections Seen in Patients with Stomatitis (*continued*)

| Infectious Organism | Appearance | Management | | Comments |
|---|---|---|---|---|
| | | **Drug** | **Dose** | |
| *Virus*<br>*Herpes simplex* | Activated by stress of disease and treatment; vesicle is painful and itchy; ruptures within 12 hrs and becomes encrusted with dry exudate; yellow-brown membrane easily dislodges, causing severe pain; regresses in 7–10 days | acyclovir 5% ointment | q 3–6 hrs while awake | Apply with gloves (topical application) |
| | | acyclovir 200 mg capsules | 1 capsule 5 times/day | Systemic therapy for diffuse herpes until shedding completed; can require 1–2 gm/day |
| | | acyclovir 5 mg/kg IV | Administer over 1 hour, q 8 hrs, for 7 days (Zinner, Belcher, and Murphy 1988) | |

*Source:* Modified from Daeffler, R.J. (1994). Protective mechanisms: Mucous membranes. In B.L. Johnson and J. Gross (eds.): *Handbook of Oncology Nursing.* Boston: Jones & Bartlett, 416–419.

Grade III stomatitis (confluent ulcerations with white patches covering > 25%) or Grade IV (hemorrhagic ulcerations), cleansing should be practiced every 2 hours: warm saline gargles alternated every 2 hours with an antifungal or antibacterial suspension, unless the patient has thick mucus or saliva. In that case, an oxidizing/mucolytic agent, such as sodium bicarbonate or hydrogen peroxide, followed by a saline rinse, is used every 4 hours. Soft sponge-tipped applicators instead of a soft toothbrush prevent pain or trauma to the fragile mucous membranes. If *Candida* persists after topical treatment, then systemic therapy with ketoconazole or amphotericin B is used.

Flossing should be discontinued if bleeding occurs or if the platelet count is less than 40,000/mm$^3$ or the white blood count is less than 1500/mm$^3$. Also at this time, soft sponge-tipped applicators should be used instead of a toothbrush.

Comfort is promoted by the use of topical anesthetics, such as viscous xylocaine, or "cocktails," such as diphenhydramine/xylocaine/ Kaopectate gargles, but systemic analgesics might be required, including morphine infusions for severe mucositis pain. Sucralfate suspension as described by Ferraro and Mattern (1984) (Table 4.7) theoretically promotes healing of oral ulcers, much as it does with duodenal and gastric ulcers, by binding to the proteinaceous exudate of the ulcer and providing protection for healing. Although the use of sucralfate suspension has not been studied prospectively to evaluate oral ulcer healing, when applied 4 times a day after meals and cleansing of the oral cavity, patients have reported decreased pain and discomfort (Wilkes 1986). Patients receiving cisplatin and 5-day 5-FU continuous infusion were studied. Patients receiving sucralfate had significantly less mucositis, and patients tended to prefer the sucralfate (Pfeiffer et al. 1990). Table 4.10 shows

**Table 4.9** Sucralfate Suspension

To prepare a concentration of 1 gm/15 ml, 120 ml bottle:

Place 8 sucralfate tablets in a clean 120 ml glass bottle.

Add 40 ml sterile water for irrigation; allow tablets to dissolve, and then shake well.

Add 40 ml of Sorbitol 70% and shake well.

Separately, mix 1–3 Ensure Vari Flavor Pacs with 10 ml sterile water for irrigation and add to the drug mixture. Add sufficient sterile water for irrigation to complete 120 ml.

Label: refrigerate, expires in 14 days.

Instructions for use: 3 tsp, swish for 2 mins, and then swallow; after post-eating mouth cleansing and at bedtime.

*Source:* Ferraro, J.M., and Mattern, J.Q.A. (1984). Sucralfate suspension for stomatitis. *Drug Intelligence and Clinical Pharmacology* 18: 153.

oral agents used to treat mucositis (Fishman and Mrozek-Orlowski 1999).

Ice has been shown to be effective in the prevention of 5-fluorouracil/leucovorin-induced oral stomatitis. Ice is applied (sucked) 20 minutes prior to chemotherapy (Mahood 1991). Table 4.11 is an example of a standardized care plan for stomatitis.

## Esophagitis

Esophagitis is inflammation of the esophageal mucosa caused by injury to basal epithelial cells of the mucosa. These cells are similar to those of the oral cavity and are histologically the same, with similar growth rates. Esophagitis occurs in about the same time frame as oral stomatitis. Cell replacement is interrupted as the basal stem cells are damaged, and the mucosa lining the esophagus becomes thin and atrophied. Painful ulceration, secondary infection, and hemorrhage may occur. Oral candidiasis can spread to the esophagus by swallowing fungal organisms and can progress to septicemia by penetration

**Table 4.10** Oral Agents Used to Treat Mucositis

| Indication | Agent | Dosage | Action |
|---|---|---|---|
| To promote cleanliness (Beck 1992) | Baking soda and H$_2$O | 1/2 tsp baking soda with 4 oz water | Debride oral mucosa |
| | Soft toothbrush and dental floss | After each meal and before bed | Debride oral mucosa and remove plaque |
| | Saline solution | 1/2 tsp salt with 8 oz water | Debride oral mucosa |
| | Fluoride | 1% sodium fluoride daily | Prevent dental caries related to radiation therapy to the head and neck |
| | Chlorhexidine | 15 cc swish and spit twice a day | May decrease risk of oral infection |
| To promote moisturizing | Saline solution | 1/2 tsp salt with 8 oz water | Moisturize oral mucosa |
| | Sugar-free candy | As needed | Stimulate production of saliva |
| | MoiStir™ | Administer topically | Salivary supplement |
| | Pilocarpine (Salagen) | 5 mg orally 3 times a day | Stimulate production of saliva 5 mg orally 3 times a day in xerostomia related to radiation therapy to head and neck. Note: contraindicated in uncontrolled asthma, narrow angle glaucoma Treat overdose with atropine 0.5–1.0 mg subcutaneous or IV |
| To maintain integrity of oral mucosa | Allopurinol (Savaris, Caragiauris, and Kosmidis 1988) | Administer topically | Unknown, but may decrease intensity of mucositis and provide comfort |
| | Sucralfate (Solomon 1986) | 1 tablet in 15 cc water to make slurry. Swish and swallow 3 times a day. | Unknown, but may involve the binding of sucralfate to damaged mucosal surface proteins, thus forming a protective coating |
| | Vitamin E and beta-carotene (Hogan 1984) | Puncture capsule and apply directly on lesions | Exert natural protective action on mucosal membranes in radiation mucositis |
| To promote comfort | | | |
| Topical anesthetics | Diclonine hydrochloride | 5–10 ml swish and spit every 3–4 hrs (Fischer et al. 1993) | Local anesthetic |
| | Viscous lidocaine (Katon 1981) | 5 cc swish and spit prior to meals or 4 times daily | Local anesthetic; may cause numbing |
| | Zilactin (Rodu, Russell, and Ray 1988) | Topical application to lesion(s) prn | Burns upon administration |
| Topical anti-inflammatory agents | Antacids | 15 cc every 2 hrs | Coat oral tissues |
| | Combinations of diphenhydramine hydrochloride elixir, viscous lidocaine, nystatin | 15 cc 4 times a day, swish and swallow | Soothing, antifungal |
| Systemic analgesics | Aspirin | 650 mg every 4 hrs | Reduce inflammation |
| | Acetaminophen | 650–1,000 mg every 4 hrs | Provide systemic pain relief |
| | Opioids (e.g., MSO4) | Varies according to drug used | Provide systemic pain relief for severe oral discomfort |

*Source:* Fishman, M., and Mrozek-Orowski, M. (1999). *Cancer Chemotherapy Guidelines and Recommendations for Practice.* 2nd ed. Pittsburgh: Oncology Nursing Press.

**Table 4.11** Standardized Nursing Care Plan for Patient Experiencing Stomatitis

| Nursing Diagnosis | Expected Outcomes | Nursing Interventions |
|---|---|---|
| I. *Potential for altered oral mucous membranes* | I. A. Oral mucosa will remain pink, moist, intact, without debris | I. A. Assess oral mucosa (baseline)<br>1. Assess history of alcohol use, smoking<br>2. Assess history of dental problems, oral hygiene practices, and prior or concurrent radiation to head or neck<br>3. Perform oral exam<br>  a. Lips<br>  b. Upper inner lip and gums<br>  c. Tongue (dorsum, lateral borders, ventral surface)<br>  d. Inner cheeks (buccal mucosa)<br>  e. Hard and soft palate<br>  f. Floor of mouth<br>  g. Oral pharynx<br>4. Assess amount, consistency of saliva<br>5. Assess condition of teeth<br>B. Assess nutritional status<br>C. Initiate and discuss dental referral as needed prior to therapy<br>D. Instruct in oral hygiene self-care measures (see IV. Potential for knowledge deficit) |
| II. *Altered oral mucous membranes,*<br>*Grade I* (generalized erythema)<br>*Grade II* (small ulceration or white patches) | II. A. Oral mucosa will be pink, moist, intact, and painless within 5–7 days | II. A. Assess oral mucosa q shift or at each clinic visit; document size and location of abnormality and intervention<br>B. Assess comfort and ability to eat, drink<br>C. Institute oral hygiene q 2 hrs during day and q 6 hrs during night<br>1. Warm normal saline rinses *unless* crusts, debris, thick mucus or saliva; then use sodium bicarbonate (1 tsp in 8 oz water) q 4 hrs alternating with warm saline rinses q 4 hrs<br>2. (Warm) sterile normal saline rinses if WBC < 1000/mm$^3$ (Daeffler 1985, 268)<br>3. Reserve hydrogen peroxide (1:4 strength) for *resistant*, thick secretions or white patches (*candida*) and resistant debris, and rinse afterward with water<br>D. Encourage flossing qd and brushing with soft-bristled brush pc and hs unless plt < 40,000/mm$^3$ or WBC < 1500/mm$^3$ (Beck 1979, 44)<br>E. Encourage pt to remove dentures during oral hygiene rinsing and if irritating mucosa<br>F. Encourage pt to moisten lips with medicated lip ointment, water-soluble lubricating jelly, or lanolin<br>G. Encourage pt to avoid citrus fruits and juices, spicy foods, hot foods, and to eat bland, cool foods<br>H. Discuss use of antifungal therapy if candidiasis present |

*(continued)*

**Table 4.11** Standardized Nursing Care Plan for Patient Experiencing Stomatitis *(continued)*

| Nursing Diagnosis | Expected Outcomes | Nursing Interventions |
|---|---|---|
| III. *Altered oral mucous membranes,* Grade III (confluent ulcerations with white patches > 25% or unable to drink liquids) Grade IV (hemorrhagic ulcerations and/or unable to drink liquids and eat solid food) | III. A. Oral mucosa will heal within 10–14 days, and white patches (*candida*) are absent | III. A. Assess oral mucosa q 4 hrs for evidence of infection, response to therapy<br>B. Assess ability to eat, drink, communicate<br>C. Assess level of comfort, discomfort<br>D. Culture ulcerated areas that appear infected<br>E. Cleanse mouth q 2 hrs while awake, q 4 hrs during night<br>  1. Alternate warm saline mouth rinse with antifungal or antibacterial oral suspension q 2 hrs<br>  2. Use sodium bicarbonate solution for thick secretions, debris; if ineffective in removing debris, use 1:4 hydrogen peroxide followed by water or saline rinse<br>F. Suggest soft sponge-tipped applicator to cleanse teeth, mouth pc and hs<br>G. Apply lip lubricant q 2 hrs |
| IV. *Potential for knowledge deficit, re risk for stomatitis and self-care management* | IV. A. Pt verbally repeats steps of self-assessment<br>B. Pt demonstrates self-care techniques (mouth rinse, brushing, flossing) | IV. A. Instruct pt in stomatitis as potential side effect of chemotherapy as appropriate<br>B. Instruct pt in daily oral exam<br>  1. Use of mirror and self-exam<br>  2. Signs and symptoms to report (burning, redness, blisters, ulcers; difficulty swallowing; swelling of lips, tongue; pain)<br>C. Instruct pt in oral care<br>  1. Remove dentures; wash and rinse mouth; and then replace<br>  2. Floss daily with unwaxed dental floss<br>  3. Brush with soft toothbrush and nonabrasive toothpaste pc and hs<br>  4. Rinse with water, saline, dilute sodium bicarbonate solution, or mouthwash without alcohol<br>  5. Avoid oral irritants (tobacco, alcohol, poorly fitting dentures, mouthwashes containing alcohol)<br>D. Instruct pt in self-care q 2 hrs if actual stomatitis occurs<br>  1. Cleansing solution of warm normal saline or sodium bicarbonate solution unless resistant thick secretions, debris; then can use 1:4 hydrogen peroxide with water rinse following<br>  2. Medication application as indicated<br>  3. High-calorie, high-protein, cool, bland foods<br>  4. Small, frequent feedings; fluids to 3 L/day |

| Nursing Diagnosis | Goals | Interventions |
|---|---|---|
| V. *Pain related to stomatitis* | V. A. Pt states relief from oral pain | V. A. Use mild analgesic q 2 hrs, timing 15 mins ac; gargles must be swished 2 min<br>1. Viscous zylocaine 2% gargles, 10–15 cc swish/spit q 3 hrs, duration 20 mins (max 120 mg/24 hrs; Brager and Yasko 1984)<br>2. Orabase emollient for local relief<br>3. 1:1:1 viscous zylocaine:diphenhydramine HCl (12.5 mg/ml): Kaopectate swish and swallow q 2–4 hrs<br>4. Benzocaine 20%—apply directly or swish and spit (duration 20 mins)<br>5. Dyclonine HCl (Dyclone) 0.5% 15 mins ac: 5–10 cc swish for 2 mins, gargle and spit, onset 10 mins, duration 1 hr<br>B. Parenteral analgesics may be necessary, including morphine infusion |
| VI. *Impaired verbal communication related to pain, increased or thickened saliva* | VI. A. Pt will communicate needs effectively | VI. A. Assess pt's ability to communicate<br>B. If secretion is thick, copious, instruct pt in tonsil-tip suctioning technique<br>C. Develop satisfactory communication tool if pt unable to talk (i.e., magic slate, writing message)<br>D. Respond promptly to pt call light |
| VII. *Potential for altered nutrition: less than body requirements related to pain of mucositis* | VII. A. Pt will regain baseline weight within 5% | VII. A. Premedicate with analgesics 15 mins ac<br>B. Encourage high-calorie, high-protein, small, frequent feedings with cool, bland liquid or pureed foods; also, creative popsicles, custards<br>C. If inability to eat persists, discuss with MD need for enteral, parenteral nutrition<br>D. Encourage popsicles, ice creams as desired<br>E. Discourage citrus juices, fruits, hot and spicy foods, rough or hard foods |
| VIII. *Potential for infection* | VIII. A. Pt will be free of infection<br>B. Infection will be detected early and treated | VIII. A. Assess oral mucosa q 4–8 hrs for s/s infection—culture any suspicious sites<br>B. Monitor vs, T q 4 hrs; if outpatient, teach pt to monitor temperature at least BID<br>C. Encourage pt to cleanse oral mucosa prior to administration of antibiotic or antifungal medication—keep NPO for 15–30 mins p medication administration<br>D. Consider administration of antifungal or antibiotic as frozen popsicle if extreme pain, as this can decrease discomfort<br>E. Administer systemic antibiotics if ordered |

*(continued)*

**Table 4.11** Standardized Nursing Care Plan for Patient Experiencing Stomatitis *(continued)*

| Nursing Diagnosis | Expected Outcomes | Nursing Interventions |
|---|---|---|
| IX. *Potential for altered tissue perfusion related to hemorrhage* | IX. A. Pt will be without oral bleeding<br>B. Bleeding will be detected early and terminated | IX. A. Assess for s/s bleeding in gingiva, mucosa<br>B. Remove dentures, partial plates<br>C. If *bleeding*, monitor platelet count, hematocrit<br>  1. Transfuse platelets as ordered<br>  2. Topical thrombin, aminocaproic acid, or microfibrillar collagen may be ordered (Peterson 1984)<br>  3. Leave clots undisturbed—discontinue mechanical oral care<br>D. Use sponge-tipped applicator rather than toothbrush if platelets < 50,000/mm³ to minimize trauma to gingiva, mucosa<br>E. Encourage liquid, cool or cold, high-calorie, high-protein supplements as tolerated; pt should be NPO if bleeding |
| X. *Xerostomia* (uncommon) | X. A. Pt will have moist mucosa with thin secretions | X. A. Encourage frequent mouth moisturizing with ice chips, artificial saliva (containing carboxymethyl cellulose)<br>B. Oral hygiene pc and hs<br>C. Encourage fluids as tolerated, offering fluids every 1–2 hrs<br>D. Discourage mucosal irritants (smoking, alcohol)<br>E. Encourage soft, moist foods with sauces<br>F. Encourage use of sugarless candy or gum to stimulate saliva production<br>G. Increase air moisture as needed by humidifier or vaporizer<br>H. Oral assessment q day, as xerostomia may precede stomatitis (erythema) |

of the esophageal mucosa (Frattore et al. 1986). Mucosal healing occurs as the bone marrow recovers and the white blood count rises (Nunnally and Donoghue 1986).

Risk factors include chemotherapy with antimetabolite drugs, and others that cause stomatitis, and concurrent or subsequent radiation therapy of the neck, chest, or upper back. Esophagitis is usually dose-limiting, and therapy is interrupted until esophagitis resolves.

Early signs and symptoms of esophagitis include discomfort or pain on swallowing (odynophagia), dysphagia of solid foods, and a sensation of having a "lump" in the throat when swallowing (Nunnally, Donoghue, and Yasko 1983). Patient problems are similar to those encountered in patients with stomatitis, and nursing care is directed toward maintaining optimal nutrition for healing, minimizing patient discomfort, and preventing secondary infection.

## Diarrhea

Diarrhea is defined by Brager and Yasko (1984) as the passage of three or more soft or liquid stools in a 24-hour period, which may occur during or after therapy. The mucosal epithelial cells lining the intestines (villi and microvilli) are characterized by rapid cell division (high mitotic rate) and a cell generation time of 24 hours, so they may replace the cells damaged by the trauma of digestion (Brager and Yasko 1984). It is estimated that 20–50 million epithelial cells are normally shed *every hour* (Culhane 1983). If these cells are not replaced, the mucosal cells atrophy and become inflamed; the villi and microvilli shorten and become denuded; and the inflamed mucosa produces large amounts of mucus, which stimulates accelerated peristalsis. The damaged villi and microvilli, together with the rapid transit time of intestinal contents, prevents absorption of nutrients, water, and electrolytes (Brager and Yasko 1984).

Diarrhea is a common and potentially severe side effect of 5-fluorouracil (5-FU). It may precede severe bone marrow depression and usually *requires* interruption of therapy. Diarrhea occurring during methotrexate therapy is not as common but requires interruption of therapy to prevent hemorrhagic enteritis or perforation (Dorr and Von Hoff 1994). Besides the previously mentioned antimetabolites, other drugs that can cause diarrhea are actinomycin-D, doxorubicin, daunomycin, cisplatin, hydroxyurea, irinotecan, and the nitrosoureas. Irinotecan (Camptosar®) has both acute (cholinergic) and delayed diarrhea. Acute diarrhea and/or diaphoresis (abdominal cramping) occurs during or immediately after drug infusion, and is treated with IV atropine 0.25 mg. Delayed diarrhea occurs on day 8–12 and can be very severe. Patients should be instructed in use of loperamide to halt diarrhea. (Wilkes et al. 1999).

Potential sequelae of diarrhea include malnutrition, fluid and electrolyte imbalance, abdominal discomfort (pain), irritated perianal mucosa or skin activity intolerance, and fatigue (see Figure 4.11). Nursing interventions are directed toward (1) patient teaching regarding high-calorie, high-protein, low-residue diet, elimination of irritating foods, and high fluid intake; (2) monitoring of fluid and electrolyte values and replacement as needed; (3) providing scrupulous perianal skin care and teaching patient to use sitz baths; and (4) administering medications as ordered to provide relief or cessation of diarrhea. Medications that may provide relief include Pepto-Bismol or Kaopectate every 4–6 hours around the clock or after every loose stool, or diphenoxylate HCl (Lomotil) or loperamide (Imodium) if diarrhea persists

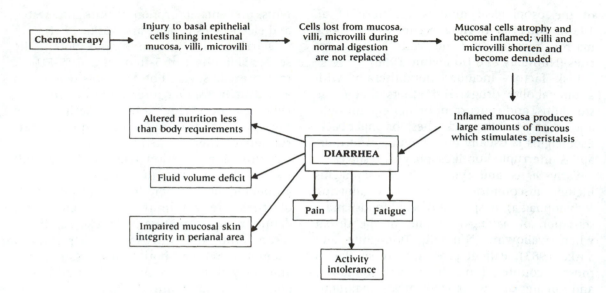

**Figure 4.11**   Potential Sequelae of Diarrhea

(Brager and Yasko 1984). Sometimes bulk-forming agents, such as methylcellulose or psyllium (i.e., Metamucil), are helpful. Table 4.12 is an example of a standardized care plan for diarrhea.

---

## III. ALOPECIA

Another rapidly proliferating normal tissue population is the hair follicles. *Alopecia*, or loss of hair, can range from hair thinning to total loss of scalp hair. The hair follicles have a growth cycle, characterized by a period of active growth (*anagen*, lasting 2–6 years) followed by a resting period (*telogen*, lasting about 3 months), then repeating the cycle (Dunagin 1984). Approximately 90% of hair follicle cells are in active growth at any one time, and exposure to chemotherapy results in destruction of

the rapidly dividing epithelial cells of the hair follicle. The stem cells at the base of the hair shaft are damaged, leading to atrophy of the hair follicle and the subsequent production of a thinner and weaker hair shaft that can break off at the scalp surface (Dunagin 1984) or that is released spontaneously from the hair follicle (Chernecky and Yasko 1986).

Hair loss usually begins 1–2 weeks after a single pulse chemotherapy dose and becomes maximal 1–2 months later (Dorr and Fritz 1980). The loss is temporary, and regrowth may begin during or shortly after therapy ends, when the drug no longer interferes with active growth. Hair regrowth might be softer in texture, curlier, and slightly different in color. The degree and duration of hair loss depends on the drug dose and the length of drug exposure (Chernecky and Yasko 1986). Drugs responsible for alopecia include alkylating agents, antimetabolites, and

**Table 4.12** Standardized Nursing Care Plan for Patient Experiencing Diarrhea

| Nursing Diagnosis | Expected Outcomes | Nursing Interventions |
|---|---|---|
| I. *Potential for altered nutrition: less than body requirements* | I. A. Pt will maintain base-line weight within 5%<br>B. Serum electrolytes will be within normal limits | I. A. Assess pt's usual weight, dietary preferences, and usual pattern of bowel elimination<br>B. Monitor intake/output, daily weight, calorie count as appropriate<br>C. Encourage high-calorie, high-protein, low-residue diet in small, frequent meals (cottage cheese, cream cheese, yogurt, broth, fish, poultry, custard, cooked cereals, peeled apples, macaroni, cooked vegetables)<br>D. If diarrhea is severe, recommend liquid diet<br>E. Discourage foods that stimulate peristalsis (bran, whole-grain bread, fried food, fruit juices, raw vegetables, nuts, rich pastry, caffeine-containing foods and drinks)<br>F. Encourage foods high in potassium as appropriate (bananas, baked potatoes, asparagus tips); monitor serum potassium, other electrolytes |
| II. *Potential for fluid volume deficit* | II. A. Pt's skin will have normal turgor<br>B. Mucous membranes will be moist | II. A. Encourage 3 liters of fluid/day, especially bouillon, Gatorade<br>B. If nutritional supplements are needed, recommend lactose-free or low-osmolality products<br>C. Monitor intake/output |
| III. *Diarrhea*<br>A. Mild/moderate (4–6 stools/day)<br>B. Severe (> 6 stools/day) | III. A. Pt will have < 4 stools/day | III. A. Assess bowel sounds and abdomen for ridigity<br>B. Assess frequency, consistency, and volume of stooling and document. Have pt maintain diary if an outpatient<br>C. Administer antidiarrheal medication as ordered; assess response to therapy; assess need for antispasmodics, antianxiety (anxiolytic) medications<br>D. Instruct pt in self-care measures<br>1. Self-administration of medications<br>2. Low-residue diet, fluids to 3 L/day<br>3. Perianal skin care<br>4. Alternate rest/activity periods<br>E. Discuss interruption of chemotherapy with physician |

*(continued)*

**Table 4.12**  Standardized Nursing Care Plan for Patient Experiencing Diarrhea *(continued)*

| Nursing Diagnosis | Expected Outcomes | Nursing Interventions |
|---|---|---|
| IV. *Potential for impaired mucosal and skin integrity, perianal skin, related to diarrhea* | IV. A. Skin and perianal mucosa will remain intact | IV. A. Assess perineal, perianal skin, and mucous membranes for integrity and for s/s irritation<br>B. Recommend sitz baths p̄ each stool, if diarrhea severe<br>C. Provide skin cleansing with water and mild soap p̄ each stool, and application of skin barrier as needed, if pt unable to perform care; otherwise instruct pt in self-care<br>D. Apply topical anesthetic as needed<br>E. Use absorbent pads under pt to prevent maceration of skin |
| V. *Potential for pain* | V. A. Pt will verbalize decreased pain | V. A. Give symptomatic treatment to minimize or alleviate pain |
| VI. *Potential for fatigue* | VI. A. Pt will verbalize decreased fatigue | VI. A. Assess energy level and help pt to plan activities when energy level is maximal<br>B. Assess for changes in lifestyle necessitated by diarrhea<br>C. Encourage pt to alternate rest and activity periods<br>D. Provide care that pt is unable to perform; encourage pt to involve family if pt is at home; consider/refer community agencies as needed (for homemaker, home health aide) if diarrhea is severe and resistant to treatment<br>E. Assist pt in determining activity priorities and measures to conserve energy |
| VII. *Potential for activity intolerance* | VII. A. Pt will participate in activities important to him or her | VII. A. Activities will be consistent with pt's level of well-being |

antibiotics (Dorr and Fritz 1980). The following drugs are associated with some degree of hair loss:

bleomycin

cisplatin

cyclophosphamide

dactinomycin

daunorubicin

docetaxel

doxorubicin

etoposide

5-fluorouracil

hydroxyurea

ifosfamide

methotrexate

mitomycin-c

mitoxantrone

melphalan

paclitaxel

topotecan

vinblastine

vincristine

vinorelbine

Drugs with long half-lives of active metabolites, such as doxorubicin, the nitrosoureas, and cyclophosphamide, produce severe hair loss (Dorr and Fritz 1980). Other factors influencing the likelihood and severity of alopecia are dose and schedule of administration. Weekly administration of lower-dose doxorubicin causes less alopecia than *pulse* doses every 3 weeks (Brager and Yasko 1984) or prolonged continuous infusion therapy (Keller and Blausey 1988). Hair follicles elsewhere on the body do not provide long hair because of a short growth phase and a long resting phase. Also, at any given time, 90% of these cells are in the resting phase so that chemotherapy does not greatly affect this growth (Dunagin 1984). If the duration of drug exposure is long, cells in the resting phase are lost, and there are no new cells in the growth phase to replace them (Dunagin 1984).

Hair preservation techniques that have been investigated over the years include peripheral scalp hypothermia and constriction. Theoretically, both prevent the chemotherapy drug from reaching the hair follicle by decreasing superficial blood flow to the hair follicle stem cells and should prevent alopecia. A scalp tourniquet decreases blood flow to the hair follicles, thus decreasing the delivery of chemotherapy agent(s). Cold temperatures used in hypothermia cause vasoconstriction and a subsequent decrease in blood flow to the scalp; also, hypothermia decreases the metabolic rate of hair follicles in active growth phase and may inactivate or decrease the uptake of temperature-dependent drugs, such as doxorubicin (Keller and Blausey 1988). Hypothermia, with or without a scalp tourniquet, may decrease hair loss when doxorubicin doses are less than 40–50 mg/m$^2$ (Dean et al. 1983). However, patients may feel chills, headache, and a feeling of pressure and may require premedication with acetaminophen 650 mg po prior to the procedure. Cooling is applied 15–20 minutes before treatment and afterward for at least 30 minutes.

Because both hypothermia and scalp constriction decrease drug concentration in the scalp, a sanctuary for micrometastatic malignant cells occurs. Therefore, patients with primary tumors that may metastasize to the skin are not appropriate candidates. These include patients with leukemia, lymphoma, sarcoma, mycosis fungoids, or cancer of the breast, lung, kidney, or stomach. Scalp constriction or a tourniquet is contraindicated in patients with hypertension or thrombocytopenia

< 50,000/mm$^3$ (Chernecky and Yasko 1986). Studies using minoxidil to accelerate scalp hair regrowth have been disappointing (Denes 1994), as have trials using intradermal (scalp) interleukin-1 (IL-1) (Jimenez et al. 1994).

Body image concerns may result from alopecia. Baxley and colleagues (1984) studied 40 male and female patients receiving chemotherapy and found that patients experiencing alopecia had lower body image scores than those who did not lose their hair. Alopecia may adversely affect perceived sexual attractiveness, self-esteem, and social activities, and for many is a visible reminder of cancer and its treatment.

Initially, prior to beginning chemotherapy, nursing assessment should determine the patient's self-perception and interaction with significant others to determine adaptive abilities (Keller and Blausey 1988). Patient teaching and emotional support help the patient first anticipate hair loss, talk about its potential impact, and learn self-care techniques, such as purchasing a wig prior to beginning therapy. After therapy begins, ongoing support often is necessary to help the patient grieve his or her loss, working through the grief reactions of shock or denial, anger, depression, and finally acceptance. Patients can support each other, with the nurse acting as a facilitator of discussion (Keller and Blausey 1988). It is important to reassure the patient that this is a temporary loss and hair will grow back. Some men prefer to shave their head once the hair has started falling out, and to wear baseball caps. Women may choose scarves or wigs. In cold climates, because up to 25% of body heat is lost through the scalp, patients should be advised to wear caps at night. Other self-care measures to reduce the mechanical damage to the hair shaft are to avoid excessive brushing or shampooing of hair; avoid electric curlers, hot dryers, and hair dyes; and use a mild, protein-based shampoo

every 3–5 days (Chernecky and Yasko 1986). Local groups, such as the American Cancer Society–sponsored program "Look Good, Feel Better" offers personalized instruction in self-care of facial skin and hair. Finally, resources often are available to help the patient purchase a wig: the local American Cancer Society (1-800-ACS-2345) and some insurance plans if the wig is prescribed by a physician as a "cranial prosthesis." For Internal Revenue Service purposes, a wig is a tax-deductible expense (Chernecky and Yasko 1986). Patient information materials are available from the Cancer Information Service, Room 307, 550 North Broadway, Baltimore, MD 21205, 1-800-4-CANCER (*Hair Care: Helpful Hints for Chemotherapy Patients*), or can be developed by enterprising nurses, as documented by Keller and Blausey (1988). Table 4.13 is an example of a standardized care plan for alopecia.

## IV. GONADAL DYSFUNCTION

The reproductive tissues are composed of rapidly dividing gonadal cells in men, whereas women are born with their full complement of ovarian follicles. Damage from chemotherapy can result in temporary or permanent sterility, irregular menses, amenorrhea, premature menopause, and alteration in libido. Which, if any, reproductive change occurs depends on the age of the patient when treated, the intensity (dose and duration) of treatment (Perry and Yarbro 1984), and, in some cases, on the drug(s) involved. In addition, many chemotherapeutic agents are *mutagenic*, causing changes in the DNA in the ova or sperm, and *teratogenic*, causing alterations in the developing fetus (Brager and Yasko 1984).

Issues of reproduction and sexuality are important because they represent basic human

**Table 4.13**  Standardized Nursing Care Plan for Patient Experiencing Alopecia

| Nursing Diagnosis | Defining Characteristics | Expected Outcomes | Nursing Interventions |
|---|---|---|---|
| I. *Potential body image disturbances related to alopecia* | I. A. Chemotherapy agents attack rapidly dividing normal as well as abnormal cells. The cells and tissues responsible for hair growth have a high mitotic rate and are sensitive to the effects of chemotherapy. The potential depends on the activity of the drug in specific phases of replication. The drugs most commonly implicated in causing alopecia because they affect the S phase of the cell cycle are<br><br>bleomycin  ifosfamide<br>cisplatin  melphalan<br>cyclophosphamide  methotrexate<br>dactinomycin  mitomycin-C<br>daunorubicin  paclitaxel<br>docetaxel  topotecan<br>doxorubicin  vinbastine<br>etoposide  vincristine<br>5-fluorouracil  vinorelbine<br>hydroxyurea<br><br>B. Doxorubicin causes alopecia in greater than 80% of pts treated, usually within 21 days. Alopecia caused from cyclophosphamide depends on dose (occurs more frequently with higher doses). Alopecia from methotrexate is also dose related. With 5-fluorouracil, thinning of eyebrows and loss of eyebrows may be observed in addition to loss of scalp hair. Range of alopecia may be from thinning of hair to a total body hair loss.<br><br>C. Regrowth depends on schedule of treatments and doses administered. Usually regrowth begins 2–3 months after cessation of therapy.<br><br>D. Whole-brain radiation (5000–7000 rads) usually results in permanent alopecia as a result of permanent damage to hair follicles. Radiation to lower levels of brain may not cause permanent alopecia. | I. A. Pt, significant other, or family member will verbalize an understanding of factors that cause alopecia (chemotherapy, radiation therapy)<br><br>B. Pt will discuss the impact of alopecia on his or her lifestyle<br><br>C. Pt will demonstrate knowledge of appropriate measures to minimize alopecia | I. A. Assess pt for being at risk for developing alopecia<br><br>B. Instruct pt about hair loss, temporary or permanent, and the effects of chemotherapy on hair follicles<br><br>C. Instruct pt on the potential for regrowth and for the potential change in color and texture<br><br>D. Assess the impact of alopecia on pt<br><br>E. Encourage verbalization of feelings<br><br>F. Encourage pt to cut long hair short so as to minimize the shock of alopecia<br><br>G. Discuss various measures to take during hair loss: wigs, scarves, hats, turban, use of makeup to highlight other features, baseball caps, cowboy hats<br><br>H. Encourage support groups with people experiencing alopecia<br><br>I. Encourage pt to help maintain personal identity by wearing own clothes in hospital and retaining social contacts<br><br>J. Instruct pt on proper scalp care<br>  1. Use baby shampoo or mild soap<br>  2. Use soft brush to minimize pulling at hair<br>  3. Use mineral oil or Vitamin A&D ointment to reduce itching<br>  4. Always use a sunscreen when exposed to sun (SPF 15 or higher)<br><br>K. If pt loses eyelashes or eyebrows instruct pt to use methods for protecting eyes (eyeglasses, hats with wide brim) |

needs. If unaddressed, they can lead to dysfunction and a decrease in self-esteem. Cancers that may be cured by chemotherapy often occur in children and young adults, such as acute lymphoblastic leukemia, Hodgkin's disease, and testicular carcinoma (Yarbro and Perry 1985). Thus, even though gonadal injury from chemotherapy does not pose a lethal threat, it is critical to address problems of reproduction and sexuality to help patients and their significant others achieve a high quality of life. Table 4.14 highlights the sexual and reproductive dysfunction caused by the administration of chemotherapeutic agents.

Female changes in reproductive function following chemotherapy treatment appear largely age related but also are influenced by drug dose intensity, duration of treatment, and previous reproductive health. Women are born with a full complement of primordial ovarian follicles, which number about 448,000 at ages 6–9 and decrease in number to 8300 at ages 40–44 (Block 1952).

Early studies on women receiving chemotherapy for Hodgkin's disease have shown that ovarian damage is more severe and permanent as the age of the woman increases. Women aged 35 and over are more apt to develop ovarian fibrosis and failure (Yarbro and Perry 1985), whereas younger women are better able to tolerate chemotherapy. However, it is not clear if these women experience early menopause. In addition, amenorrhea in young women in their 20s is usually reversible but becomes irreversible after age 30 (Yarbro and Perry 1985). It appears that the ovarian damage is progressive, and women aged 20–30 receiving aggressive chemotherapy often develop complete ovarian failure in their 30s (Chapman 1984). Alkylating agents are the most threatening agents, causing a loss of ova and an increase in mutation rate of ova (Kaempfer 1981). Women with ovarian failure

experience symptoms of premature menopause such as hot flashes, amenorrhea, vaginal dryness, and dyspareunia (Yarbro and Perry 1985). Other events that may occur are atrophy of the endometrial lining of the uterus, irregular menses or amenorrhea, temporary sterility, spontaneous abortions, and stillbirths (Yasko 1983). However, normal-appearing children have been born to mothers who have received chemotherapy, but these children require close follow-up by a pediatrician and an oncologist (Yasko 1983; Kreuser et al. 1988).

German investigators studying reproductive and endocrine gonadal function in young adults receiving chemotherapy for acute lymphoblastic or acute undifferentiated leukemia found that all male patients (aged 14–38 years) had azoospermia, with recovery of spermatogenesis in the second year of maintenance therapy. Women in this study (aged 14–36) did not show any reproductive dysfunction, as evidenced by intact ovarian follicle function and ovulation, or endocrine dysfunction, as evidenced by normal serum levels of gonadal steroids and gonadotrophins. Drugs administered during induction, consolidation, and maintenance therapy were prednisone, vincristine, daunorubicin, L-asparaginase, cyclophosphamide, mercaptopurine, dexamethasone, vincristine, doxorubicin, thioguanine, and methotrexate. However, the median age of women studied was 23; most of the drugs used were antimetabolites, which have less gonadal toxicity; and the total cyclophosphamide dose was 2.6 $gm/m^2$ versus the higher doses used in treatment of Hodgkin's disease of 6–12 $gm/m^2$ (Kreuser et al. 1988).

Chemotherapy-induced gonadal dysfunction in men manifests as damage to the germinal epithelium and stem cell depletion of the seminiferous tubules. This results in severe oligospermia (few sperm) or azoospermia

**Table 4.14**  Sexual and Reproductive Dysfunction Caused by the Administration of Chemotherapeutic Agents

| Dysfunction | Gender | Causative Factors |
|---|---|---|
| I. *Altered sexuality patterns related to body image changes and decreased level of sexual excitement* | Male and female | A. Side effects of chemotherapy: alopecia, weight loss related to nausea/vomiting, diarrhea, fatigue, decreased libido |
| II. *Alterations in the ability to achieve sexual fulfillment* | Female | A. Side effects of chemotherapy: dryness of vaginal mucosa secondary to decreased estrogen levels, inflammation and ulceration of vaginal mucosa (mucositis) secondary to stem cell injury<br>B. Other possible factors: altered role function, fear, fatigue, anxiety, lack of privacy, anger, medications/alcohol/analgesics, nausea/vomiting, pain |
|  | Male | A. Side effects of chemotherapy: temporary impotence possibly related to fatigue, pain<br>B. Other possible factors: altered role function, fear, fatigue, anxiety, lack of privacy, anger, medications/alcohol/analgesics, nausea/vomiting, pain |
| III. *Sexual dysfunction* | Female | A. Side effects of chemotherapy<br>  1. Temporary or permanent sterility<br>    a. Ovarian fibrosis with decrease in estrogen levels, decrease in number of available ova, especially with higher-dose alkylating agents and age over 30<br>    b. Atrophy of endometrial lining of uterus<br>    c. Irregular menses or amenorrhea (may be reversible under 30 years of age)<br>  2. Potential for mutation of available ova (especially by alkylating agents)<br>    a. Spontaneous abortion, stillbirth, birth defects<br>    b. May have normal children who should be followed by pedioncologist |
|  | Male | A. Side effects of chemotherapy<br>  1. Temporary or permanent sterility<br>    a. Damage and destruction of testicular germ cells and epithelium of seminiferous tubules<br>    b. Oligospermia or azoospermia 90–120 days after treatment begins; normal sperm levels may be achieved several years after therapy<br>    c. Testosterone levels not altered<br>  2. Possible sperm mutation<br>    a. Spontaneous abortion, stillbirth, birth defects<br>    b. Normal children have been fathered; child should be closely followed by pedioncologist |
| IV. *Alterations in fetal development* |  | A. Possible side effects of chemotherapy<br>  1. Drugs cross placental barrier<br>  2. Antimetabolites (e.g., MTX) and alkylating agents most harmful<br>  3. 1st trimester: Drugs can cause cellular damage and destruction leading to spontaneous abortion<br>  4. 2nd, 3rd trimester: Cellular destruction leads to low birth weight or premature infant, stillbirth, birth defects, great potential for development of malignancy; there may be mutation of ova of female child |

*Source:* Modified from Yasko, J.M. (1983). Sexual and reproductive dysfunction. In J.M. Yasko (ed.): *Guidelines for Cancer Care: Symptom Management.* Reston, Vir.: Reston Publishing Co., 269–290.

(absence of sperm) (Yarbro and Perry 1985) occurring 90–120 days after initiation of chemotherapy (Yasko 1983). Some drugs, such as the antimetabolites, are relatively nontoxic to gonadal cells, whereas others, such as the alkylating agents, are very toxic. Damage from alkylating agents is reversible up to a certain threshold (e.g., chlorambucil 400 mg, cyclophosphamide 6–10 gm), and becomes irreversible beyond this (Perry and Yarbro 1984). However, for many patients damage is reversible, with recovery of spermatogenesis occurring within 2 years of cessation of therapy (Drasga et al. 1983; Kreuser et al. 1988).

In advanced Hodgkin's disease, it was found that the risk of gonadal damage using MOPP (mechlorethamine hydrochloride [nitrogen mustard], Oncovin, prednisone, procarbazine) was quite high: at least 80% of men were likely to develop azoospermia, germinal aplasia, and testicular atrophy (Sherins and DeVita 1973). More recently, researchers have determined that apparently equal tumor response with less gonadal dysfunction can be achieved using ABVD (Adriamycin, bleomycin, vinblastine, and dacarbazine) (Bonfante et al. 1985). Patients receiving combined pelvic radiation and alkylating chemotherapy appear to have a high incidence of gonadal failure (Chapman 1984). Finally, treatment for prostate cancer using estrogen is likely to result in impotence.

In summary, whether a patient receiving chemotherapy will develop sterility is unpredictable. The risk in females appears to be largely age related, with women older than age 30 at greatest risk of developing ovarian failure. Failure is also related to specific drug and dose intensity.

In men, damage to the germ cells and stem cells of the seminiferous tubules may induce temporary sterility. If damage is not permanent, normal spermatogenesis returns within 2 years of termination of therapy. In addition, most men receiving anti-androgen therapy develop decreased libido and many cannot attain/maintain an erection. Nursing care focuses initially on accurate patient assessment of coping strategies, body image changes, self-esteem, self-concept issues, sexual identity, role relationships, and support of both the patient and significant other. More obvious drug side effects, such as alopecia, nausea and vomiting, and weight loss or gain can alter one's body image and alter normal sexual patterns. Nursing interventions to explore the impact on the individual, to encourage the patient to verbalize feelings, and to provide emotional support are helpful, as are specific suggestions for coping with altered sexuality.

The role of the nurse as an educator is a critical one, as this will help the patient "live" with the treatment. The patient should be taught the actual and potential risks of chemotherapy as they relate to sexual and reproductive health. Male patients may choose to use a sperm bank, and referral should be made *prior* to the initiation of chemotherapy so that functional, dense sperm can be collected. In addition, new techniques for assisted reproduction are available (Sweet 1996). A list of Human Semen Cryobanks can be obtained from the American Fertility Society, 1608 13th Avenue S, Birmingham, AL 35256. Some patients may have depressed sperm counts prior to therapy, related to disease such as testicular, lymphoma, or hematologic malignancies, and be unable to produce an adequate specimen for preservation. Kaempfer and colleagues (1985) surveyed cancer patients who had banked sperm for a 10-year period (1974–1984): of 24 patients, 3 had withdrawn samples for artificial insemination, and there was 1 confirmed pregnancy, with delivery of healthy twins. One patient had fathered two children after discontinuing chemotherapy.

Birth control practices are recommended by most practitioners for 2 years following chemotherapy (Kaempfer et al. 1985), as this provides for evaluation of disease response, avoidance of possible teratogenic drug effects, and, in male patients, recovery of spermatogenesis. An assessment of the patient's current birth control practices should be explored and alternatives discussed as necessary (i.e., patients with hormonally dependent tumors should not use oral contraceptives) (Kaempfer et al. 1985).

Smith (1989) recommends using the PLIS-SIT model for sexual rehabilitation, developed by Jack Annon, and describes the levels as follows:

1. Permit the patient to express sexual concerns (95% of problems can be dealt with at this level).
2. Provide limited information regarding the consequences of disease or therapy on sexual functioning.
3. Provide specific suggestions for alternative methods of sexual expression.
4. Refer for intensive therapy, either surgical or psychosexual.

Glasgow, Halfin, and Althausen (1987) suggest that couples who have satisfactory sexual relationships prior to cancer diagnosis and treatment are able to find a satisfactory relationship afterward, whereas those experiencing problems have dysfunction. Two excellent patient/significant other booklets are available without charge from the American Cancer Society, written by Leslie Schorer, PhD, Section Head of Psychosexual Disorders, Dept. of Psychiatry and Urology, Cleveland Clinic Foundation: *Sexuality and Cancer: For the Woman Who Has Cancer and Her Partner* and *Sexuality and Cancer: For the Man Who Has Cancer and His Partner*. Table 4.15 is an example of a standardized care plan for the patient experiencing sexual dysfunction.

## Section B. *Nausea and Vomiting*

Nausea and vomiting are common following chemotherapy and pose a significant challenge to patients and to nurses caring for them. Nausea or vomiting can be *acute*, occurring soon after drug administration, such as with nitrogen mustard; *subacute*, occurring 6–12 hours later, as with cyclophosphamide; *delayed*, occurring 2–3 days later, as with cisplatin; and *anticipatory*, a conditioned response to past experience of nausea or vomiting after chemotherapy administration. It is estimated that 25–50% of patients with cancer delay one or more scheduled courses of therapy (Lazlo 1983) and that up to 10% of patients with cancer refuse further chemotherapy, even curative treatment, because of the distress related to nausea and vomiting (Siegel and Longo 1981). Other potential complications of nausea and vomiting include esophageal tears (Mallory-Weiss syndrome), fractures, prolonged anorexia, malnutrition, metabolic abnormalities, and volume depletion (Craig and Powell 1987). Fortunately, progress has been made in the control of nausea and vomiting related to chemotherapy. Figure 4.12 illustrates the potential sequelae of nausea and vomiting in a nursing diagnostic framework.

*Nausea* refers to a vague, wavelike sensation and conscious need to vomit; *vomiting* refers to the actual forceful expulsion of gastric contents through the mouth; *retching* is the rhythmic contraction of respiratory muscles, causing up and down movement of gastric contents into the esophagus.

The vomiting or emetic center coordinates the reflex act of vomiting and is located in the lateral reticular formation of the medulla

**Table 4.15** Standardized Nursing Care Plan for the Patient Experiencing Sexual Dysfunction

| Nursing Diagnosis | Defining Characteristics | Expected Outcomes | Nursing Interventions |
|---|---|---|---|
| I. *Sexual dysfunction related to disease process, treatment, or infertility* | I. A. Cancer pts often experience some sexual alteration as a result of physical or psychological insults by the disease process, diagnosis, side effects of chemotherapy, surgical intervention, or radiation<br>B. Some chemotherapy causes sexual infertility:<br>    chlorambucil<br>    cyclophosphamide<br>    doxorubicin<br>    cytarabine<br>    procarbazine<br>    vinblastine<br>C. Dimensions altered by cancer therapy may affect behavior used to express sexual identity | I. A. Pt will demonstrate knowledge of factors that may potentially affect sexuality<br>B. Pt will verbalize the potential impact of diagnosis on sexual activity<br>C. Pt will maintain satisfying sex role and sexual self-image<br>D. Pt will identify strategies used to minimize sexual dysfunction<br>E. Pt or significant other will identify other measures used for sexual expression | I. A. Establish a trusting relationship with the pt<br>B. Assess pt's knowledge regarding the effects of the disease and treatment on sexuality<br>C. Provide a comfortable, relaxed environment in which to discuss with pt the effects of disease and treatment on sexuality<br>D. Allow pt and significant other to verbalize perceptions of how disease and treatment will affect sexual function and sexuality<br>E. Discuss strategies to minimize sexual dysfunction<br>  1. Alternative forms of sexual expression<br>  2. Alternative positions to decrease pain and prevent injury<br>  3. Encourage sexual activity when energy levels are highest (in morning, after naps)<br>  4. Help pt to recognize sexual feelings and urges<br>  5. Include sexual partner in counseling and teaching<br>  6. Explain effects of drugs and treatment on fertility<br>  7. Refer for further counseling, if necessary<br>F. Discuss options regarding alternative methods of family planning<br>  1. Foster parenthood<br>  2. Adoption<br>  3. Provide information on sperm banking |

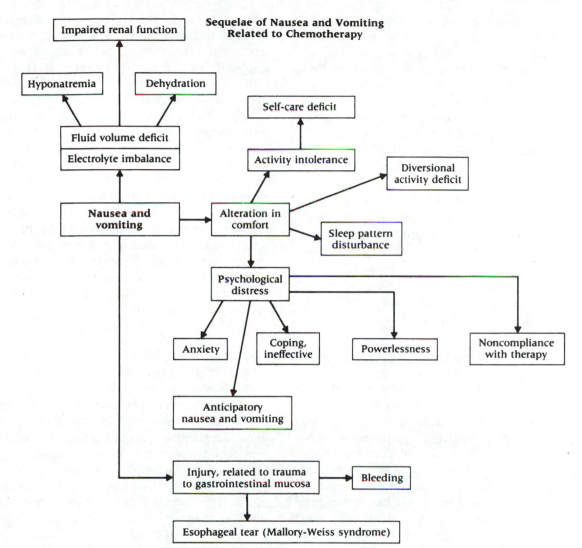

Figure 4.12 Potential Patient Problems Related to Nausea and Vomiting

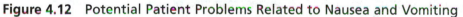

oblongata, close to the reflex centers controlling cardiovascular and respiratory function. Thus, shared efferent pathways bring about signs and symptoms of tachycardia; diaphoresis; weakness or dizziness during nausea; bradycardia and decreased blood pressure during vomiting; and increased rate and depth of respi-

ration (Borison and McCarthy 1984). The vomiting center receives stimulation from five areas (Yasko 1985):

1. Intestinal tract through the vagus nerve (vagal visceral afferents), stimulated by delayed gastric emptying or GI distention

2. Cortical pathway via hypothalamus (cerebral cortex and limbic system), stimulated by anxiety or increased intracranial pressure; the cortical pathway is probably responsible for anticipatory nausea and vomiting

3. Vestibular pathway via labyrinth system and vagus nerve, stimulated by rapid position changes; the pathway does not play a significant role in chemotherapy-induced emesis

4. Peripheral pathways via sympathetic visceral afferents from the GI tract, heart, and kidneys, stimulated by irritation or spasm

5. Chemoreceptor trigger zone (CTZ), stimulated by blood-borne toxins, drugs such as chemotherapy, and altered hormones of pregnancy

The CTZ contains receptors for histamine (H1 and H2), dopamine, acetylcholine, and opiates, but the actual neurochemical physiology of chemotherapy-induced nausea and vomiting is not well known (Craig and Powell 1987). Blood-borne chemotherapy appears to stimulate the CTZ, which then stimulates the vomiting center, probably via dopaminergic and serotonin pathways. The vomiting center has muscarinic (cholinergic) and histamine receptors, as do the vestibular and efferent vagal motor nuclei (Goodman 1987). Prostaglandins may also play a role in the stimulation of nausea and vomiting, and it is postulated that prostaglandin A2 may be released by trauma to the GI mucosa by chemotherapy (Ignoffo 1983). Figure 4.13 illustrates multiple pathways of stimulation for nausea and vomiting. However, it appears that the most significant mechanism for acute chemotherapy-induced nausea and vomiting is the peripheral pathway mediated by the vagal and splanchnic afferent nerves. Chemotherapy causes mucosal injury to the mucosal surfaces of the small intestines (enterochromaffin cells), which then release serotonin (5-hydroxytryptamine, 5-HT3) as well as other neurotransmitters. Following release, serotonin (5-HT3) then stimulates 5-HT3 receptors on the GI vagal afferent fibers, stimulating the vomiting center. The 5-HT3 receptor appears to have two sections, one of which, when stimulated, causes the release of additional serotonin. While the serotonin antagonists have afforded significant prevention and control of acute chemotherapy-induced nausea and vomiting, these agents are not as successful in preventing delayed nausea and vomiting. This suggests that delayed nausea and vomiting have a different mechanism of action, likely mediated via a dopamine pathway. The most effective antiemetic regimens include drugs that act on some or all of the different pathways. Although it is quite likely that nausea and vomiting occurring after chemotherapy administration are related to the drugs given, it is important to exclude other potential causes. These include bowel obstruction or peritonitis, CNS metastasis, drugs such as narcotics, fluid and electrolyte imbalance, hepatic metastasis, infections (local or systemic), radiation therapy, and uremia.

Psychogenic factors can influence the occurrence of nausea and vomiting, and thus it is crucial to try to prevent this from occurring with the first treatment cycle. Anticipatory nausea and vomiting (ANV) refers to the learned conditioned response of nausea and vomiting when triggered by the memory or reminder of chemotherapy administration, such as the smell of alcohol or the sight of the chemotherapy nurse. The vomiting center is stimulated by higher cortical areas (limbic system) resulting in pretreatment nausea or vomiting. Anticipatory nausea and vomiting usually develops after the third or fourth cycle of therapy and may affect as many as 33% of patients (Nicholas 1982).

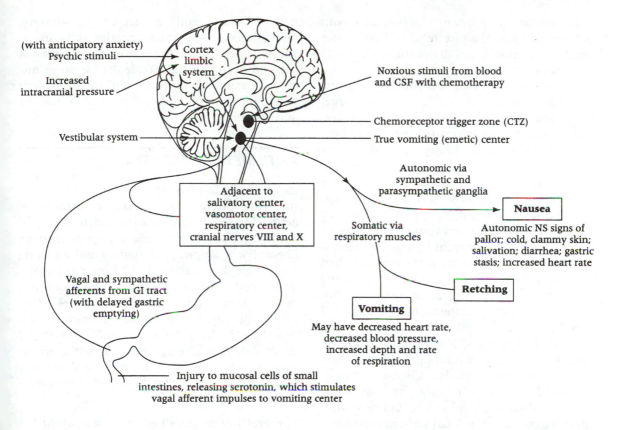

(with anticipatory anxiety)
Psychic stimuli

Cortex
limbic
system

Noxious stimuli from blood
and CSF with chemotherapy

Increased
intracranial pressure

Vestibular system

Chemoreceptor trigger zone (CTZ)

True vomiting (emetic) center

Autonomic via
sympathetic and
parasympathetic ganglia

Adjacent to
salivatory center,
vasomotor center,
respiratory center,
cranial nerves VIII and X

**Nausea**

Autonomic NS signs of
pallor; cold, clammy skin;
salivation; diarrhea; gastric
stasis; increased heart rate

Somatic via
respiratory muscles

**Retching**

Vagal and sympathetic
afferents from GI tract
(with delayed gastric
emptying)

**Vomiting**

May have decreased heart rate,
decreased blood pressure,
increased depth and rate
of respiration

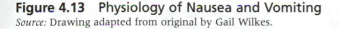

Injury to mucosal cells of small
intestines, releasing serotonin, which stimulates
vagal afferent impulses to vomiting center

**Figure 4.13** Physiology of Nausea and Vomiting
*Source:* Drawing adapted from original by Gail Wilkes.

Studies have shown that behavioral techniques may be useful in decreasing the distress and degree of ANV. These techniques include hypnosis with guided imagery, systematic desensitization, and progressive muscle relaxation, where relaxation becomes the conditioned response. In addition, the drug lorazepam, with its amnesiac quality, helps to decrease ANV. According to Morrow (1982), patients at risk for developing ANV experience the triad of warm/hot sensation, severe nausea/vomiting, and diaphoresis following treatment. Yasko (1985) suggests increased risk in patients who

experience a metallic taste after treatment, have anxiety or depression, and are less than 50 years old. Cotanch and Strum (1987) use five specific patient instructions together with behavioral techniques prior to chemotherapy administration. The patient is told that he or she will feel (1) restful sleep, (2) relinquishment of control, (3) swift passage of time, (4) thirst upon awakening but will fall back asleep again, and (5) satisfaction upon completion of therapy.

In contrast to ANV patients, who have great difficulty tolerating treatment due to nausea and vomiting, it appears that patients with histories of alcohol abuse tend to have better results with antiemetics than other patients do (Hesketh et al. 1988).

The degree of nausea and vomiting and the duration of distress are related to the drug, dose, frequency, and method of administration, where the risk is greater with IV administration than with oral dosing and with shorter infusion than when the drug is administered over a longer time. Also affecting the degree and duration of emesis is the delayed excretion of the drug or drug metabolites, which may cause delayed nausea and vomiting. For example, it is possible to prevent nausea and vomiting during cisplatin administration and then have the patient develop nausea and vomiting 24–48 hours after drug administration. This occurs in 30–60% of patients and lasts up to 7 days (Strum et al. 1985; Rhodes, Watson, and Johnson 1985). Thus, it is important to continue antiemetic protection post-cisplatin therapy to prevent emesis. Cisplatin causes decreased gastric emptying, and metoclopramide often is useful in combination with dexamethasone for 3–5 days after chemotherapy (Wickham 1999). Although mild antiemetics are helpful in preventing emesis from low to moderate emetogenic drug combinations, aggressive, multidrug combinations are necessary for preventing emesis from highly emetogenic drugs such as high-dose cisplatin or DTIC (see Table 4.16).

The nurse's prechemotherapy assessment should include hydration and electrolyte status, and these should be corrected prior to chemotherapy administration. Anxiety can be reduced by supportive and empathetic communication with the patient to explore concerns or provide distraction as appropriate, technical expertise of the nurse, and consistency of care providers between successive courses of therapy. Nursing care is directed toward preventing

nausea and vomiting, decreasing anxiety, increasing comfort, and promoting self-care, as shown in the standardized nursing care plan at the end of this section. Table 4.17 is an example of a standardized care plan for the patient experiencing chemotherapy-induced nausea and vomiting.

## ANTIEMETIC TREATMENT

In designing antiemetic treatment, antiemetics must be administered or have a duration of action for the period of expected nausea and vomiting from the specific chemotherapeutic agent. For example, peak nausea and vomiting from cyclophosphamide is 12 hours; therefore, antiemetic coverage should extend beyond this period. Drug administration schedules often begin the night before drug administration, especially if the patient has ANV. Antiemetic drugs should be given prior to chemotherapy so that receptors in the CTZ can be effectively blocked, thus preventing the stimulation of nausea and vomiting:

- oral antiemetics should be given 30–40 minutes before treatment

- when administered rectally, up to 60 minutes before

- by IM injection 20–30 minutes before

- IV dosing should be given 10–20 minutes prior to treatment

In this way, the blockade is in place before the chemotherapy drug enters the bloodstream. In general, antiemetics should be administered prior to chemotherapy administration and regularly after treatment for at least 24 hours for drugs that have moderate to high emetogenic potential (Yasko 1985).

The past 15 years have seen many studies conducted in the search for more effective

**Table 4.16**  Emetic Potential of Chemotherapy Drugs

| High (> 80% Incidence) | Antiemetic Regimen |
|---|---|
| cisplatin<br>cyclophosphamide, high-dose<br>cytosine arabinoside, high-dose<br>dacarbazine (DTIC)<br>irinotecan<br>mechlorethamine (nitrogen mustard)<br>melphalan, high-dose<br>methotrexate, high-dose<br>mitomycin C<br>nitrosoureas (BCNU, CCNU)<br>topotecan | Aggressive combination antiemetics (i.e., granisetron or ondansetron), metoclopramide, or high-dose phenothiazine with dexamethasone ± lorazepam |
| **Moderate (50%)** | |
| carboplatin<br>cyclophosphamide<br>dactinomycin<br>daunorubicin<br>doxetaxel<br>doxorubicin<br>etoposide<br>ifosfamide<br>hexamethylmelamine<br>mitoxantrone<br>procarbazine | Moderately aggressive therapy with IV phenothiazines (perphenazine, prochlorperazine) ± decadron, lorazepam |
| **Low (< 25%)** | |
| bleomycin<br>carboplatin<br>chlorambucil<br>cytosine arabinoside (Ara-C)<br>etoposide<br>5-fluorouracil (5-FU)<br>hydroxyurea<br>L-asparaginase<br>melphalan<br>methotrexate<br>paclitaxel<br>6-mercaptopurine<br>tamoxifen<br>teniposide<br>thioguanine<br>thiotepa<br>vinblastine<br>vincristine | Oral phenothiazines |

*Source:* Modified by permission of the publisher from Dorr, R.T., and Fritz, W. (1980). *Cancer Chemotherapy Handbook.* Reprinted by permission of Elsevier Science Publishing Company, Inc.

**Table 4.17** Standardized Nursing Care Plan for Patient Experiencing Nausea and Vomiting

| Nursing Diagnosis | Expected Outcomes | Nursing Interventions |
| --- | --- | --- |
| I. *Potential for altered nutrition, less than body requirements* | I. A. Pt will maintain weight within 5% of baseline<br><br>B. Pt will be without nausea and vomiting and, if it occurs, it is minimal | I. A. Administer antiemetics prior to chemotherapy, and then regularly through expected duration of nausea and vomiting (depending on specific chemotherapeutic agent)<br><br>1. Evaluate past effectiveness of antiemetic regime<br><br>2. Evaluate need for continuing antiemetics 12–24 hrs after treatment<br><br>3. Attempt to prevent nausea and vomiting during first treatment cycle to prevent anticipatory nausea and vomiting<br><br>B. Administer chemotherapy at night or late afternoon if possible<br><br>C. Experiment with eating patterns: suggest pt avoid eating prior to, during, and immediately after initial treatment to assess tolerance; discourage heavy, greasy, fatty, sweet, and spicy foods<br><br>D. Encourage small, frequent, bland meals on day of therapy (if tolerates eating day of therapy) and increase fluid intake to 3 quarts/day<br><br>E. Encourage pt to suck hard candy during therapy<br><br>F. Provide environment that is clean, quiet, subdued, without odors<br><br>G. Encourage weekly weighings; if pt unable to stabilize weight, refer to dietitian for intensive counseling, together with person responsible for doing the cooking<br><br>H. Teach pt self-care measures<br><br>1. Self-administration of antiemetics, including indications, dose, schedule, and potential side effects<br><br>2. Dietary counseling encouraging bland, cool foods, cottage cheese, toast, if experiencing nausea and vomiting<br><br>3. Encourage favorite high-calorie, high-protein, small, frequent feedings as tolerated; encourage fluids to 3 quarts/day, including chicken soup, Gatorade, sherbet, ginger ale |

4. Give pt copy of *Eating Hints* (NCI free publication), with ideas such as whole milk plus 1–2 T powdered milk in eggnogs, snacks to increase protein, calorie intake

| | | |
|---|---|---|
| II. *Potential for comfort alteration related to nausea and vomiting* | II. A. Pt will verbalize decreased anxiety and increased physical comfort | II. A. Encourage pt to verbalize feelings re: prior treatments, if any, and significance of treatment to the pt |
| | | B. Provide emotional support |
| | | C. Consider anxiety-reducing drugs in antiemetic regime, such as lorazepam |
| | | D. Minimize time pt is in waiting room or chemotherapy room |
| | | E. Provide distraction using VCR/TV or radio as pt desires; for some pts, having a chaplain read the Psalms during therapy can be quite therapeutic |
| | | F. Teach pt progressive muscle relaxation exercises and help pt to imagine peaceful past experiences; encourage fresh air |
| | | G. Keep emesis basin within reach, provide cloth for face and hands if pt vomits |
| | | H. Assist pt with mouth care after emesis |
| | | I. Telephone pt, if treated as an outpt, the evening of or the day after chemotherapy administration to assess tolerance and comfort |
| III. *Potential powerlessness* | III. A. Pt will have control over self-care activities | III. A. Pt and family teaching re: potential side effects and self-care measures; offer pt and family *Chemotherapy and Use: A Self-Help Guide* (free NCI publication) |
| | | B. Encourage pt to live as normal a lifestyle as possible, going out and engaging in usual activities; often doing something "nice" for oneself *after* treatment helps to minimize the distress and increase control |
| | | C. Involve pt and family in appropriate decisions in treatment |

*(continued)*

**Table 4.17** Standardized Nursing Care Plan for Patient Experiencing Nausea and Vomiting (*continued*)

| Nursing Diagnosis | Expected Outcomes | Nursing Interventions |
|---|---|---|
| IV. *Potential for knowledge deficit of self-care measures* | IV. A. Pt will verbally repeat self-care measures and schedule for carrying them out | IV. A. Instruct pt and family member in self-care measures<br>1. Self-administration of antiemetics postchemotherapy<br>2. Drink 3 quarts fluids per day, especially chicken soup, etc.<br>3. Bland, cool, frequent, high-calorie, high-protein foods as tolerated<br>4. Call health care provider for persistent nausea and vomiting > 3 times/day, inability to keep fluids down<br>B. Use a positive approach in teaching re the potential side effect of nausea and vomiting, stressing efforts to prevent nausea and vomiting from occurring<br>C. If nausea and vomiting occur, reassure pt that there are other antiemetic regimens that can be used to control, and hopefully prevent, it for the next cycle |
| V. *Potential for injury related to nausea and vomiting (esophageal tears, bleeding)* | V. A. Pt will be free from injury<br>B. Injury, if it occurs, will be detected early | V. A. Reinforce teaching to call clinic or health care provider if persistent nausea and vomiting occur, as well as if pain, bleeding, or any other abnormality occurs<br>B. If pt is taking steroids as part of chemotherapy or antiemetic regimen, teach pt to take pills with food |

antiemetic regimens. Craig and Powell (1987) identify key elements to look for when reviewing antiemetic studies:

1. Is the study randomized and double-blind? Is it a parallel or crossover study, which reduces bias? A crossover design allows the patient to act as his or her own control.
2. Are there comparable, randomized patient populations in which it is the first treatment cycle for all patients and patients are not taking any other medications that may have antiemetic potential? Are the patients receiving equally emetogenic chemotherapy drugs, and are they in the same treatment setting (i.e., inpatient or ambulatory setting)?
3. Is there a clear definition of response? Is there a distinction between nausea and vomiting? Is patient preference evaluated? Is the number of vomiting episodes measured in a given period of time? Are the same outcomes measured? How is complete response defined?
4. Is there an adequate sample to make a valid statistical statement?

As oncology nurses administering chemotherapy, it is essential to remain knowledgeable about current antiemetic research findings. Certain patients may not respond to standard antiemetic regimens, and it is important to be a patient advocate, discussing with the physician alternative antiemetic regimens that may be more effective.

## PHARMACOLOGY OF ANTIEMETICS

The following eight groups of antiemetic drugs—serotonin (5-HT$_3$) antagonists, phenothiazines, butyrophenones, substituted benzamides, benzodiazepines, glucocorticosteroids, cannabinoids, and antihistamines—commonly are used in antiemetic therapy for cancer chemotherapy

side effects. This section presents information on selected drugs within each group.

## Serotonin (5-HT$_3$) Antagonists

These agents have become the most effective agents in the prevention and control of acute nausea and vomiting related to moderately to severely emetogenic drugs (i.e., cisplatin); the likelihood of complete protection from cisplatin-induced nausea and vomiting is increased by the addition of dexamethasone.

| Drug | Dose/Schedule | Comments |
|---|---|---|
| granisetron (Kytril) | *PO:* 1 mg bid or 2 mg single dose beginning 30–60 mins prior to chemotherapy *IV:* 1 mg (10 µg/kg) IV over 5 mins | Half-life is 9 hrs Half-life is 2.5 hrs Continue oral dosing for 2 days after cisplatin |
| ondansetron (Zofran) | *PO:* 8 mg PO TID; first dose 30 mins before chemotherapy, then at 4 and 8 hrs after first dose, then TID *IV:* 32 mg IV over 15–30 mins or 0.15 mg/kg q 4 hrs × 3 beginning 30 mins before chemotherapy | Zofran dose titrated to emetogenicity of chemotherapy (Hesketh et al. 1994) |
| dolasetron (Anzemet) | *PO:* 100 mg PO one hour prechemotherapy *IV:* 1.8 mg/kg (or 100 mg fixed dose) 30 mins prechemotherapy | Oral peaks in 1hr, IV peaks in 30 mins |

*Action:* Blocks serotonin (5-HT$_3$) receptors on the abdominal vagal afferent nerve fibers (peripheral) and in or around the CTZ (central), thus preventing stimulation of the vomiting center.

*Efficacy:* Granisetron (Kytril) and dolasetron are at least as effective as ondansetron (Zofran), resulting in 50–60% complete protection against nausea and vomiting caused by high-dose cisplatin (100 mg/mm). Both are superior to all other antiemetics. When dexamethasone is added, complete protection may approach 90%.

**Side Effects:** Mild: constipation, diarrhea, headache. In general, does not cause extrapyramidal side effects. Rare, with rapid infusion of ondansetron: orthostatic hypotension, dizziness, transient blindness—resolving within minutes to hours. All rarely cause prolongation of QT interval on EKG.

## Phenothiazines

These agents have been the mainstay of antiemetic therapy since the 1950s. Phenothiazines with a piperazine side-chain are more effective antiemetics (e.g., perphenazine, prochlorperazine) than those with an alkyl group (e.g., chlorpromazine).

| Drug | Dose/Schedule | Comments |
|------|---------------|----------|
| prochlorperazine (Compazine) | *PO:* 5, 10, 25 mg q 4–6 hrs<br>*Slow-release PO:* 10, 15, 30, 75 mg q 12 hrs<br>*PR:* 25 mg q 4–6 hrs<br>*IM/IV:* 5–40 mg q 3–4 hrs mix in 50 cc D₅W or NS and give over 20–30 mins (Carr et al. 1985) | |
| perphenazine (Trilafon) | *PO:* 4 mg q 4–6 hrs maximum 30 mg in 24 hrs for inpatients, 15 mg for outpatients<br>*IM/IV:* 5 mg IVB q 4–6 hrs or then infusion at 1 mg/hr for 10 hrs (Smaglia 1984) | |

**Action:** Blocks dopamine receptors in CTZ; also decreases vagal stimulation of vomiting center by peripheral afferents. Effective for low-emetogenic drugs (e.g., methotrexate, 5-FU, low-dose cyclophosphamide) at usual doses and more emetogenic chemotherapy agents at higher doses.

**Efficacy:** Prochlorperazine equally effective as droperidol and low-dose metoclopramide against cisplatin-containing chemotherapy, but less effective than cannabinoids, corticosteroids, and high-dose metoclopramide (Bakowski 1984). Carr and colleagues (1985) studied high-dose prochlorperazine and found increased effectiveness against cisplatin without increased toxicity when diphenhydramine was given. Prochlorperazine and perphenazine were found equally effective against cisplatin when equal doses were given (loading and continuous infusion) (Smaglia 1984).

**Side Effects:** Sedation, hypotension, and extrapyramidal side effects, especially dystonia. Rarely, can cause lowering of seizure thresholds, skin reactions, agranulocytosis, cholestatic jaundice, and increased prolactin levels.

## Butyrophenones

These are potent neuroleptics. They are major tranquilizers used as antiemetics.

| Drug | Dose/Schedule | Comments |
|------|---------------|----------|
| droperidol (Inapsine) | *IM/IV:* 0.5–2.5 mg q 4–6 hrs or drip, but reports suggest large loading dose, then intermittent IVB or continuous infusion for 6–10 hrs (Citron et al. 1984; Wilson et al. 1981) | Caution in patients with cardiac dysfunction on anticonvulsants |
| haloperidol (Haldol) | *PO:* 3–5 mg q 2 hrs × 3–4 doses, beginning 30 mins before chemotherapy<br>*IM:* 0.5–2 mg | Oral well absorbed |

**Action:** Dopamine antagonists that suppress the CTZ and vomiting center; considered more potent than the phenothiazines. Also decreases stimulation of the vomiting center along vestibular pathway.

*Efficacy:* Droperidol appears to require higher doses to provide adequate protection against cisplatin-containing regimens. Citron and colleagues (1984) suggest a loading dose of 5–15 mg IVB, then 5–7.5 mg IV every 2 hours for 6–8 hours (Wilson et al. 1981). Haloperidol IM or PO was shown to be equivalent to tetrahydrocannabinoid and superior to phenothiazines when tested against non-cisplatin-containing regimens. IV haloperidol was not as effective as high-dose metoclopramide against cisplatin (Greenberg et al. 1984; Neidhart et al. 1981).

*Side Effects:* Sedation, restlessness, extrapyramidal reactions (less severe than with phenothiazines), and tardive dyskinesia may occur in older patients. Can induce respiratory depression when used with narcotic analgesics.

## Substituted Benzamides

The only substituted benzamide with antiemetic potential is metoclopramide (Reglan), which is a procainamide derivative without cardiac effects.

| Drug | Dose/Schedule | Comments |
|---|---|---|
| metoclopramide hydrochloride (Reglan) | *IV:* 1–3 mg/kg IV 30 mins before chemotherapy administration, then repeat q 2 hrs for 2-4 doses *PO:* For delayed nausea and vomiting, 20–40 mg q 4 hrs × 24 hrs or 0.5 mg/kg qid × 4 days beginning 24 hrs after cisplatin together with dexamethasone 8 mg bid d 1–2, 4 mg bid d 3–4 (Kris and Gralla 1986) | Dosage of 2 mg/kg every 2 hrs for 3–5 doses is appropriate for high-dose CDDP (120 mg/m²). PO route may result in increased number of stools. |

*Action:* Acts both centrally and peripherally. Dopamine antagonist blocking CTZ; also stimulates upper GI tract motility, thus increasing gastric emptying, and opposes retrograde peristalsis of retching (Goodman 1987).

*Efficacy:* Dose related, with 60% effectiveness against high-dose cisplatin and increased to 66% with the addition of steroids, lorazepam (Strum et al. 1984). As a single agent, metoclopramide is superior to placebo, THC, dexamethasone, prochlorperazine, and haldol in controlling cisplatin-induced nausea and vomiting, and prevents all vomiting in 40% of patients (Gralla et al. 1984). Lower doses (1 mg/kg) appear equally effective as higher doses in patients receiving cisplatin < 75mg/m² (Raila et al. 1985). High-dose oral and continuous infusion administration appears equally effective as intermittent bolus administration (Craig and Powell 1987).

*Side Effects:* Sedation, akathesia (restlessness), other extrapyramidal side effects, especially in patients younger than 30 years, where the incidence is 30%, versus 1.8% in older adults (Allen et al. 1985). Diarrhea occurs in about 30% of patients and is well controlled by antidiarrheal medication or may be prevented by the addition of dexamethasone to the regimen.

## Benzodiazepines

These CNS depressants decrease anxiety (anxiolytic), increase sedation, and cause anterograde amnesia, so that if nausea or vomiting occur, they are not remembered.

| Drug | Dose/Schedule | Comments |
|---|---|---|
| lorazepam (Ativan) | *IV:* 0.5-1.5 mg/m² to 4 mg total dose* IVP or in 50 cc D$_5$W or NS over 10 mins, 30 mins prior to chemotherapy, q 4–6 hrs postchemotherapy *PO:* 1–3 mg 30 mins prior to chemotherapy, q 4–6 hrs postchemotherapy | Have someone accompany patient home if outpatient. Dosage should be titrated to induce arousable sleep state. Should be mixed immediately prior to administration. |

*Dose reduced in elderly, debilitated patients; patients with severe hepatic dysfunction (bilirubin > 2 mg%) or serum albumin < 2 mg%; and in patients with severe COPD where respiratory center depression is inadvisable.

*Action:* May work by blocking cortical pathways to the vomiting center, and thus may be useful in controlling anticipatory nausea and vomiting when begun the night before treatment. It is 90% absorbed from GI tract within 30 minutes of administration.

*Efficacy:* Lorazepam has been shown to be an effective addition to antiemetic regimens. A study by Gagen and colleagues (1984) comparing the effectiveness of metoclopramide to lorazepam and dexamethasone demonstrated that not only was the second combination more effective but patients preferred the lorazepam combination 70–12% (Laszlo et al. 1985). However, lorazepam is most commonly used in combination with more active agents such as high-dose metoclopramide. Sublingual administration achieves peak and plasma levels similar to IV administration (Caille, Speneid, and Lacasse 1983).

*Side Effects:* Arousable sedation but may occasionally be profound; prolonged amnesia; hypotension; perceptual disturbances; urinary incontinence.

*Drug Interactions:* CNS depression when given with alcohol, phenothiazines, barbiturates, MAO inhibitors, and other depressants. Increased sedation when combined with scopalamine.

## Glucocorticosteroids

Glucocorticosteroids usually are used in conjunction with other antiemetic therapy.

*Action:* May inhibit prostaglandin release by stabilizing lysosomal membranes, thereby theoretically interrupting hypothalamic prostaglandin release and subsequent stimulation of nausea and vomiting (Goodman 1987).

*Efficacy:* Used in combination with other antiemetic agents, high doses of dexamethasone

(oral or parenteral) have been effective in preventing nausea and vomiting in many patients (70–80% overall responses), especially in previously untreated patients (Markman et al. 1984). Also, the addition of high-dose dexamethasone in combination with high-dose metoclopramide significantly decreases the incidence of diarrhea from metoclopramide, as well as increasing the effectiveness of the antiemetic action of metoclopramide in some studies (Gralla et al. 1987). As a single agent, corticosteroids are effective against low to moderate emetogenic agents.

| Drug | Dose/Schedule | Comments |
| --- | --- | --- |
| dexamethasone (Decadron) | *IV:* 10–20 mg begin 30 mins before chemotherapy, then q 4–6 hrs *PO:* 4 mg q 4 × 4 doses beginning 1–8 hrs before chemotherapy (Goodman 1987) | Use with caution in diabetics |
| methylprednisolone (Solu-Medrol) | *IV:* 125–250 mg beginning 30 mins before chemotherapy, then q 4 × 3 more doses (Mason, Dambra, and Grossman 1982) | |
| prednisone | *PO:* 25–50 mg 4 hrs before chemotherapy and q 4 × 8 doses (Goodman 1987) | |

*Side Effects:* During IVP administration, may have brief, intense perineal burning or pruritis, which is prevented by infusion. Immediate vomiting has been reported and is self-limiting (Goodman 1987). Other side effects include lethargy, weakness, mood changes, hyperglycemia, leukocytosis secondary to demargination of WBC, and insomnia and agitation the evening following therapy. Side effects are usually mild, as the drug is given for only short periods. High-dose steroids should be avoided in patients with a history of psychosis.

## Cannabinoids

Synthetic preparations of marijuana have been proven effective in preventing or minimizing the nausea and vomiting that occur as side effects of chemotherapy.

| Drug | Dose/Schedule | Comments |
|------|---------------|----------|
| dronabinol (Marinol) | *PO:* 5–7.5 mg/m$^2$ 1–3 hrs before chemo-therapy, then 2–4 hrs postchemotherapy for 4–6 doses per day | If ineffective and no toxicity, can increase by 2.5 mg/m$^2$ increments to max 15 mg/m$^2$ dose (Sargeant and Fisher 1986) |

*Action:* Active ingredient is delta-9-tetra-hydro-cannabinol (THC). Its mechanism of action is unclear but probably relates to CNS depression and may involve disruption of higher cortical input or inhibition of prostaglandin synthesis. Or it may bind to opiate receptors in the brain to indirectly block the vomiting center.

*Efficacy:* More effective than placebo, in some cases equal to or better than prochlorperazine (Compazine). However, not shown to be effective in patients receiving cisplatin (Gralla et al. 1984). It is an expensive drug, has high potential for abuse, and is indicated for patients who have failed standard antiemetics. Complete responses in 20–25%, partial responses in 40–55% against low-emetogenic drugs (Sargeant and Fisher 1986).

*Side Effects:* Mood changes, disorientation, drowsiness, muddled thinking, dizziness; brief impairment of perception, coordination, and sensory functions. Rarely, dry mouth, increased appetite, general increase in central sympathomimetic activity with increased heart rate, and postural hypotension. Increased CNS toxicity in the elderly (up to 35%).

## Antihistamines

These play a major role in preventing extrapyramidal side effects of dopamine antagonists.

*Action:* Diphenhydramine (Benadryl) inhibits histamine and has slight, if any, antiemetic activity by blocking the CTZ and decreasing vestibular stimulation.

| Drug | Dose/Schedule | Comments |
|------|---------------|----------|
| diphenhydramine (Benadryl) | *IV:* 50 mg before chemotherapy or 25 mg q 4 hrs × 4 during metoclopramide or Trilafon (perphenazine) dosing, beginning prior to antiemetic *PO:* 25–50 mg q 4 *IM:* 25–50 mg q 4 | Sedate to desired degree of sedation without compromising antiemetic activity |

*Efficacy:* Limited role in antiemesis but highly effective in the prevention or resolution of extrapyramidal side effects.

*Side Effects:* Drowsiness, dry mouth, dizziness.

## EXTRAPYRAMIDAL SIDE EFFECTS: ASSESSMENT AND INTERVENTION

The most effective antiemetics to date seem to work by blocking or antagonizing dopamine receptors in the CTZ. All of these agents also have the potential to cause extrapyramidal side effects. Diphenhydramine (Benadryl) 50 mg IVP is rapidly effective in resolving acute dystonic reactions. If the symptoms are less acute, 50 mg IM usually brings relief within 15 minutes.

Symptoms of extrapyramidal reactions are:

- tongue protrusion, neck dystonia (disordered muscle tone)
- opisthotonus (spasm where the head and heels are bent backward and the body bowed forward)

- trismus (spasm of chewing muscles so that mouth cannot open)
- oligogyric crisis (movement of the eye around the anteroposterior axis, together with laryngeal and pharyngeal spasm, can cause respiratory distress and ultimately anoxia)
- limb dystonia (spasm of muscles of head, neck, back, which may resemble seizures)
- akathesia (involuntary feeling of restlessness)
- tremor
- anxiety
- insomnia
- dizziness

*Extrapyramidal* side effects are so called because they result from excessive cholinergic activity in the extrapyramidal tract of the nervous system, caused by an unintentional blockade of the postsynaptic dopamine receptors by the antiemetic drug. Motor neurons, which are responsible for movement, lie in bundles located within tracts in the brain. Those that pass through a pyramid-shaped area and that allow for direct cortical control and initiation and patterning of skilled movement are called the *pyramidal tracts*. Those lying outside of this area are called the *extrapyramidal tracts*, and these are involved in motor activities, such as the control and coordination of posture and locomotion. The extrapyramidal tracts inhibit muscle contractions that are "coordinated" by the cholinergic receptors in the pyramidal system. The pyramidal tracts are also able to inhibit cholinergic stimulation. The antiemetic drugs that work by blocking dopamine receptors (dopamine antagonists) also block postsynaptic dopamine receptors, preventing completion of the nervous stimulation in the pyramidal tract. This imbalance leads to disinhibition of the extrapyramidal cholinergic receptors, with resulting excessive cholinergic activity, as seen in the extrapyramidal side effects (Bickal 1987).

Dystonic reactions occur twice as commonly in young males and in individuals younger than 35 years old (Gralla et al. 1987). Numerous studies have shown that adding diphenhydramine or lorazepam as part of combined antiemetics can prevent the development of this side effect in many cases. For example, diphenhydramine 50 mg can be given prior to initial metoclopramide dose. Lorazepam is especially effective in preventing akathesia (restlessness), as well as the other extrapyramidal symptoms (Kris et al. 1985).

In summary, prophylactic combination antiemetics should be given prior to all moderate and highly emetogenic chemotherapy agents. Combinations containing a serotonin antagonist and dexamethasone offer the best antiemetic protection to date for highly emetogenic chemotherapy. Antiemetics should be continued for 4–7 days after cisplatin to prevent delayed nausea and vomiting. Delayed nausea and vomiting following cisplatin appears to be mediated by a dopinergic pathway, so dopamine antagonists (e.g., phenothiazines) are as effective and less expensive than serotonin-antagonists. Delayed emesis protocols often contain dexamethasone 4 mg po bid and metoclopramide 10 mg po QID × 3–5 days after cisplatin chemotherapy. The use of metoclopramide plus dexamethasone orally has been shown in a study by Kris and colleagues (1989) to be superior to dexamethasone alone or placebo to prevent or control delayed nausea and vomiting. In providing antiemetic protection for moderately emetogenic chemotherapy, either metoclopramide or a phenothiazine plus dexamethasone are effective and should be continued for 24 hours post-chemotherapy by either oral or IV route. For chemotherapeutic agents with low emetogenic potential, phenothiazine or dexamethasone alone, or no initial therapy, should be adequate.

It is critical to attempt to prevent nausea and vomiting at the first chemotherapy treatment, for only then can anticipatory nausea and vomiting be prevented. However, if ANV does occur, the use of intensive antiemetics, including lorazepam prior to therapy, and behavioral techniques may be helpful. If patients experience nausea and vomiting despite standard antiemetic therapy, they may benefit from tetrahydrocannabinol (synthetic derivative Marinol) together with a phenothiazine to minimize CNS side effects (Craig and Powell 1987). Despite the best efforts using combination antiemetics, 10–30% of patients may experience nausea and vomiting related to chemotherapy. Serotonin-antagonist antiemetics have significantly improved control of *acute* chemotherapy-induced emesis, and as our understanding of serotonin-mediated pathways expands, newer antagonists will become available. However, the problem of *delayed* nausea and vomiting continues, and clinical research in this area is critical.

## Section C. *Toxicity to Other Organ Systems*

### INTRODUCTION

The following section addresses chemotherapy-related toxicities in other organ systems: systems that do not have a rapid cell proliferation rate but that attract specific anticancer drugs. Consequently, damage may result from drug binding to tissue, such as doxorubicin and heart muscle myofibrils, when these cells have no affinity to other chemotherapeutic agents. Toxicity may be found in certain organs responsible for drug elimination and excretion, such as the liver, kidneys, lungs, or sweat glands (Yasko 1983). The onset and degree of organ toxicity depend on the specific drug, dose received, and, in many cases, the administration schedule (Yasko 1983).

Knowledge of drug-induced organ toxicity is critical to the oncology nurse administering chemotherapy. Certain tests must be performed prior to initial drug treatment and periodically during treatment to identify early organ damage before symptoms become apparent. Although the ordering of these tests is the physician's responsibility, it is the nurse's responsibility to be certain the tests are performed and the results are within safe limits, prior to administering the drug. Also prior to drug administration, the nurse assesses the patient for signs or symptoms of early organ toxicity.

### I. CARDIOTOXICITY OF ANTINEOPLASTIC DRUGS

The most well known antineoplastic agents with cardiotoxicity potential are the anthracyclines, doxorubicin and daunorubicin, and their analogues. These drugs are used widely in the treatment of breast and ovarian cancers, lymphomas and leukemias, and osteosarcomas. Often the patient with cancer is older and may have pre-existing heart disease, so a careful cardiovascular assessment must be performed prior to drug administration. Cardiotoxicity can be (1) *acute*, occurring soon after drug administration and manifested by EKG abnormalities (Tokaz and Von Hoff 1984); (2) *subacute*, fibrinous pericarditis with myocardial dysfunction, occurring during the first 4–5 weeks of therapy (Kaszyk 1986); and (3) *cardiomyopathy*, usually occurring within months of treatment (Tokaz and Von Hoff 1984). The incidence of EKG abnormalities occurring during or soon after drug administration is estimated at 0–41% (Ali et al. 1979). EKG abnormalities most often are benign and reversible, and they do not prevent further drug administration: these include nonspecific ST-T wave changes, sinus tachycardia, and premature atrial and ventricular contractions (Tokaz and Von Hoff 1984). However, a decrease in QRS voltage may occur, which often is irreversible and may be associated with total dose of drug received (Cortes et al. 1975). Finally, there have been reports of sudden death and life-threatening arrythmias during or just after drug administration, so caution is still important (Tokaz and Von Hoff 1984). It is not customary to use cardiac monitoring or serial EKGs during or after administration of anthracyclines.

The more serious, dose-limiting cardiomyopathy that may develop is related to cumulative drug dose and high peak serum levels of bolus injection. Myofibril damage and degeneration are gradual, and if the patient becomes symptomatic while receiving treatment, maximum drug damage will not be seen for weeks to months after the last drug dose (Kaszyk 1986). However, most commonly, if patients do develop symptomatic cardiomyopathy, it occurs a week to 2 1/2 months after the final dose of doxorubicin (Saltiel and McGuire 1983). When total dose of doxorubicin is controlled at < 550 mg/m$^2$, resultant cardiomyopathy is 1–5% in comparison to 30% in patients receiving doxorubicin at a cumulative dose > 550 mg/m$^2$ (Tokaz and Von Hoff 1984). The pathophysiologic process centers on damage to the myofibril, the contractile element of the myocyte (Kaszyk 1986). Several drugs have been developed to try to duplicate the effectiveness of doxorubicin, without the cardiotoxicity (e.g., liposomal doxorubcin or Doxil).

Within the myocyte, the sarcoplasmic reticulum swells, and then damage to the myofibril results in the degeneration of the mitochondria (energy storehouse) and nucleus and loss of contractility of the myofibril (Kaszyk 1986). Another biochemical change caused by doxorubicin that may increase myocyte damage is a decrease in cardiac glutathione peroxidase (the enzyme that converts toxic substances into harmless ones), resulting in damage to the heart cell membranes by destructive free radicals (Bristow 1982). It is suggested that there is preferential binding to heart cell mitochondria, causing damage and possible alterations in calcium channel flow within the membrane (Kaszyk 1986). As more myofibrils are lost, the heart muscle has to work harder to compensate for the loss of pumping ability, the heart enlarges (hypertrophy), and there is increased oxygen demand. The degree of damage can range from minor EKG changes to severe congestive heart failure (CHF), requiring digitalis and diuretics.

Early detection of cardiomyopathy is difficult without the use of invasive or noninvasive scans. The most precise measure of myocardial damage is endomyocardial biopsy, with quantification of damage using the Billingham scale of anthracycline damage (Bristow 1982). However, radionuclide angiography (gated blood pool scan), which measures left ventricular ejection fraction (pumping effectiveness), is noninvasive and correlates well with cardiac damage and toxicity (Taylor, Applefeld, and Wiernik 1984).

Nursing assessment is aimed at identification of patients at risk for developing cardiomyopathy, examination for signs and symptoms of CHF, and knowledge of gated blood scan results.

Factors that appear to increase the *risk* of cardiomyopathy are as follows:

1. *Total cumulative drug dose:* A dose >550 mg/m$^2$ increases risk, or doses >400 mg/m$^2$ when concurrent chemotherapy is given with drugs such as cyclophosphamide or if the patient has received prior mediastinal irradiation (Tokaz and Von Hoff 1984). Because not all patients develop the same cardiac damage at the same dose, risks and benefits must be weighed. Daunorubicin-related CHF is 1.5% at total dose of 600 mg/m$^2$ and 12% at 1 gm/m$^2$ (Von Hoff et al. 1977).

2. *Dosing schedule:* Apparent high peak serum drug levels, such as IV bolus drug administered every 3 weeks, increase risk over schedules of low weekly dosing and continuous infusion (Legha et al. 1982).

3. *Age:* Young children and persons aged 50 or older. The higher incidence with increasing age > 50 may be related to the increased incidence of preexisting myocardial damage (Tokaz and Von Hoff 1984).

4. *Preexisting myocardial damage:* Abnormal EKG, hypertension.

5. Concurrent combination chemotherapy: Probable potentiation of risk with cyclophosphamide; possible risk with Actinomycin D, Mitomycin C, or dacarbazine (Tokaz and Von Hoff 1984).

6. *Prior radiation* (XRT) therapy to the mediastinum potentiates myocardial damage induced by anthracyclines.

Early signs and symptoms of CHF may be a non-specific dry cough or tachycardia (Kaszyk 1986). As the cardiomyopathy progresses, the patient may be dyspneic at rest and feel "winded." Physical exam may reveal an S$_4$ gallop heart rhythm on auscultation, distended neck veins, pedal edema, hepatomegaly, and cardiomegaly (Kaszyk 1986). Obviously, at the first sign of CHF, doxorubicin would be discontinued pending further investigation. Recovery, if it occurs, is dependent on patient compensatory cardiac functions, and treatment is symptomatic with digoxin and diuretics.

Lastly, baseline and subsequent radionuclide angiography or gated blood pool scans (GBPS) should be done to identify early changes in myocardial function. A GBPS indicates the left ventricular ejection fraction, which shows the heart's pumping ability. Most chemotherapy protocols will determine frequency of testing, but in general, in addition to a baseline study prior to the first dose, GBPS is repeated after the patient has received 200 mg/m$^2$ of doxorubicin. If the ejection fraction drops significantly, then a GBPS is performed prior to each dose of the drug. In certain circumstances, the drug is withheld, and a myocardial biopsy may be performed (Kaszyk 1986).

Other chemotherapeutic agents that may induce cardiac damage are shown in Table 4.18.

Research currently is being conducted to develop new drugs with less risk of cardiotoxicity; to develop and utilize other drugs to block cardiotoxic damage; and to evaluate different administration schedules. Dorr and Lasel (1994) reported significant cardioprotective effects against doxorubicin and daunorubicin cardiotoxicity using amifostine (WR-2721) and its metabolite WR-1065. Protection from damage appears to be due to the drugs' ability to scavenge chemotherapy-induced oxygen free radicals. Zinecard (dexrazone ICRF-187) has been approved for use in women with metastatic breast cancer who have received a cumulative doxorubicin dose of 300 mg/m$^2$ and who would benefit from continuing doxorubicin therapy. Studies have demonstrated significantly lower risks and incidences of congestive heart failure and cardiac events in women receiving cumulative

**Table 4.18** Chemotherapeutic Agents Associated with Cardiac Toxicities

| Drug | Dosage | Cardiac Toxicity | Occurrence | Comments |
|---|---|---|---|---|
| aminoglutethimide | 250 mg po qid | Hypotension, tachycardia | 10% | Can occur at any time during treatment. |
| amsacrine (AMSA) | 100 mg/m² IV qd × 3 or 75–150 mg/m² IV qd × 5 | Ventricular fibrillation Cardiomyopathy | 5% | Risk is increased by accumulative dose of greater than 900 mg/m² or greater than 200 mg/m² of AMSA in 48 hrs. Increased incidence with previous anthracycline exposure. Cardiac toxicity is enhanced by preexisting hypokalemia. |
| cisplatin | Unknown | Cardiac ischemia | Rare | |
| cisplatin-based combination therapy | Unknown | Arterial occlusion events, MI, CVA | Rare | Reports of myocardial infarction (MI), cerebrovascular accident (CVA) after treatment with cisplatin, velban, bleomycin, etoposide. |
| cyclophosphamide | 120–270 mg/kg × 1–4 days | Hemorrhagic myocardial necrosis | Rare | Occurs with induced myelosuppression for bone marrow transplantation. Potentiates anthracycline-induced cardiomyopathy. |
| dactinomycin | 0.25 mg/m² × 5 days | Cardiomyopathy | Rare | Seen with previous anthracycline exposure. |
| daunorubicin | 400–550 mg/m² (lifetime dose) | Transient EKG changes Cardiomyopathy | 0–41% 1.5% | Increased risk with concomitant cyclophosphamide or previous chest irradiation. Young children and the elderly are most susceptible. |
| diethylstilbestrol (DES) | 5 mg q d | Thromboembolic myocardial infarction | CVA, frequent | Risk decreased by decreasing dose to 1 mg qd. |
| doxorubicin | 450–550 mg/m² (lifetime dose) | Transient EKG changes Cardiomyopathy | 2.2% 1–5% | Same as for daunorubicin. |
| doxydoxorubicin (DXDX; synthetic anthracycline) | 25–30 mg/m² | CHF (cumulative dose-related cardiotoxicity with 250 mg/m²) | Rare | Radionuclide ejected fraction performed after pt receives 150 mg/m² cumulative dose. Repeat at each dose of 250 mg/m². |
| 4'-epidoxorubicin (anthracycline analogue) | 100mg/m² q 3 wks or 60 mg/m² dl, 8 q 28 days; 900mg/m² (lifetime dose) | Transient EKG changes, ventricular extrasystole CHF | 1% | Spectrum of activity is similar to doxorubicin. Incidence of CHF is 1.6% when cumulative when doses of 700 mg/m² are given. |
| estramustine | 600 mg/m² po in 3 divided doses | Hypertension, angina, myocardial infarction, arrhythmias, pulmonary emboli | 10–15% | Increased risk with history of cardiovascular disease. |

| Agent | Dose | Cardiac Toxicity | Incidence | Comments |
|---|---|---|---|---|
| estrogens | 5 mg qd | CHF with ischemic heart disease, thromboembolic CVA | 39% | Increased risk with history of cardiovascular disease. |
| etoposide (VP-16) | Unknown | Myocardial infarction | Rare | May be worsened with prior mediastinal XRT and preexisting coronary artery disease. |
| fluorouracil | 12–15 mg/kg q wk; 1000 mg/m² qd 1–4 days as continuous infusion | Angina 3–18 hrs after drug administered; or during high-dose continuous infusion | Rare | Not necessarily with preexisting cardiovascular disease. Can recur with subsequent doses. Cardiac enzymes are normal. |
| mithramycin | 25–50 mg/kg IV qod × 3–8 days | Cardiomyopathy | Rare | Exacerbates subclinical anthracycline-induced cardiotoxicity. |
| mitomycin | 15 mg/m² q 6–8 wks | Cardiomyopathy | Rare | Increased risk with previous chest irradiation or anthracycline exposure. Synergistic with anthracyclines. |
| mitoxantrone | a. 12–14 mg/m² q 3 wks b. 100 mg/m² lifetime dose with prior exposure to anthracyclines c. 160 mg/m² lifetime dose without prior exposure to anthracyclines | a. Transient EKG changes b. Decreased ejection fraction c. CHF | a. 28% b. 44% c. 2.1–12.5% | Increased risk of cardiomyopathy with previous anthracycline exposure, chest irradiation, or cardiovascular disease. CHF has occurred in pts who have not received prior anthracycline therapy. |
| paclitaxel | 135 mg/m² or higher | Asymptomatic bradycardia; rarely may progress to heart block Rarely, chest pain, brief ventricular tachycardia or supraventricular tachycardia | 29% | Asymptomatic bradycardia may occur during or up to 8 hrs after paclitaxel infusion; one fatal myocardial infarction has been reported. |
| vincristine and vinblastine | Unknown | Myocardial infarction | Rare | Phenomena not well described. |

*Source:* Adapted with permission from Kaszyk, L.K. (1986). Cardiac toxicity associated with cancer therapy. *Oncology Nursing Forum 13*(4): 81–88.

doses of doxorubicin $> 300$ mg/m$^2$. Zinecard should not be used with the first cycle of doxorubicin therapy as it may diminish antitumor effects. Side effects of Zinecard include enhanced myelosuppression (more severe granulocytopenia and thrombocytopenia) and pain on injection. The dosage regimen is a 10:1 ratio (e.g., Zinecard 500 mg, doxorubicin 50 mg) given slow IVP or IVB within 30 minutes prior to the doxorubicin. The drug requires chemotherapy safety precautions during handling (Pharmacia, package insert 1995).

## II. PULMONARY TOXICITY

Pulmonary toxicity is another dose-limiting potentially lethal toxicity of certain chemotherapeutic agents, generally manifested as pulmonary fibrosis. The most well known of the drugs that may cause toxicity are bleomycin and the nitrosoureas (carmustine and busulfan). Others are listed in Table 4.19.

Bleomycin is preferentially distributed to the skin and lungs, and thus both these areas show drug toxicity. In the lungs, there is a decrease in type I pneumocytes and an increase and redistribution of type II pneumocytes into the alveolar spaces. There may be symptoms of pneumonitis. The alveolar septas become thickened and decreased in number, and there is an increase in the amount of collagen secreted by the interstitial fibroblasts, with resulting generalized interstitial fibrosis of the lung (Ginsberg and Comis 1984). If damage continues, end-stage interstitial fibrosis reveals obliteration of the alveoli and dilated air spaces, followed by a thickened, stiff interstitium (Seltzer, Goldstein, and Herman 1983). Pulmonary dysfunction is restrictive, with functionally decreased lung volume,

increased work of breathing, and impaired gas exchange (Wickham 1986). The incidence of bleomycin-induced pulmonary toxicity is 5–11% (Ginsberg and Comis 1984).

Nursing assessment features are (1) patients at risk for developing pulmonary toxicity, (2) signs and symptoms of dysfunction, and (3) evaluation of pulmonary function tests to identify early dysfunction.

Identified risk factors for bleomycin-induced pulmonary toxicity are the following:

1. *Age:* Risk increases with age, with risk 5% until age 70, then increasing to 15% after age 70 (Wickham 1986).

2. *Prior pulmonary or thoracic radiation:* Radiotherapy potentiates toxicity, and 35–55% of patients develop severe bleomycin toxicity (over 50% of these patients die of this toxicity). *Concurrent* radiotherapy and low-dose bleomycin cannot be safely given simultaneously due to the high incidence of pneumonitis and respiratory failure (Einhorn et al. 1976; Ginsberg and Comis 1984).

3. *Total cumulative dose:* Increased risk when $> 400–500$ units of bleomycin are administered. Overall, cumulative dose of $< 450$ units had an incidence of 3–5%, 450 units had 13% incidence, and 550 units had 17% incidence (10% mortality). However, this is unpredictable, and toxicity has occurred at lower cumulative doses (i.e., 50–60 units) (Blum, Carter, and Agre 1973).

4. *High peak serum levels:* Higher IV bolus administration of bleomycin ($25 \pm 2$ U/wk) had greater decreases in pulmonary function than lower doses ($16 \pm 1.6$ U/wk) (Comis et al. 1979). *Continuous infusion* of bleomycin appears to decrease the risk of pulmonary toxicity (Carlson and Sikic 1983).

5. *Preexisting lung disease:* Not well studied but requires careful administration; also, if patient smokes or has a smoking history, risk may increase (Yasko 1983).

6. *Receiving combination chemotherapy* with another potentially pulmonary toxic drug, such as cyclophosphamide (Yasko 1983).

7. *Exposure to high oxygen concentrations after bleomycin treatment:* There is a synergistic effect of toxicity—therefore, care must be taken to use $FiO_2$ << 100% during anesthesia for patients who have received bleomycin (Ginsberg and Comis 1984).

Early physical findings include dry hacking cough, fine bibasilar rales with dyspnea upon exertion, and decrease in DLCO (diffusion capacity). Chest X-ray often has only minimal changes but may show fine reticular bibasilar infiltrate (Ginsberg and Comis 1984).

Later signs are dyspnea at rest, tachypnea, fever, coarse rales, chest X-ray changes with consolidation, significant decrease in DLCO, and hypoxemia.

Pulmonary function tests are performed routinely *prior* to the initial dose of bleomycin to establish a baseline, and then are repeated serially during treatment. Diffusion capacity is the most sensitive indicator of injury (Wickham 1986). Bleomycin therapy should be discontinued if DLCO falls to ≤ 40% of initial testing, if FVC (forced vital capacity) falls to < 25% of initial testing, or if symptoms or physical findings indicating bleomycin toxicity are found (Ginsberg and Comis 1984). A correction factor is used if anemia is present.

It appears that if pulmonary function is identified early (i.e., when physical findings are minimal), and the patient has normal resting arterial oxygenation ($PO_2$), progressive pulmonary failure does not occur. However, if signs and symptoms of severe dysfunction occur—dyspnea at rest, hypoxemia ($PO_2$ < 55 mmHg), tachypnea, coarse rales, consolidation on chest X-ray—then

pulmonary injury usually is irreversible and progressive (Ginsberg and Comis 1984).

Acute hypersensitivity pulmonary toxicity may occur with a number of antineoplastic agents, including bleomycin, and is characterized by fever, diffuse infiltrates on chest X-ray, and eosinophilia. The condition appears to respond to steroid therapy (Ginsberg and Comis 1984). It is important to distinguish between the agents; steroids are of questionable value in treating bleomycin toxicity. Doses of steroids may vary and generally are 20–160 mg/day (Wickham 1986). Pulmonary toxicity related to other antineoplastic agents is shown in Table 4.19.

The nursing goal is to identify early dysfunction and discontinue the drug to prevent progressive pulmonary toxicity.

## III. HEPATOTOXICITY

The liver is an important site of cancer chemotherapy drug metabolism, yet it withstands significant damage from most of the drugs due to the slow growth of hepatocytes (Perry 1984). Drugs metabolized by the liver are alkylating agents (e.g., cyclophosphamide), nitrosoureas (e.g., BCNU, CCNU), plant alkaloids (e.g., vincristine), antimetabolites (e.g., 5-fluorouracil, cytosine arabinoside, methotrexate), antibiotics (e.g., doxorubicin), and miscellaneous drugs such as procarbazine. However, certain drugs are hepatotoxic, as shown in Table 4.20.

Factors that increase the risk of hepatotoxicity when potentially hepatotoxic drugs are given are as follows (Goodman 1987):

1. previous or concurrent hepatic irradiation (vincristine and abdominal radiation)
2. concurrent administration of other hepatotoxic drugs (e.g., 6-mercaptopurine and doxorubicin; cyclophosphamide and methotrexate)
3. active hepatitis

**Table 4.19  Drugs That Can Induce Pulmonary Toxicity**

| Drug | Risk Factors | Signs and Symptoms/Comments |
|------|--------------|------------------------------|
| *Incidence: Frequent* | | |
| bleomycin | Age > 70<br>Dose: At 400–500 U constant low rate, at 500 U rate increases but can occur at low doses<br>High $O_2$ exposure, thoracic radiation, and renal dysfunction | Dry cough, dyspnea, tachypnea, fever, and rales, which can progress to coarse rhonchi and occasional pleural friction rub<br><br>Incidence: 5–11% |
| carmustine (BCNU) | Preexisting lung disease, tobacco use, industrial exposure, possible synergism with cyclophosphamide and thoracic radiation<br>Dose: > 1000 mg/m², linear toxicity effect | Variable, none to dyspnea; dry cough; bibasilar crepitant rales<br>Incidence: 20–30%<br>Mortality: 24–80% |
| *Incidence: Moderate* | | |
| busulfan | Thoracic radiation: 500 mg may be threshhold dose for toxicity | Insidious onset; dyspnea, dry cough, and fever progressive over weeks to months; bilateral basilar crepitant rales and tachypnea |
| methotrexate delayed | Daily and weekly schedules most likely to result in toxicity | Prodromal symptoms; headache and malaise, dyspnea, dry cough, and fever for days to weeks; tachypnea, cyanosis, rales, skin eruptions—16%; eosinophilia—50%; steroid therapy may be helpful |
| *Incidence: Moderate to low* | | |
| cyclophosphamide | None identified, but frequently reported in patients with Hodgkin's and non-Hodgkin's lymphoma; possibly related to concurrent bleomycin | Dyspnea, fever, dry cough, tachypnea, scattered rales, rarely chest pain or pleural rub |
| mitomycin | High concentration of $O_2$ | Progressive dyspnea, nonproductive cough, bibasilar rales; may occur with low doses and after first dose; may be associated with renal toxicity |
| fludarabine | Concurrenent administration with pentostatin (deoxycofomycin) has resulted in fatal pulmonary toxicity | Pneumonia occurs in 16–22% of patients. Pulmonary hypersensitivity is characterized by dyspnea, cough, interstitial pulmonary infiltrate |
| *Incidence: Low* | | |
| chlorambucil | None identified; duration of therapy 6 mos to > 2 yrs; total dose > 2 gm | Dyspnea, dry cough, fever developing over 1–2 mos; bibasilar rales, anorexia, fatigue |
| cytosine arabinoside | None identified | Dyspnea and tachypnea develop during or after therapy, associated with GI lesions; rare pulmonary edema |
| melphalan | None identified; total dose 80 mg to > 3 gm; duration of therapy 2–83 mos | Rapid progressive dyspnea and fever over 2–10 days; tachypnea, rales common |

*(continued)*

**Table 4.19**  Drugs That Can Induce Pulmonary Toxicity *(continued)*

| Drug | Risk Factors | Signs and Symptoms/Comments |
|---|---|---|
| *Incidence: Rare* | | |
| Chlorozotocin | None identified | Exertional dyspnea, rales, fatigue |
| etoposide | Questionable synergism with methotrexate | Fever, dyspnea, cough, dry rales, cyanosis, tachypnea |
| lomustine | Dose: > 1100 mg/m$^2$ Questionable synergism with other pulmonary-toxic chemotherapy | Dyspnea, tachypnea, weight loss, anorexia |
| mercaptopurine | None identified | Acute respiratory distress |
| methotrexate | | Pulmonary edema, acute onset of dyspnea, tachypnea 6–12 hrs after oral or intrathecal (IT) drug administration |
| procarbazine | None identified; potential risk for hypersensitivity-prone individuals | Fever, chills, eosinophilia, rash, cough, dyspnea, progressive pulmonary insufficiency; rapid recovery after discontinuation of drug |
| semustine | None identified | Exertional dyspnea, rales, pleural friction rub |
| Spirogermanium | None identified: potential risk for patients previously treated with other chemotherapy or thoracic radiation | Progressive cough, dyspnea, fatigue, and fever; onset of symptoms insidious |
| teniposide | Previous treatment with XRT to spinal axis and BCNU | Dyspnea, cyanosis, tachypnea |
| vindesine and vinblastine | Seen in patients treated simultaneously with mitomycin | Acute onset; dyspnea and cough, tachypnea, rales |
| Zinostatin | None identified | Dry cough, hemoptysis, progressive pulmonary insufficiency |

*Source:* Modified from Wickham, R. (1986). Pulmonary toxicity secondary to cancer treatment. *Oncology Nursing Forum* 13(5): 69–76.

Injury to the hepatocytes is first manifested by elevations of liver function tests (LFTs): serum glutamic oxaloacetic transaminase (SGOT) and serum glutamic pyruvic transaminase (SGPT), bilirubin, lactic dehydrogenase (LDH), and alkaline phosphatase (Goodman 1987). Alterations in these LFTs can be temporary and transient or progress to hepatic cirrhosis when the drug (e.g., methotrexate, mercaptopurine) is used continuously on a long-term basis (Dorr and Fritz 1981). Certain drugs, such as L-asparaginase and mithramycin, can cause acute injury to the liver and require dose modifications. Liver function tests should be monitored when mithramycin is used in low doses for management of hypercalcemia. Other drugs produce more delayed or chronic injury as shown in Table 4.21. A recent cause of hepatotoxicity is veno-occlusive disease of the liver, and as more bone marrow transplantations are performed, it is expected that this complication will increase. Veno-occlusive disease and subsequent hepatotoxicity have been reported after treatment with mitomycin C, carmustine, cytosine arabinoside, busulfan, and cyclophosphamide (Perry 1984).

The taxanes, paclitaxel and docetaxel, as well as the antimetabolite capecitabine can cause elevations in bilirubin and alkaline phosphatase. These drugs should not be given if severe hyperbilirubinemia develops (Wilkes et al. 1999).

Nursing management issues concern pretreatment and post-treatment analysis: (1) identifying the drugs that are potentially hepatotoxic, identifying patient risk factors, such as preexisting liver disease or history of alcohol abuse, and monitoring the patient's baseline and pretreatment liver function values; and (2) assessment of the patient's hepatic function prior to subsequent drug administration. An abnormal liver test should be investigated to determine whether it is drug related and the patient may require a liver biopsy, abdominal ultrasound, or abdominal CT.

Finally, because it is clear that many antineoplastic drugs are metabolized by the liver, if

**Table 4.20   Potential Hepatotoxicity of Chemotherapeutic Agents**

| Drug | Toxicity | Comments |
|---|---|---|
| amsacrine (investigational) | Mild increase in bilirubin in 20–40% patients; rare hepatic failure | |
| *Nitrosoureas* | | |
| (carmustine, lomustine) | Increased LFTs, normalize in 1 wk Rare veno-occlusive disease in BMT | Appears dose related; hold drug for prolonged elevations |
| streptozocin | Increased LFTs (in ~ 15% patients) | Occurs with usual and high doses; does not usually require treatment |
| *Antimetabolites* | | |
| methotrexate | Increased SGOT, LDH (short, frequent doses or high doses); fibrosis, cirrhosis (long-term use) | Resolve within 1 mo after treatment stops; avoid use in patients with Laennec's cirrhosis or preexisting liver disease |
| 6-mercaptopurine | Increased bilirubin, SGOT, alkaline phosphatase; cholestasis, necrosis | Usually not given to patients with preexisting liver disease; discontinue drug if increased LFTs occur—usually related to doses > 2 mg/kg/day |
| cytosine arabinoside | Increased LFTs | |
| hydroxyurea | Rare increase in LFTs, hepatitis | |
| capecitabine | Increase in bilirubin, alkaline phosphatase | Dose reduce for hyperbilirubinemia |
| *Antibiotics* | | |
| mithramycin | Acute necrosis, altered LFTs, clotting factors | Stop drug or reduce dose |
| Bisantrene | Rare hepatitis | |
| *Enzymes* | | |
| L-asparaginase | Fatty changes, with decreased albumin, clotting factor synthesis; impaired handling of lipids | Usually improves after treatment stopped, resolving over days to weeks |
| *Miscellaneous* | | |
| dacarbazine | Transient increase in SGPT, SGOT, bilirubin (diffuse hepatocellular dysfunction); also reported venoocclusive disease—rare | Treatment not usually necessary |
| *Alkylating agents* | | |
| chlorambucil | Hepatitis, dysfunction | Stop drug |
| cisplatin | Steatosis and cholestasis | |
| busulfan | Cholestatic jaundice | |
| *Plant alkaloids* | | |
| paclitaxel | Usually mild increase in LFTs | Incidence 7–22%; dose reduce if severe toxicity |
| doxetaxel | Increased bilirubin and aklkaline phosphatase | Stop drug if severe toxicity |

*Sources:* Perry, M.C. (1984). Hepatotoxicity. In M.C. Perry and J.W. Yarbro (eds.): *Toxicity of Chemotherapy*. Orlando: Grune and Stratton, 297–312; Dorr, R.T., and Fritz, W.L. (1981). *Cancer Chemotherapy Handbook*. New York: Elsevier, 130–133; Goodman, M.S. (1987). *Cancer: Chemotherapy and Care*. Evansville, Ind.: Bristol-Myers USP&NG, 32–33.

**Table 4.21**  Suggested Dose Modification with Hepatic Dysfunction (% of usual dose to administer, if any, on the day of treatment)

| Drug | Bili < 1.5% and SGOT < 60 IU | Bili = 1.5–3.0 SGOT = 60–180 | Bili = 3.1–5.0 or SGOT > 180 | Bili > 5.0 |
|---|---|---|---|---|
| 5-fluorouracil | 100% | 100% | 100% | Omit |
| cyclophosphamide | 100% | 100% | 75% | Omit |
| methotrexate | | | 75% | Omit |
| mitoxantrone | 100% | 75% | 50% | Omit |
| daunorubicin | 100% | 75% | 50% | Omit |
| doxorubicin | 100% | 50% | 25% | Omit |
| vinblastine | 100% | 50% | Omit | Omit |
| vincristine | 100% | 50% | 25%* | Omit |
| VP-16 | 100% | 50% | 25%* | Omit |
| VM-26 | 100% | 50% | 25% | Omit |

*Source:* Modified from Perry, M.C. (1984). Hepatotoxicity. In M.C. Perry and J.W. Yarbro (eds.): *Toxicity of Chemotherapy.* Orlando: Grune and Stratton, 297–312. Fischer D.S., and Knobf, M.T. (1989). *The Cancer Chemotherapy Handbook.* 3rd ed. Chicago: Year Book Medical Publishers.

hepatic dysfunction occurs, certain drug dosages must be adjusted, as shown in Table 4.21. Otherwise, as the drug has a decreased rate of metabolic breakdown and excretion, circulating serum levels of the drug would be higher than normal, increasing drug toxicity. The nurse should discuss dose modification with the physician prior to drug administration.

## IV. NEPHROTOXICITY

Chemotherapy-induced renal damage can occur directly, via direct injury to renal cells by specific chemotherapeutic agents, (e.g., cisplatin, methotrexate), or indirectly, by metabolic changes following treatment (e.g., hyperuricemic nephropathy related to rapid tumor cell lysis) (Yasko 1983). Renal toxicity may be acute, chronic, or delayed. The usual signs are increased blood urea nitrogen (BUN), increased serum creatinine (Cr), and decreased renal clearance of creatinine. Risk factors are preexisting renal disease, volume depletion, and concomitant use of nephrotoxic drugs.

Specific drugs that are potential nephrotoxins are cisplatin, methotrexate, and the nitrosoureas, as shown in Table 4.22.

*Cisplatin*, a heavy metal with an alkylating action, can cause proximal and distal renal tubular necrosis (Schilsky 1984) and can decrease the ability of the renal tubules to resorb magnesium and calcium (Lydon 1986). Nephrotoxicity is a dose-limiting toxicity; it is mild and reversible with low doses but may become severe and permanent with high doses and multiple courses of therapy (Lydon 1986). Abnormalities include increased BUN and creatinine, decreased creatinine clearance, hypomagnesemia, hypocalcemia, and proteinuria. On a cellular level, focal degeneration of basement membrane, hyaline droplets in renal tubules, and tubular necrosis can occur (Dentino et al. 1978). Newer platinum analogues, such as carboplatin, are not nephrotoxic and often replace cisplatin use.

Renal toxicity is minimized by vigorous saline hydration of at least 100–150 cc/hr (cisplatin reabsorption by the kidney is prevented by a platinum-chloride complex formation), to provide a urine output of at least 100 cc/hr. In some settings, mannitol is used to mobilize extracellular fluid into the vascular space and increase renal blood flow and filtration, or Lasix is used for similar purposes. Research has shown that mannitol and Lasix are equal in their protection (Ostrow et al. 1981), but it is not clear that saline and diuretics are superior to saline hydration alone (Lydon 1986). Also, hypertonic saline and longer infusion time appear to decrease nephrotoxicity (Ozols et al. 1982). It appears that cisplatin is unstable in low chlorine concentrations, exchanging a chloride group for a hydroxyl or $H_2O$ group, and the resulting molecule is felt to be the nephrotoxic element (Lydon 1986). Hypertonic (3%) saline decreases the formation of these molecules, and thus decreases cisplatin-induced nephrotoxicity (Ozols et al. 1982). Risk factors that increase toxicity are preexisting renal dysfunction and administration of concurrent nephrotoxic antibiotics. Magnesium repletion is usually required and can be given in the hydration fluid.

*Methotrexate*, an antimetabolite, is excreted via the kidneys, with 90% of conventional doses excreted unchanged in the urine (Schilsky 1984). It may cause injury by crystallizing or precipitating in the tubules and collecting ducts, causing subsequent obstructive nephropathy (Abelson and Garnick 1982). Precipitation is increased in an acid environment. Damage is rare and reversible with short-term low-dose treatment, but the patient's BUN and Creatinine should be monitored prior to treatment. Incidence is high with high-dose methotrexate (1–15 gm/m$^2$) and can be permanent, but it can be prevented by (1) vigorous hydration before, during, and after treatment (100 ml/m$^2$/hr) to produce a diuresis of at least 150 cc/hr; (2) alkalinization of the urine with sodium bicarbonate or diamox, as this decreases drug precipitation in

the renal tubule; (3) close monitoring of serum methotrexate levels; and (4) administration of calcium leucovorin rescue doses exactly on time (Lydon 1986). Risk factors increasing nephrotoxicity include preexisting renal dysfunction; pleural and other effusions in which the drug can be sequestered and released slowly into the systemic circulation; dehydration or volume depletion; concomitant use of salicylates, sulfonamides, and probenecid, which displace drugs from albumin; and increased circulating serum levels of methotrexate.

In the event of renal dysfunction resulting from high-dose methotrexate (HDMTX) therapy, renal excretion of the drug is decreased and systemic serum levels of the drug are elevated. This causes more severe systemic toxicity, such as mucositis and bone marrow depression. Therefore, nursing care of patients receiving HDMTX therapy is quite precise and demands scrupulous attention to details to prevent nephrotoxicity.

In caring for patients receiving nephrotoxic drugs, assessment *must* include renal function, electrolyte balance, and degree of hydration (Goodman 1987). Drug administration may have to wait until these are corrected.

Assessment of renal function is essential prior to administration of any drug that is excreted by the kidneys. If there is compromised renal function, then the drug dose is often reduced or discontinued until renal function improves. These drugs include bleomycin, cisplatin, cyclophosphamide, methotrexate, mithramycin, and the nitrosoureas.

The *nitrosoureas* include streptozocin. Streptozocin may cause tubulointerstitial nephritis and tubular atrophy, resulting in (1) electrolyte imbalance (hypophosphatemia, hypokalemia, hyperchloremia) and (2) renal dysfunction (elevated BUN and creatinine, decreased creatinine clearance, with urinary wasting of protein, glucose, phosphorus, and

**Table 4.22**  Relative Risks of Chemotherapeutic Agents: Nephrotoxicity

| Drug | Pathophysiology | Laboratory Abnormalities | Nursing Interventions |
|---|---|---|---|
| *I. High risk of immediate nephrotoxicity* | | | |
| A. cisplatin | A. Proximal and distal renal tubule injury produces tubular necrosis, focal degeneration of basement membrane, hyaline droplet deposits in renal tubules<br>1. *Mild*, reversible with low doses<br>2. *Severe*, permanent damage with high doses and multiple courses | A. ↑ BUN and creatinine, ↓ creatinine clearance, azotemia, ↓ serum magnesium, ↓ serum calcium; renal wasting with hypermagnesuria, hypercalcuria, proteinuria, enzymuria | A. 1. Saline hydration at least 100–150 ml/hr<br>2. Diuresis with mannitol or furosemide<br>3. Post-treatment hydration of at least 3 L/day<br>4. Prevent dehydration and vomiting |
| B. High-dose methotrexate | B. Drug crystallizes or precipitates in renal tubules and collecting ducts; directly affects renal tubular cells; directly affects afferent vascular supply, resulting in ↓ glomerular filtration rate (GFR)<br>1. Rare and reversible with short-term low doses<br>2. Occasional long-term, low-dose permanent dysfunction<br>3. High incidence with high dose, usually reversible but with significant systemic drug toxicity | B. ↑ BUN and creatinine, oliguria/anuria, azotemia, acidosis, hypokalemia, anemia, osteomalacia, hypophosphatemia, aminoaciduria | B. 1. Vigorous hydration to maintain high urine flow<br>2. Alkalinize urine to pH ≥ 7.0<br>3. Prevent dehydration, vomiting<br>4. Prevent systemic drug toxicity<br>  a. Leucovorin rescue *exactly* on time until methotrexate level < 5 × $10^{-8}$M (Shilsky 1984)<br>  b. Effusions should be drained *prior to* drug administration<br>  c. Eliminate concomitant administration of sulfonamides, salicylates, probenecid |
| C. streptozocin | C. 10–20% of intact, active drug is excreted by kidneys, with primary injury on renal tubules and glomeruli, resulting in tubular interstitial nephritis and tubular atrophy<br>1. Low doses produce transient, reversible damage<br>2. Continued therapy can lead to severe and permanent chronic renal failure<br>3. Dose-limiting factor | C. ↑ BUN and creatinine, ↓ creatinine clearance, hypophosphatemia, hypokalemia, hyperchloremia, proteinuria, glycosuria, aminoaciduria, phosphaturia | C. 1. Adequate hydration during and 24 hrs after treatment<br>2. Prevent vomiting, dehydration<br>3. Assess 24-hr urine creatinine clearance before treatment |

*(continued)*

**Table 4.22  Relative Risks of Chemotherapeutic Agents: Nephrotoxicity (continued)**

| Drug | Pathophysiology | Laboratory Abnormalities | Nursing Interventions |
|---|---|---|---|
| D. High-dose mithramycin | D. Direct damage to renal tubules, causing distal and proximal tubule necrosis<br>1. Rare with low dose<br>2. High incidence with high dose and may be permanent | D. ↑ BUN and serum creatinine, azotemia, proteinuria, hypophosphatemia, hypomagnesemia, hypokalemia, hypocalcemia | D. 1. Monitor renal function<br>2. No prevention strategies; however, high doses rarely administered |
| E. ifosfamide | E. Renal toxicity incidence ~ 6%, apparently related to tubular damage<br>1. Laboratory abnormalities usually transient<br>2. Bladder irritation, consisting of hemorrhagic cystitis, dysuria, and urinary frequency, occurs in 6–92% of patients without uroprotection<br>3. Urotoxicity is dose dependent | E. ↑ BUN and serum creatinine, ↓ urine creatinine clearance, rare proteinuria, acidosis<br>1. Microscopic hematuria | E. 1. Monitor kidney function (laboratory tests), vigorous hydration<br>2. Uroprotector must be administered with ifosfamide (i.e., mesna)<br>  a. Assess urine for presence of RBC prior to subsequent dosing<br>  b. Manufacturer recommends urinalysis be assessed prior to each drug dose<br>    1) If microscopic hematuria present (> 10 RBC/high power field), dose should be held until complete resolution<br>    2) Further drug administration should be given with vigorous oral/parenteral hydration |
| II. *High risk of nephrotoxicity from long-term use* | | | |
| A. nitrosoureas (BCNU, CCNU, MeCCNU) | A. Postulated that drug binds irreversibly to amino acid residues → glomerular and tubular damage, decrease in kidney size<br>1. Uncommon with doses < 1000 mg/m² <br>2. In high dose, chronic renal failure may occur | A. ↑ BUN and serum creatinine, ↓ glomerular filtration rate (GFR), azotemia, proteinuria | A. 1. No prevention strategies; suggest hydration during and after drug administration (oral fluids to 3 L/day for 24 hrs)<br>2. Frequent long-term follow-up, as renal failure may occur up to 5 years later |
| B. mitomycin C | B. Postulated drug interferes with DNA synthesis and induces immune complex deposits, damaging glomeruli and tubules<br>1. Cumulative toxicity<br>2. Mild and reversible to fatal renal failure (i.e., if hemolytic uremic syndrome [HUS] develops) | B. 1. ↑ BUN, azotemia, proteinuria<br>2. HUS: hypertension, hematuria, anemia, thrombocytopenia | B. 1. No prevention strategies<br>2. Suggest hydration during and 24 hrs post-treatment<br>3. Assess renal function |

3. Renal vasculitis may be increased with concurrent 5-fluorouracil administration

III. *Moderate risk of nephrotoxicity*

A. cyclophosphamide

   1. Drug metabolites may injure collecting ducts and distal renal tubules, causing impaired water excretion and dilutional hyponatremia (SIADH) at high doses (> 50 mg/kg)

   2. Drug metabolites irritate stretched bladder capillaries, causing hemorrhagic cystitis

   3. Preventable

   4. Dose-limiting

B. Low-dose methotrexate — See pathophysiology—high-dose methotrexate

C. 5-azacytidine (investigational) — Tubular damage and renal insufficiency possible when given in combination with other drugs

D. High-dose 6-thioguanine — High dose (oral or IV) appears to induce reversible toxicity, possibly by inhibiting purine metabolism

E. L-asparaginase — Prerenal azotemia

A. SIADH: Lab values of water intoxication: serum hyponatremia, ↑ urine osmolality ↓ serum osmolality, ↓ urinary output

  A. 1. Monitor electrolytes, treat SIADH if it occurs

    2. Prevent by aggressive hydration (at least 3 L/day)

    3. Encourage pt to void at least q 2–3 hrs

    4. Do not administer at noc

B. Hemorrhagic cystitis: urinary frequency, urgency, dysuria, hematuria

  B. No nursing interventions

C. ↑ BUN and creatinine, azotemia, acidosis, hyperphosphatemia, hypomagnesemia, hypocalcemia, glycosuria, sodium wasting, aminoaciduria

  C. No prevention strategies known; assess renal function prior to each dose

D. ↑ BUN and creatinine, azotemia

  D. No prevention strategies; monitor renal function studies prior to each dose

E. ↑ BUN

  E. Use cautiously with nephrotoxic antibiotics; monitor renal function studies

IV. *Low-risk of nephroxoticity*

A. Anthracyclines (doxorubicin in high doses, daunorubicin)

B. Low-dose mithramycin

C. Tenoposide (VM-26)

D. 5-fluorouracil

E. vincristine (SIADH, ↓ serum Na⁺⁺, inappropriate urinary sodium wasting)

F. 6-mercaptopurine (hematuria, requires dose reduction)

G. carboplatin (rare tubular damage)

H. hydroxyurea (mild, reversible, requires dosage reduction)

*Source:* Modified from Lydon, J. (1986). Nephrotoxicity of cancer treatment. *Oncology Nursing Forum* 13(2): 68–77.

amino acids) (Lydon 1986). Injury to the renal tubules and glomeruli is transient and reversible with low doses, but with continued therapy it often causes chronic interstitial nephritis with progressive renal failure, which continues after treatment is stopped (Perry and Yarbo 1984). Hydration during and 24 hours after therapy is important, as well as pretreatment BUN and creatinine and 24-hour creatinine determination. The other nitrosoureas (BCNU, CCNU, and MeCCNU) cause glomerular and renal tubule damage at cumulative doses above 1000 mg/m$^2$. Hydration is important, but renal failure can develop up to 5 years after treatment is completed, and long-term renal follow-up is essential.

Indirect injury to the kidneys can occur when there is rapid tumor lysis. Patients with large, bulky chemosensitive tumors or rapidly proliferating tumors, such as acute leukemia, Burkitt's lymphoma, and diffuse histiocytic lymphomas, are at risk to develop hyperuricemic nephropathy and renal failure. With the destruction (lysis) of large numbers of malignant cells, there is a release of excessive amounts of nucleic acids, which are converted to uric acid. In an acid environment, uric acid is less soluble, and the high concentration of uric acid to be excreted may lead to precipitation of uric acid crystals in the distal nephron, especially the collecting ducts, where urine concentration is maximal (Fields, Josse, and Bergsagel 1982). Signs and symptoms are characteristic of acute renal failure, with oliguria or anuria, hyperuricemia (> 8 mg/dl), and often uric acid crystals in the urine. Without intervention, this progresses to uremia. Rapid reversal of renal failure usually occurs with the administration of allopurinol but may require hemodialysis (Schilsky 1984). Early recovery is manifested by the onset of diuresis (Fields et al. 1982).

The most important intervention is the *prevention* of acute hyperuricemic nephropathy, using the following treatment (Schilsky 1984):

1. *Intravenous hydration* to produce a urinary output of at least 100 cc/hr (requires > 3 L/24 hrs) to increase renal tubular filtration.

2. *Urinary alkalinization* to increase urine pH ≥ 7.0, thus increasing uric acid solubility (requires adding NaHCO$_3$ 50–100 mg to each liter of IV fluid, or administration of acetazolamide 250–500 mg/day (if not contraindicated).

3. *Allopurinol* administration to decrease the formation of uric acid (requires 500 mg/m$^2$ for 2–3 days, and then reduced to 200 mg/m$^2$/day). Allopurinol inhibits xanthine oxidase, an enzyme that is essential to the degradation of nucleic acid (purines) to uric acid.

Hyperuricemic nephropathy may occur as a separate entity or, if accompanied by the rapid release of intracellular ions, is called *tumor lysis syndrome* (TLS). This syndrome is considered a metabolic emergency. Patients at risk for both TLS and hyperuricemic nephropathy are those with large, rapidly proliferating tumors (i.e., lymphomas with LDH > 1500, leukemias, and small cell lung cancer). Also at risk are patients with preexisting renal dysfunction with creatinine ≥ 1.6 mg/dl and uric acid ≥ 8 mg/dl (Moore 1985).

Symptoms are characteristic of the metabolic abnormalities and include:

- weakness
- confusion
- irritability
- numbness, tingling
- muscle cramping

Preventive treatment should begin 12-24 hours prior to chemotherapy administration in high-risk patients, as previously discussed (Schilsky 1984): (1) vigorous hydration, (2) urinary alkalinization, (3) administration of allopurinol. During the first 24–48 hours of therapy, serum electrolytes, calcium, phosphorus, and creatinine should be assessed every 6–8 hours (Schilsky 1984). In addition, the nurse should strictly monitor (1) intake and output, total body fluid balance, and daily weights to identify fluid overload or retention or inadequate renal flow; (2) vital signs to assess circulatory tolerance of hydration and the development of arhythmias; and (3) urine for pH $\geq 7.0$ and assess for the presence of uric acid crystals. The risk period of rapid tumor cell lysis lasts 5–7 days after chemotherapy administration, and usually the above measures are adequate to prevent TLS. However, if severe

**Table 4.23**  Nursing Protocol for the Management of Tumor Lysis Syndrome

| Problem | Intervention |
|---|---|
| Fluid balance | Administer IV hydration. Monitor weight, I&O, response to diuretics. Observe for signs of fluid overload, especially patients with potential or preexisting cardiac damage. |
| Electrolyte balance | Monitor electrolytes q day or q 6–12 hrs as indicated. Correct imbalances as prescribed. |
| | Observe for signs of hyperkalemia: weakness, flaccid paralysis, EKG changes, cardiac arrest. |
| Potential renal failure | Monitor $Ca^{++}$, $PO4^+$, uric acid, BUN, and creatinine daily for the 5–7-day period of cytolysis. |
| | Maintain hydration, especially if preexisting renal insufficiency (creatinine > 1.6 mg/dL, uric acid $\geq 8$ mg/dL), and monitor urinary output. |
| | Administer allopurinol 300–800 mg PO q day. |
| | Monitor urine pH: maintain $\geq 7$ by administering IV $NaHCO_3$ as prescribed. |
| | Report decreased urine output, lethargy. |
| | Prepare to manage patient on temporary hemodialysis if renal failure develops. |
| Potential effects of drug therapy | Observe for side effects from allopurinol: skin rashes, GI disturbances, fever (rarely), vasculitis, and blood dyscrasias. |
| | Decrease doses of 6-MP and azathioprine if given concurrently with allopurinol. |
| Potential cardiac irritability | Monitor lab values for increased K+ and decreased $Ca^{++}$. |
| | Check pulse rate and rhythm frequently. Report irregularity. |
| | Observe for EKG changes, cardiac arrest. |
| Potential neuromuscular irritability | Monitor serum $Ca^{++}$ level. |
| | Observe for symptoms of hypocalcemia: tetany, positive Chvostek's and Trousseau's signs. |

*Source:* Adapted from  Moore, J. (1985). Metabolic emergencies: Tumor lysis syndrome. In B.L. Johnson and J. Gross (eds.): *Handbook of Oncology Nursing.* New York: John Wiley and Sons, 470–476.

$Ca^{++}$ = ionized calcium; K+ = ionized potassium; 6-MP = 6-mercaptopurine; $NaHCO_3$ = sodium bicarbonate; PO4$^+$ = phosphate ion(s).

metabolic derangements occur, hemodialysis may be necessary. See Table 4.23 for nursing interventions.

# V. NEUROTOXICITY

Neurotoxicity may occur following specific drug treatment, but, as neurologic signs and symptoms usually occur at some time during the course of malignancy, it is important to distinguish those related to drug toxicity (Kaplan and Wiernik 1984). Injury can be to the central nervous system, with resulting acute or chronic encephalopathies, or to peripheral nerves, producing neuropathies related to demyelination and axonal degeneration (Goodman 1986; Holden and Felde 1987). Toxicity can occur soon after drug administration or up to years after treatment (Yasko 1983). The potential neurotoxicities that can occur are summarized in Table 4.24. Table 4.25 describes the specific drug-related neurotoxicities.

## Central Nervous System (CNS) Toxicity

Chemotherapy may be toxic to the central nervous system through a number of different mechanisms. This section describes specific drugs, their associated neurological toxicities, and nursing implications.

Following intrathecal administration of drugs such as methotrexate and cytosine arabinoside to treat or prevent CNS metastasis, there may be signs of arachnoiditis or meningial irritation. These signs include stiff neck, headache, nausea and vomiting, fever, and lethargy. They begin 2–4 hours after drug administration and last 12–72 hours (Kaplan and Wiernik 1984). The incidence of arachnoiditis is significantly reduced by (1) the use of *preservative-free* drug and diluent (if the nurse assists the physician in intrathecal drug administration, it is imperative to ensure that

this is used) and (2) delivery of small doses of drug over several days, perhaps via an Ommaya reservoir, rather than large, intermittent doses (Kaplan and Wiernik 1984).

Both methotrexate and cytosine arabinoside in high doses effectively cross the blood-brain barrier, and it is therefore critical that these drugs be reconstituted with a preservative-free diluent, again to prevent arachnoiditis.

Chronic encephalopathies may occur with intraventricular or intrathecal methotrexate administration and can be either subacute and transient or chronic. Radiation increases the risk of CNS damage when given in combination with intrathecal methotrexate or if radiotherapy to the CNS is given prior to methotrexate (Kaplan and Wiernik 1984). One syndrome is necrotizing leukoencephalopathy, which is characterized by demyelination, multifocal white matter necrosis, and damage to the nerve axons (Kaplan and Wiernik 1984). Signs and symptoms include confusion, drooling, somnolence or irritability, ataxia, tremors, dementia, spasticity, quadraparesis, and slurred speech.

Cytosine arabinoside in high doses (greater than 3 gm/m$^2$ times 4–8 doses for treatment of adult acute myelocytic leukemias) has resulted in dose-limiting acute encephalopathies characterized by somnolence, altered personality, difficulty carrying out calculations, headaches, or seizures. This was seen frequently with cerebellar dysfunction, and the severity was parallel. Age over 50 was an increased risk factor (Herzig et al. 1987).

An acute cerebellar syndrome may occur after high-dose bolus injection of 5-fluorouracil, believed related to high peak plasma levels of the drug (Goodman 1987). Signs include dysmetria (difficulty controlling muscle movement), ataxia of trunk or extremities, unsteady gait, slurred speech, nystagmus, dizziness, and oculomotor disturbances (Kaplan and Wiernik

**Table 4.24** Possible Neurologic Syndromes Caused by Antineoplastic Agents

| Acute Encephalopathies | Chronic Encephalopathies |
|---|---|
| Intrathecal methotrexate (MTX)—XRT | Necrotizing leukoencephalopathy |
| Radiotherapy (XRT) ± intrathecal (IT) MTX |   Radiotherapy—IT MTX |
| High-dose MTX ("stroke-like") |   IT or IV MTX |
| asparaginase (early and late) |   IT cytosine arabinoside (Ara-C) |
| hexamethylmelamine | Mineralizing microangiopathy |
| 5-fluorouracil (with allopurinol) |   XRT ± IT MTX |
| procarbazine | Cerebral atrophy |
| BCNU (intracarotid) |   IT MTX ± XRT |
| cisplatin (intracarotid) |   IT Ara-C ± XRT |
| cyclophosphamide | Pontine myelinolysis |
| 5-azacytidine |   XRT ± IT MTX |
| High-dose cytosine arabinoside (Ara-C) | |

| Arachnoiditis/Myelopathy | Acute Cerebellar Syndromes/Ataxia | Cerebral (Mental Status) Changes |
|---|---|---|
| Encephalomyelopathy | 5-fluorouracil | L-asparaginase |
|   IT or intraventricular | procarbazine | cisplatin |
|   MTX or high-dose MTX | hexamethylmelamine | carboplatin |
|   IT Ara-C | BCNU | ifosfamide |
|   IT thiotepa | | pentostatin |

**Neuropathies**

| Peripheral | Cranial | Ototoxicity |
|---|---|---|
| *Axonal degeneration* | vinca alkaloids | cisplatin |
| vinca alkaloids | cisplatin | misonidazole |
| misonidazole | 5-fluorouracil | |
| | carboplatin | |
| *Demyelination* | cyclophosphamide | |
| cisplatin | Levamisole | |

| *Sensory* | *Sensorimotor* | |
|---|---|---|
| vinca alkaloids | vinca alkaloids | |
| carboplatin | paclitaxel | |
| cisplatin | hexamethylmelamine | |
| cytarabine | docetaxel | |
| procarbazine | 5-azacytidine | |
| etaposide | | |
| misonidazole | *Uncertain* | |
| paclitaxel | hexamethylmelamine | |
| docetaxel | procarbazine | |
| | 5-azacytadine | |
| | VP-16 | |

*Source:* Modified from Kaplan, R.S., and Wiernik, P.H. (1984). Neurotoxicity of antitumor agents. In M.C. Perry and J.W. Yarbro (eds.): *Toxicity of Chemotheraphy*. Orlando: Grune and Stratton, 365–431.

**Table 4.25** Neurotoxicity of Anticancer Agents

| Drug | Incidence | Signs/Symptoms | Crosses BBB | Onset/Resolution | Dose Relation |
|---|---|---|---|---|---|
| *Plant alkaloids* | | | | | |
| vincristine | Common, dose-limiting | Paresthesias, constipation, loss of deep tendon reflexes (DTR), weakness, SIADH | – | 1–2 weeks to 1–3 months | High dose (> 2 mg/dose) and high cumulative doses |
| vinblastine | Rare, dose-limiting | Same as vincristine | – | Same as vincristine | Same as vincristine |
| etoposide | Rare (10–20%) | Peripheral neuropathy CNS: confusion, somnolence, seizures | – | Reversible | Increased incidence with high dose |
| paclitaxel | Common | Sensorimotor peripheral neuropathy | – | Within 24 hrs with high dose; usually after several doses | Dose dependent |
| docetaxel | Common (40%) | Sensorimotor peripheral neuropathy | – | After several doses | Does dependent |
| *Alkylating agents* | | | | | |
| ifosfamide | Rare | CNS: lethargy, confusion, seizures, ataxia, stupor, weakness | + | 1–8 hrs, spontaneously reversible | High doses; uncommon at usual dosing |
| nitrogen mustard (mechlorethamine hydrochloride) | Rare (intra-arterial, toxic IV doses) | Tinnitus, coma, seizures, death | + high dose | Immediate to rapidly progressive | Toxic in high IV doses; normal intra-arterial doses |
| chlorambucil | Rare | Hypersensitivity, coma, seizures | + high dose | Immediate with rapid recovery | Accidental overdose |
| *Nitrosoureas* | | | | | |
| lomustine (CCNU) | Rare | Confusion, lethargy, ataxia | + + | Delayed (days to weeks) | Usual doses |
| semustine (MeCCNU) | Very rare | Acute metabolic encephalopathy | + + | 2 days → 2 weeks | |
| carmustine (BCNU) | Very rare | Optic neuroretinitis | + + | Onset 8 days → slow resolution | Unknown |
| *Antimetabolites* | | | | | |
| 5-fluorouracil | Very rare (< 1%) | Ataxia, cerebellar dysfunction | + | Immediate to 1 week with slow recovery | Variable |
| methotrexate | Common with intrathecal dose but preventable using *preservative-free* diluent | Stiff neck, headache, meningismus, rare seizures | Low dose – high dose + (IV) | 2–4 hrs onset, 12–72 hrs duration | Large IT doses or prolonged therapy |

|  |  |  |  |  |  |
|---|---|---|---|---|---|
| cytosine arabinoside (Ara-C) | Rare IT | Meningismus, headache, vomiting | Low dose – high dose + + | Immediate to 1 hr, lasting 12 hrs–2 days | ↑ with larger doses |
| High-dose cytosine arabinoside | 0–25% | Cerebellar dysfunction, somnolence, dysarthria, ataxia Encephalopathy: confusion, impaired cognition and memory, seizures | + + | Improvement in 4–7 days but may be permanent | Doses > 36 gm/m² |
| 5-azacytidine | Rare | Some cases of myalgia leading to somnolence and coma | + | During weeklong infusions | Dose dependent |
| *Others* |  |  |  |  |  |
| L-asparaginase | Common, 30–60% incidence; may be dose-limiting | Somnolence, lethargy, personality changes | – | Within the first day to 1–3 days after drug cessation | None |
| corticosteroids | 10–60% | CNS: depression, delirium, ↓ memory, ↓ concentration, emotional lability, tremor, sleep disturbances, proximal muscle weakness and atrophy | – | Reversible | Increases with dose > 40 mg prednisone per day and with long-term therapy |
| procarbazine | Infrequent (po), 8–30% incidence; dose-limiting when given IV | Optic neuroretinitis, somnolence, CNS depression, manic psychosis, peripheral neuropathies, paresthesias, ↓ reflexes | + + | Onset in 8 days with slow resolution when oral dosing Onset immediate with rapid recovery with IV dosing | Unknown in high doses |
| hexamethyl-melamine | 10–25% | Peripheral neuropathy (paresthesias, weakness, impaired sensation) CNS: depression, hallucinations, ataxia, confusion, petit mal seizures | ± | Reversible | Increased incidence with high dose |
| cisplatin | Common | Unilateral or bilateral ototoxicity, peripheral neuropathy | Unknown | Rapid onset; unknown recovery | Dose related |
| mitotane | 40% of patients | Lethargy, sedation, vertigo | + + | Rapid onset with slow resolution | May be related to cumulative dose |

*Source:* Modified by permission of the publisher from Dorr, R.T., and Fritz, W.L. (1980). *Cancer Chemotherapy Handbook.* New York: Elsevier, 120–122. Reprinted with permission from Elsevier Science Publishing Company, Inc.

1984). The syndrome is reversible within 1–6 weeks of drug discontinuance. This toxicity has not been seen with continuous infusion therapy (120 hours) despite the fact that higher doses are administered. Hexamethylmelamine may cause CNS symptoms with continuous high-dose oral administration, characterized by depression, hallucinations, somnolence or insomnia, dysphagia, questionable seizures, prominent ataxia, and tremors (Kaplan and Wiernik 1984).

Procarbazine is a weak monoamine oxidase inhibitor that rapidly crosses the blood-brain barrier and can cause altered levels of consciousness and, rarely, ataxia, which is reversible (Kaplan and Wiernik 1984). It is important to remember that procarbazine potentiates the effects of phenothiazines, barbiturates, and narcotics, so concurrent administration of these medications should be done with caution.

The Syndrome of Inappropriate Antidiuretic Hormone (SIADH) occurs rarely following administration of the vinca alkaloids (vincristine, vinblastine) or cyclophosphamide. Kaplan and Wiernik (1984) describe the hyponatremia related to the vinca alkaloids as moderate to severe, developing within 10 days of drug administration and resolving in 1–2 weeks. It is believed that there is a direct drug effect on the hypothalamus, neurohypophyseal tract, or posterior pituitary (Stuart et al. 1975). It is possible that rare mental changes, confusion, delirium, and seizures reported after vincristine administration may be due to SIADH-induced hyponatremia (Kaplan and Wiernik 1984). Cyclophosphamide-induced SIADH appears related to a transient decrease in free-water clearance and urine volume, as active metabolites of the drug are excreted in the urine and there is a consequent fall in serum sodium concentration 4–12 hours after drug infusion, lasting up to 20 hours (DeFronzo et al. 1973). It is possible that slower infusion of cyclophosphamide may minimize neurotoxic reactions (Kaplan and Wiernik 1984).

## Neuropathies

The drugs most commonly associated with neuropathies are the vinca alkaloids and cis-platin, and they will be discussed in detail. Of the three vinca alkaloids, vincristine has the greatest potential to cause neurotoxicity because it has been shown to be rapidly taken up by unsheathed nerves and is extensively tissue bound, leading to prolonged exposure of neural tissue (Nelson, Dyke, and Root 1980). However, vindesine and vinblastine may cause similar toxicity. An early sign of vincristine neurotoxicity is the loss of the Achilles tendon reflex, and with continued treatment, the other deep tendon reflexes may be lost even though the patient is asymptomatic (Sandler, Tobin, and Henderson 1969). The most common symptom is paresthesia of the hands or feet, occurring in up to 57% of patients, which may progress to muscle pain, weakness, gait disturbance, and sensory impairment with continued drug dosing (Kaplan and Wiernik 1984). However, neurotoxic drugs are not usually discontinued unless there is loss of deep tendon reflexes. Loss of dorsiflexion reflexes of the foot leads to distressing foot drop or a slapping gait, and then may continue to severe muscle weakness (Weiss, Walker, and Wiernik 1974). The sensory and motor impairment is symmetrical and appears to be dose related, although patients with lymphoma appear to develop neuropathies earlier in the treatment course (Kaplan and Wiernik 1984). If treatment is stopped when loss of reflexes or paresthesia is first identified, then recovery occurs in

1–3 months; in contrast, if vincristine is continued, loss of deep tendon reflexes may be permanent (Kaplan and Wiernik 1984).

Cisplatin is a compound that contains a heavy metal and appears to act as an alkylating agent. Neuropathy is an increasingly more common side effect as higher doses of cisplatin are administered, and the impact on the patient can be devastating. The neuropathy is generally dose dependent, but there is much variability in symptoms. Patients first experience numbness and tingling of the extremities and may have decreased vibratory sensation and decreased deep tendon reflexes. This progresses to impaired position sense, and in some to sensory ataxia (Mollman et al. 1988). Because cisplatin-induced nephropathy is easily preventable, neuropathy is now becoming the dose-limiting factor. In an effort to try to decrease the neurotoxicity of cisplatin, Mollman and colleagues (1988) used the radioprotective agent amifostine (Etyol) and showed a significantly lower incidence of neuropathy in a study of 69 patients receiving cisplatin-containing chemotherapy regimens. They also found the highest incidence of severe peripheral neuropathy at cisplatin doses of 40 mg/m$^2$ on 5 consecutive days repeated monthly, while in another report by Legha and Dimery (1985), the median cumulative dose of cisplatin was 775 mg/m$^2$ in patients developing neurotoxicity.

Damage to cranial nerves can occur in up to 10% of patients receiving vincristine, and damage is usually reversible when treatment is interrupted (Kaplan and Wiernik 1984). The signs of damage to cranial nerves are as follows:

- recurrent laryngeal nerve→vocal cord paresis or paralysis
- oculomotor nerve→bilateral ptosis, diplopia
- rare optic neuropathy→transient cortical blindness
- trigeminal nerve→severe jaw pain after first dose

## Sensory/Perceptual Impairment

Holden and Felde (1987) describe five categories of sensory-perceptual losses. The first, *auditory*, includes the ototoxicity experienced by many patients receiving high-dose cisplatin. It is estimated that reversible tinnitus occurs in about 9% of patients receiving doses up to 60 mg/m$^2$; symptomatic hearing loss occurs in about 6%; and audiogram abnormalities (high-frequency puretone hearing loss) occur in at least 24% and may not be reversible (Kaplan and Wiernik 1984). As higher doses of cisplatin are administered, these percentages increase. Audiograms should be performed prior to cisplatin therapy and repeated if the patient develops impaired speech perception; at that time, a decision based on potential risks and benefits would be made about continuing therapy (Kaplan and Wiernik 1984).

The second loss is *visual loss*, and patients might experience blurred vision and impaired color vision (color saturation and discrimination along the blue-yellow axis) (Wilding et al. 1985). In Holden and Felde's survey (1987), the loss of precise color vision was most distressing to patients. Other changes, although rare, are similar to heavy metal poisoning, such as papilledema and retrobulbar neuritis (see Table 4.26). Patient problems include mistaken colors, potential for injury, and decreased appreciation for food and environment related to loss of color discrimination.

*Taste changes* occur but may be related to other factors and often involve hypersensitivity to red meat.

*Tactile changes* are distressing and develop as bilateral, symmetrical paresthesias and dysethesias in a stocking-and-glove

**Table 4.26** Ocular Toxicity

| Drug | Direct Effect |
| --- | --- |
| busulfan | Cataracts |
| chlorambucil | Rare diplopia, papilledema, retinal hemorrhage |
| cisplatin | Rare papilledema, blurry vision, retrobulbar neuritis |
| cytosine arabinoside (high dose) | Increased lacrimation, conjunctivitis as drug is excreted in tears |
| corticosteroids | Cataracts |
| cyclophosphamide | Rare blurred vision |
| doxorubicin | Rare conjunctivitis |
| 5-fluorouracil | Increased lacrimation, blurred vision, photophobia (drug excreted in tears) |
| methotrexate | Rare ocular irritation (some drug found in tears) |
| nitrosoureas | Rare optic neuroretinitis, loss of depth perception, blurred vision, retinopathy |
| procarbazine | Rare retinal hemorrhage, nystagmus, diplopia, photophobia |
| tamoxifen (high dose) | Decreased visual acuity, retinopathy, corneal opacities |
| vinca alkaloids | Ptosis, diplopia, nerve palsies, photophobia, optic neuropathy |

*Source:* Modified from Brager, B.L., and Yasko, J.M. (1984). *Care of the Client Receiving Chemotherapy*. Reston, Vir.: Reston Publishing Co. and Vizel, M., and Oster, M. (1982). Ocular side effects of cancer chemotherapy. *Cancer* 49: 1999–2002.

distribution (Kaplan and Wiernik 1984), from fingertips to wrist and toes to knees. Vibration sense is often disturbed, as well as fine motor movement. Patient problems include the potential for injury related to insensitivity to temperature.

*Proprioceptive losses* can be devastating due to the loss of ability to determine the position of body parts without visual cues. Patients might have gait disturbances and difficulty with handwriting (Kaplan and Wiernik 1984). Patient problems may include alterations in role and self-esteem, if proprioceptive and sensory changes require changes in occupation, and altered ability to perform activities of daily living.

Lastly, autonomic neuropathy is very common, especially constipation and colicky abdominal pain. This occurs in 33–46% of patients and may precede the onset of paresthesias or diminished deep tendon reflexes (Kaplan and Wiernik 1984). Nurses should make certain that patients receiving vinca alkaloids are receiving a bowel regimen containing stool softeners and laxatives as needed to *prevent* constipation, as this can lead to adynamic ileus and severe morbidity.

Amifostine has shown usefulness in preventing the development of peripheral neuropathy in patients receiving cisplatin without affecting tumor effectiveness. (Hausheer et al. 1998). It appears that amifostine also can be used to treat/reverse periperal neuropathy when given at low doses 3 ×/week. This is currently being studied by the Gynecology Oncology Group.

Table 4.27 an example of a standardized care plan for the patient experiencing neuropathy. The role of the oncology nurse for neurological, as well as other side effects secondary to chemotherapy is symptom management, minimizing injury and improving quality of life for the person with cancer.

**Table 4.27** Standardized Nursing Care Plan for the Patient Experiencing Neuropathy

| Nursing Diagnosis | Expected Outcomes | Nursing Interventions |
|---|---|---|
| I. *Potential for injury related to* ↓ *sensitivity to temperature, gait disturbance,* ↓ *proprioception* | I. A. Pt will be without injury<br>B. Pt will report changes in tactile and proprioceptive function<br>C. Pt will develop safe measures to compensate for losses | I. A. Assess integrity of *tactile* and *proprioceptive* functions<br>   1. Sensory perception to light touch, pinprick, vibration, temperature; vision, color vision<br>   2. Pt's ability to tolerate light touch, cool water, presence of numbness and tingling, presence of painful sensations<br>   3. Proprioception testing of station, gait, deep tendon reflexes, muscle weakness or atrophy, and balance<br>   4. Pt's ability to sense placement of body parts, ability to write, evidence of muscle weakness<br>B. Discuss alterations in sensation, proprioception, and impact on ability to do activities of daily living (ADLs)<br>C. Discuss alternative strategies to prevent injury<br>   1. Instruct pt in safety measures and use of visual cues<br>   2. Encourage pt to take time to complete activities, focus attention to task<br>   3. Use potholder when cooking<br>   4. Use gloves when washing dishes, gardening<br>   5. Inspect skin for cuts, abrasions, burns daily, especially arms, legs, toes, fingers<br>D. Refer as appropriate for occupational or physical therapy, diagnostic testing using EMG<br>E. If pt presents with S/S of peripheral neuropathy, hold chemotherapy and discuss with physician |
| II. *Potential for impaired self-care related to tactile and proprioception dysfunction* | II. A. Pt will identify activities of self-care that are difficult<br>B. Pt will identify strategies to meet needs | II. A. Assess pt's ability to perform ADLs such as eating, hygiene, dressing, walking, and handwriting<br>B. Discuss and develop strategies to meet self-care needs<br>   1. Referral to occupational therapy for splint, etc.<br>   2. Involve family members in care planning<br>   3. Community resource referral as appropriate (homemaker, home health aide, visiting nurse) |
| III. *Potential for alteration in comfort related to painful paresthesias* | III. A. Pt will have decreased pain | III. A. Assess comfort level and presence of severe tingling or prickling sensation, cramping or burning<br>B. Assess intensity, quality, and frequency of discomfort<br>C. Identify precipitating factors, such as warm or cold stimulation, and develop realistic plan to avoid precipitating factors<br>D. Consider adjunctive analgesics with neurologic action for dysaesthetic pain: amitriptyline HCl (Elavil), phenytoin sodium (Dilantin)<br>E. Consider nonpharmacologic intervention: teach pt guided imagery, progressive muscle relaxation, massage, etc. |

*(continued)*

**Table 4.27** Standardized Nursing Care Plan for the Patient Experiencing Neuropathy (*continued*)

| Nursing Diagnosis | Expected Outcomes | Nursing Interventions |
|---|---|---|
| IV. *Impaired mobility related to decreased proprioception, muscle dysfunction* | IV. A. Pt will ambulate safely | IV. A. Assess pt's level of activity, muscle strength, and mobility level prior to chemotherapy, then prior to each treatment, and at each visit once therapy is completed<br>B. Encourage pt to use visual cues to determine position of body parts<br>C. Teach measures to prevent injury<br>D. Refer for physical, occupational therapy and assistive devices as needed |
| V. *Potential for sexual dysfunction related to altered tactile sensation, muscle weakness, changes in role* | V. A. Pt and significant other will identify alterations in sexual expression<br>B. Pt and significant other will identify alternative methods of sexual expression | V. A. Discuss with pt the impact of treatment-related dysfunction on sexuality, social role, and self-esteem<br>B. Discuss appropriate alternative means of sexual expression<br>C. Refer for specific sexual counseling if diminished ability to have erection<br>D. Observe for changes in needs related to affection and emotional support |
| VI. *Potential for role change with changes and alterations in self-esteem and self-concept related to sensory/perceptual dysfunction, changes in social function, changes in ability to perform occupational role* | VI. A. Pt and family will demonstrate positive coping strategies | VI. A. Assess impact of sensory/perceptual dysfunction on social and work roles: ability to meet role expectations of self and family<br>B. Discuss modifications in job and role, as appropriate and available<br>C. Refer pt to OT/PT to see if appliances available to foster rehabilitation (braces, etc.)<br>D. Encourage independence and provide positive reinforcement for accomplishments<br>E. Support pt as he or she grieves loss(es); assess need for support groups or counseling<br>F. Support pt and family by providing information to help explain these behavioral responses to treatment-related dysfunction |
| VII. *Potential for alteration in nutrition: less than body requirements related to taste distortions, anorexia, hypersensitivity to foods* | VII. A. Pt will eat balanced diet from four food groups<br>B. Pt will attain ideal body weight following completion of treatment | VII. A. Assess dietary preferences, changes in food tolerances<br>B. Teach pt to select high-calorie, high-protein foods<br>C. Suggest dietary modifications based on taste changes (e.g., Crazy Jane Salt and spices if foods are tasteless)<br>D. Perform periodic weights prior to each treatment cycle<br>E. Evaluate pt's ability to do fine-motor movement to feed self, cook<br>F. Refer to nutritionist or dietitian as needed<br>G. Monitor laboratory values, especially magnesium and calcium, on cisplatin therapy |

VIII. *Potential for constipation related to autonomic neuropathy (vinca alkaloids)*

VIII. A. Pt will move bowels at least every other day

VIII. A. Assess normal elimination pattern
B. Encourage pt to drink at least 3 liters of fluid/day
C. Encourage daily exercise
D. Teach pt to include bulky, high-fiber foods in diet
E. Teach pt to self-administer stool softeners and laxatives as needed

IX. *Knowledge deficit related to self-care measures related to neuropathic changes*

IX. A. Pt will identify risk of development of neuropathy
B. Pt will identify signs and symptoms to report to health care provider

IX. A. Teach pt re potential side effect(s) of neuropathy
1. Constipation
2. Numbness/tingling in hands/feet
3. Motor weakness
a. Gait changes (e.g., foot drop)
b. Loss of fine-motor movement (buttoning shirt, picking up dime)
4. Inability of males to have erection
5. Difficulty urinating
B. Teach pt to report the occurrence of signs and symptoms of neuropathies

*Sources:* Ogrinc, M. (1985). Sensory/perceptual alterations related to peripheral neuropathy. In J.C. McNally, J.C. Stair, and E.T. Somerville (eds.): *Guidelines for Cancer Nursing Practice.* Orlando: Grune and Stratton, 185–188; Holden, S., and Felde, G. (1987). Nursing care of patients experiencing cisplatin-related peripheral neuropathies. *Oncology Nursing Forum* 14(1): 13–19; Brager, B.L., and Yasko, J.M. (1984). *Care of the Client Receiving Chemotherapy.* Reston, Vir.: Reston Publishing Co.; Kaplan, R.S., and Wiernik, P.H. (1984). Neurotoxicity of antitumor agents. In M.C. Perry and J.W. Yarbro (eds.): *Toxicity of Chemotherapy.* Orlando: Grune and Stratton, 365–431.

## *BIBLIOGRAPHY*

### Bone Marrow Depression

Antman, K.D., Griffin, J.D., Elias, A., et al. (1988). Effect of recombinant human granulocyte-macrophage colony stimulating factor on chemotherapy-induced myelosuppression. *New England Journal of Medicine* 319(10): 593–598.

Bergsagel, D.E. (1971). Assessment of massive dose chemotherapy of malignant disease. *Canadian Medical Association Journal* 104: 31–36.

Blesch, K.S. (1988). The normal physiological changes of aging and their impact on the response to cancer treatment. *Seminars in Oncology Nursing* 4(3): 178–188.

Bodey, G.P. (1984). Current status of prophylaxis of infection with protected environments. *American Journal of Medicine* 76: 678–684.

Bodey, G.P., Buckley, M., Sathe, Y.S., et al. (1966). Quantitative relationship between circulating leukocytes and infections in patients with acute leukemia. *Annals of Internal Medicine* 64(2): 328–340.

Brager, B.L., and Yasko, Y.M. (1984). *Care of the Client Receiving Chemotherapy*. Reston, Vir.: Reston Publishing Co., 96, 106, 178, 180.

Braine, H.G. (1980). Infectious complications of granulocytopenia after cancer chemotherapy. In M.D. Abeloff (ed.): *Complications of Cancer: Diagnosis and Management*. Baltimore/London: Johns Hopkins University Press, 152.

Brandt, B. (1984). A nursing protocol for the client with neutropenia. *Oncology Nursing Forum* 11(2): 24–28.

Carlson, A.C. (1985). Infection prophylaxis in the patient with cancer. *Oncology Nursing Forum* 12(3): 60.

Cheung, W.K., Goon, B.L., Guilfoyle, M.S., and Wacholtz, M.C. (1998). Pharmacokinetics and pharmacodynamics of recombinant human erythropoietin after single and subcutaneous doses to healthy people. *Clinical Pharmacology and Therapeutics* 64(4): 412–420.

Dorr, R.T., and Fritz, W.L. (1980). *Cancer Chemotherapy Handbook*. New York: Elsevier.

Dorr, R.T., and Von Hoff. D.D. (1994). *Cancer Chemotherapy Handbook*. 2nd ed. Norwalk, Conn.: Appleton and Lange.

Fox, L.S. (1981). Granulocytopenia in the adult cancer patient. *Cancer Nursing* (December): 24.

Freifeld, A.G., Walsh, J.T., and Pizzo, P.A. (1997). Infections in the cancer patient. In V.T. DeVita, Jr., S. Hellman, and S.A. Rosenberg (eds.): *Cancer: Principles and Practice of Oncology*. 5th ed. Philadelphia: Lippincott, 2662.

Golden, W. (1971). Routine protective isolation: Worth the trouble in neutropenic patients. *Journal of the American Medical Association* 242(19): 2045.

Heyman, M.R., and Schiffer, C.A. (1990). Platelet transfusion therapy for the cancer patient. *Seminars in Oncology* 17: 198–209.

Haeuber, D., and Spross, J. (1994). Protective mechanisms: Bone marrow. In B.L. Johnson and J. Gross (eds.): *Handbook of Oncology Nursing*. Boston: Jones & Bartlett, 373–399.

McConnell, E.A. (1986). Leukocyte studies: What the counts can tell you. *Nursing 86* (March): 42–43.

Medical Economics Company. (1998). *Physicians' Desk Reference*. Oradell, N.J.: Medical Economics Company.

Neuseff, W., and Maki, D. (1981). A study of the value of simple protective isolation in patients with granulocytopenia. *New England Journal of Medicine* 304(8): 448–453.

Pizzo, P.A. (1989). Combating infections in neutropenic patients. *Hospital Practice* 22: 93–110.

Pizzo, P.A. (1993). Management of fever in patients with cancer and treatment of treatment induced neutropenia. *New England Journal of Medicine* 328: 1323–1332.

Rodriguez, V., and Ketchel, S.J. (1981). Acute infections in patients with malignant disease. In J.W. Yarbro and R.S. Bornstein (eds.): *Oncologic Emergencies*. New York: Grune and Stratton.

Schimpff, S.C., Young, V.M., Green, W.H., et al. (1972). Origin of infection in acute ANLL: Significance of hospital acquisition of pathogens. *Annals of Internal Medicine* 77: 707–714.

Wilkes, G.M., Ingwersen, K., and Barton-Burke, M. (1999). *Oncology Nursing Drug Reference*. Sudbury, Mass.: Jones & Bartlett, 464.

Wroblewski, S.S., and Wroblewski, S.H. (1981). Caring for the patient with chemotherapy-induced thrombocytopenia. *American Journal of Nursing* 81(4): 746.

Zaia, J.A. (1990). Viral Infections associated with bone marrow transplantation. *Hematology and Oncology Clinics of North America* 7: 293–315.

## Stomatitis

Adrian, R.M., Hood, A.F., and Skarin, A.T. (1980). Mucocutaneous reactions to antineoplastic agents. *Cancer Journal for Clinicians* 30: 142–157.

Beck, S. (1979). Impact of a systemic oral care protocol on stomatitis after chemotherapy. *Cancer Nursing* 2 (June): 186.

Beck, S., and Yasko, J.M. (1984). *Guidelines for Oral Care*. Cary, Ill.: Sage Products.

Bersani, G., and Carl, W. (1983). Oral care for cancer patients. *American Journal of Nursing* 83: 533.

Brager, B.L., and Yasko, J.M. (1984). *Care of the Client Receiving Chemotherapy*. Reston, Vir.: Reston Publishing Co.

Capizzi, R.L., DeConti, R.C., Marsh, J.C., et al. (1970). Methotrexate therapy of head and neck cancer: Improvement in therapeutic index by the use of leucovorin rescue. *Cancer Research* 30: 1783.

Chi, K.H., Chen, S.Y., Chan, W.K., et al. (1994). Effect of granulocyte macrophage colony stimulating factor (GM-CSF) on oral mucositis in head and neck cancer patients with cisplatin, 5-FU and leucovorin therapy. *Proceedings of the American Society of Clinical Oncologists* 13: 428.

Daeffler, R.J. (1994). Protective mechanisms: Mucous membranes. In B.L. Johnson and J. Gross (eds.): *Handbook of Oncology Nursing*. Boston: Jones & Bartlett, 399–421.

Dreizen, S., Boday, G., and Rodriguez, V. (1975). Oral complications of cancer chemotherapy. *Postgraduate Medicine* 58: 76.

Dudjak, L.A. (1987). Mouth care for mucositis due to radiation therapy. *Cancer Nursing* 10(3): 131–140.

Engelking, C. (1988). Managing stomatitis: A nursing process approach. In *Supportive Care for the Patient with Cancer*. Richmond, Vir.: A.H. Robins, 20–28.

Fardal, O., and Turnbull, R.S. (1986). A review of the literature on use of chlorhexidine in dentistry. *Journal of the American Dental Association* 112 (June): 863–869.

Ferraro, J.M., and Mattern, J.Q.A. (1984). Sucralfate suspension for stomatitis. *Drug Intelligence and Clinical Pharmacology* 18: 153.

Ferretti, G.A. (1990). Chlorhexidine prophylaxis for chemotherapy and radiation induced stomatitis: A randomized clinical trial. *Oral Surgery, Oral Medicine, Oral Pathology* 69: 331–338.

Ferretti, G.A., Ash, R.C., Brown, A.T., et al. (1987). Chlorhexidine for prophylaxis against oral infections and associated complications in patients receiving bone marrow transplants. *Journal of the American Dental Association* 114 (April): 461–467.

Ferretti, G.A., Hanse, I.A., Whittenburg, K., et al. (1987). Therapeutic use of chlorhexidine in bone marrow transplant patients: Case studies. *Oral Surgery* 63: 683–687.

Ferretti, G.A., Raybould, T., Whittenberg, A., et al. (1987). Effect of chlorhexidine mouthrinse on mucositis in patients receiving intensive chemotherapy. *Journal of Dental Research* 66 (Special Issue): 342.

Fishman, M., and Mrozek-Orowski, M. (1999). *Cancer Chemotherapy Guidelines and Recommendations for Practice*. 2nd ed. Pittsburgh: Oncology Nursing Press.

Frattore, L., Larson, R.A., and Mostofi, R.S. (1986). Dental management of cancer patients receiving chemotherapy. *Illinois Medical Journal* 169: 223–227.

Goodman, M.S., and Stoner, C. (1991). Mucous membrane integrity, impairment of stomatitis. In J.C. McNally, J.C. Stair, and E.T. Somerville (eds.): *Guidelines for Cancer Nursing Practice*. Philadelphia: Saunders, 241–246.

Lavalle, C., and Proctor, D. (1978). *Clinical Pathology of the Oral Mucosa*. Hagerstown, Md.: Harper and Row.

Lockhart, P., and Sonis, S. (1979). Relationship of oral complications to peripheral blood leukocyte and platelet counts in patients receiving cancer chemotherapy. *Oral Surgery* 48: 21–28.

Mahood, D., Dose, A.M., Loprinzi, C., et al. (1991). Inhibition of fluorouracil-induced stomatitis by oral cryotherapy. *Journal of Clinical Oncology* 9: 449–452.

McGaw, W.T., and Belch, A. (1985). Oral complications of acute leukemia: Prophylactic impact of a chlorhexidine mouth rinse regimen. *Oral Surgery, Oral Medicine, Oral Pathology* 60(3): 275–280.

National Institutes of Health Consensus Development Panel (1990). Consensus Statement: Oral complications of cancer therapies. *NCI Monographs* 9: 3–8.

National Institutes of Health (1989). Oral complications of cancer therapies: Diagnosis, prevention, and treatment. *NIH Consensus Development Conference on Stomatitus* 7: 7.

Nieweg, R., Van Tinteren, H., Poelhuis, E.K., and Abraham-Inpijn, L. (1992). Nursing care for oral complications associated with chemotherapy: A survey among members of the Dutch Nursing Society. *Cancer Nursing* 15: 313–321.

Peterson, D.E., and Schubert, M.M. (1992). Oral toxicity. In M.C. Perry (ed.): *The Chemotherapy Source Book*. Baltimore: Williams and Wilkins, 508–528.

Pfeiffer, P., Madsen, E.L., Hansen, O., et al. (1990). Effect of prophylactic sucrarfate suspension on stomatitis induced by cancer chemotherapy. *Acta Oncology* 29: 171–173.

Poland, J.M. (1991). Prevention and treatment of oral complications of the cancer patient. *Oncology* 5: 45–50.

———. (1987). Comparing Moie-stir to lemon glycerine swabs. *American Journal of Nursing* 87: 87.

Siena, S., et al. (1988). Amelioration of severe mucositis by misoprostol following total body irradiation and high dose melphalan with autologous bone marrow transplantation. *Gastroenterology International* 1(Suppl): 1044.

Sonis, S.T., Sonis, A.L., and Lieberman, A. (1978). Oral complications in patients receiving treatment for malignancies other than head and neck. *Journal of the American Dental Association* 97: 468–472.

Western Consortium on Cancer Nursing Research (1991). Development of a staging system for chemotherapy induced stomatitis. *Cancer Nursing* 14: 6–12.

Wilkes, G.M. (1986). Sucralfate suspension for mucositis. *Oncology Nursing Forum* 13: 71–72.

Yasko, J.M. (ed.). (1983). *Guidelines for Cancer Care: Symptom Management.* Reston, Vir.: Reston Publishing Co.

Zinner, S.H., Belcher, A.E., and Murphy, C. (1988). *Assessing the Risk of Herpes in Immunocompromised Patients.* Research Triangle Park, N.C.: Burroughs Wellcome.

## Esophagitis and Diarrhea

Brager, B.L., and Yasko, J.M. (1984). *Care of the Client Receiving Chemotherapy.* Reston, Vir.: Reston Publishing Co., 247–255.

Culhane, B. (1983). Diarrhea. In J. Yasko (ed.): *Guidelines for Cancer Care: Symptom Management.* Reston, Vir.: Reston Publishing Co.

Daeffler, R.J. (1985). Mucous membranes. In B.L. Johnson and J. Gross (eds.): *Handbook of Oncology Nursing.* New York: John Wiley and Sons, 253–274.

Davis, M. (1985). Bowel elimination, alterations in: diarrhea. In J.C. McNally, J.C. Stair, and E.T. Somerville (eds.): *Guidelines for Cancer Nursing Practice.* Orlando: E.L. Grune and Stratton, 239–242.

Dorr, R.T., and Fritz, W.L. (1980). *Cancer Chemotherapy Handbook.* New York: Elsevier.

Dorr, R.T., and Von Hoff, D.D. (1994). *Cancer Chemotherapy Handbook.* 2nd ed. Norwalk, Conn.: Appleton and Lange.

Frattore, L., Larson, R.A., and Mostofi, R. S. (1986). Dental management of cancer patients receiving chemotherapy. *Illinois Medical Journal* 169: 223–227.

Kris, M.G., Gralla, R.J., Clark, R.A., et al. (1988). Control of chemotherapy-induced diarrhea with the synthetic enkephalin BW 942C: A randomized trial with placebo in patients receiving cisplatin. *Journal of Clinical Oncology* 6(4): 663–669.

Nunnally, C., and Donoghue, M. (1986). Nursing management of gastrointestinal dysfunction. In J.M. Yasko (ed.): *Nursing Management of Symptoms Associated with Chemotherapy.* Columbus, Ohio: Adria Laboratories.

Nunnally, C., Donoghue, M., and Yasko, J.M. (1983). Esophagitis. In J.M. Yasko (ed.): *Guidelines for*

*Cancer Care: Symptom Management.* Reston, Vir.: Reston Publishing Co.

Perry, M.C., and Yarbro, J.W. (1984). *Toxicity of Chemotherapy.* New York: Grune and Stratton.

Ropka, M.E. (1985). Nutrition. In B.L. Johnson and J. Gross (eds.): *Handbook of Oncology Nursing.* New York: John Wiley and Sons, 205.

Wilkes, G.M., Ingwersen, K., and Barton-Burke, M. (1999). *1999 Oncology Nursing Drug Handbook.* Sudbury, Mass.: Jones & Bartlett, 150–151.

## Alopecia

Baxley, K.O., Erdman, L.K., Henry, E.B., et al. (1984). Alopecia: Effect on cancer patients' body image. *Cancer Nursing* 7(6): 499–502.

Brager, B.L., and Yasko, J.M. (1984). *Care of the Client Receiving Chemotherapy.* Reston, Vir.: Reston Publishing Co., 247–255.

Chernecky, C.C., and Yasko, J.M. (1986). Alopecia. In J.M. Yasko (ed.): *Nursing Management of Symptoms Associated with Chemotherapy.* Columbus, Ohio: Adria Labs.

Cline, B.W. (1984). Prevention of chemo-induced alopecia: A review of the literature. *Cancer Nursing* 7(3): 221–228.

Dean, J.C., Griffith, K.S., Cetus, T.C., et al. (1983). Scalp hypothermia: A comparison of ice packs and the kold kap in the prevention of doxorubicin-induced alopecia. *Journal of Clinical Oncology* 1(1): 33–37.

Denes, A.E. (1994). Failure of topical minoxidil to accelerate hair growth following chemotherapy. *Proceedings of the American Society of Clinical Oncologists* 13: 446.

Dorr, R.T., and Fritz, W.L. (1980). *Cancer Chemotherapy Handbook.* New York: Elsevier, 107–109.

Dunagin, W.G. (1984). Dermatologic toxicity. In M.C. Perry and J.W. Yarbro (eds.): *Toxicity of Chemotherapy.* Orlando: Grune and Stratton.

Jimenez, J.J., Maharaj, D., Guerra, M., et al. (1994). Phase I trial of intracutaneous IL-I for the prevention of chemotherapy-induced alopecia. *Proceedings of the American Society of Clinical Oncologists* 13: 417.

Keller, J.F., and Blausey, L.A. (1988). Nursing issues and management in chemotherapy-induced alopecia. *Oncology Nursing Forum* 15(5): 603–607.

Lindsey, A.M. (1985). Building the knowledge base for practice: Alopecia, self-breast exam and other human responses. Part 2. *Oncology Nursing Forum* 12(2): 27–34.

Parker, R. (1987). The effectiveness of scalp hypothermia in preventing cyclophosphamide-induced alopecia. 14(6): 49–55.

Perez, J.E., Macchiavelli, M., Leone, B.A., et al. (1986). High-dose alpha-tocopherol as a preventative of doxorubicin-induced alopecia. *Cancer Treatment Reports* 70(10): 1213–1214.

## Gonadal Dysfunction

Block, E. (1952). Quantitative morphological investigations of the follicular system in women, variations at different ages. *Acta Anatomy* 14: 108–123.

Bonfante, V., Santoro, A., Bajetta, E., et al. (1985). Hodgkin's disease: An overview and ABVD studies in Milan. In B.I. Sikic, M. Rozencweig, and S.K. Carter (eds.): *Bleomycin Chemotherapy.* New York: Academic Press.

Brager, B.L., and Yasko, J. (1984). *Care of the Client Receiving Chemotherapy.* Reston, Vir.: Reston Publishing Co.

Chapman, R.M. (1984). Effect of cytotoxic therapy on sexuality and gonadal function. In M.C. Perry and J.W. Yarbro (eds.): *Toxicity of Chemotherapy.* Orlando: Grune and Stratton, 343–365.

Chapman, R.M., Sutcliffe, S.B., and Malpas, J.S. (1979). Cytoxic-induced ovarian failure in females with Hodgkin's disease. Part I: Hormone function. *Journal of the American Medical Association* 242: 1877–1881.

Drasga, R.E., Einhorn, L.H., Williams, S.D., et al. (1983). Fertility after chemotherapy for testicular cancer. *Journal of Clinical Oncology* 1: 179–183.

Fisher, S.G. (1983). The psychosexual effects of cancer and cancer treatment. *Oncology Nursing Forum* 10(2): 63–68.

Glasgow, M., Halfin, V., and Althausen, A. (1987). Sexual response and cancer. *CA—A Cancer Journal for Clinicians* 37(6): 322–333.

Howard-Ruben, J. (1985). Sexual dysfunction related to disease process and treatment. In J.C. McNally, J.C. Stair, and E.T. Somerville (eds.): *Guidelines for Cancer Nursing Practice.* Orlando: Grune and Stratton, 268–277.

Kaempfer, S. (1981). The effect of cancer chemotherapy on reproduction—A review of the literature. *Oncology Nursing Forum* 8: 11–18.

Kaempfer, S.H., Wiley, F.M., Hoffman, D.J., et al. (1985). Fertility considerations and procreative alternatives in cancer care. *Seminars of Oncology Nursing* 1(1): 25–34.

Kreuser, E.D., Hetzel, W.D., Heit, W., et al. (1988). Reproductive and endocrine gonadal function in adults following multidrug chemotherapy for acute lymphoblastic or undifferentiated leukemia. *Journal of Clinical Oncology* 6(4): 588–596.

Perry, M.C., and Yarbro, J.W. (1984). *Toxicity of Chemotherapy*. New York: Grune and Stratton.

Santoro, A., Viviani, S., Zucoli, R., et al. (1983). Comparable results and toxicity of MOPP vs ABVD combined with radiotherapy in PS IIB, III(A&B) HD. *Proceedings of the American Society of Clinical Oncologists* 2: 583.

Sherins, R.J., and DeVita, V.T. (1973). Effects of drug treatment of lymphoma on male reproductive capacity. *Annals of Internal Medicine* 79: 216–220.

Smith, D.B. (1989). Sexual rehabilitation of the cancer patient. *Cancer Nursing* 12(1): 10–15.

Sweet, V., Servy, E.J., and Karow, A.M. (1996). Reproductive issues for men with cancer: Technology and nursing management. *Oncology Nursing Forum* 23: 51–58.

Tarpy, C.C. (1985). Birth control considerations during chemotherapy. *Oncology Nursing Forum* 12(2): 75–78.

Viviani, S., Santoro, A., Ragni, G., et al. (1985). Gonadal toxicity after combination chemotherapy for Hodgkin's disease. Comparative results of MOPP vs. ABVD. *European Journal of Cancer Clinical Oncology* 21: 601–605.

Yarbro, C.H., and Perry, M.C. (1985). The effect of cancer therapy on gonadal function. *Seminars in Oncology Nursing* 1(1): 3–8.

Yasko, J.M. (1983). Sexual and reproductive dysfunction. In J.M. Yasko (ed.): *Guidelines for Cancer Care: Symptom Management*. Reston, Vir.: Reston Publishing Co., 269–290.

## Nausea and Vomiting

Allen, T.C., Gralla, R., Reilly, L., et al. (1985). Metoclopramide: Dose-related toxicity and preliminary antiemetic studies in children receiving cancer chemotherapy. *Journal of Clinical Oncology* 3: 1136–1141.

Bakowski, M. (1984). Advances in antiemetic therapy. *Cancer Treatment Reviews* 11: 237–256.

Batton, D. (1990). Recent development in the management of emesis with the 5-HT$_3$ antagonist granisetron. *Journal of Oncology* 6(4) (Suppl 1): 14–20

Bickal, T. (1987). A protocol for the diagnosis and treatment of extrapyramidal symptoms of neuroleptic drugs. *Nurse Practitioner* 12(1): 25–38.

Borison, H., and McCarthy, L. (1984). Neuropharmacology of chemotherapy-induced emesis. *Drugs* 25(Suppl 1): 8–17.

Caille, G., Speneid, J., and Lacasse, J. (1983). Pharmacokinetics of two lorazepam formations, oral and sublingual, after multiple doses. *Biopharm Drug Dispos* 4: 31–42.

Carr, B., Blayney, D., Leong, L., et al. (1985). A prospective, double-blind dose-response study of prochlorperazine therapy for cisplatin-induced emesis. *Proceedings of the American Association of Clinical Oncologists* 4: 268.

Citron, M., Johnson-Early, A., Boyer, M., et al. (1984). Droperidol: Optimal dose and time of initiation. *Proceedings of the American Society of Clinical Oncologists* 3: 106.

Costall, B., Domeney, A.M., Gunning, S.T., et al. (1987). GR 38032F: A potent and novel inhibitor of cisplatin-induced emesis in the ferret. *British Journal of Pharmacology* 90: 90.

Cotanch, P.M., and Strum, S. (1987). Progressive muscle relaxation as antiemtic therapy for cancer patients. *Oncology Nursing Forum* 14(1): 33–37.

Craig, J.B., and Powell, B.L. (1987). Review: The management of nausea and vomiting in clinical oncology. *American Journal of Medical Sciences* 293(1): 34–41.

Cunningham, D., Pople, A., Ford, H.T., et al. (1987). Prevention of emesis in patients receiving cytotoxic drugs by GR38032F, a selective 5-HT$_3$ receptor antagonist. *Lancet* 27(June): 1461–1462.

Dilly, S. (1992). Are granisetron and ondansetron equivalent in the clinic? *European Journal of Cancer* 28(Suppl): 532–535.

Dorr, R.T., and Fritz, W. (1980). *Cancer Chemotherapy Handbook*. New York: Elsevier, 103–104.

Fiore, J.J., and Gralla, R.J. (1984). Pharmacologic treatment of chemotherapy-induced nausea and vomiting. *Cancer Investigation* 2(5): 351–361.

Gagen, M., Gochnour, D., Young, D., et al. (1984). A randomized trial of metoclopramide and a combination of dexamethasone and lorazepam for prevention of chemotherapy-induced vomiting. *Journal of Clinical Oncology* 2: 696–701.

Goodman, M. (1987). Management of nausea and vomiting induced by outpatient cisplatin therapy. *Seminars in Oncology Nursing* 3(1) (Suppl 1): 23–35.

Gralla, R.J., Tyson, L., Bordin, L., et al. (1984). Antiemetic therapy: A review of recent studies and a report of a random assignment trial comparing metoclopramide with delta-9-tetrahydrocannabinol. *Cancer Treatment Reports* 68(1): 163–172.

Gralla. R.J., Tyson, L.B., Kris, M.G., et al. (1987). The management of chemotherapy-induced nausea and vomiting. *Medical Clinic of North America* 71(2): 294–297.

Greenberg, S., Gala, K., Lampenfeld, M., et al. (1984). Comparison of the antiemetic effect of high-dose metoclopramide and high-dose IV haloperidol. *Journal of Clinical Oncology* 21: 782–783.

Hesketh, P.J., Beck, T.M., Uhlenhoop, M. et al. (1994). Adjusting the dose of IV ondansetron plus dexamethasone to the emetogenic potential of the chemotherapy regimen. *Proceedings of the American Society of Clinical Oncologists* 13: 433.

Hesketh, P.J., Murphy, W.K., Khojasten, A., et al. (1988). GR-C507175 (GR38032F): A novel compound effective in the treatment of cisplatin induced nausea and vomiting. *Proceedings of the American Society of Clinical Oncologists* 7: 280.

Hesketh, P.J., Murphy, W.K., Lester, E.P., et al. (1988). GR38032F (GR-C507/75): A novel compound effective in the prevention of acute cisplatin-induced emesis. *Proceedings of the American Society of Clinical Oncologists* 7: 280.

Ignoffo, R.J. (1983). Conversations with the pharmacist. *Highlights on Antineoplastic Drugs* (August): 3.

Kris, M.G. et al. (1985). Consecutive dose-finding trials adding lorazepam to the combination of metoclopramide plus dexamethasone: Improving subjective effectiveness over the combination of diphenhydramine plus metoclopramide plus dexamethasone. *Cancer Treatment Reports* 69: 1257–1262.

Kris, M., and Gralla, R. (1986). Antiemetic trials to control delayed vomiting following high-dose cisplatin. *Proceedings of the American Society of Clinical Oncologists* 5: 1005.

Kris, M.G., Gralla, R.J., Tyson, L.B., et al. (1989). Controlling delayed vomiting: Double-blind, randomized trial comparing placebo, dexamethasone alone, and metoclopramide plus dexamethasone in patients receiving cisplatin. *Journal of Clinical Oncology* 7(1): 108–114.

Laszlo, J. (1983). Nausea and vomiting as major complications of cancer chemotherapy. *Drugs* 25 (Suppl 1): 1–7.

Laszlo, J., Clark, R.A., Harrison, D.C., et al. (1985). Lorazepam in cancer patients treated with cisplatin: A drug having antiemetic, amnesic and anxiolytic effects. *Journal of Clinical Oncology* 3: 864–869.

Levitt, M.L., Warr, D., Yelle, L., et al. (1993). Ondansetron compared with dexamethasone and metoclopramide as antiemetics with CMF. *New England Journal of Medicine* 328: 547–550.

Markman, M., Scheidler, V., Ettinger, D.S., et al. (1984). Antiemetic efficacy of dexamethasone. *New England Journal of Medicine* 311: 549–552.

Mason, B.A., Dambra, J., and Grossman, B. (1982). Effective control of cisplatin-induced nausea using HD steroids and droperidol. *Cancer Treatment Reports* 66(2): 243–245.

Morrow, G.A. (1982). Clinical characteristics associated with the development of anticipatory nausea and vomiting in cancer patients undergoing chemotherapy treatment. *Journal of Clinical Oncology* 2(10): 1170.

Neidhart, J., Gagen, M., Wilson, H., et al. (1981). Comparative trial of antiemetic effects of THC and haloperidol. *Journal of Clinical Pharmacology* 21: 385–390.

Nicholas, D. (1982). The prevalence of anticipatory nausea and emesis in cancer chemotherapy patients. *Journal of Behavioral Medicine* 5(3): 461–463.

Raila, F., Tonato, M., Basusto, C., et al. (1985). Antiemetic activity of two different high doses of metoclopramide in cisplatin-treated cancer patients. *Cancer Treatment Report* 69: 1353–1357.

Rhodes, V.A., Watson, P.M., and Johnson, M.H. (1985). Patterns of nausea and vomiting in chemotherapy patients: A preliminary study. *Oncology Nursing Forum* 12(3): 42–48.

Roxane Laboratories (1986). Marinol (dronabinol) Manufacturer's Information Sheet. Roxane Laboratories.

Sargeant, K.S., and Fisher, J.M. (1986). Delta-9-tetrahydrocannabinol as antiemetic. *Drug Intelligence and Clinical Pharmacology* 20: 271–272.

Siegel, L.J., and Longo, D.L. (1981). The control of chemotherapy-induced emesis. *Annals of Internal Medicine* 95: 352–359.

Smaglia, R.A. (1984). Antiemetic effect of perphenazine versus prochlorperazine intravenously before cisplatin therapy. *American Journal of Hospital Pharmacology* 41 (March): 560.

Strum, S., McDerned, H.M., Abrahano-Umali, R., et al. (1985). Management of platinum-induced delayed onset nausea and vomiting: Preliminary results with two drug regimens. *Proceedings of the American Sociecty of Clinical Oncologists* 4: 263.

Strum, S.B., McDermed, J.E. Pileggi, J., et al. (1984). Intravenous metoclopramide: Prevention of chemotherapy-induced nausea and vomiting. *Cancer* 53(6): 1432–1439.

Wickham, R. (1999). Nausea and vomiting. In C.H. Yarbro, M.H. Frogge, and M. Goodman (eds.): *Cancer Symptoms Management*. Sudbury, Mass.: Jones & Bartlett, 228–264.

Wilson, J.M., Weltz, M., Solimando, D., et al. (1981). Continuous infusion droperidol: Antiemetic therapy for Cis-Platinum toxicity. *Proceedings of the American Society of Clinical Oncologists* 22: 421.

Yasko, J.M. (1985). Holistic management of nausea and vomiting caused by chemotherapy. *Topics in Clinical Nursing* (5): 26–29.

## Cardiac Toxicity

Ali, M.K., Soto, A., Maroongronge, D., et al. (1979). Electrocardiographic changes after Adriamycin chemotherapy. *Cancer* 43: 465–471.

Bristow, M.R. (1982). Toxic cardiomyopathy due to doxorubicin. *Hospital Practices* (December): 102–111.

Cortes, E.P., Lutman, G., Wanka, J., et al. (1975). Adriamycin cardiotoxicity: A clinicopathologic correlation. *Cancer Chemotherapy Report* Part 3, 6(2): 215–225.

Doll, D.C., List, A.F., Greco, A., et al. (1986). Acute vascular ischemic events after cisplatin-based combination chemotherapy for germ-cell tumors of the testes. *Annals of Internal Medicine* 105: 48–51.

Doll, D.C., Ringenberg, Q.S., and Yarbro, J.W. (1986). Vascular toxicity associated with antineoplastic agents. *Journal of Clinical Oncology* 4(9): 1450–1417.

Dorr, R.T., and Lasel, K.E. (1994). Anthracycline cardioprotection by amifostine (WR-2721) and its active metabolite (WR-1065) in vitro. *Proceedings of the American Society of Clinical Oncologists* 13: 435.

Druck, M.N., Gulenchyn, K.Y., Evans, W.K., et al. (1984). Radionucleotide angiography and endomyocardial biopsy in the assessment of doxorubicin cardiotoxicity. *Cancer* 53(8): 1667–1674.

Kaszyk, L.K. (1986). Cardiac toxicity associated with cancer therapy. *Oncology Nursing Forum* 13(4): 81–88.

Legha, S., Benjamin, R.S., MacKay, B., et al. (1982). Reduction of doxorubicin cardiotoxicity by prolonged continuous intravenous infusion. *Annals of Internal Medicine* 96: 133–139.

Minow, R.A., Benjamin, R.S., and Gottlieb, J.A. (1975). Adriamycin cardiomyopathy—An overview with determination of risk factors. *Cancer Chemotherapy Reports* 6: 195–201.

Saltiel, E., and McGuire, W. (1983). Doxorubicin cardiomyopathy. *Western Journal of Medicine* 139(3): 332–341.

Taylor, A.L., Applefeld, M.M., and Wiernik, P.H. (1984). Acute anthracycline cardiotoxicity: Comparative morphologic study of 3 analogues. *Cancer* 53(8): 1660–1666.

Tokaz, L.K., and Von Hoff, D.D. (1984). The toxicity of anticancer agents. In M.C. Perry and J.W. Yarbro (eds.): *Toxicity of Chemotherapy*. Orlando: Grune and Stratton, 199–226.

Tomitotti, M., Riundi, R., Pulici, S., et al. (1984). Ischemic cardiomyopathy from cis-diammine dichloroplatinum (CDDP). *Tumori* 70: 235–236.

Von Hoff, D., Rozencweig, M., Layard, M., et al. (1977). Daunomycin-induced cardiotoxicity in children and adults: A review of 110 cases. *American Journal of Medicine* 62: 200–208.

Yasko, J.M. (1983). *Guidelines for Cancer Care: Symptom Management*. Reston, Vir.: Reston Publishing Co.

Zinecard. (1995). Package Insert. Columbus, Ohio: Pharmacia, Inc.

## Pulmonary Toxicity

Blum, R.H., Carter, S.K., and Agre, K. (1973). A clinical review of bleomycin—A new antineoplastic agent. *Cancer* 31(4): 903–914.

Carlson, R.W., and Sikic, B.I. (1983). Continuous infusion or bolus injection in cancer chemotherapy. *Annals of Internal Medicine* 99(6): 823–833.

Comis, R.L., Kuppinger, M.S., Ginsberg, S.G., et al. (1979). Role of single-breath carbon monoxide diffusion capacity in monitoring the pulmonary efforts of bleomycin in germ cell tumor patients. *Cancer Research* 39(12): 5078–5080.

Einhorn, L., Krause, M., Hornbach, N., et al. (1976). Enhanced pulmonary toxicity with bleomycin and radiotherapy in oat cell lung cancer. *Cancer* 37(5): 2414–2416.

Ginsberg, S.J., and Comis, R.L. (1984). The pulmonary toxicity of antineoplastic agents. In M.C. Perry and J.W. Yarbro (eds.): *Toxicity of Chemotherapy*. New York: Grune and Stratton, 227–268.

Goodman, M.S. (1987). *Cancer: Chemotherapy and Care*. Evansville, Ind.: Bristol-Myers USP&NG, 33–34.

Holoyl, P.Y., Luna, M.A., Mackay, B., et al. (1978). Bleomycin hypersensitivity pneumonitis. *Annals of Internal Medicine* 88: 47–49.

Iacovino, J.R., Leitner, J., Abbas, A., et al. (1976). Fatal pulmonary reaction from low doses of bleomycin. *Journal of the American Medical Association* 235(12): 1253–1255.

Kriesman, H., and Wolkave, N. (1992). Pulmonary toxicity of antineoplastic therapy. In M.C Perry (ed.): *The Chemotherapy Source Book*. 2nd ed. Baltimore: Williams and Wilkins, 598–619.

Seltzer, S.E., Goldstein, J.D., and Herman, P.G. (1983). Iatrogenic thoracic complications induced by drugs. In P. Herman (ed.): *Iatrogenic Complications*. New York: Springer-Verlag, 1–8.

Wickham, R. (1986). Pulmonary toxicity secondary to cancer treatment. *Oncology Nursing Forum* 13(5): 69–76.

Yasko, J.M. (1983). *Guidelines for Cancer Care: Symptom Management*. Reston, Vir.: Reston Publishing Co.

## Hepatotoxicity

Dorr, R.T., and Fritz, W.L. (1981). *Cancer Chemotherapy Handbook*. New York: Elsevier, 130–133.

Fischer, D.S., and Knobf, M.T. (1989). *The Cancer Chemotherapy Handbook*. 3rd ed. Chicago: Year Book Medical Publishers.

Goodman, M.S. (1987). *Cancer: Chemotherapy and Care*. Evansville, Ind.: Bristol-Myers USP&NG, 32–33.

Menard, D.B., Gisselbrecht, C., Marty, M., et al. (1980). Antineoplastic agents and the liver. *Gastroenterology* 78: 142–164.

Perry, M.C. (1984). Hepatotoxicity. In M.C. Perry and J.W. Yarbro (eds.): *Toxicity of Chemotherapy*. Orlando: Grune and Stratton, 297–312.

Wilkes, G.M., Ingwersen, K., and Barton-Burke, M. (1999). *Oncology Nursing Drug Handbook*. Sudbury, Mass.: Jones & Bartlett, 60–186.

Woods, W.G., Denner, L.P., Nesbit, M.E., et al. (1980). Fatal veno-occlusive disease of the liver following high-dose chemotherapy, irradiation, and bone marrow transplantation. *American Journal of Medicine* 68: 285–290.

Zafrani, E.S., Pinaudeau, Y., and Dhumeaux, D. (1983). Drug-induced vascular lesions of the liver. *Archives of Internal Medicine* 143: 495–502.

## Nephrotoxicity

Abelson, H.T., and Garnick, M.D. (1982). Renal failure induced by cancer chemotherapy. In R.E. Rieselbach and M.B. Garnick (eds.): *Cancer and the Kidney*. Philadelphia: Lea and Febriger.

Cohen, D. (1983). Metabolic complications of induction therapy for leukemia and lymphoma. *Cancer Nursing* 6: 307.

Dentino, M., Luft, F.C., Yum, M.N., et al. (1978). Long-term effect of Cis-diammine-dichloro-platinum (CDDP) on renal function and structure in man. *Cancer* 41(4): 1224–1281.

Fields, A.L.A., Josse, R.G., and Bergsagel, D.E. (1982). Metabolic emergencies. In V.T. DeVita, Jr., S. Hellman, and S.A. Rosenberg (eds.): *Cancer: Principles and Practice of Oncology.* Philadelphia: Lippincott.

Garnick, M., and Mayer, R. (1978). Acute renal failure associated with neoplastic disease and its treatment. *Seminars in Oncology* 5(2): 155.

Goodman, M.S. (1987). *Cancer: Chemotherapy and Care.* Evansville, Ind.: Bristol-Myers USP&NG.

Lydon, J. (1986). Nephrotoxicity of cancer treatment. *Oncology Nursing Forum* 13(2): 68–77.

Moore, J. (1985). Metabolic emergencies: Tumor lysis syndrome. In B.L. Johnson and J. Gross (eds.): *Handbook of Oncology Nursing.* New York: John Wiley and Sons, 470–476.

Ostrow, S., Egorin, M.J., Hahn, D., et al. (1981). High-dose cisplatin therapy using mannitol vs. furosemide diuresis: Comparative pharmacokinetics and toxicities. *Cancer Treatment Reports,* 65(1–2): 73–78.

Ozols, R.F., Javadpour, N., Messerschmidt, G.L., et al. (1982). Poor prognosis non-seminomatous testicular cancer: An effective high-dose Cis-Platinum regimen without increased renal toxicity. *Proceedings of the American Society of Clinical Oncologists* 1: 113.

Perry, M.C., and Yarbro, J.W. (1984). *Toxicity of Chemotherapy.* New York: Grune and Stratton.

Schilsky, R.L. (1984). Renal and metabolic toxicities of cancer treatment. In M.C. Perry and J.W. Yarbro (eds.): *Toxicity of Chemotherapy.* Orlando: Grune and Stratton, 317–333.

Weiss, R.B., and Poster, D.S. (1982). The renal toxicity of cancer chemotherapy agents. *Cancer Treatment Reviews* 9(1): 37–56.

Yasko, J.M. (1983). *Guidelines for Cancer Care: Symptom Management.* Reston, Vir.: Reston Publishing Co.

## Neurotoxicity

Brager, B.L., and Yasko, J.M. (1984). *Care of the Client Receiving Chemotherapy.* Reston, Vir.: Reston Publishing Co.

DeFronzo, R.A., Braine, H., Colvin, O.M., et al. (1973). Water intoxification in man after cyclophosphamide therapy. *Annals of Internal Medicine* 78: 861–869.

Dorr, R.T., and Fritz, W.L. (1980). *Cancer Chemotherapy Handbook.* New York: Elsevier, 120–122.

Dorr, R.T., and Von Hoff, D.D. (1994). *Cancer Chemotherapy Handbook.* 2nd ed. Norwalk, Conn.: Appleton and Lange.

Furlong, T.G. (1993). Neurologic complications of immunosuppressive cancer therapy. *Oncology Nursing Forum* 20(9): 1337–1352.

Goodman, M.S. (1987). *Cancer: Chemotherapy and Care.* Evansville, Ind.: Bristol Myers USP&NG.

Hausheer, F.H., Kanter, P., Cao, S., et al. (1998). Modulation of platinum-induced toxicities and therapeutic index: Mechanistic insights and first and second generation protecting agents. *Seminars in Oncology* 25: 584–599.

Herzig, R.H., Herzig, G.P., Wolff, S.N., et al. (1987). Gentral nervous system effects of high-dose cytosine arabinoside. *Seminars in Oncology* 14(2) (Suppl 1): 21–24.

Holden, S., and Felde, G. (1987). Nursing care of patients experiencing cisplatin-related peripheral neuropathies. *Oncology Nursing Forum* 14(1): 13–19.

Kaplan, R.S., and Wiernik, P.H. (1984). Neurotoxicity of antitumor agents. In M.C. Perry and J.W. Yarbro (eds.): *Toxicity of Chemotherapy.* Orlando: Grune and Stratton, 365–431.

Legha, S.S., and Dimery, I.W. (1985). High-dose cisplatin administration without hypertonic saline: Observation of disabling neurotoxicity. *Journal of Clinical Oncology* 3: 1373–1378.

Maciewicz, R., Bouckoms, A., and Martin, J. (1985). Drug therapy of neuropathic pain. *Journal of Pain* 1(1): 39–49.

Mollman, J.E., Glover, D.J., Hogan, M., et al. (1988). Cisplatin neuropathy: Risk factors, prognosis, and protection by WR-2721. *Cancer* 56(8): 1934–1939.

Nelson, R.L., Dyke, R.W., and Root, M.A. (1980). Comparative pharmacokinetics of vindesine, vincristine, and vinblastine in patients with cancer. *Cancer Treatment Review* 7 (Suppl): 17–24.

Ogrinc, M. (1985). Sensory/perceptual alterations related to peripheral neuropathy. In J.C. McNally, J.C. Stair, and E.T. Somerville (eds.): *Guidelines for Cancer Nursing Practice*. Orlando: Grune and Stratton, 185–188.

Sandler, S.G., Tobin, W., and Henderson, E.S., (1969). Vincristine-induced neuropathy: A clinical study of fifteen leukemic patients. *Neurology* (Minn) 19: 367–374.

Schaefer, S.D., Post, J.D., Close, L.G., et al. (1985). Ototoxicity of low-and moderate-dose cisplatin. *Cancer* 56(8): 1934–1939.

Seifert, P., Baker, L.H., Reed, M.L., et al. (1975). Comparison of continuously infused 5-fluorouracil with bolus injection in treatment of patients with colorectal adenocarcinoma. *Cancer* 36: 123–128.

Stuart, M.J., Cuaso, C., Miller, M., et al. (1975). Syndrome of recurrent increased secretion of antidiuretic hormone following multiple doses of vincristine. *Blood* 45: 315–320.

Weiss, H.D., Walker, M.D., and Wiernik, P.H. (1974). Neurotoxicity of commonly used anticancer agents. *New England Journal of Medicine* 291: 75–81.

Wilding, G., Caruso, R., Lawrence, T., et al. (1985). Retinal toxicity after high-dose cisplatin therapy. *Journal of Clinical Oncology* 3(12): 1683–1689.

Vizel, M., and Oster, M. (1982). Ocular side effects of cancer chemothrapy. *Cancer* 49: 1999–2002.

Yasko, J.M. (1983). *Guidelines for Cancer Care: Symptom Management*. Reston, Vir.: Reston Publishing Co.

# Chapter 5

# Chemotherapeutic Agents

## Standardized Nursing Care Plans to Minimize Toxicity

## INTRODUCTION

The nursing process forms the basis for nursing practice. This chapter integrates the nursing process into the activities of chemotherapy administration. The content of both the drug information forms and the care plans is meant to be information that the nurse needs to know at the time of administration in order to give the medication safely. The information is not meant to replace any hospital formulary or manufacturer information. The writers and publisher of this book have made every effort to ensure that the dosage regimens set forth in the text are accurate and in accord with current labeling at the time of publication. However, in view of the constant flow of information resulting from ongoing research and clinical experience, as well as changes in government regulations, nurses are urged to check the package insert of each drug they plan to administer to be certain that changes have not been made in its indications or contraindications or in the recommended dosage for each use. This is particularly important when a drug is new or infrequently used.

The following information is a synthesis of many sources reviewed by the authors. In-depth drug information can be gathered from the sources at the back of the chapter and from the numerous books that are available solely on cancer chemotherapy. The drug care plans are meant to be shorthand for the larger side-effect care plans that are in Chapters 4 and 9.

The nursing diagnoses used in this chapter are analogous to the NANDA-approved nursing diagnoses. These diagnoses occur when a patient receives the specific chemotherapeutic agent. At times these diagnoses seem repetitive (as do the nursing interventions), but the reader will notice that the defining characteristics are always individualized to the specific drug. The nursing interventions should be individualized to the specific patient being cared for, using the plan as a basis for care.

Patient education is an integral part of all nursing care. The authors have included aspects of patient education under specific nursing interventions, rather than separating patient education into a specific nursing diagnosis of its own.

# Acridinyl anisidide
## (AMSA, M-AMSA)

*Class:* Investigational

## MECHANISM OF ACTION

Cell cycle phase–specific—S phase. The primary mechanism of action is not yet clearly understood. It is believed that AMSA binds with DNA by intercalating between base pairs and thus prohibiting RNA synthesis.

## METABOLISM

Broken down into metabolites in the liver and excreted in the bile and urine. The initial half-life of AMSA is 12 minutes; the half-life of the metabolites is 2.5 hours.

## DOSAGE/RANGE

Drug is undergoing clinical trials. Consult individual protocol for specific dosages.

## DRUG PREPARATION

AMSA is available as two sterile liquids: one ampule with an orange-red solution of AMSA; a second with the dilutant L-lactic acid.

The solution, once mixed, is chemically stable for 48 hours. It should be discarded after 8 hours because of lack of bacteriostatic preservatives.

AMSA is not stable in sodium chloride-containing solutions. Precipitates form. Only 5% dextrose solutions should be used.

## DRUG ADMINISTRATION

Dilute the AMSA solution further in $D_5W$ and infuse over 1 hour unless contraindicated.

## SPECIAL CONSIDERATIONS

Drug is a vesicant.

Drug is investigational.

No anaphylaxis reported.

Do not dilute AMSA with chloride-containing solutions.

Impaired liver function may require dose modifications.

Drug is orange-red when reconstituted.

## Acridinyl anisidide

| Nursing Diagnosis | Defining Characteristics | Expected Outcomes | Nursing Interventions |
|---|---|---|---|
| I. *Altered nutrition, less than body requirements related to* A. Nausea and vomiting | I. A. The frequency and severity of the nausea or vomiting is dose dependent; only occurs in ~10% of pts and lasts only a few hours | I. A. Pt will be without nausea and vomiting; nausea and vomiting, if they occur, will be minimal | I. A. 1. Premedicate with antiemetics and continue prophylactically × 24 hrs to prevent nausea and vomiting, at least first treatment 2. Encourage small, frequent feedings of cool, bland foods and liquids |
| B. Stomatitis | B. Mild to moderate | B. Oral mucous membranes will remain intact without infection | B. 1. Teach pt oral assessment 2. Encourage pt to report early stomatitis 3. Teach pt oral hygiene 4. See sec. on stomatitis, Chapter 4 |
| C. Diarrhea | C. Infrequent and mild | C. Pt will have minimal diarrhea | C. 1. Encourage pt to report onset of diarrhea 2. Administer or teach pt to self-administer antidiarrheal medications 3. See sec. on diarrhea, Chapter 4 |
| D. Hepatic dysfunction | D. Hepatitis is rare but may occur; also, disturbances in liver function studies, especially elevated serum alkaline phosphatase and serum bilirubin | D. Hepatic dysfunction will be identified early | D. 1. Monitor LFTs (i.e., alkaline phosphatase and bilirubin), periodically during treatment 2. Monitor pt for any elevations 3. Dose modifications may be necessary if LFT elevation occurs |

*(continued)*

## Acridinyl anisidide (*continued*)

| Nursing Diagnosis | Defining Characteristics | Expected Outcomes | Nursing Interventions |
|---|---|---|---|
| II. *Infection and bleeding related to bone marrow depression* | II. A. Hematologic toxicity is the dose-limiting toxicity<br>B. Leukopenia nadir 7–14 days with recovery by day 25<br>C. Relatively platelet-sparing with only mild thrombocytopenia except in pt with history of radiation to major marrow-producing sites<br>D. Mild anemia | II. A. Pt will be without s/s of infection or bleeding<br>B. Early s/s of infection or bleeding will be identified | II. A. Monitor CBC, platelet count prior to drug administration as well as s/s of infection and bleeding<br>B. Instruct pt in self-assessment of s/s of infection and bleeding<br>C. Dose reduction necessary with compromised bone marrow function<br>D. Refer to sec. on bone marrow depression, Chapter 4 |
| III. *Alteration in cardiac output related to high-dose AMSA* | III. A. Pts have developed ventricular fibrillation when the serum potassium level was low<br>B. CHF has been reported in pt with prior history of antitumor antibiotics (e.g., doxorubicin or daunorubicin)<br>C. Cardiac arrest has been reported during amsacrine infusions | III. A. Early s/s of CHF and cardiac irregularities will be identified | III. A. Assess pt for s/s of CHF and quality/regularity of heartbeat<br>B. Monitor I&O<br>C. Discuss gated blood pool scans with MD<br>D. Instruct pt to report dyspnea, shortness of breath, palpitations, swelling in extremities<br>E. Check potassium levels; monitor for cardiac irregularities associated with low serum potassium levels |

| Nursing diagnosis | Assessment data | Expected outcomes | Interventions |
|---|---|---|---|
| IV. *Impaired skin integrity related to phlebitis* | IV. A. Pain may occur if drug is not properly diluted<br>B. Skin discoloration (yellow-orange) has been reported in 10% of pts | IV. A. AMSA will be diluted according to manufacturer's recommendations<br>B. Pt will verbalize any pain related to chemotherapy administration<br>C. Phlebitis will be identified early and treated to minimize adverse effects | IV. A. Follow manufacturer's recommendations for drug preparation<br>B. Assess pt for s/s of immediate or late pain/phlebitis<br>C. Teach pt s/s of phlebitis and to report any symptoms early<br>D. Discuss with pt potential skin discoloration and strategies to minimize distress |
| V. *Potential for injury related to*<br>A. Hypersensitivity reactions | V. A. Range from transient skin rashes to anaphylactic reactions in ~0.4% of patients | V. A. Early s/s of hypersensitivity will be identified | V. A. 1. Teach pt about the potential of a hypersensitivity reaction and to report any unusual symptoms<br>2. Obtain baseline vital signs and note pts mental status<br>3. Assess pt for s/s of a reaction: localized flare reaction—anaphylaxis. See sec. on reactions, Chapter 9<br>4. Administer therapy in case of reaction according to MD orders |
| B. Neurological reactions | B. At very high doses of AMSA, transient paresthesias, hearing loss, and seizure activity have been reported | B. Early s/s of paresthesias and seizure activity will be identified | B. 1. Teach pt the potential of neurologic reactions and to report any unusual symptoms<br>2. Obtain baseline neurologic mental and hearing functions<br>3. Assess pt for any unusual neuro symptoms and report changes to MD |

## Adrenocorticoids
(Cortisone, Hydrocortisone, Dexamethasone, Methylprednisone, Methylprednisolone, Prednisone, Prednisolone)

*Class:* Hormones

### MECHANISM OF ACTION

Cause lysis of lymphoid cells, which led to their use against lymphatic leukemia, myeloma, malignant lymphoma. May also recruit malignant cells out of $G_0$ phase, making them vulnerable to damage caused by cell cycle phase–specific agents.

### METABOLISM

Metabolized by the liver, excreted in urine. Prednisone is activated by the liver in its active form, prednisolone.

### DOSAGE/RANGE

Varies according to which preparation is used. Dexamethasone is 25 times the potency of hydrocortisone.

Sample doses:

| | |
|---|---|
| Cortisone | 25 mg |
| Hydrocortisone | 20 mg |
| Prednisone, prednisolone | 5 mg |
| Methylprednisone, Methylprednisolone | 4 mg |
| Dexamethasone | 0.75 mg |

### DRUG PREPARATION

None

### DRUG ADMINISTRATION

Oral

### SPECIAL CONSIDERATIONS

Chronic steroid use is associated with numerous side effects. Intermittent therapy is safer and in some conditions just as effective as daily therapy.

# Adrenocorticoids

ADRENOCORTICOIDS **193**

| Nursing Diagnosis | Defining Characteristics | Expected Outcomes | Nursing Interventions |
|---|---|---|---|
| I. *Altered nutrition, less than body requirements related to* <br> A. Gastric irritation | I. A. 1. Steroids may cause increase in secretion of hydrochloric acid and decreased secretion of protective gastric mucus <br> 2. May exacerbate existing gastric ulcer | I. A. Gastric irritation will be avoided/minimized | I. A. 1. Administer drug with meals, antacid, or $H_2$ blocker. Instruct pt in optimal schedule for drug administration <br> 2. Instruct pt to report evidence of gastric distress immediately |
| B. Decreased carbohydrate metabolism; hyperglycemia | B. Steroids are insulin antagonists and may cause gluconeogenesis | B. Blood sugar will remain within normal limits | B. 1. Obtain baseline glucose levels; monitor blood sugar periodically throughout therapy <br> 2. Teach pt to recognize s/s of hyperglycemia (polyuria, polydipsia, polyphagia) and to report these to doctor or nurse <br> 3. Dipstick urine for glucose |
| II. *Potential for injury related to* <br> A. Sodium and water retention | II. A. Occurs occasionally | II. A. Fluid and electrolyte balance will be maintained | II. A. 1. Identify pts at risk for complications associated with fluid/sodium retention (pts with preexisting cardiac, renal, hepatic dysfunction) <br> 2. Inform pts of potential for sodium/water retention, of s/s to watch for, and to report to MD <br> 3. Assess pt daily (if inpatient) for s/s of fluid/electrolyte imbalance |

*(continued)*

## Adrenocorticoids (continued)

| Nursing Diagnosis | Defining Characteristics | Expected Outcomes | Nursing Interventions |
|---|---|---|---|
| II. *Potential for injury related to* B. Hypokalemia/ hypocalcemia | II. B. 1. Causes increased excretion of potassium, calcium 2. Osteoporosis may occur with long-term therapy | II. B. Potassium and calcium levels will remain within normal limits | II. B. 1. Teach pt to report s/s of hypocalcemia (leg cramps, tingling in fingertips, muscle twitching) 2. Instruct pt to report s/s hypokalemia (weakness, ileus) 3. Monitor eletrolytes on a regular basis; report abnormal values and replace as needed with supplements 4. Encourage high-potassium, high-calcium diet; if indicated, discuss supplements 5. Instruct pt in safety measures to avoid injury |
| C. Steroid-induced immunosuppression | C. 1. Increases susceptibility to infections, tuberculosis 2. May mask or aggravate infection 3. May prolong or delay healing of injuries | C. Pt will remain free of infection | C. 1. Instruct pt to report slow healing of wounds and signs of infection (inflammation, redness, soreness, etc) or colds 2. Instruct pt in hygiene regimens: mouth, perineal, foot care |
| III. *Potential sensory/ perceptual alterations* | III. A. Cataracts or glaucoma may develop with prolonged steroid use B. Increased risk of ocular infections resulting from viruses or fungi | III. A. Pts vision will remain at baseline levels | III. A. Opthalmoscopic exams recommended every 2–3 months B. Instruct pt to report s/s eye infection (discharge, vision changes), or decreased vision |

IV. *Potential for body image disturbance*

IV. A. Cushingoid state may occur with prolonged use
B. Every other day therapy may reduce Cushingoid changes
C. May include acne, moonface, striae, purpura, hirsutism

IV. A. Pt will verbalize feelings about altered body image and identifies strategies for coping with changes

IV. A. Discuss possible body changes with pt and emphasize that they will resolve when therapy is discontinued
B. Assess pt for Cushingoid features
C. Offer emotional support
D. Administer drug in early morning with breakfast

V. *Potential alteration in behavior*

V. A. Commonly causes behavioral changes, which include emotional lability, insomnia, mood swings, psychosis, increased appetite

V. A. Pt will avoid significant changes in behavior
B. Behavioral changes, should they occur, will be tolerable to pt

V. A. Inform pt and family that behavioral changes may occur and that they will resolve when therapy is discontinued
B. Encourage pt to report troublesome behavioral changes to physician

VI. *Potential for immobility*

VI. A. Loss of muscle mass may occur with chronic use and may be serious enough to impair walking
B. Muscle cramping can occur with discontinuation of treatment

VI. A. Pt will maintain baseline mobility

VI. A. Inform pt that muscle weakness may occur with therapy and that muscle cramping may occur on discontinuation of therapy
B. Encourage pts to report weakness, cramping; weakness may necessitate discontinuation of therapy, as recovery is not always complete

# Amifostine for injection
(Ethyol, WR-2721)

*Class:* Free-radical scavenger, metabolized to a free thiol that can neutralize cisplatin in normal cells

## MECHANISM OF ACTION

Drug is phosphorylated by alk phos, producing free thiol. Inside the cell, the free thiol binds to reactive cisplatin, thus neutralizing the platinum in normal tissues so that cellular DNA and RNA are not damaged. Normal cells are protected because of differences in cell physiology (alkaline phosphate concentrations and tissue pH) and transport that promote the preferential uptake of free thiol into normal tissues.

## METABOLISM

Drug is rapidly metabolized to an active freethiol metabolite and cleared from the plasma, so the drug should be administered 30 minutes prior to drug dose.

## DOSAGE/RANGE

910 mg/m$^2$ administered intravenously (IV) 30 minutes prior to beginning cisplatin-based therapy, but some investigators suggest initial dose of 740 mg/m$^2$.

If patient is unable to receive the full dose because infusion was stopped for hypotension and not resumed, the next dose and subsequent doses should be reduced to 740 mg/m$^2$.

## DRUG PREPARATION

Available in 10-ml vials containing 500 mg of drug; store at room temperature.

Use only 0.9% sodium chloride.

Reconstitute vial with 9.7 ml of sterile 0.9% sodium chloride.

Further dilute with sterile 0.9% sodium chloride to total 50 ml.

Stable at 5 mg/ml to 40 mg/ml for 5 hours at room temperature, and for 24 hours if refrigerated.

## DRUG ADMINISTRATION

Hypertension medicines should be stopped 24 hours prior to drug administration.

Place patient in supine position.

Administer combination antiemetics.

Infuse amifostine IV over 15 minutes, beginning 30 minutes prior to cisplatin.

## SPECIAL CONSIDERATIONS

Patients unable to tolerate cessation of antihypertensive medications are not candidates for the drug.

Drug is indicated to reduce the cumulative renal toxicity from cisplatin in patients with advanced ovarian cancer or non-small-cell lung cancer.

Studies have shown no decrease in drug efficacy when given with first-line therapy in ovarian cancer.

No evidence exists that drug interferes with tumor response from chemotherapy in other cancers, but research is ongoing.

Offers significant protection of kidneys.

Offers protection of bone marrow and nerves.

Drug has been shown to protect skin, mucous membranes, and bladder and pelvic structures against late moderate to severe radiation reactions.

## Amifostine for injection (Ethyol, WR-2721)

| Nursing Diagnosis | Defining Characteristics | Expected Outcomes | Nursing Interventions |
|---|---|---|---|
| I. *Alteration in nutrition, less than body requirements, related to nausea and vomiting, hypocalcemia* | I. A. Nausea and vomiting are common, and may be severe. These are preventable using serotonin antagonist and dexamethasone<br>B. Drug has a known hypocalcemic effect but not at this dose. Incidence is < 1% | I. A. Pt will be without nausea and vomiting<br>B. Nausea/vomiting will be minimized<br>C. Serum calcium will remain within normal limits | I. A. Administer serotonin antagonist (e.g. granisetron, ondansetron, or dolasetron) and dexamethasone 20 mg IV prior to amifostine<br>B. Encourage small, frequent meals of cool, bland foods and liquids<br>C. Teach pt self-management tips and to avoid greasy or heavy foods<br>D. Teach pt to maintain oral hydration as tolerated<br>E. Monitor calcium and albumin, both before and during treatment. Repeat as necessary |
| II. *Alteration in oxygenation related to hypotension potential* | II. A. Drug causes transient, reversible hypotension in 62% of pts | II. A. Pt will maintain systolic BP greater than recommended threshold (see below) | II. A. Antihypertensives should be stopped 24 hrs prior to drug administration<br>B. Assess baseline systolic BP (SBP) and heart rate<br>C. Place pt in supine position: monitor SBP every 5 mins during infusion, and 5 mins postinfusion. Stop infusion temporarily if SBP falls below threshold. BP should normalize within 5 mins (if not, terminate infusion, give IV hydration, and place pt in Trendelenburg, if necessary). Restart infusion if SBP recovers within 5 mins<br>D. Administer drug over 15 mins, increases in side effects have been noted with longer infusions |

*(continued)*

## Amifostine for injection (Ethyol, WR-2721) (continued)

| Nursing Diagnosis | Defining Characteristics | Expected Outcomes | Nursing Interventions |
| --- | --- | --- | --- |
| III. Alteration in comfort related to flushing, chills, dizziness, somnolence, hiccups, and sneezing | III. A. These effects may occur during or after drug infusion and are mild<br>B. Allergic reactions are rare, ranging from skin rash to rigors, but anaphylaxis has not been reported | III. A. Pt will report comfort throughout infusion | III. A. Assess comfort level, and ask pt to report above symptoms<br>B. Treat side effects per physician order<br>E. Manufacturer recommends the following guidelines: |

| Baseline Systolic BP (SBP) | Threshold SBP in mm Hg |
| --- | --- |
| < 100 | < 80 |
| 100–119 | 75–94 |
| 120–139 | 90–109 |
| 140–179 | 100–139 |
| ≥ 180 | ≥ 130 |

# 9-aminocamptothecin
(9-AC)

*Class:* Topoisomerase inhibitor

## MECHANISM OF ACTION

Induces protein-linked DNA single-strand breaks and blocks DNA and RNA synthesis in dividing cells, preventing cells from entering mitosis. Cell cycle specific.

## METABOLISM

32% of the drug is excreted in the urine as unchanged drug at 96 hours.

## DOSAGE/RANGE

35 µg/m$^2$/hour every 2 weeks or 45 µg/m$^2$/hr every 3 weeks (Phase II trials) as 72-hour infusion.

Prolonged infusion studies under way.

## DRUG PREPARATION

Per protocol

## DRUG ADMINISTRATION

IV infusion over 72 hours

## SPECIAL CONSIDERATIONS

Neutropenia is dose-limiting toxicity.

## 9-aminocamptothecin (9-AC)

| Nursing Diagnosis | Defining Characteristics | Expected Outcomes | Nursing Interventions |
|---|---|---|---|
| I. *Infection and bleeding related to bone marrow depression* | I. A. May cause neutropenia (dose-limiting), thrombocytopenia, and anemia | I. A. Pt will be without s/s of infection or bleeding<br>B. Signs of infection and/or bleeding will be identified and reported early | I. A. Monitor Hct, WBC with differential, and platelets prior to drug administration. Discuss any abnormalities with physician (drug should not be given if ANC is < 750 cells/mm$^3$)<br>B. Drug dose to be reduced with renal impairment: if creatinine is greater than 3 mg/dl, reduce dose by 50%<br>C. Drug dose to be reduced with hepatic dysfunction: 50% reduction if serum bilirubin is greater than 3 mg/dl, 25% reduction if serum bilirubin is 1.2–3.0 mg/dl<br>D. Assess for s/s infection and bleeding, and instruct patient in self-assessment and to report s/s immediately<br>E. Teach pt self-care measures to minimize risk of infection and bleeding, including avoidance of OTC aspirin-containing medications<br>F. Refer to section on bone marrow depression, Chapter 4 |
| II. *Alteration in nutrition, less than body requirements, related to nausea and vomiting, diarrhea* | II. A. Nausea, vomiting, diarrhea, mucositis may occur | II. A. Patient will be without nausea or vomiting<br>B. Nausea/vomiting will be minimized | II. A. Premedicate with antiemetics and continue for 24 hrs to prevent nausea and vomiting<br>B. Encourage small, frequent feedings of cool, bland foods and liquids<br>C. Instruct pt in oral self-care measures, and to report nausea/vomiting and diarrhea to health care providers<br>D. Teach self-administration of prescribed antidiarrheals, and self-care techniques for discomfort and maintenance of mucosal integrity |

| | | E. Refer to clinical protocol for more details |
| | | F. Refer to section on nausea/vomiting and diarrhea, Chapter 4 |
| *III. Alteration in skin integrity related to alopecia* | III. A. Alopecia may occur | III. A. Teach pt about possible side effect and self-care measures, including obtaining a wig or cap as appropriate prior to hair loss |
| | III. A. Pt will verbalize understanding of possibility of alopecia and self-care measures to minimize distress | B. Identify pt resources to help coping with loss |
| | | C. Encourage pt to verbalize feelings and provide emotional support |
| *IV. Potential for activity intolerance related to fatigue* | IV. A. Fatigue and anemia are common | IV. A. Teach pt to report increasing fatigue, signs of severe anemia (shortness of breath, chest pain/angina, headaches). Discuss self-care measures to minimize fatigue |
| | IV. A. Pt will verbalize understanding of need to report fatigue, of self-care measures to minimize fatigue | B. Monitor hemoglobin/hematocrit; discuss transfusion with physician if signs/symptoms develop or hematocrit falls (refer to protocol) |

# Aminoglutethimide
(Cytadren, Elipten)

*Class:* Adrenal steroid inhibitor

## MECHANISM OF ACTION

Causes "chemical adrenalectomy." Blocks adrenal production of steroids, reducing levels of glucocorticoids, mineralocorticoids, and estrogens. Also inhibits peripheral aromatization of androgens to estrogens.

## METABOLISM

Well absorbed orally. Hydroxylated in liver, undergoes enterohepatic circulation. Most of drug is excreted in urine.

## DOSAGE/RANGE

750–2000 mg orally daily in divided doses
40 mg hydrocortisone daily given to replace glucocorticoid deficiencies

## DRUG PREPARATION

None

## DRUG ADMINISTRATION

Oral

## SPECIAL CONSIDERATIONS

Skin rash may develop within 5–7 days, lasting 8 days, often with malaise and fever (100°–102°F; 37.5°–39°C). If not resolved in 7–14 days, drug should be discontinued.

Adjuvant corticosteroids need to be administered.

# Aminoglutethimide

| Nursing Diagnosis | Defining Characteristics | Expected Outcomes | Nursing Interventions |
|---|---|---|---|
| I. *Impairment of skin integrity related to rash* | I. A. Seen within 1 week of treatment and disappears in 5–8 days<br>B. If rash does not disappear within expected time, drug may be discontinued<br>C. May be accompanied by malaise and low-grade fever<br>D. Symptoms may include erythema, pruritis, and unexplained dermatitis | I. A. Pt will verbalize feelings regarding changes in skin and identifies s/s of potential alterations | I. A. Assess skin for any cutaneous changes, including location and description<br>B. Instruct pt in self-care measures<br>1. Avoid abrasive products, clothing<br>2. Avoid tight-fitting clothing<br>3. Avoid scratching involved areas |
| II. *Sensory/perceptual alteration related to chemotherapy* | II. A. Lethargy common<br>B. Other s/s include somnolence, visual blurring, vertigo, ataxia, and nystagmus<br>C. Symptoms may be general and transient | II. A. Sensory-perceptual neurological disturbances will be identified early | II. A. Obtain baseline neurologic/motor function prior to administering chemotherapy<br>B. Teach pt self-assessment techniques and risks of disturbances<br>C. Encourage pt to report any disturbances early<br>D. Further dose reductions may be necessary |
| III. *Infection related to myelosuppression* | III. A. Leukopenia is rare | III. A. Pt will be without infection<br>B. Early s/s of infection will be identified | III. A. Monitor CBC, including WBC, differential prior to drug administration<br>B. Drug dosage may be reduced or held for lower than normal blood values<br>C. See sec. on bone marrow depression, Chapter 4 |

*(continued)*

## Aminoglutethimide (*continued*)

| Nursing Diagnosis | Defining Characteristics | Expected Outcomes | Nursing Interventions |
|---|---|---|---|
| IV. *Altered nutrition, less than body requirements related to* A. Nausea and vomiting | IV. A. Nausea and vomiting usually mild | IV. A. Pt will be without nausea or vomiting; nausea or vomiting, if they occur, will be minimal | IV. A. 1. Premedicate with antiemetics and continue prophylactically × 24 hrs to prevent nausea and vomiting at least for first treatment 2. Encourage small, frequent feedings of cool, bland foods and liquids |
| B. Anorexia | B. Mild | B. Pt will maintain baseline weight ± 5% | B. 1. Encourage small, frequent feedings of favorite foods, especially high-calorie, high-protein (HCHP) foods 2. Encourage use of spices 3. Weekly weights 4. Nutritional consult as needed |
| V. *Alteration in fluid/ electrolyte balance* | V. A. Possible with higher doses of aminoglutethimide B. Symptoms of hyponatremia include headache, nausea/vomiting, muscle weakness, lethargy C. Symptoms of hyperkalemia include abdominal cramping, muscle weakness, tingling, cardiac irregularities, mental status changes | V. A. Fluid and electrolyte balance will be maintained | V. A. Monitor patient for weight gain, edema with daily weights B. Monitor I&O C. Check electrolytes daily, monitor for clinical s/s of imbalance |

VI. *Potential for endocrine dysfunction related to adrenal insufficiency*

VI. A. Causes reversible chemical adrenalectomy (adrenal insufficiency) by blocking synthesis of all steroid hormones

B. Additional s/s of cortisol insufficiency

C. Hyponatremia, postural hypotension (aldosterone), possible hypothyroidism

D. Possible ovarian malfunction, resulting in virilization

VI. A. Pt will verbalize feelings regarding sexual dysfunction and body image changes due to hormonal alterations

B. Side effects from corticosteroid replacement therapy will be identified early

VI. A. Educate pt and significant other in self-administration of hormone replacement therapy (i.e., preferred time of administration, potential side effects, tapering schedule)

B. Encourage pt to report any untoward effects, especially while on steroid replacement

C. Monitor electrolytes, especially Na+, K+, Ca++

D. Encourage diet high in carbohydrates and protein

E. Weekly weight

F. Assess for s/s of infection

G. Monitor I&O

H. Assess pt for behavioral changes

I. Assess pt for Addisonian/adrenal crisis

J. As appropriate, explore with pt and significant other reproductive and sexuality patterns and impact chemotherapy may have; see sec. on gonadal dysfunction, Chapter 4

# Anastrozole
## (Arimidex)

*Class:* Nonsteroidal aromatase inhibitor

## MECHANISM OF ACTION

Inhibits the enzyme aromatase. Aromatase is one of the P-450 enzymes and is involved in estrogen biosynthesis. Circulating estrogen in postmenopausal women (mainly estradiol) arises from the aromatase-mediated conversion of androstenedione (made by the adrenals) to estrone, then estrone to estradiol, in the peripheral tissues, such as adipose tissue. Anastrozole is highly selective for this enzyme and does not affect steroid synthesis, so that estradiol synthesis is potently suppressed (to undetectable levels) while cortisol and aldosterone levels are unchanged.

## METABOLISM

Extensively metabolized, with 85% of the drug metabolized by the liver. About 10% of the unchanged drug and 60% of the drug as metabolites are excreted in the urine within 72 hours of drug administration.

## DOSAGE/RANGE

1 mg PO qd. No dosage adjustment required for mild to moderate hepatic impairment

## DRUG PREPARATION

None. Available as 1-mg tablet

## DRUG ADMINISTRATION

Take orally with or without food, at approximately the same time daily

## SPECIAL CONSIDERATIONS

Second-line therapy for postmenopausal women with advanced breast cancer.

Well-tolerated with low toxicity profile.

Coadministration of corticosteroids is not necessary.

Absolutely contraindicated during pregnancy.

## Anastrozole

| Nursing Diagnosis | Defining Characteristics | Expected Outcomes | Nursing Interventions |
|---|---|---|---|
| I. Sexual dysfunction related to decreased estrogen levels | I. A. Hot flashes (12%), asthenia or loss of energy (16%), and vaginal dryness may occur | I. A. Pt will verbalize understanding of the possibility of side effects affecting sexual function, and strategies to cope with changes | I. A. As appropriate, explore with pt and partner patterns of sexuality, and impact therapy may have  B. Discuss strategies to preserve sexual health  C. Teach pt that the vaginal dryness may be from menopause (and not the drug), and she should avoid estrogen creams, but should use some lubrication |
| II. Potential alteration in cardiac output related to thrombophlebitis | II. A. Thrombophlebitis may occur, but is uncommon | II. A. Cardiac output will remain at baseline | II. A. Identify pts at risk for thromboembolic complications  B. Teach pts to report/come to emergency room for pain, redness, or marked swelling in arms or legs, or if shortness of breath or dizziness occur |
| III. Alteration in comfort related to headaches, weakness | III. A. Headaches are mild and occur in about 13% of patients  B. Decreased energy and weakness is common  C. Mild swelling of arms/legs may occur and is mild | III. A. Pt will report comfort throughout treatment process | III. A. Teach pt to take OTC analgesics for headache, and to report headaches that are unrelieved by them  B. Elevate extremities when at rest, as needed |

(continued)

## Anastrozole (continued)

| Nursing Diagnosis | Defining Characteristics | Expected Outcomes | Nursing Interventions |
|---|---|---|---|
| IV. *Potential alteration in nutrition, less than body requirements, related to nausea, diarrhea* | IV. A. Nausea is mild, with a 15% incidence. Diarrhea is uncommon and mild | IV. A. Pt will be without nausea or diarrhea | IV. A. Determine baseline weight, and monitor at each visit<br>B. Teach pt about the possibility of nausea, and measures that may be used to alleviate it, including diet and dosing time<br>C. Assess for changes in bowel pattern, and teach pt to report diarrhea<br>D. Instruct pt in administration of antidiarrheal medications (Kaopectate, loperamide, etc.), and in reporting unrelieved diarrhea |

# Androgens
testosterone propionate (Neohombreol, Oreton), fluoxymesterone (Halotestin, Ora-Testryl), testolactone (Teslac)

*Class:* Hormones

## MECHANISM OF ACTION

Has stimulatory effect on red blood cells that results in an increased hematocrit. Other mechanism of action unknown.

## METABOLISM

Metabolized by the liver; excreted in the urine and feces.

## DOSAGE/RANGE

Testosterone propionate 50–100 mg IM 3 times weekly

Fluoxymesterone 10–30 mg orally daily (3–4 divided doses)

Testolactone 100 mg IM 3 times weekly or 250 mg orally 4 times daily

## DRUG PREPARATION

Drug comes in ready-to-use vials or tablets.

## DRUG ADMINISTRATION

Before IM administration, shake vial vigorously and give injection immediately to avoid solution settling.

## SPECIAL CONSIDERATIONS

Fluoxymesterone may increase sensitivity to oral anticoagulants. Should be administered in divided doses because of its short action.

## Androgens

| Nursing Diagnosis | Defining Characteristics | Expected Outcomes | Nursing Interventions |
|---|---|---|---|
| I. *Altered nutrition, less than body requirements related to* A. Nausea and vomiting | I. A. Uncommon but may occur | I. A. Pt will be without nausea and vomiting | I. A. 1. Inform pt that nausea and vomiting can occur; encourage patient to report nausea or vomiting <br> 2. Encourage small, frequent feedings of cool, bland foods and liquids <br> 3. Refer to sec. on nausea and vomiting, Chapter 4 |
| II. *Potential for injury related to* A. Sodium and water retention | II. A. Occur occasionally and may imply need for dose reduction or diuretic therapy | II. A. Fluid and electrolyte balance will be maintained | II. A. 1. Identify pts at risk for complications associated with fluid/sodium retention: cardiac history, renal or hepatic disease, low serum protein <br> 2. Inform pt of potential for sodium/water retention, of s/s to watch for, and to report to MD <br> 3. Assess pt daily (if inpatient) for s/s of fluid/electrolyte imbalance |
| B. Hypercalcemia | B. 1. Uncommon in everyone except those patients with bony metastases <br> 2. Risk is highest during induction therapy | B. 1. Serum calcium will remain within normal limits <br> 2. Hypercalcemia will be identified and treated early | B. 1. Identify pts at risk and monitor serum calcium closely during the first few weeks of therapy; hypercalcemia is an indication to discontinue treatment <br> 2. Teach pt s/s of hypercalcemia (drowsiness, increased thirst, constipation, increased urine output); instruct pt to notify MD if s/s occur |

| | | | |
|---|---|---|---|
| C. Obstructive jaundice | C. Has occurred with methyltestosterone, fluoxymesterone, and oxymethalone | C. LFTs will remain within normal limits | C. 1. Teach pt to report GI distress, diarrhea, onset of jaundice<br>2. Monitor LFTs |
| III. *Sexual dysfunction related to masculinization* | III. A. Occurs commonly in women; increased risk when therapy duration exceeds 3 months; prolonged use may cause irreversible masculinization<br>B. Symptoms include increased libido, deepening of voice, excessive body hair growth (especially noticeable on face), acne, clitoral hypertrophy<br>C. In men, drug may cause priapism (sustained and often painful erections) and reduced ejaculatory volume | III. A. Pt will report onset of changes in sexual characteristics<br>B. Pt and significant other will verbalize understanding of changes in sexuality that may occur<br>C. Pt and significant other identify strategies to cope with sexual dysfunction | III. A. Instruct pt to report onset of symptoms, indicating changes in sexual characteristics, functioning; those symptoms may necessitate terminating therapy<br>B. As appropriate, explore with pt and significant other issues of reproductive and sexuality patterns and the impact therapy may have on them<br>C. Discuss strategies to preserve sexual and reproductive health<br>D. See sec. on gonadal dysfunction, Chapter 4 |

# 5-Azacytidine
(Azacytidine, 5AZ)

*Class:* Investigational

## MECHANISM OF ACTION

Interferes with nucleic acid metabolism by acting as a false metabolite when incorporated into DNA and RNA; cell cycle phase specific for S phase.

## METABOLISM

90% of the total administered dose is excreted in the urine during the first 24 hours. Drug half-life depends on the route of administration: SQ 3.5 hours, IV 4.2 hours.

## DOSAGE/RANGE

100–400 mg/m² daily, weekly, biweekly, or continuous infusion schedule. Consult individual clinical trials protocol for specific dose.

## DRUG PREPARATION

This drug is supplied by the National Cancer Institute. The powder is reconstituted with sterile water for injection. *Do not reconstitute with 5% dextrose.*

## DRUG ADMINISTRATION

SQ administration may be painful and may result in a brownish discoloration at the injection site.

IV bolus or continuous infusion.

This drug is rapidly metabolized, and once reconstituted it decomposes quickly. The infusion bottles need to be changed every 3–4 hours due to drug decomposition. Stable in lactated Ringer's solution for 4 hours.

## SPECIAL CONSIDERATIONS

Patients develop side effects as a result of nephrotoxicity, hepatotoxicity, and CNS involvement.

Thromboembolic phenomena may occur.

## 5-Azacytidine

| Nursing Diagnosis | Defining Characteristics | Expected Outcomes | Nursing Interventions |
|---|---|---|---|
| I. *Altered nutrition, less than body requirements related to* | | | |
| A. Nausea and vomiting | I. A. 1. Dose related with a frequency of about 75% <br> 2. Usually occurs 1–3 hours after administration <br> 3. Symptoms are worse the first 2 days of infusion and lessen as infusion progresses | I. A. 1. Pt will be without nausea and vomiting <br> 2. Nausea and vomiting, should they occur, will be minimal | I. A. 1. Premedicate with antiemetics and continue prophylactically × 24 hrs to prevent nausea and vomiting <br> 2. Encourage small, frequent feedings of cool, bland foods and liquids <br> 3. If vomiting occurs, assess for s/s of fluid/electrolyte imbalance; monitor I&O, daily weights, lab results <br> 4. Refer to sec. on nausea and vomiting, Chapter 4 |
| B. Diarrhea | B. Develops in about 50% of pts | B. Pt will have minimal diarrhea | B. 1. Encourage pt to report onset of diarrhea <br> 2. Administer or teach administration of antidiarrheal medications <br> 3. Check all stools for blood <br> 4. If diarrhea is protracted, ensure adequate hydration, monitor I&O and electrolytes, and teach perineal hygiene regimen <br> 5. See sec. on diarrhea, Chapter 4 |
| C. Stomatitis | C. Rare | C. Oral mucous membranes will remain intact and without infection | C. 1. Teach pt oral assessment and mouth care regimen <br> 2. Encourage pt to report early stomatitis <br> 3. Provide pain relief measures, if indicated <br> 4. See sec. on stomatitis, Chapter 4 |

*(continued)*

## 5-Azacytidine (continued)

| Nursing Diagnosis | Defining Characteristics | Expected Outcomes | Nursing Interventions |
|---|---|---|---|
| | D. 1. Develops in a small percentage of pts<br>2. Marked by abnormal LFTs | D. Hepatic dysfunction will be identified early | D. 1. Monitor SGOT, SGPT, LDH, alkaline phosphatase, and bilirubin periodically during treatment<br>2. Notify MD about any changes |
| II. *Infection and bleeding related to bone marrow depression* | II. A. Leukopenia, thrombocytopenia, and anemia all occur<br>B. Leukopenia nadir days 14–17; lasts 2 weeks; recovery in 14 days | II. A. Pt will be without s/s of infection or bleeding<br>B. S/s of infection or bleeding will be identified early | II. A. Monitor CBC, platelet count prior to drug administration, as well as s/s of infection or bleeding<br>B. Instruct pt in self-assessment of s/s infection or bleeding<br>C. Refer to sec. on bone marrow depression, Chapter 4 |
| III. *Sensory/perceptual alterations* | III. A. Neurologic syndrome has been observed, characterized by lethargy, myalgia, and coma<br>B. Most likely to occur on the 2nd or 3rd day of therapy | III. A. Neurotoxicity will be identified early<br>B. Pt safety will be assured | III. A. Teach pt s/s of neurotoxicity: encourage pt to report s/s early<br>B. Assess for neurotoxicity; notify MD if it occurs<br>C. Institute safety precautions when warranted; explain precautions to pt |
| IV. *Impairment of skin integrity* | IV. A. Pruritic, follicular skin rash occurs in about 2% of pts<br>B. Usually transient, does not require dose reduction | IV. A. Skin integrity will be maintained | IV. A. Assess and teach pt to assess skin for rash, other dermatologic changes<br>B. Administer antihistamines/ antipruritic medication as ordered |
| V. *Alteration in comfort* | V. A. Fever can occur within 1–2 hrs after infusion (rare), up to 24 hrs later<br>B. Hypotension (rare)<br>C. Fever and hypotension have been associated with rapid IV infusion | V. A. Fever will be recognized early and treated<br>B. Pt will maintain adequate blood pressure | V. A. Monitor temp frequently after drug given<br>B. Report fever to MD<br>C. Administer antipyretic medications and measures as ordered<br>D. Monitor BP during and after infusion; report changes to MDs |

# Aziridinylbenzaquinone
(AZQ, Diaziquone)

*Class:* Investigational

## MECHANISM OF ACTION

Structure suggests alkylating activity and is also a class of drug that cross-links DNA. Lipid-soluble synthesized drug designed to penetrate CNS.

## METABOLISM

Excreted by the kidney. Extra precautions should be taken with patients with impaired renal function. Cleared rapidly from plasma, with a terminal half-life of 30 minutes. Crosses the blood-brain barrier.

## DOSAGE/RANGE

Dosages still under investigation, but 24–28 mg/m$^2$/day for 5 days has been reported.

## DRUG PREPARATION

AZQ should be mixed in 0.9% sodium chloride or lactated Ringer's. AZQ is less stable in a 5% dextrose solution. For continuous infusion, dilute drug in 1 liter NS daily.

## DRUG ADMINISTRATION

IV infusion. Administer immediately after reconstitution, as there is 25% loss of potency after 3 hours. Continuous infusion for 3–5 days.

## SPECIAL CONSIDERATIONS

Dosages may vary with individual protocols, so protocol should be checked for specific dosage ranges.

Anaphylaxis was noted in one patient who had a history of multiple drug allergies.

## Aziridinylbenzaquinone

| Nursing Diagnosis | Defining Characteristics | Expected Outcomes | Nursing Interventions |
|---|---|---|---|
| I. Infection, bleeding, and anemia related to bone marrow depression | I. A. 33% of pts experience leukopenia/ thrombocytopenia<br>B. Bone marrow depression is dose-limiting toxicity<br>C. Leukopenia nadir 2–3 weeks after treatment, lasting 1–3 weeks<br>D. Thrombocytopenia is rarer, with a nadir comparable to leukopenia<br>E. Anemia occasionally occurs<br>F. Severe leukopenia, thrombocytopenia have been reported<br>G. Recovery of peripheral blood counts is late—average 48 days after therapy | I. A. Pt will be without s/s of infection, anemia, or bleeding<br>B. Early s/s of infection, anemia, or bleeding will be identified | I. A. Monitor CBC, platelet count prior to drug administration, as well as s/s of infection, bleeding, anemia<br>B. Instruct pt in self-assessment of s/s of infection, bleeding, anemia<br>C. Dose reduction often necessary with compromised bone marrow function<br>D. Transfuse with red cells, platelets per MD order<br>E. Administer growth factors (erythropoietin and GCSF) as ordered<br>F. Refer to sec. on bone marrow depression, Chapter 4 |
| II. Altered nutrition, less than body requirements related to<br>A. Nausea and vomiting | II. A. 1. Occurs in 75% of pts and may be severe<br>2. Nausea and vomiting start within 1–3 hrs after injection; moderate, more common at 28 mg dose; abate in 3–4 hrs; usually by 10 days after injection has completely subsided | II. A. 1. Pt will be without nausea/vomiting<br>2. Nausea/vomiting, if they occur, will be minimal<br>3. Pt will maintain baseline weight ± 5% | II. A. 1. Premedicate with antiemetics 24–48 hrs before treatment and continue prophylactically to prevent nausea/vomiting, especially for first treatment<br>2. Encourage small, frequent feedings of cool, bland foods<br>3. I&O, daily weights if inpatient (assess for s/s of fluid and electrolyte imbalance)<br>4. Refer to sec. on nausea and vomiting, Chapter 4 |

| | | | |
|---|---|---|---|
| B. Stomatitis | B. Stomatitis moderate to severe | B. Oral mucous membranes will remain intact and without infection | B. 1. Assess oral cavity every day; teach pt to do own oral assessment and oral hygiene regimen<br>2. Encourage pt to report early stomatitis<br>3. Pain relief measures, if indicated<br>4. See sec. on stomatitis/mucositis, Chapter 4 |
| C. Diarrhea | C. 1 Occurs in 50% of pts and may be severe<br>2. Starts 2–3 days after treatment and subsides spontaneously | C. Pt will have minimal diarrhea | C. 1. Encourage pt to report onset of diarrhea<br>2. Administer or teach pt to self-administer antidiarrheal medications<br>3. See sec. on diarrhea, Chapter 4 |
| D. Hepatic dysfunction | D. 1. Rare but may be serious<br>2. S/s may include changes in LFTs to hepatic coma<br>3. AZQ contraindicated in pts with hepatic metastasis or elevated albumin levels | D. Hepatic dysfunction will be identified early | D. 1. Monitor SGOT, SGPT, LDH, alkaline phosphatase, and bilirubin periodically during treatment<br>2. Notify MD of any elevations |

*(continued)*

## Aziridinylbenzaquinone (continued)

| Nursing Diagnosis | Defining Characteristics | Expected Outcomes | Nursing Interventions |
|---|---|---|---|
| III. *Potential for injury, hypersensitivity reactions* | III. A. Rare<br>B. Transient fevers lasting 24 hrs after treatment<br>C. Hypotension | III. A. Early s/s of hypersensitivity will be identified | III. A. Teach pt about the potential of a hypersensitivity reaction and to report any unusual symptoms<br>B. Obtain baseline vital signs and note pt's mental status<br>C. Assess pt for s/s of a reaction; see sec. on reactions, Chapter 9<br>D. Administer therapy for reactions according to MD orders |
| IV. *Impaired skin integrity related to dermatitis* | IV. A. Rare<br>B. Transient pruritic rash | IV. A. Pt will identify any changes in the skin | IV. A. Assess pt for changes in skin<br>B. Discuss with pt impact of changes and strategies to minimize distress<br>C. Topical medications as ordered |
| V. *Potential for injury related to neuromuscular complications* | V. A. Rare<br>B. Onset of symptoms likely within 2–3 days of treatment<br>C. Symptoms range from lethargy, muscle pain, tenderness, or weakness to confusion or somnolence | V. A. Pt will identify s/s of neuromuscular changes early | V. A. Teach pt about the potential for injury due to neuromuscular changes and to report any unusual symptoms<br>B. Teach pt self-assessment techniques<br>C. Obtain baseline physical, muscular, and mental status<br>D. Assess pt for s/s of any complications<br>E. Administer therapy as ordered |

# Bicalutamide
(Casodex)

*Class:* Nonsteroidal antiandrogen

## MECHANISM OF ACTION

Binds to androgen receptors in the prostate; affinity is four times greater than that of flutamide.

## METABOLISM

Extensively metabolized in the liver. Decreased drug excretion in patients with moderate to severe hepatic dysfunction.

## DOSAGE/RANGE

50 mg po qd

## DRUG PREPARATION

None

## DRUG ADMINISTRATION

Orally

## SPECIAL CONSIDERATIONS

Use cautiously in patients with moderate to severe hepatic dysfunction. Observe closely for toxicity, as dosage adjustment may be required.

No dose modification needed for renal dysfunction.

In a study comparing castration to bicalutamide 50 mg/day, there was no difference in time to disease progression or subjective tolerance, but overall health of group receiving castration was better (Kaisery 1994).

# Bicalutamide

| Nursing Diagnosis | Defining Characteristics | Expected Outcomes | Nursing Interventions |
|---|---|---|---|
| I. Alteration in comfort, related to gynecomastia and hot flashes | I. Gynecomastia occurs in 23% of pts, breast tenderness in 26%, and hot flashes in 9.3% | I. Pt will report comfort throughout treatment course | I. Teach pt about possibility of these side effects, and discuss measures that may offer symptomatic reliefs |
| II. Alteration in nutrition, less than body requirements, related to nausea | II. A. Nausea may occur in 6% of pts | II. A. Pt will be without nausea | II. A. Teach pt that nausea may occur, and to report it if it does B. Determine baseline weight, and monitor at each visit C. Discuss strategies to minimize nausea, including diet modification and time of dosing |
| III. Alteration in elimination, related to constipation or diarrhea | III. A. Incidence of constipation is 6%, while that of diarrhea is 2.5% | III. A. Pt will maintain baseline elimination pattern | III. A. Assess baseline elimination pattern B. Teach pt that alterations may occur, and to report them if changes do not respond to OTC medications and dietary modifications |

# Bleomycin sulfate
## (Blenoxane)

*Class:* Antitumor antibiotic—isolated from fungus *Streptomyces verticullus.* Possesses both antitumor and antimicrobial actions

## MECHANISM OF ACTION

Primary action of bleomycin is to induce single-strand and double-strand breaks in DNA. DNA synthesis is inhibited. The action of drug is not exerted against RNA.

## METABOLISM

Excreted via the renal system. About 70% is excreted unchanged in urine; 30–60 minutes after IV infusion, urine levels are 10 times the serum level.

## DOSAGE/RANGE

5–20 U/m$^2$ once a week

10–20 U/m$^2$ twice a week

(frequency and schedule may vary according to protocol and age)

## DRUG PREPARATION

Dilute powder in normal saline or sterile water.

## DRUG ADMINISTRATION

IV, IM, or SC doses may be administered. Some clinical trials may utilize 24-hour infusions. There is a risk for anaphylaxis and hypotension with some diseases and with higher doses of drug. It may be recommended that a test dose be given before the first dose to detect hypersensitivity.

## SPECIAL CONSIDERATIONS

Because of pulmonary toxicities with increasing dose, PFTs and CXR should be obtained before each course or as outlined by protocol.

Incidence of anaphylaxis increases over the age of 70.

May cause chemical fevers up to 103°–105°F, 39.5°–40.5°C (60%). May need to administer premedications such as acetaminophen, antihistamines, and in some cases steroids.

Watch for signs/symptoms of hypotension and anaphylaxis. Test dose needed.

May cause irritation at site of injection (is considered an irritant, not a vesicant).

Maximum cumulative lifetime dose: 400 U.

Decreases the oral bioavailability of digoxin when given together.

Decreases the pharmacologic effects of phenytoin when given in combination.

# Bleomycin sulfate

| Nursing Diagnosis | Defining Characteristics | Expected Outcomes | Nursing Interventions |
|---|---|---|---|
| I. *Potential alteration in comfort related to* | | | |
| A. Fever and chills | I. A. 1. Fever and chills occur in 60% of pts 4–10 hrs after drug dose, persisting up to 24 hrs<br>2. Severity of reaction decreases with successive doses | I. A. Pt will remain comfortable during therapy | I. A. 1. Assess pt for these symptoms during the hour following treatment<br>2. Discuss with MD premedication with acetaminophen, antihistamines, or steroids<br>3. Evaluate the effectiveness of the symptomatic relief that is prescribed<br>4. Monitor the quantity of cumulative dose |
| B. Pain at tumor site | B. Pain at tumor site due to chemotherapy-induced cellular damage | B. Pt will be supported during therapy | B. 1. Offer emotional support to pt<br>2. Reinforce information on the action and side effects of bleomycin<br>3. Discuss with MD medicating with acetaminophen |
| II. *Potential for impaired skin integrity related to* | | | |
| A. Alopecia | II. A. Usually occurs late, 3–4 weeks after dose | II. A. Pt will verbalize feelings re hair loss and identifies strategies to cope with changes in body image | II. A. 1. Discuss with pt impact of hair loss<br>2. Suggest wig as appropriate prior to actual hair loss<br>3. Explore with pt response to actual hair loss and plan strategies to minimize distress (e.g., wig, scarf, cap)<br>4. Refer to sec. on alopecia, Chapter 4 |
| B. Skin changes | B. Skin changes occur in 50% of pts (e.g., striae, pruritis, skin peeling—fingertips, hyperpigmentation, and hyperkeratosis) | B. 1. Skin discomfort will be minimized and skin will remain intact | B. 1. Skin changes are not an indication to stop the drug |

| | | 2. Discuss with MD symptomatic management of skin changes<br>3. Reinforce pt teaching on the action and side effects of bleomycin<br>4. Offer emotional support |
| | 2. Pt will verbalize feelings re skin changes | |
| C. Skin eruptions | C. Macular rash (hands and elbows), urticaria, and vesicles are the type of eruptions most likely to be seen | C. 1. Skin eruptions are not an indication to stop the drug<br>2. Discuss with MD symptomatic management<br>3. Reinforce pt teaching on the action and side effects of bleomycin<br>4. Offer emotional support |
| | C. 1. Skin discomfort will be minimized, and skin will remain intact<br>2. Pt will verbalize feelings re skin changes | |
| D. Nail changes | D. Nail changes and possible nail loss can occur | D. 1. Nail changes are not an indication to stop the drug<br>2. Discuss with MD symptomatic management<br>3. Reinforce pt teaching on the action and side effects of bleomycin<br>4. Offer emotional support |
| | D. Pt will verbalize feelings about nail changes and identify strategies to cope with loss | |
| III. *Potential alteration in nutrition related to*<br>A. Nausea and vomiting | III. A. Nausea and vomiting are rare | III. A. 1. Premedicate with antiemetic if needed and continue prophylactically to prevent nausea and vomiting<br>2. Encourage small, frequent feedings of favorite foods, especially high-calorie, high-protein foods<br>3. Refer to sec. on nausea and vomiting, Chapter 4 |
| | III. A. Pt will be without nausea and vomiting; if either occurs, it will be minimal | |

*(continued)*

**Bleomycin sulfate** (*continued*)

| Nursing Diagnosis | Defining Characteristics | Expected Outcomes | Nursing Interventions |
|---|---|---|---|
| B. Anorexia and weight loss | B. Anorexia and weight loss may occur and may be prolonged | B. Pt will maintain baseline weight ± 5% | B. 1. Encourage small, frequent feedings of favorite foods, especially high-calorie, high-protein foods<br>2. Encourage use of spices<br>3. Weekly weights |
| C. Stomatitis | C. Stomatitis may decrease ability and desire to eat | C. Oral mucous membranes will remain intact and without infection | C. 1. Teach pt oral assessment<br>2. Encourage pt to report early stomatitis<br>3. Teach pt oral hygiene<br>4. Medicate for pain as needed<br>5. See sec. on stomatitis, Chapter 4 |
| IV. *Potential for impaired gas exchange related to pulmonary toxicity* | IV. A. Incidence 8–10%: pneumonitis (rales, dyspnea, infiltrate) may progress to irreversible pulmonary fibrosis; PFTs decrease before X-ray changes<br>B. High risk<br>1. Age > 70 years old<br>2. Dose > 150 U (maximum lifetime dose is 400 U)<br>3. XRT to chest (prior to chemotherapy or concomitantly) | IV. A. Early s/s or pulmonary toxicity will be identified | IV. A. Discuss with MD the need for pulmonary function tests and CXR prior to beginning therapy<br>B. Assess lung sounds prior to drug administration<br>C. Instruct pt to report cough, dyspnea, shortness of breath<br>D. See sec. on pulmonary toxicity, Chapter 4 |
| V. *Potential for sexual dysfunction* | V. A. Drug is mutagenic and probably teratogenic | V. A. Pt and significant other will understand needs for contraception | V. A. 1. As appropriate, explore with pt and significant other issues of reproductive and sexuality pattern and impact chemotherapy may have on them |

| | | |
|---|---|---|
| | B. Pt and significant other will identify strategies to cope with sexual dysfunction | 2. Discuss strategies to preserve sexual and reproductive health (e.g., sperm banking, contraception)<br>3. See sec. on gonadal dysfunction, Chapter 4 |
| VI. *Potential for injury related to anaphylaxis* | VI. A. Early s/s of hypersensitivity will be identified | VI. A. 1% of lymphoma pts experience anaphylaxis<br>B. S/s include tachycardia, wheezing, hypotension, facial edema | VI. A. Review standing orders for management of pt in anaphylaxis and identify location of anaphylaxis kit containing epinephrine 1:1000, hydrocortisone sodium succinate (Solucortef), diphenhydramine HCL (Benadryl), Aminophylline, $H_2$ blockers and others<br>B. Prior to drug administration, obtain baseline vital signs and record mental status<br>C. Observe for following s/s during infusion, usually occurring within first 15 mins of start of infusion:<br>1. *Subjective*<br>a. generalized itching<br>b. nausea<br>c. chest tightness<br>d. crampy abdominal pain<br>e. difficulty speaking<br>f. anxiety<br>g. agitation<br>h. sense of impending doom<br>i. uneasiness<br>j. desire to urinate or defecate |

*(continued)*

## Bleomycin sulfate (continued)

| Nursing Diagnosis | Defining Characteristics | Expected Outcomes | Nursing Interventions |
|---|---|---|---|
| | | | k. dizziness |
| | | | l. chills |
| | | | 2. *Objective* |
| | | | a. flushed appearance (angioedema of face, neck, eyelids, hands, feet) |
| | | | b. localized or generalized urticaria |
| | | | c. respiratory distress ± wheezing |
| | | | d. hypotension |
| | | | e. cyanosis |
| | | | D. If reaction occurs, stop infusion and notify MD |
| | | | E. Place pt in supine position to promote perfusion of visceral organs |
| | | | F. Monitor vital signs until stable |
| | | | G. Provide emotional reassurance to pt and family |
| | | | H. Maintain pt airway and have CPR equipment ready if needed |
| | | | I. Document incident |
| | | | J. Discuss with MD desensitization versus drug discontinuance for further dosing |
| | | | K. See sec. on reactions, Chapter 9 |

# Busulfan
(Myleran)

*Class:* Alkylating agent

## MECHANISM OF ACTION

Forms carbonium ions through the release of a methane sulfonate group. This results in the alkylating of DNA. Acts primarily on granulocyte precursors in the bone marrow and is cell cycle phase–nonspecific.

## METABOLISM

Well absorbed orally; almost all metabolites are excreted in the urine. Has a very short half-life.

## DOSAGE/RANGE

2–10 mg/day po for 2–3 weeks initially, then maintenance dose of 2–6 mg/m$^2$ po qd or 0.05 mg/kg po qd. Dose titrated to WBC counts.

## DRUG PREPARATION

None

## DRUG ADMINISTRATION

Available in 2-mg scored tablets given po

## SPECIAL CONSIDERATIONS

If WBC is high, patient is at risk for hyperuricemia. Allopurinol and hydration may be indicated.

Follow weekly CBC and platelet count initially, then monthly. Dose is decreased to maintenance when leukocyte count falls below 50,000 mm$^3$.

Hyperpigmentation of skin creases may occur due to increased melanin production.

If given according to accepted guidelines, patient should have minimal side effects.

## Busulfan

| Nursing Diagnosis | Defining Characteristics | Expected Outcomes | Nursing Interventions |
|---|---|---|---|
| I. *Potential for infection*<br>A. Myelosuppression<br>B. Delayed, refractory pancytopenia | I. A. Nadir 11–30 days, with recovery occurring over 24–54 days<br>B. Delayed, refractory pancytopenia has occurred | I. A. Pt will have normal recovery of bone marrow function<br>B. Pt will be without infection, bleeding | I. A. Monitor CBC weekly initially, then at least monthly<br>B. Monitor WBC closely: drug dose adjustment or discontinuance is based on WBC |
| II. *Potential for impaired gas exchange related to interstitial pulmonary fibrosis (rare)* | II. A. Rare complication; may occur within a year of beginning therapy, but usually occurs after long-term therapy<br>B. Symptoms may be delayed and usually occur after 4 years: anorexia, cough, rales, dyspnea, fever<br>C. Usually fatal due to rapid diffuse fibrosis; high-dose corticosteroids may be helpful | II. A. Pulmonary dysfunction will be identified early | II. A. Carefully assess pulmonary function of pts receiving long-term therapy<br>1. Breath sounds and presence of dyspnea<br>2. Periodic pulmonary function studies<br>B. Assess for underlying conditions (opportunistic infections, leukemic infiltrates)<br>C. Lung biopsy may be needed to diagnose "busulfan lung"; drug should be stopped *immediately* if this occurs |
| III. *Potential for sexual dysfunction* | III. A. Testicular atrophy, impotence, and amenorrhea may occur<br>B. Successful pregnancies have been described after and during treatment with busulfan<br>C. Men may experience gynecomastia<br>D. Drug is potentially teratogenic | III. A. Pt will understand potential dysfunction and that sterility may occur<br>B. Pt and significant other will discuss potential impact of sterility on their lives<br>C. Pt will understand importance of birth control if appropriate | III. A. Prechemo assessment of sexual patterns and function; institute patient and significant other teaching<br>B. Facilitate discussion between pt and partner re reproductive issues. Provide information, support counseling, and referral as needed<br>C. As appropriate, discuss birth control measures |

# Busulfan injection
(Busulfex)

*Class:* Alkylating agent

## MECHANISM OF ACTION

Forms carbonium ions through the release of a methane sulfonate group. This results in the alkylating of DNA. Acts primarily on granulocyte precursors in the bone marrow and is cell cycle phase–nonspecific.

## METABOLISM

Thirty percent of drug is excreted in the urine over 48 hours: negligible amounts have been recovered in feces.

## DOSAGE/RANGE

0.8 mg/kg of ideal body weight (IBW) or actual body weight (whichever is lower) q 6 hours as a 2-hour infusion for a total of 16 doses, followed by cytoxan

## DRUG PREPARATION

Dilute with NS or $D_5W$.

Diluent quantity should be ten times the volume of Busulfex so that the final concentration of the drug is 0.5 mg/ml.

Open ampule, withdraw drug using the filter needle provided, remove the needle, and inject the drug into the IV bag, which already contains the correct amount of fluid.

## DRUG ADMINISTRATION

Administer using an IV pump over 2 hours.

When mixed in NS, is stable (refrigerated) for 12 hours. In $D_5W$, is stable at room temperature for 8 hours. Infusion must be completed within these 2 time frames.

## SPECIAL CONSIDERATIONS

Profound myelosuppression occurs in all patients. Drug is currently indicated ONLY for patients who are getting conditioning regimen for hematopoetic progenitor cell transplantation.

Diluted drug must be used within 8 (if mixed in $D_5W$) or 12 (if mixed in NS) hours of reconstitution.

Crosses the blood-brain barrier. Patients should be premedicated with phenytoin before drug administration.

Probable increased risk of hepatic veno-occlusive disease with patients who have history of XRT or greater than 3 cycles of chemotherapy or prior progenitor cell transplantation. Elevated LFTs are common.

**Busulfan injection**

| Nursing Diagnosis | Defining Characteristics | Expected Outcomes | Nursing Interventions |
|---|---|---|---|
| I. *Alteration in cardiac output* | I. A. Mild to moderate tachycardia noted in 50% of patients; various other rhythm abnormalities occurred in less than 10% of patients<br>B. Mild to moderate thrombosis, usually associated with central venous catheter<br>C. Hypertension noted in 25% of pts<br>D. Vasodilation occurred in 23% of pts, with 17% experiencing hypotension | I. A. Patient will maintain baseline cardiac function<br>B. Changes in cardiac function will be identified early | I. A. Assess baseline cardiac status, including HR, BP, EKG, etc<br>B. Monitor pt for changes in cardiac parameters throughout treatment course; report changes<br>C. Monitor central venous lines for patency; watch for symptoms of venous thrombosis |
| II. *Infection and bleeding related to bone marrow depression* | II. A. At the indicated doses, busulfan injection produces profound myelosuppression in all pts. Severe leukopenia occurs in 100% of pts, thrombocytopenia in 86%, and anemia 50% of pts | II. A. Pt will be without s/s of infection or bleeding<br>B. Signs of infection and/or bleeding will be identified and reported, and treated early | II. A. Monitor Hct, WBC with differential, and platelets prior to drug administration. Discuss any abnormalities with physician<br>B. Monitor continuously for s/s of infection and bleeding; instruct patient in self-assessment and to report s/s immediately<br>C. Teach pt self-care measures to minimize risk of infection and bleeding, including avoidance of OTC aspirin-containing medications<br>D. Monitor CBC at least daily (more often if s/s of bleeding occur)—transfuse with PRBCs and platelets per protocol and physician order<br>E. Refer to section on bone marrow depression, Chapter 4 |

| III. Alteration in nutrition related to GI disturbances | III. A. Mild to moderate nausea/vomiting occurs in greater than 90% of patients<br>B. Stomatitis common; is mild–moderate in most pts, but severe in 13% of patients<br>C. Hyperglycemia occurs in over half of pts<br>D. Anorexia and dyspepsia common, usually mild–moderate in severity<br>E. Diarrhea and constipation both occur | III. A. Pt will be without nausea or vomiting<br>B. Nausea/vomiting will be minimized<br>C. Serum glucose will remain within normal limits<br>D. Pt will maintain weight within 5% of baseline<br>E. Pt will maintain baseline patterns of elimination | III. A. Premedicate with antiemetics and continue for 24 hrs to prevent nausea and vomiting<br>B. Encourage small, frequent feedings of cool, bland foods and liquids<br>C. Instruct pt in oral self-care measures, and to report nausea/vomiting to health care providers<br>D. Refer to sec. on nausea/vomiting, Chapter 4<br>E. Weigh pt each day. Dietary consult prior to treatment to determine pt preferences and educate pt in low-bacteria diet<br>F. Follow serum glucose; report abnormal values<br>G. Monitor bowel elimination pattern: use dietary measures, antidiarrheals or laxatives to maintain pts baseline pattern |
| IV. Potential for impaired gas exchange related to pulmonary toxicities | IV. A. Dyspnea occurs in 22% of pts<br>B. Mild/moderate rhinitis and cough observed in 44% of pts<br>C. Less frequent side effects include hyperventilation, respiratory failure, alveolar hemorrhages, asthma, pleural effusion, and hypoxia | IV. A. Pt will maintain pulmonary function within baseline limits<br>B. Pulmonary side effects will be identified and treated early | IV. A. Assess baseline pulmonary function<br>B. Monitor pt throughout treatment course for objective and subjective changes in breathing and lung sounds<br>C. Assess for underlying conditions (infection, effusions, leukemic infiltrates)<br>D. Report changes in pulmonary function |

*(continued)*

**Busulfan injection** (*continued*)

| Nursing Diagnosis | Defining Characteristics | Expected Outcomes | Nursing Interventions |
|---|---|---|---|
| V. *Alteration in comfort related to neurologic toxicities* | V. A. Anxiety and insomnia occur frequently<br>B. Mild/moderate headache occurs in 65% of pts, unspecified pain in 40%<br>C. Dizziness and depression noted in over 20% of pts<br>D. Less frequent side effects, occurring in less than 10% of pts, include nervousness, delirium, agitation | V. A. Pt will report relative comfort, adequate coping throughout treatment | V. A. Explain to pt that neurologic toxicities may occur, to report discomfort and changes in neuro functioning<br>B. Medicate for symptoms above, report all changes<br>C. Relaxation/meditation as able |
| VI. *Alteration in skin integrity related to rash* | VI. A. 50% of pts experience mild/moderate rash, 29% pruritis | VI. A. Pt's skin will remain intact throughout treatment course | VI. A. Assess pt q day for changes in skin<br>B. Inform pt about possibility of skin changes, to report them when they occur<br>C. Topical agents as ordered, antipruritic agents as needed |

# Capecitabine
(Xeloda, N4-pentoxycarbonyl-5-deoxy-5-fluorocytidine)

*Class:* Fluoropyrimidine carbamate

## MECHANISM OF ACTION

Metabolites bind to thymidylate synthetase, inhibiting the formation of uracil from thymidylate, and reducing the cell's ability to produce DNA. It also prevents cell division by hindering the formation of RNA, by causing nuclear transcription enzymes to mistakenly incorporate its metabolites in the process of RNA transcription.

## METABOLISM

Absorbed from the intestinal mucosa as an intact molecule, metabolized in the liver to intermediary metabolite, and then in the liver and tumor tissue to 5-FU precursor. It is then converted through catalytic activation to 5-FU at the tumor site. Metabolites are cleared in the urine.

## DOSAGE/RANGE

2500 mg/m$^2$ po in two divided doses with food for 2 weeks. Treatment followed by a 1-week rest period. Treatment repeated every 3 weeks.

## PREPARATION/ADMINISTRATION

Oral

Administer after meals with plenty of water.

Divide daily dose in half; take 12 hours apart.

## SPECIAL CONSIDERATIONS

Monitor bilirubin baseline and before each cycle, as dose modifications are necessary with hyperbilirubinemia.

Folic acid should be avoided while taking drug.

**Capecitabine**

| Nursing Diagnosis | Defining Characteristics | Expected Outcomes | Nursing Interventions |
|---|---|---|---|
| I. *Potential for infection and bleeding related to bone marrow depression* | I. A. Commonly causes anemia, neutropenia, and thrombocytopenia | I. A. Pt will be without s/s of infection or bleeding<br>B. Signs of infection and/or bleeding will be identified and reported early | I. A. Monitor Hct, WBC with differential, and platelets prior to drug administration. Discuss any abnormalities with physician<br>B. Assess for s/s infection and bleeding, and instruct pt in self-assessment and to report s/s immediately<br>C. Teach pt self-care measures to minimize risk of infection and bleeding, including avoidance of OTC aspirin-containing medications<br>D. Refer to section on bone marrow depression, Chapter 4 |
| II. *Altered nutrition, less than body requirements, related to nausea and vomiting, stomatitis, and diarrhea* | II. A. Nausea and vomiting occur in 30–50% of pts<br>B. Stomatitis and diarrhea also occur in about 50% of pts | II. A. Pt wil be without nausea, vomiting, stomatitis, and diarrhea | II. A. Premedicate with antiemetics and continue for 24 hrs to prevent nausea and vomiting<br>B. Encourage small, frequent feedings of cool, bland foods and liquids<br>C. Instruct pt in oral self-care measures, and to report nausea/vomiting to health care providers<br>D. Refer to sec. on nausea/vomiting, Chapter 4 |
| III. *Alteration in skin integrity/ comfort related to hand/foot syndrome* | III. Hand/foot syndrome occurs in more than half of pts and is characterized by tingling, numbness, pain, erythema, dryness, rash, swelling, and/or pruritus of hands and feet | III. Pt will verbalize understanding of informing physician if hand/foot syndrome occurs | III. Teach pt about the possibility of this side effect, and to inform physician immediately should it occur |

# Carboplatin
## (Paraplatin)

*Class:* Alkylating agent (heavy metal complex)

## MECHANISM OF ACTION

A second-generation platinum analog. The cytotoxicity is identical to that of the parent, *Cis*-platinum. Cell cycle phase nonspecific. Reacts with nucleophilic sites on DNA, causing predominantly intrastrand and interstrand cross-links rather than DNA-protein cross-links. These cross-links are similar to those formed with *Cis*-platinum but are formed later.

## METABOLISM

At 24 hours post-administration, approximately 70% of carboplatin is excreted in the urine. The mean half-life is roughly 100 minutes.

## DOSAGE/RANGE

As a single agent, 360 mg/m$^2$ on day 1, cycle repeated every 4 weeks; *or* 300 mg/m$^2$ on day 1 combined with cyclophosphamide for advanced ovarian cancer, cycle repeated every 4 weeks. Drug administration may have to be delayed if neutrophil count is less than 2000 mm$^3$ or platelet count is less than 100,000 mm$^3$.

Drug dose reduction for urine creatinine clearance < 60 ml/minute. Since carboplatin has predictable pharmacokinetics based on the drug's excretion by the kidneys, area under the curve (AUC) dosing is now recommended for this drug. The Calvert formula is used where the total dose (mg) = (target AUC) × (glomerular filtration rate [GFR] + 25).

The GFR is approximated by the urine creatinine clearance, either estimated or actual. AUC dose is determined by the physician based on the treatment plan, and for previously treated patients receiving single-agent carboplatin, is 4–6 mg/ml/min (see package insert).

## DRUG PREPARATION

Available as a white powder in amber vial.

Reconstitute with sterile water for injection, D$_5$W, or NS.

Dilute further in D$_5$W or normal saline.

The solution is chemically stable for 24 hours; discard solution after 8 hours because of the lack of bacteriostatic preservative.

## DRUG ADMINISTRATION

Administered by IV bolus over 30 minutes to 1 hour.

May also be given as a continuous infusion over 24 hours.

## SPECIAL CONSIDERATIONS

Does not have the renal toxicity seen with Cis-platinum.

Monitor urine creatinine clearance.

# Carboplatin

| Nursing Diagnosis | Defining Characteristics | Expected Outcomes | Nursing Interventions |
|---|---|---|---|
| I. *Potential for infection and bleeding related to bone marrow depression* | I. A. Myelosuppression is major dose-limiting toxicity<br>B. Thrombocytopenia nadir 14–21 days, with recovery by day 28<br>C. Leukopenia nadir usually follows thrombocytopenia by 1 week but may take 5–6 weeks to recover<br>D. Mild anemia frequently observed | I. A. Pt will be without s/s of infection or bleeding<br>B. S/s of infection or bleeding will be identified early | I. A. Monitor CBC, platelet count prior to drug administration, as well as s/s of infection or bleeding<br>B. Instruct pt in self-assessment of s/s of infection or bleeding<br>C. Dose reduction often necessary (35–50%) if bone marrow function is compromised<br>D. Refer to sec. on bone marrow depression, Chapter 4 |
| II. *Altered nutrition, less than body requirements related to*<br>A. Nausea and vomiting | II. A. 1. Nausea and vomiting begin 6+ hrs after dose and usually last for < 24 hrs<br>2. 80% of pts experience some nausea or vomiting but often mild to moderate in severity | II. A. 1. Pt will be without nausea and vomiting<br>2. Nausea and vomiting, should they occur, will be minimal | II. A. 1. Premedicate with antiemetics and continue prophylactically × 24 hrs to prevent nausea and vomiting<br>2. Encourage small, frequent feedings of cool, bland foods and liquids<br>3. If vomiting occurs, assess for s/s of fluid/electrolyte imbalance: monitor I&O, daily weights, lab results<br>4. Refer to sec. on nausea and vomiting, Chapter 4 |
| B. Anorexia | B. Somewhat common but usually lasts for less than 1 day | B. Pt will maintain baseline weight ± 5% | B. 1. Encourage small, frequent feedings of favorite foods, especially high-calorie, high-protein foods<br>2. Encourage use of spices<br>3. Weekly weights<br>4. Dietary consult as needed |

| | | | |
|---|---|---|---|
| C. Stomatitis | C. Occurs in ~10% of pts but usually mild | C. Oral mucous membranes will remain intact and without infection | C. 1. Teach pt oral assessment and oral hygiene regimen<br>2. Encourage pt to report early stomatitis<br>3. See sec. on stomatitis, Chapter 4 |
| D. Diarrhea | D. Occurs in ~10% of pts but is usually mild | D. Pt will have minimal diarrhea | D. 1. Encourage pt to report onset of diarrhea<br>2. Administer or teach pt to self-administer antidiarrheal medications<br>3. See sec. on diarrhea, Chapter 4 |
| E. Hepatic dysfunction | E. Mild to moderate reversible disturbances in liver function studies, especially alkaline phosphatase and SGOT, rarely SGPT and bilirubin | E. Hepatic dysfunction will be identified early | E. 1. Monitor LFTs (i.e., alkaline phosphatase, SGOT, SGPT, and bilirubin) periodically during treatment<br>2. Monitor pt for any elevations in LFTs<br>3. Dose modifications may be necessary if elevation occurs |
| III. *Altered urinary elimination related to nephrotoxicity* | III. A. Does not have the renal toxicity seen with Cis-platinum<br>B. Minimal diuresis and hydration needed; if occurs, usually mild | III. A. Pt will be without renal dysfunction<br>B. Early s/s of renal dysfunction will be identified | III. A. Monitor BUN and creatinine prior to initiating drug administration, as drug is excreted by the kidneys<br>B. Check parameters of BUN and creatinine established in protocol, as myelotoxicity is directly related to renal function status<br>C. Dose modifications may be made for renal impairment based on urine creatinine clearance |

*(continued)*

## Carboplatin (continued)

| Nursing Diagnosis | Defining Characteristics | Expected Outcomes | Nursing Interventions |
|---|---|---|---|
| IV. Potential for sensory/ perceptual alterations due to high-dose carboplatin | IV. A. Neurotoxicity and ototoxicity rare; similar to those seen with Cis-platinum (but not as severe)<br>B. Neurotoxicity: peripheral neuropathies, reversible confusion and dementia<br>C. Ototoxicity: transient | IV. A. Neuropathies and ototoxicities will be identified early | IV. A. If pt is to receive high-dose carboplatin, obtain baseline neurological and auditory test<br>B. Assess pt for changes during treatment course<br>C. Teach pt the potential for neurologic toxicity problems and to report any changes |
| V. Potential for sexual dysfunction | V. A. Drug is mutagenic and probably teratogenic | V. A. Pt and significant other will understand needs for contraception<br>B. Pt and significant other will identify strategies to cope with sexual dysfunction | V. A. As appropriate, explore with pt and significant other issues of reproductive and sexuality pattern and impact chemotherapy will have<br>B. Discuss strategies to preserve sexual and reproductive health (sperm banking, contraception)<br>C. See sec. on gonadal dysfunction, Chapter 4 |
| VI. Potential for injury related to hypersensitivity reactions | VI. A. Anaphylaxis or anaphylactic-like reactions have been reported (reactions similar to parent drug cisplatin)<br>1. Tachycardia<br>2. Wheezing<br>3. Hypotension<br>4. Facial edema | VI. A. Early s/s of hypersensitivity will be identified | VI. A. Teach pt about the potential of a hypersensitivity reaction and ask pt to report any unusual s/s |

B. Occurs within a few minutes of initiating the drug and usually responds to steroid, epinephrine, or antihistamines

B. Assess baseline mental status
C. Adverse reaction kit with epinephrine in room
D. *If reaction occurs*, administer treatment per MD orders
E. Document anaphylactic incident
F. Discuss with MD precautionary measures to be taken before next drug dose is given *or* drug discontinuance
G. See section on hypersensitivity reactions, Chapter 9

# Carmustine
## (BiCNU, BCNU)

*Class:* Nitrosoureas

## MECHANISM OF ACTION

Alkylates DNA in the same manner as classic mustard agents—by causing cross-strand breaks. Also, carbamoylates cellular proteins of nucleic acid synthesis. Is cell cycle phase–nonspecific.

## METABOLISM

Rapidly distributed and metabolized, with a plasma half-life of 1 hour; 70% of IV dose is excreted in urine within 96 hours. Significant concentrations of drug remain in CSF for 9 hours due to lipid solubility of drug.

## DOSAGE/RANGE

75–100 mg/m² IV/day × 2 days
   *or*
200–225 mg/m² every 6 weeks
   *or*
40 mg/m² day on 5 successive days

## DRUG PREPARATION

Add sterile alcohol (provided with drug) to vial, then add sterile water for injection.

May be further diluted with 100–250 ml $D_5W$ or NS.

## DRUG ADMINISTRATION

Discard solution 2 hours after mixing.

Administer via volutrol over 45–120 minutes as tolerated by patient.

## SPECIAL CONSIDERATIONS

Drug is an irritant; avoid extravasation.

Pain at the injection site or along the vein is common. Treat by applying ice pack above the injection site and decreasing the infusion flow rate.

Patient may act inebriated due to the alcohol diluent and may experience flushing.

Increased myelosuppression when given with cimetidine.

Can decrease the pharmacologic effects of phenytoin.

# Carmustine

| Nursing Diagnosis | Defining Characteristics | Expected Outcomes | Nursing Interventions |
|---|---|---|---|
| I. Potential for infection related to myelosuppression | I. A. Nadir: 3–5 weeks after dose, persists 1–3 weeks longer<br>B. Myelosuppression is cumulative and may be delayed | I. A. Pt will be without infection<br>B. Early s/s of infection will be identified | I. A. Monitor CBC, including WBC differential, prior to drug administration<br>B. Drug dosage may be reduced or held for lower than normal blood values<br>C. See sec. on bone marrow depression, Chapter 4 |
| II. Alteration in comfort related to drug administration<br>A. Pain along vein | II. A. 1. Drug diluent is absolute alcohol<br>2. Drug is an irritant and can cause pain along a vein<br>3. True thrombophlebitis is rare<br>4. Venospasms commonly occur during rapid infusion | II. A. Pt will be without pain or will have minimal discomfort during infusion | II. A. 1. Administer drug in 100–250 ml $D_5W$ or NS over 45–120 mins<br>2. Use ice pack above injection site, decrease infusion rate, further dilute drug if pain occurs |
| B. Flushing of skin or burning of eyes | B. Occurs with rapid drug infusion | B. Pt will be without flushing or burning of eyes | B. Administer drug slowly; if symptoms occur, slow rate of infusion |

(continued)

## Carmustine (continued)

| Nursing Diagnosis | Defining Characteristics | Expected Outcomes | Nursing Interventions |
|---|---|---|---|
| III. *Altered nutrition, less than body requirements related to* <br> A. Nausea and vomiting | III. A. Severe nausea and vomiting may occur 2 hrs after administration and last 4–6 hrs | III. A. 1.Pt will be without nausea and vomiting <br> 2. Nausea and vomiting, if they occur, will be minimal | III. A. 1. Premedicate with antiemetics and continue prophylactically × 24 hrs to prevent nausea and vomiting, at least for first treatment <br> 2. Encourage small, frequent feedings of cool, bland foods and liquids |
| B. Liver dysfunction (rare) related to subacute hepatitis | B. Abnormal SGOT, alkaline phosphatase, and serum bilirubin have occurred; also painless jaundice and hepatic coma, usually reversible | B. Laboratory abnormalities will be identified early | B. 1. Monitor LFTs (SGOT, SGPT, LDH, alkaline phosphatase, bilirubin) during treatment <br> 2. Notify MD of elevations |
| IV. *Altered urinary elimination related to nephrotoxicity* | IV. A. Increased BUN occurs in ~10% of treated pts, usually reversible | IV. A. Pt will be without renal dysfunction <br> B. Early s/s of renal dysfunction will be identified | IV. A. Monitor BUN and creatinine prior to initiating drug dose, as drug is excreted by the kidneys <br> B. Check parameters of BUN and creatinine established in protocol, as myelotoxicity is directly related to renal function <br> C. Dose modifications may need to be made for renal impairment |

V. *Potential for impaired gas exchange related to pulmonary fibrosis*

V. A. Presents as insidious cough and dyspnea or sudden onset of respiratory failure
B. CXR shows interstitial infiltrates
C. Pulmonary function tests show hypoxia with diffusion and restrictive defects
D. Risk may increase with concurrent cyclophosphamide
E. Risk increases as dose exceeds gm/m$^2$
F. Incidence 20–30% with mortality of 24–80%

V. A. Early dysfunction will be identified

V. A. Assess pts at risk
1. Cumulative dose 1 gm/m$^2$
2. Preexisting lung disease
3. Concurrent cyclophosphamide therapy or thoracic irradiation
B. Assess breath sounds and presence of dyspnea
C. Monitor pulmonary function studies periodically for evidence of pulmonary dysfunction

VI. *Potential for sexual dysfunction*

VI. A. Drug is teratogenic

VI. A. Pt and significant other understand need for contraception

VI. A. 1. As appropriate, explore with pt and significant other issues of reproductive and sexuality pattern and impact chemotherapy may have
2. Discuss strategies to preserve sexual and reproductive health (e.g., sperm banking, contraception)
3. See sec. on gonadal dysfunction, Chapter 4

# Chlorambucil
(Leukeran)

*Class:* Alkylating agent

## MECHANISM OF ACTION

Alkylates DNA by causing strand breaks and crosslinks in the DNA. Is a derivative of a nitrogen mustard

## METABOLISM

Pharmacokinetics are poorly understood. Is well absorbed orally, with a plasma half-life of 1.5 hours. Degradation is slow; appears to be eliminated by metabolic transformation with 60% of drug excreted in urine in 24 hours.

## DOSAGE/RANGE

0.1–0.2 mg/kg/day (equals 4–8 mg/m$^2$/day) to initiate treatment

*or*

14 mg/m$^2$/day × 5 days with a repeat every 21–28 days depending upon platelet count and WBC

## DRUG PREPARATION

None

## DRUG ADMINISTRATION

Oral

## SPECIAL CONSIDERATIONS

Simultaneous administration of barbiturates may increase toxicity of chlorambucil due to hepatic drug activation.

# Chlorambucil

| Nursing Diagnosis | Defining Characteristics | Expected Outcomes | Nursing Interventions |
|---|---|---|---|
| I. *Potential for infection related to myelosuppression* | I. A. WBC decreases for 10 days after last dose<br>B. Neutropenia, thrombocytopenia occur with prolonged use and may be irreversible<br>C. Secondary malignancies have been reported (acute myelogenous leukemia)<br>D. Increased toxicity may occur with prior barbiturate use | I. A. Pt will be without infection<br>B. Early s/s of infection will be identified | I. A. Monitor CBC, including WBC differential, prior to drug administration<br>B. Drug dosage may be reduced or held for lower than normal blood values<br>C. See sec. on bone marrow depression, Chapter 4 |
| II. *Potential for sexual dysfunction* | II. A. Drug is mutagenic and teratogenic and suppresses gonadal function, with consequent sterility (permanent or temporary)<br>B. Amenorrhea<br>C. Oligospermia | II. A. Pt and significant other will understand need for contraception<br>B. Pt and significant other will discuss strategies to cope with change in sexual function | II. A. As appropriate, explore with pt and significant other issues of reproductive and sexuality pattern and impact chemotherapy will have<br>B. Discuss strategies to preserve sexual and reproductive health (e.g., sperm banking, contraception)<br>C. See sec. on gonadal dysfunction, Chapter 4 |

*(continued)*

## Chlorambucil (continued)

| Nursing Diagnosis | Defining Characteristics | Expected Outcomes | Nursing Interventions |
|---|---|---|---|
| III. *Potential alteration in nutrition related to* | | | |
| A. Nausea and vomiting | III. A. Nausea and vomiting are rare | III. A. 1. Pt will be without nausea and vomiting 2. If they occur, they are minimal | III. A. 1. Premedicate with antiemetic if ordered and continue prophylactically to prevent nausea and vomiting 2. Encourage small, frequent feedings of cool, bland foods and liquids 3. Administer oral dose on an empty stomach 4. Refer to sec. on nausea and vomiting, Chapter 4 |
| B. Anorexia and weight loss | B. Anorexia and weight loss may occur and be prolonged | B. Pt will maintain baseline weight ± 5% | B. 1. Encourage small, frequent feedings of favorite foods, especially high-calorie, high-protein foods 2. Encourage use of spices 3. Weekly weights |
| C. Hepatic dysfunction | C. Hepatitis is rare but may occur (also disturbances in liver function) | C. Hepatic dysfunction will be identified early | C. 1. Monitor LFTs (i.e., alkaline phosphatase and bilirubin) periodically during treatment 2. Monitor pt for any elevations 3. Dose modifications may be necessary if elevation occurs |

| | | | |
|---|---|---|---|
| IV. *Potential for impaired skin integrity* | IV. A. Dermatitis and urticaria may occur (rarely)<br>B. Cross-hypersensitivity may exist between Alkeran and chlorambucil (skin rash) | IV. A. Skin will remain intact<br>B. Early skin impairment will be identified | IV. A. 1. Assess skin for integrity<br>2. If symptoms are severe, discuss drug discontinuance with MD |
| V. *Potential for impaired gas exchange related to pulmonary fibrosis* | V. A. Alveolar dysplasia and pulmonary fibrosis may occur with long-term use<br>B. Infrequent | V. A. Early dysfunction is identified | V. A. Assess pts at risk<br>1. Cumulative dose 1 gm/m$^2$<br>2. Preexisting lung disease<br>3. Concurrent cyclophosphamide or thoracic irradiation<br>B. Assess breath sounds and presence of dyspnea<br>C. Monitor pulmonary function studies periodically for evidence of pulmonary dysfunction |
| VI. *Potential for sensory/perceptual alterations (rare)* | VI. A. Ocular disturbances may occur<br>1. Diplopia<br>2. Papilledema<br>3. Retinal hemorrhage | VI. A. Visual disturbances will be identified early | VI. A. Assess vision before giving treatment<br>B. Encourage pt to report any visual changes |

# Cisplatin
(*Cis*-Platinum, CDDP, Platinum, Platinol)

*Class:* Heavy metal that acts like alkylating agent

## MECHANISM OF ACTION

Inhibits DNA synthesis by forming interstrand and intrastrand cross-links and by denaturing the double helix, preventing cell replication. Is cell cycle phase–nonspecific. Has chemical properties similar to that of bifunctional alkylating agents.

## METABOLISM

Rapidly distributed to tissues (predominantly the liver and kidneys), with less than 10% in plasma 1 hour after infusion. Clearance from plasma proceeds slowly after the first 2 hours due to platinum's covalent bonding with serum proteins; 20–74% of administered drug is excreted in the urine within 24 hours.

## DOSAGE/RANGE

50–120 mg/m$^2$ every 3–4 weeks
  *or*
15–20 mg/m$^2$ × 5 repeated every 3–4 weeks

## DRUG PREPARATION

10-mg and 50-mg vials. Add sterile water to develop a concentration of 1 mg/ml.

Further dilute solution with 250 ml or more of NS or $D_5W$ $^1/_2$ NS. Never mix with $D_5W$, as a precipitate will form.

Refrigerate lyophilized drug, but *not* reconstituted drug, as a precipitate will form.

## DRUG ADMINISTRATION

Avoid aluminum needles when administering, as precipitate will form.

## SPECIAL CONSIDERATIONS

Hydrate vigorously before and after administering drug. Urine output should be at least 100–150 ml/hr. Mannitol or furosemide diuresis may be needed to ensure this output.

Hypersensitivity reactions have occurred, manifested by wheezing, flushing, hypotension, tachycardia. Usually occur within minutes of starting infusion. Treat with epinephrine, corticosteroids, antihistamines.

Decreases the pharmacologic effects of phenytoin.

## Cisplatin

| Nursing Diagnosis | Defining Characteristics | Expected Outcomes | Nursing Interventions |
|---|---|---|---|
| I. Potential alteration in urinary elimination | I. A. Drug accumulates in kidney, causing necrosis of proximal and distal renal tubules<br><br>B. Is a dose-limiting toxicity and is cumulative with repeated doses<br><br>C. Damage to distal renal tubules prevents reabsorption of Mg, Ca, K, with resultant decreased serum levels<br><br>D. Peak detrimental effect usually occurs 10–20 days after treatment and is reversible<br><br>E. Hyperuricemia may occur due to impaired tubular transport of uric acid but is responsive to allopurinol | I. A. Pt will maintain normal renal function as evidenced by BUN < 20, creatinine < 1.5<br><br>B. Mg, K, Ca levels will be normal<br><br>C. Pt will maintain baseline weight ± 5% | I. A. Prevent nephrotoxicity with vigorous hydration and diuresis to produce urinary output of at least 100 cc/hr during treatment infusion<br><br>B. A typical hydration schedule is NS or $D_5W\,{}^1/_2$ NS at 250 cc/hr for 3 hrs prior to cisplatin and for 5 hrs after; outpatient hydration would be over 1–2 hrs; diuresis is induced by the use of lasix or mannitol given prior to cisplatin administration<br><br>C. Monitor BUN and creatinine prior to initiating drug dose, as drug is excreted by the kidneys<br><br>D. Check parameters of BUN and creatinine established in protocol<br><br>E. Dose modifications may be made for renal impairment<br><br>F. Concurrent use of aminoglycosides is not recommended |

*(continued)*

## Cisplatin (continued)

| Nursing Diagnosis | Defining Characteristics | Expected Outcomes | Nursing Interventions |
|---|---|---|---|
| II. *Altered nutrition, less than body requirements related to*<br>A. Nausea and vomiting | II. A. Nausea and vomiting may be severe; begins 1 + hrs after dose, lasts 8–24 hrs, and may recur 48–72 hrs after dose | II. A. 1. Pt will be without nausea and vomiting<br>2. Nausea and vomiting, if they occur, will be minimal | II. A. 1. Premedicate with antiemetics and continue prophylactically × 24 hrs to prevent nausea and vomiting, at least for first treatment; continue antiemetic for 3–5 days after treatment ends<br>2. Encourage small, frequent feedings of cool, bland foods and liquids<br>3. Infuse cisplatin over at least 1 hr to minimize nausea and vomiting<br>4. Refer to sec. on nausea and vomiting, Chapter 4 |
| B. Taste alteration | B. Taste alterations can occur with long-term use | B. Pt will eat adequate calories, proteins, minerals | B. 1. Suggest increased use of spices as tolerated<br>2. Help pt or significant other develop menu based on past favorite foods<br>3. Dietary consultation as needed |
| III. *Potential for injury related to anaphylaxis* | III. A. Anaphylactic hypersensitivity reactions have occurred (infrequently) following IV drug administration to previously treated pts<br>B. Tachycardia, wheezing, hypotension, facial edema<br>C. Usually controlled by corticosteroids, epinephrine, antihistamines | III. A. If anaphylaxis occurs, pt will maintain vital signs within normal limits | III. A. Have anaphylaxis tray with corticosteroids, antihistamines, epinephrine ready in clinic or unit where chemotherapy is administered<br>B. Discuss with physician the development of standing orders in case anaphylaxis occurs<br>C. Monitor and observe pt closely during cisplatin infusions<br>D. Refer to sec. on reactions, Chapter 9 |

| | | |
|---|---|---|
| IV. *Infection and bleeding related to bone marrow depression* | IV. A. Bone marrow depression mild with low to moderate doses<br>B. High-dose nadir is 2–3 weeks, with recovery in 4–5 weeks<br>C. Concurrent low-dose cisplatin and radiotherapy may result in bone marrow depression | IV. A. Pt will be without s/s of infection or bleeding | IV. A. Monitor CBC, platelet count prior to drug administration, as well as s/s infection and bleeding<br>B. Administer growth factors (erythropoietin and GCSF) as ordered<br>C. Refer to sec. on bone marrow depression, Chapter 4 |
| V. *Potential for activity intolerance related to anemia-induced fatigue* | V. A. Cisplatin may interfere with renal erythropoietin, causing subsequent late anemia | V. A. Pt will be able to do desired activities<br>B. Early fatigue related to anemia will resolve | V. A. Monitor hemoglobin, hematocrit<br>B. Transfuse per MD for hematocrit < 25, s/s of severe anemia<br>C. Teach pt about high-iron diet |
| VI. *Potential for sensory/perceptual alterations related to neurological toxicity* | VI. A. Neurotoxicity and ototoxicity may be severe<br>1. Neurotoxicity: glove and stocking distribution neuropathy, with numbness, tingling, and sensory loss in arms and legs<br>2. Ototoxicity: high-frequency hearing loss above frequency of normal speech, affecting > 30% of pts<br>B. 1. May be preceded by tinnitis<br>2. Appears dose related and can be unilateral or bilateral<br>3. Results from the destruction of hair cells lining organ of Corti<br>4. Damage is cumulative and may be permanent | VI. A. Neurotoxicity and ototoxicity will be identified early<br>B. If ototoxicity occurs, pt will verbalize feelings of discomfort and loss of function and identify alternative coping strategies | VI. A. Assess motor and sensory function prior to therapy, and at regular intervals after each dose is given<br>B. Encourage pt to verbalize feelings regarding discomfort and sensory loss |

*(continued)*

## Cisplatin (continued)

| Nursing Diagnosis | Defining Characteristics | Expected Outcomes | Nursing Interventions |
|---|---|---|---|
| | | | C. Help pt discuss alternative coping strategies |
| | | | D. See sec. on neurotoxicity, Chapter 4 |
| | | | E. Baseline audiogram if high-dose platinum to be administered |
| | | | F. Repeat audiogram if pt complains of tinnitus, feeling underwater, or auditory discomfort |
| | | | G. If audiogram reveals hearing decline, discuss with pt and MD benefits/risks of further cisplatin therapy |
| VII. *Potential for sexual dysfunction* | VII. A. Drug is mutagenic and probably teratogenic | VII. A. Pt and significant other will understand need for contraception<br>B. Pt and significant other will identify strategies to cope with sexual dysfunction | VII. A. As appropriate, explore with pt and significant other issues of reproductive and sexuality pattern and impact chemotherapy may have<br>B. Discuss strategies to preserve sexual and reproductive health (e.g., sperm banking, contraception)<br>C. See sec. on gonadal dysfunction, Chapter 4 |

# Cladribine
(Leustatin, 2-CdA)

*Class:* Antimetabolite

## MECHANISM OF ACTION

A chlorinated purine nucleoside that selectively damages normal and malignant lymphocytes and monocytes that have large amounts of deoxycytidine kinase but small amounts of deoxynucleotidase. The drug enters passively through the cell membrane, is phosphorylated into the active metabolite 2-CdATP, and accumulates in the cell. 2-CdATP interferes with DNA synthesis and prevents repair of DNA strand breaks in both actively dividing and normal cells. Process may also involve programmed cell death (apoptosis).

## METABOLISM

Drug is 20% protein bound and is cleared from the plasma within 1–3 days after cessation of treatment.

## DOSAGE/RANGE

0.09 mg/kg/day IV as a continuous infusion × 7 days for one course of therapy (hairy cell leukemia)

## DRUG PREPARATION

Available in 10-mg/10-ml preservative-free, single-use vials (1 mg/ml), which must be further diluted in 0.9% sodium chloride injection. Diluted drug stable at room temperature for at least 24 hours in normal light. Once prepared, solution may be refrigerated up to 8 hours prior to use.

*Single daily dose:* Add calculated drug dose to 500 ml of 0.9% sodium chloride injection, USP.

*7-day continuous infusion by ambulatory infusion pump:* Add calculated drug dose for 7 days to infusion reservoir using a sterile 0.22-micron hydrophilic syringe filter. Then add, again using a sterile 0.22-micron filter, sufficient sterile bacteriostatic 0.9% sodium chloride injection containing 0.9% benzyl alcohol to produce 100 ml in the infusion reservoir.

## DRUG ADMINISTRATION

Administer as a continuous IV infusion for 7 days.

## SPECIAL CONSIDERATIONS

Indicated for the treatment of active hairy cell leukemia, Waldenstrom's macroglobulinemia, CLL.

Unstable in 5% dextrose, so do not use $D_5W$ as diluent.

Store unopened vials in refrigerator and protect from light.

Drug may precipitate when exposed to low temperatures. Allow solution to warm to room temperature and shake vigorously. *Do not heat or microwave.*

Drug structurally similar to pentostatin and fludarabine.

Contraindicated in patients who are hypersensitive to the drug.

Administer with caution in patients with renal or hepatic insufficiency.

Embryotoxic, so women of childbearing age should use contraception.

## Cladribine

| Nursing Diagnosis | Defining Characteristics | Expected Outcomes | Nursing Interventions |
|---|---|---|---|
| I. *Infection and bleeding related to bone marrow depression* | I. A. Neutropenia occurs in 70% of pts, with nadir 1–2 weeks after infusion and recovery by weeks 4–5; incidence of infection 28%, with 40% due to bacterial etiology<br>   1. Prolonged bone marrow hypocellularity occurs in 34% of pts, lasting at least 4 months<br>   2. Infections most common in pts with pancytopenia and lymphopenia due to hairy cell leukemia<br>   3. Most common sites are lungs and venous access site<br>B. Lymphopenia common, with decreased CD4 (helper T-cells) and CD8 (suppressor T-cells) and recovery by weeks 26–34<br>   1. Incidence of infection 34%<br>   2. Of these, 20% have viral etiology and 20% fungal etiology<br>C. Thrombocytopenia occurs commonly, along with purpura (10%), petechia (8%), and epistaxis (5%)<br>   1. 12–14% of pts require platelet transfusion<br>   2. Recovery by day 12 | I. A. Pt will be without s/s of infection or bleeding | I. A. Monitor Hct, WBC with differential, and platelets prior to drug administration. Discuss any abnormalities with physician<br>B. Assess for s/s of infection and bleeding, and instruct pt in self-assessment and to report s/s immediately<br>C. Teach pt self-care measures to minimize risk of infection and bleeding, including avoidance of OTC aspirin-containing medications<br>D. Transfuse PRBCs and platelets per physician order<br>E. Administer, teach self-administration of erythropoietin per physician orders<br>F. Instruct pt in energy conservation and stress-reduction measures aimed at reducing fatigue<br>G. Refer to section on bone marrow depression, Chapter 4 |

II. *Fatigue related to anemia*

II. A. Fatigue occurs in 45% of pts
   B. Anemia
      1. Approximately 37–44% of pts require red blood cell transfusion
      2. Red cell recovery by week 8
   C. Asthenia occurs in 9% of pts

II. A. Pt will manage fatigue

II. A. Monitor hemoglobin and hematocrit and transfuse per MD order or administer erythropoietin per MD order
   B. Teach pt to alternate rest and activity
   C. Teach diet
   D. Teach stress reduction/relaxation techniques
   E. Exercise may improve energy level
   F. Refer to sec. on bone marrow depression, Chapter 4

III. *Alteration in comfort*

III. A. Fever (> 100°F, 37.5°C) occurs in 66% of pts during the month following treatment
      1. May be related to infection (47%)
      2. May be related to release of endogenous pyrogen from lysed lymphocytes
    B. Other symptoms: chills (9%), diaphoresis (9%), malaise (7%), dizziness (9%), insomnia (7%), myalgia (7%), arthralgias (5%)
    C. Headache occurs in 22% of pts

III. A. Pt will be comfortable

III. A. Assess pt for fever, chills, diaphoresis during visits; assess for s/s of infection
     B. Teach pt self-assessment, how to report this, and measures to reduce fever
     C. Anticipate laboratory and X-ray tests to rule out infection and perform according to MD order

*(continued)*

## Cladribine (continued)

| Nursing Diagnosis | Defining Characteristics | Expected Outcomes | Nursing Interventions |
|---|---|---|---|
| IV. *Potential impairment of skin integrity* | IV. A. Rash occurs in 27–50% of pts<br>B. Other symptoms: pruritis (6%), erythema (6%)<br>C. Injection site reactions include erythema, swelling and pain (2%), phlebitis (2%) | IV. A. Pt will verbally report changes in skin and describes self-care measures | IV. A. Assess skin for any cutaneous changes, such as rash or changes at injection site, and any associated symptoms such as pruritis; discuss with MD<br>B. Instruct pt in self-care measures<br>  1. Avoid abrasive skin products, clothing<br>  2. Avoid tight-fitting clothing<br>  3. Use of skin emollients appropriate for skin alteration<br>  4. Measures to avoid scratching involved areas<br>C. Consider venous access device if skin is at risk for reaction |
| V. *Alteration in nutrition* | V. A. Nausea is mild and occurs in 28% of pts<br>B. Vomiting occurs in 13% of pts, and if antiemetics are required, it is easily controlled by phenothiazines<br>C. Renal and hepatic function studies are rarely affected | V. A. Pt will be without nausea and vomiting<br>B. Pt will maintain weight within 5% of baseline | V. A. Premedicate with antiemetics; if nausea and vomiting occur, teach pt to self-medicate with antiemetics per MD order<br>B. Encourage small, frequent feedings of cool, bland foods and liquids<br>C. Teach pt to record diet history for 2–3 days and weekly weights<br>D. Refer to sec. on nausea and vomiting, Chapter 4<br>E. If pt has decreased appetite, assess food preferences (encourage or discourage) and suggest use of spices |

| | | | |
|---|---|---|---|
| VI. *Alteration in elimination* | VI. A. Diarrhea occurs in 10% of pts<br>B. Constipation occurs in 9% of pts<br>C. Abdominal pain occurs in 6% of pts | VI. A. Pt will have minimal diarrhea<br>B. Pt will have minimal constipation | VI. A. Encourage pt to report onset of change in bowel habits (diarrhea or constipation)<br>B. Assess factors contributing to change in bowel habits<br>C. Administer or teach pt self-administration of antidiarrheal medication or cathartic as ordered<br>D. Teach pt diet modification regarding foods that minimize diarrhea or constipation |
| VII. *Potential for impaired gas exchange* | VII. A. Cough (10%), abnormal breath sounds (11%) may occur<br>B. Shortness of breath (7%) | VII. A. Early abnormalities in respiratory pattern will be identified | VII. A. Assess baseline pulmonary status, including breath sounds, presence of cough, shortness of breath<br>B. Instruct pt to report symptoms (i.e., cough or shortness of breath)<br>C. Refer to sec. on pulmonary toxicity, Chapter 4 |
| VIII. *Potential alteration in cardiac output* | VIII. A. Rare<br>B. Edema (6%), tachycardia (6%) | VIII. A. Early signs of alterations in cardiac function will be identified | VIII. A. Assess baseline cardiac status, including apical heart rate, presence of peripheral edema<br>B. Teach pt to report rapid heartbeat or swelling of ankles |

# Cyclophosphamide
(Cytoxan, Endoxan, Endoxana, Neosar)

*Class:* Alkylating agent

## MECHANISM OF ACTION

Causes cross-linkage in DNA strands, thus preventing DNA synthesis and cell division. Cell cycle phase–nonspecific.

## METABOLISM

Inactive until converted by microsomes in liver and serum enzymes (phosphamidases). Both cyclophosphamide and its metabolites are excreted by the kidneys. Plasma half-life is 6–12 hours, with 25% of drug excreted by 8 hours. Prolonged plasma half-life in pts with renal failure results in increased myelosuppression.

## DOSAGE/RANGE

400 mg/m$^2$ IV × 5 days
100 mg/m$^2$ po × 14 days
500–1500 mg/m$^2$ IV q 3–4 weeks

## DRUG PREPARATION

Dilute vials with sterile water. Shake well. Allow solution to clear if lyophilized preparation is not used. Do not use solution unless crystals are fully dissolved. Available in 25- and 50-mg tablets.

## DRUG ADMINISTRATION

PO: administer in morning or early afternoon to allow adequate excretion time. Should be taken with meals.

IV: for doses greater than 500 mg, prehydration and hemorhagic cystitis. Administer Mesna with high-dose cyclophosphosphamide. Administer drug over at least 20 minutes for doses greater than 500 mg.

Solution is stable for 24 hours at room temperature, 6 days if refrigerated.

Rapid infusion may result in dizziness, nasal stuffiness, rhinorrhea, or sinus congestion during or soon after infusion.

## SPECIAL CONSIDERATIONS

Metabolic and leukopenic toxicity are increased by simultaneous administration of barbiturates, corticosteroids, phenytoin, and sulfonamides.

Activity and toxicity of both cyclophosphamide and the specific drug may be altered by allopurinol, chloroquine, phenothiazines, potassium iodide, chloramphenicol, imipramine, vitamin A, warfarin, succinylcholine, digoxin, and thiazide diuretics.

Test urine for occult blood.

High-dose cyclophosphamide therapy may require catheterization and constant bladder irrigation.

## Cyclophosphamide

| Nursing Diagnosis | Defining Characteristics | Expected Outcomes | Nursing Interventions |
|---|---|---|---|
| I. *Altered nutrition, less than body requirements related to* | | | |
| A. Nausea and vomiting | I. A. Nausea and vomiting begin 2–4 hrs after dose, peak in 12 hrs, and may last 24 hrs | I. A. 1. Pt will be without nausea and vomiting<br>2. Nausea and vomiting, if they occur, will be minimal | I. A. 1. Premedicate with antiemetics and continue prophylactically × 24 hrs to prevent nausea and vomiting, at least for first treatment<br>2. Encourage small, frequent feedings of cool, bland foods and liquids |
| B. Anorexia | B. Commonly occurs | B. Pt will maintain baseline weight ± 5% | B. 1. Encourage small, frequent feedings of favorite foods, especially high-calorie, high-protein foods<br>2. Encourage use of spices<br>3. Weekly weights<br>4. Nutritional consultation as needed |
| C. Stomatitis | C. Mild | C. Oral mucous membranes will remain intact and without infection | C. 1. Teach pt oral assessment<br>2. Encourage pt to report early stomatitis<br>3. Teach pt oral hygiene regimen<br>4. See sec. on stomatitis, Chapter 4 |
| D. Diarrhea | D. Infrequent and mild | D. Pt will have minimal diarrhea | D. 1. Encourage pt to report onset of diarrhea<br>2. Administer or teach pt to self-administer antidiarrheal medications<br>3. See sec. on diarrhea, Chapter 4 |

*(continued)*

## Cyclophosphamide (continued)

| Nursing Diagnosis | Defining Characteristics | Expected Outcomes | Nursing Interventions |
|---|---|---|---|
| E. Hepatotoxicity | E. Rare | E. Early hepatotoxicity will be identified | E. 1. Monitor LFTs (i.e., alkaline phosphatase and bilirubin) periodically during treatment<br>2. Monitor pt for any elevations<br>3. Dose modifications may be necessary if elevation occurs |
| II. *Infection and bleeding related to bone marrow depression* | II. A. Leukopenia nadir 7–14 days, with recovery in 1–2 weeks<br>B. Less frequent thrombocytopenia<br>C. Mild anemia<br>D. Potent immunosuppressant | II. A. Pt will be without s/s of infection or bleeding<br>B. Early s/s of infection or bleeding will be identified | II. A. Monitor CBC, platelet count prior to drug administration and monitor for s/s of infection and bleeding<br>B. Instruct pt in self-assessment of s/s of infection and bleeding<br>C. Dose reduction often necessary (35–50%) if compromised bone marrow function<br>D. Administration of GCSF often necessary with high-dose therapy<br>E. See sec. on bone marrow depression, Chapter 4 |
| III. *Potential for injury related to*<br>A. Acute water intoxication (SIADH) | III. A. May occur with high-dose administration (> 50 mg/kg) | III. A. SIADH will be identified early | III. A. 1. If high-dose cytoxan administered, monitor serum sodium, osmolality, and urine electrolytes and osmolality<br>2. Strictly monitor I&O and total body balance<br>3. Daily weights<br>4. Water restrictions as ordered |
| B. Second malignancy (bladder cancer, acute leukemia) | B. Prolonged therapy may cause bladder cancer (related to local toxicity of drug metabolites) and acute leukemia (related to prolonged bone marrow toxicity) | B. Malignancy, if it occurs, will be identified early | B. Pts receiving prolonged therapy should be screened |

| | | |
|---|---|---|
| IV. *Altered urinary elimination related to hemorrhagic cystitis* | IV. A. Metabolites of cyclophosphamide, if allowed to accumulate in bladder, irritate bladder wall capillaries, causing hemorrhagic cystitis<br>B. Sterile chemical cystitis occurs in 5–10% of pts<br>C. Evidenced by hematuria, gross or microscopic (> 20 RBC)<br>D. Mesna frequently used to avoid hemorrhagic cystitis<br>E. Can also cause bladder fibrosis | IV. A. Pt will be without hemorrhagic cystitis | IV. A. Monitor BUN and creatinine prior to drug dose, as drug is excreted by kidneys<br>B. Provide or instruct pt in hydration of at least 3 liters of fluid/day<br>C. Encourage voiding to empty bladder at least q 2–3 hours and at bedtime<br>D. Assess pt for s/s and instruct pt to report hematuria, urinary frequency, dysuria<br>E. Instruct pt that oral cyclophosphamide should be taken early in day to prevent accumulation of drug in the bladder<br>F. Administer Mesna as ordered |
| V. *Alteration in cardiac output related to high-dose cyclophosphamide* | V. A. Cardiomyopathy may occur with high doses; also, potentiates cardiotoxicity of doxorubicin (Adriamycin) | V. A. Early s/s of cardiomyopathy will be identified | V. A. If pt is receiving high-dose cyclophosphamide, assess for s/s of cardiomyopathy<br>B. Gated blood pool scan (GBPS) or echocardiogram often used to check LVEF (left ventricular ejection fraction)<br>C. Assess quality and regularity of heartbeat<br>D. Instruct pt to report dyspnea, shortness of breath |
| VI. *Potential for impaired gas exchange related to pulmonary toxicity* | VI. A. Rare, but may occur with prolonged, high-dose therapy or continuous low-dose therapy<br>B. Appears as interstitial pneumonitis and onset insidious | VI. A. Early s/s of pulmonary toxicity will be identified | VI. A. If pt is receiving high-dose or continuous low-dose cyclophosphamide, assess for s/s of pulmonary dysfunction<br>B. Discuss pulmonary function studies to be performed periodically with MD |

*(continued)*

## Cyclophosphamide (continued)

| Nursing Diagnosis | Defining Characteristics | Expected Outcomes | Nursing Interventions |
|---|---|---|---|
| | IV. C. May respond to steroids | | IV. C. Assess lung sounds prior to drug administration |
| | | | D. Instruct pt to report cough or dyspnea |
| VII. *Altered body image related to* | | | |
| A. Alopecia | VII. A. 1. Occurs in 30–50% of pts, especially with IV dosing | VII. A. Pt will verbalize feelings re hair loss and identify strategies to cope with change in body image | VII. A. 1. Assess pt for s/s of hair loss |
| | 2. Some degree of hair loss expected in all pts | | 2. Discuss with pt impact of hair loss and strategies to minimize distress (i.e., wig, scarf, cap) |
| | 3. Begins after 3+ weeks and may grow back while on therapy | | 3. Begin discussion before therapy has been initiated |
| | 4. May be slight to diffuse thinning | | 4. See sec. on alopecia, Chapter 4 |
| B. Changes in nails, skin | B. Hyperpigmentation of nails and skin, transverse ridging of nails ("banding") may occur | B. Pt will verbalize feelings re changes in nail or skin color or texture and identify strategies to cope with change in body image | B. 1. Assess pt for changes in skin, nails |
| | | | 2. Discuss with pt impact of changes and strategies to minimize distress (i.e., wearing nail polish, long sleeves) |
| VIII. *Sexual dysfunction* | VIII. A. Drug is mutagenic and teratogenic | VIII. A. Pt and significant other will understand need for contraception | VIII. A. As appropriate, explore with pt and significant other issues of reproductive and sexuality pattern and the impact chemotherapy will have |
| | B. Testicular atrophy sometimes occurs with reversible oligo- and azoospermia | B. Pt and significant other will identify strategies to cope with sexual dysfunction | B. Discuss strategies to preserve sexual and reproductive health (e.g., sperm banking, contraception) |
| | C. Amenorrhea often occurs in females | | C. See sec. on gonadal dysfunction, Chapter 4 |
| | D. Drug is excreted in breast milk | | |

# Cytarabine, cytosine arabinoside
## (Ara-C, Cytosar-U, Arabinosyl Cytosine)

*Class:* Antimetabolite

## MECHANISM OF ACTION

Antimetabolite (pyrimidine analogue) that is incorporated into DNA, slowing its synthesis and causing defects in the linkages in new DNA fragments. Also, cells exposed to cytarabine in the S phase reinitiate DNA synthesis when the drug is removed, resulting in erroneous duplication of the early portions of the DNA strands. Most effective when cells are undergoing rapid DNA synthesis .

## METABOLISM

Inactivated by liver enzymes in biphasic manner: half-lives 10–15 minutes and 2–3 hours. Crosses the blood-brain barrier with CSF concentration of 50% that of plasma; 70% of dose excreted in urine as Ara-U; 4–10% excreted 12–24 hours after administration.

## DOSAGE/RANGE

Leukemia: 100 mg/m$^2$ day IV continuous infusion × 5–10 days
100 mg/m$^2$ every 12 hours × 1–3 weeks IV or SQ
Head and neck: 1 mg/kg every 12 hours × 5–7 days IV or SQ
High dose: 2–3 mg/m$^2$ IV
Differentiation: 10 mg/m$^2$ SQ every 12 hours × 15–21 days
Intrathecal: 20–30 mg/m$^2$

## DRUG PREPARATION

100-mg vials: Add water with benzyl alcohol, then dilute with NS or D$_5$W.

500-mg vials: Add water with benzyl alcohol, then dilute with NS or D$_5$W.

For intrathecal use and high dose: Use preservative-free diluent.

Reconstituted drug is stable 48 hours at room temperature and 7 days refrigerated.

## DRUG ADMINISTRATION

Doses of 100–200 mg can be given SQ.

Doses less than 1 gm: Administer via volutrol over 10–20 minutes.

Doses over 1 gm: Administer over 2 hours.

## SPECIAL CONSIDERATIONS

Thrombophlebitis or pain at the injection site should be treated with warm compresses.

Dizziness has occurred with too-rapid IV infusions.

Use with caution if hepatic dysfunction exists.

May decrease bioavailability of digoxin when given in combination.

## Cytarabine, cytosine arabinoside

| Nursing Diagnosis | Defining Characteristics | Expected Outcomes | Nursing Interventions |
|---|---|---|---|
| I. Altered nutrition, less than body requirements related to | | | |
| A. Nausea and vomiting | I. A. 1. Occurs in 50% of pts<br>2. Dose related<br>3. Lasts for several hours | I. A. 1. Pt will be without nausea or vomiting<br>2. Nausea and vomiting, if they occur, will be minimal | I. A. 1. Premedicate with antiemetics and continue prophylactically × 24 hrs to prevent nausea and vomiting, at least for first treatment<br>2. Encourage small, frequent feedings of cool, bland foods and liquids<br>3. I&O, daily weights if inpatient (assess for s/s of fluid and electrolyte imbalance)<br>4. Refer to sec. on nausea and vomiting, Chapter 4 |
| B. Anorexia | B. Commonly occurs | B. Pt will maintain baseline weight ± 5% | B. 1. Encourage small, frequent feedings of favorite foods, especially high-calorie, high-protein foods<br>2. Encourage use of spices<br>3. Weekly weights, daily if inpatient |
| C. Stomatitis | C. Occurs 7–10 days after therapy is initiated in about 15% of pts | C. Oral mucous membranes will remain intact and without signs of infection | C. 1. Assess oral cavity every day: teach pt to do own oral assessment and oral hygiene regimen<br>2. Encourage pt to report early stomatitis<br>3. Pain relief measures, if indicated<br>4. See sec. on stomatitis/mucositis, Chapter 4 |
| D. Diarrhea | D. Infrequent and mild | D. Pt will have minimal diarrhea | D. 1. Encourage pt to report onset of diarrhea<br>2. Administer or teach pt to administer antidiarrheal medication<br>3. See sec. on diarrhea, Chapter 4 |

| | | | |
|---|---|---|---|
| E. Hepatotoxicity | E. Usually mild and reversible, but drug should be used cautiously in pts with hepatic dysfunction | E. Early hepatotoxicity will be identified | E. 1. Monitor LFTs prior to drug dose, especially with high drug doses<br>2. Assess pt prior to and during treatment for s/s hepatotoxicity |
| II. *Infection and bleeding related to bone marrow depression* | II. A. Related to dose and duration of therapy | II. A. Pt will be without s/s of infection or bleeding | II. A. Monitor CBC, platelet count prior to drug administration, as well as s/s of infection and bleeding |
| | B. Leukopenic nadir 7–14 days after drug administration; recovery in 3 weeks | B. Early s/s of bleeding and infection will be identified | B. Assess pt q day for s/s of infection and bleeding; instruct pt in self-assessment |
| | C. Thrombocytopenia common | | C. Transfuse as necessary with red cells, platelets |
| | D. Megaloblastic changes in the marrow are common | | D. Administer growth factors (erythropoietin & GCSF) as ordered |
| | E. Anemia seen frequently | | |
| | F. Potent but transient suppression of primary and secondary antibody responses | | |
| III. *Impaired skin integrity related to alopecia* | III. A. Occurs frequently | III. A. Pt will verbalize feelings re hair loss and identify strategies to cope with change in body image | III. A. Pt will verbalize feelings re hair loss and identify strategies to cope with change in body image |
| | | | B. Discuss with pt impact of hair loss and strategies to minimize distress (i.e., wig, scarf, cap); begin before therapy is initiated |
| | | | C. See sec. on alopecia, Chapter 4 |

*(continued)*

IV. *Potential for injury related to*
A. Neurotoxicity

IV. A. 1. Can occur with high doses
2. Cerebellar toxicity is indication for immediate cessation of therapy
3. Lethargy, somnolence have resulted from too-rapid infusions of drug

IV. A. 1. Early cerebellar toxicity will be recognized and reported
2. Neurotoxicity will be minimized

IV. A. 1. Assess pt q shift and before administering drug for cerebellar toxicity
2. Instruct pt in self-assessment of cerebellar function; encourage pt to report changes in coordination, control of eye movement, etc.
3. Report changes in cerebellar function
4. Administer drug according to established guidelines; monitor pt during infusion for lethargy, somnolence
5. See sec. on neurotoxicity, Chapter 4

B. Tumor lysis syndrome (TLS), hyperuricemia

B. 1. TLS may develop secondary to rapid lysis of tumor cells
2. Usually begins 1–5 days after initiation of chemotherapy

B. Serum uric acid, potassium, and phosphorus will remain within normal limits

B. 1. Monitor BUN, creatinine, potassium, phosphorus, uric acid, and calcium
2. Monitor I&O
3. Monitor for renal, cardiac, neuromuscular s/s of TLS
4. Administer allopurinol, fluids as ordered
5. See sec. on nephrotoxicity, Chapter 4

# Cytarabine liposome injection
(DepoCyt)

*Class:* Antimetabolite

## MECHANISM OF ACTION

Drug is converted to the metabolite ara-CTP intracellularly. Ara-CTP is thought to inhibit DNA polymerase, thereby affecting DNA synthesis. Incorporation into DNA and RNA may also contribute to cytarabine cellular toxicity.

## METABOLISM

With systemically administered cytarabine, the drug is metabolized to an inactive compound, ara-U, and is then renally excreted. In the CSF, however, conversion to the ara-U is negligible, because CNS tissue and CSF lack the enzyme necessary for the conversion to occur.

## DOSAGE/RANGE

Indicated for the intrathecal treatment of lymphomatous meningitis only. To be given as follows:

Induction therapy: DepoCyt, 50 mg, administered intrathecally (intraventricular or lumbar puncture) every 14 days for 2 doses (weeks 1 and 3).

Consolidation therapy: DepoCyt, 50 mg, administered intrathecally (intraventricular or lumbar puncture) every 14 days for 3 doses (weeks 5, 7, and 9) followed by 1 additional dose at week 13.

Maintenance therapy: DepoCyt, 50 mg, administered intrathecally (intraventricular or lumbar puncture) every 28 days for 4 doses (weeks 17, 21, 25, and 29).

If drug-related neurotoxicity develops, the dose should be reduced to 25 mg. If toxicity persists, treatment with DepoCyt should be terminated.

## DRUG PREPARATION/ADMINISTRATION

Drug is supplied in single-use vials and comes as a white to off-white suspension in 5 ml of fluid.

Drug is to be withdrawn immediately before use and should not be used later than 4 hours from the time of withdrawal from vial.

DepoCyt should be administered directly into the CSF over 1–5 minutes. Pts should lie flat for 1 hour after administration.

Pts should be started on dexamethasone 4 mg bid either PO or IV for 5 days beginning on the day of DepoCyt injection.

## SPECIAL CONSIDERATIONS

Do not use inline filters with DepoCyt: administer directly into CSF.

Must be administered with concurrent dexamethasone as described above.

## Cytarabine liposome injection

| Nursing Diagnosis | Defining Characteristics | Expected Outcomes | Nursing Interventions |
|---|---|---|---|
| I. *Alteration in nutrition, less than body requirements, related to nausea and vomiting* | I. A. Nausea, vomiting, and headache are common, and are physical manifestations of chemical arachnoiditis | I. A. Nausea/vomiting will be avoided or minimized | I. A. Administer dexamethasone throughout treatment course as described above<br>B. Observe pt for at least 1 hr after administration for toxicity<br>C. Administer antiemetics as ordered. Teach pt to report nausea/vomiting and to self-administer antiemetics<br>D. Encourage small, frequent feedings of cool, bland foods<br>E. Refer to sec. on nausea and vomiting, Chapter 4 |
| II. *Alteration in comfort related to headache, neck and/or back pain, fever* | II. A. Some degree of chemical arachnoiditis is expected in about a third of pts: incidence approaches 100% of pts when dexamethasone is NOT given with DepoCyt<br>B. Causes headache, neck pain and/or rigidity, back pain, fever | II. A. Pt will report comfort throughout treatment course<br>B. Discomfort will be identified early and treated effectively | II. A. Instruct pt in dexamethasone self-administration and to report to MD if oral doses are not tolerated<br>B. Pts should lie flat for 1 hr after lumbar puncture and should be observed for immediate toxic reactions<br>C. Administer medications to treat pain |

# Dacarbazine
(DTIC-Dome, Imidazole carboximide)

*Class:* Alkylating agent

## MECHANISM OF ACTION

Unclear, but appears to be an agent that methylates nucleic acids (particularly DNA), causing cross-linkage and breaks in DNA strands. This inhibits RNA and DNA synthesis. Also interacts with sulf-hydryl groups in proteins. Generally, cell cycle phase nonspecific.

## METABOLISM

Thought to be activated by liver microsomes. Excreted renally, with a plasma half-life of 0.65 hour, and terminal half-life of 5 hours.

## DOSAGE/RANGE

375 mg/m² every 3–4 weeks

*or*

150–250 mg/m² day × 5 days, repeat every 3–4 weeks

*or*

800–900 mg/m² as a single dose every 3–4 weeks

## DRUG PREPARATION

Add sterile water or NS to vial.

## DRUG ADMINISTRATION

Administer via volutrol over 20 minutes or give via IV push over 2–3 minutes.

Stable for 8 hours at room temperature, 72 hours if refrigerated. Store lyophilized drug in refrigerator and protect from light. Drug decomposition is denoted by a change in color from yellow to pink.

## SPECIAL CONSIDERATIONS

Irritant—avoid extravasation.

Pain may occur above site. Usually unrelieved by slowing IV, but may be relieved by applying ice to painful area. May cause venospasm; slow rate if this occurs.

Anaphylaxis has occurred with infusion of dacarbazine.

Drug interactions: increased drug metabolism with concurrent administration of dilantin, phenobarbital; potential increased toxicity with Imuran and 6-MP.

# Dacarbazine

| Nursing Diagnosis | Defining Characteristics | Expected Outcomes | Nursing Interventions |
|---|---|---|---|
| I. *Altered nutrition, less than body requirements related to* A. Nausea and vomiting | I. A. 90% incidence of nausea and vomiting, moderate to severe, beginning 1–3 hrs after dose; tolerance develops when given over several days, so nausea and vomiting are less severe | I. A. 1. Pt will be without nausea and vomiting 2. Nausea and vomiting, if they occur, will be minimal | I. A. 1. Premedicate with antiemetic 2. Help pt relax using distraction, progressive muscle relaxation, imagery; teach pt how to induce relaxation 3. Infuse drug slowly over 1 hr to decrease nausea and vomiting 4. Refer to sec. on nausea and vomiting, Chapter 4 |
| B. Diarrhea | B. Uncommon | B. Diarrhea, if it occurs, will abate | B. 1. Assess pt for evidence of diarrhea 2. Administer antidiarrheal medication or teach pt to self-administer |
| C. Anorexia | C. Commonly occurs; may also cause metallic taste sensation | C. Pt will maintain baseline weight ± 5% | C. 1. Encourage small, frequent feedings of favorite foods, especially high-calorie, high-protein foods 2. Encourage use of spices 3. Weekly weight |
| D. Hepatotoxicity | D. Rare; however, hepatic veno-occlusive disease has been described (hepatic vein thrombosis and hepatocellular necrosis) | D. Hepatocellular dysfunction, if it occurs, will be identified early | D. 1. Monitor LFTs prior to treatment 2. If LFTs are elevated, discuss withholding medication with MD |
| II. *Infection and bleeding related to bone marrow depression* | II. A. Nadir 14–28 days following treatment B. Anemia may occur with long-term treatment | II. A. Pt will be without s/s of infection or bleeding B. Early s/s of infection or bleeding will be identified | II. A. Monitor CBC, platelet count prior to drug administration, as well as s/s of infection and bleeding B. Instruct pt in self-assessment of s/s of infection and bleeding C. Transfuse with red cells, platelets per MD order D. Refer to sec. on bone marrow depression, Chapter 4 |

III. *Potential for injury related to anaphylaxis*

III. A. Anaphylaxis may occur rarely, with fever, confusion, urticaria, wheezing, or hypotension

III. A. Allergic reaction or anaphylaxis, if it occurs, will be detected early
B. Airway will remain patent
C. BP will remain within 20 mmHg of baseline

III. A. Review standing orders for management of pt in anaphylaxis and identify location of anaphylaxis kit containing epinephrine 1:1000, hydrocortisone sodium succinate (Solucortef), diphenhydramine HCl (Benadryl), Aminophylline, and others

B. Prior to drug administration, obtain baseline vital signs and record mental status

C. Observe for following s/s during infusion, usually occurring within first 15 mins of start of infusion

D. Future allergic responses will be prevented
1. *Subjective*
   a. generalized itching
   b. chest tightness
   c. difficulty speaking
   d. agitation
   e. uneasiness
   f. dizziness
   g. nausea
   h. crampy abdominal pain
   i. anxiety
   j. sense of impending doom
   k. desire to urinate/defecate
   l. chills
2. *Objective*
   a. flushed appearance (angioedema of face, neck, eyelids, hands, feet)
   b. localized or generalized urticaria
   c. respiratory distress ± wheezing
   d. hypotension
   e. cyanosis

E. If reaction occurs, stop infusion and notify MD

(continued)

# Dacarbazine

| Nursing Diagnosis | Defining Characteristics | Expected Outcomes | Nursing Interventions |
|---|---|---|---|
| | | | F. Place pt in supine position to promote perfusion of visceral organs |
| | | | G. Monitor vital signs until stable |
| | | | H. Provide emotional reassurance to pt and family |
| | | | I. Maintain patent airway and have ready equipment for CPR if needed |
| | | | J. Document incident |
| | | | K. Discuss with MD desensitization versus drug discontinuance for further dosing |
| | | | L. See sec. on reactions, Chapter 9 |
| IV. *Alteration in comfort related to* A. "Flu-like syndrome" | IV. A. 1. Influenza-like syndrome characterized by malaise, headache, myalgia, chills, and hypotension <br> 2. May occur up to 7 days after first dose, last 7–21 days, and recur with subsequent doses | IV. A. Pt will verbalize increased comfort | IV. A. 1. Discuss possibility of flu-like syndrome occurring <br> 2. Suggest symptom management with acetaminophen as needed <br> 3. Encourage fluids orally ≥ 3 L/day, rest <br> 4. Encourage pt to verbalize feelings and give other emotional support |
| B. Pain at injection site | B. Drug is an *irritant* and may cause phlebitis of vein | B. Pain will be minimized | B. 1. Assess pt for appropriateness of central venous access device, especially if pt will receive successive treatments <br> 2. Administer DTIC in 100–250 cc IV fluid and infuse slowly over 1 hr <br> 3. Consider premedication and discuss with MD: <br>   a. Apply ice or heat above injection site to reduce venous burning |

| Nursing Diagnosis | Defining Characteristics | Expected Outcomes | Nursing Interventions |
|---|---|---|---|
| | | | b. Premedicate with hydrocortisone IVP, lidocaine 1–2% IVP, or heparin IVP to minimize trauma to vein prior to DTIC infusion (DTIC forms precipitate with hydrocortisone sodium succinate [Solucortef] but not with hydrocortisone) |
| V. *Impaired skin integrity related to* | | | |
| A. Alopecia | V. A. Causes alopecia in 90% of pts, with obvious impact on body image | V. A. Pt will verbalize expected side effects relating to hair loss and strategies to minimize distress related to these side effects | V. A. 1. Encourage pt to obtain wig prior to hair loss<br>2. Encourage pt to verbalize feelings re anticipated or actual hair loss and discuss strategies to minimize impact of alopecia<br>3. Provide emotional support<br>4. Refer to sec. on alopecia, Chapter 4 |
| B. Facial flushing, erythema, and urticaria | B. Facial flushing occurs rarely and is self-limiting; erythema and urticaria are rare but may occur around injection site | B. Pt will verbalize feelings re changes in skin and identify strategies to cope with these changes | B. 1. Assess pt for changes in skin<br>2. Discuss with pt impact of changes and strategies to minimize distress |
| VI. *Potential for sensory/ perceptual alterations* | VI. A. Facial paresthesia, photosensitivity | VI. A. Pt will verbalize expected side effects and self-care measures | VI. A. Instruct pt in self-care measures if sensory changes occur<br>1. To report facial paresthesias to nurse<br>2. To avoid strong sunlight, wear sunscreen on skin and protective clothing and hat |
| VII. *Potential for sexual dysfunction* | VII. A. Drug is teratogenic | VII. A. Pt and significant other will verbalize importance of and need for contraception | VII. A. As appropriate, discuss birth control measures<br>1. Discuss reproductive goals, hopes, and impact contraception will have<br>2. Provide teaching booklets<br>3. See sec. on gonadal dysfunction, Chapter 4 |

# Dactinomycin
## (Actinomycin D, Cosmegan)

*Class:* Antitumor antibiotic isolated from *streptomyces* fungus

## MECHANISM OF ACTION

Binds to guanine portion of DNA and blocks the ability of DNA to act as a template for both DNA and RNA. At lower drug doses, the predominant action inhibits RNA, whereas at higher doses both RNA and DNA are inhibited. Cell cycle–specific for $G_1$ and S phases.

## METABOLISM

Most of drug is excreted unchanged in bile and urine. There is a rapid clearance of drug from plasma (approximately 36 hours). Dose reduction in the presence of liver or renal failure may be needed.

## DOSAGE/RANGE

10–15 µg/kg/day × 5 days every 3–4 weeks

15–30 µg/kg/week, 400–600 µg/m² day for 5 days IV

Frequency and schedule may vary according to protocol and age.

## DRUG PREPARATION

Add sterile water for a concentration of 500 µg/ml. Use preservative-free water, as precipitate may develop otherwise.

## DRUG ADMINISTRATION

Usually given IV push via sidearm of running IV

## SPECIAL CONSIDERATIONS

Drug is a vesicant. Give through a running IV to avoid extravasation, which may develop into ulceration, necrosis, and pain.

Skin changes—radiation recall phenomenon. Skin discoloration along vein used for injection.

## Dactinomycin

| Nursing Diagnosis | Defining Characteristics | Expected Outcomes | Nursing Interventions |
|---|---|---|---|
| I. *Potential for infection and bleeding related to bone marrow depression* | I. A. Onset 7–10 days, nadir 14–21 days, with recovery 21–28 days<br>B. Anemia is delayed<br>C. Myelosuppression may be dose limiting and severe | I. A. Pt will be without infection or bleeding<br>B. Early s/s of infection and bleeding will be identified | I. A. Monitor CBC, platelet count prior to drug administration<br>B. Assess pt and teach pt self-assessment for s/s of infection and bleeding<br>C. Transfuse red cells, platelets per MD order<br>D. Drug dosage should be reduced for lower than normal blood values<br>E. Administer growth factors as ordered<br>F. See sec. on bone marrow depression, Chapter 4 |
| II. *Alteration in nutrition*<br>A. Nausea and vomiting | II. A. Beginning 2–5 hrs after dose, may last 24 hrs | II. A. 1. Pt will be without nausea and vomiting<br>2. Nausea and vomiting, if they occur, will be minimal | II. A. 1. Premedicate with antiemetics and continue prophylactically × 24 hrs to prevent nausea and vomiting, at least first treatment<br>2. Encourage small, frequent feedings of cool, bland foods and liquids<br>3. Administer oral dose on an empty stomach<br>4. Refer to sec. on nausea and vomiting, Chapter 4 |
| B. Diarrhea, cramps | B. 30% incidence | B. Pt will have minimal diarrhea | B. 1. Encourage pt to report onset of diarrhea<br>2. Administer or teach pt to self-administer antidiarrheal medication<br>3. See sec. on diarrhea, Chapter 4 |

*(continued)*

## Dactinomycin (continued)

| Nursing Diagnosis | Defining Characteristics | Expected Outcomes | Nursing Interventions |
|---|---|---|---|
| C. Anorexia | C. Occurs frequently | C. Pt will maintain baseline weight ± 5% | C. 1. Encourage small, frequent feedings of favorite foods, especially high-calorie, high-protein foods<br>2. Encourage use of spices<br>3. Weekly weights |
| III. *Alteration in mucous membranes, including stomatitis, esophagitis, proctitis* | III. A. There is an incidence of irritation of mucous membranes lining the entire gastrointestinal tract | III. A. 1. Oral mucous membranes will remain intact and without infection<br>2. The gastrointestinal toxicity will be minimal | III. A. Teach pt oral assessment and oral hygiene regimen<br>B. Encourage pt to report early stomatitis<br>C. Teach pt importance of stomatitis and the entire gastrointestinal system<br>D. Administer pain medications/topical anesthetics as needed<br>E. Guaiac all stools<br>F. Refer to sec. on stomatitis, mucositis, Chapter 4 |
| IV. *Impaired skin integrity* | IV. A. Radiation recall at previously irradiated skin site<br>B. Acne-like rash and alopecia can occur in 47% of pts<br>C. Drug is a vesicant | IV. A. Pt will verbalize feelings re changes in nail or skin color, texture<br>B. Identify strategies to cope with change in body image<br>C. Extravasation, if it occurs, will be detected early with early intervention<br>D. Skin and underlying tissue damage will be minimized | IV. A. 1. Assess pt for changes in skin, nails, and hair loss<br>2. Discuss with pt impact of changes and strategies to minimize distress<br>3. See sec. on reactions, Chapter 4<br>B. 1. Discuss skin changes as they relate to changes in body image<br>2. See sec. on alopecia, Chapter 4<br>C. 1. Careful technique is used during venipuncture. See sec. on intravenous administration, Chapter 4<br>2. Administer vesicant through freely flowing IV, constantly monitoring IV site and pt response |

3. Nurse should be *thoroughly* familiar with institutional policy and procedure for administration of a vesicant agent

4. If vesicant drug is administered as a continuous infusion, drug must be given through a patent central line

5. If extravasation is suspected:

   a. Stop drug being administered

   b. Aspirate any residual drug and blood from IV tubing, IV catheter/needle, and IV site if possible

   c. If antidote exists, instill antidote into area of apparent infiltration as per MD orders and institutional policy and procedure

   d. Apply cold or topical medication as per MD order and institutional policy and procedure

6. Assess site regularly for pain, progression of erythema, induration, and evidence of necrosis

7. When in doubt about whether drug is infiltrating, *treat as infiltration*

8. Teach pt to assess site and notify MD if condition worsens

*(continued)*

## Dactinomycin (continued)

| Nursing Diagnosis | Defining Characteristics | Expected Outcomes | Nursing Interventions |
|---|---|---|---|
| | | | 9. Arrange next clinic visit for assessment of site depending on drug, amount infiltrated, extent of potential injury, and pt variables |
| | | | 10. Document in pts record as per institutional policy and procedure; see sec. on reactions, Chapter 9 |
| V. *Alteration in comfort* | V. A. Flu-like symptoms may occur, including symptoms of malaise, myalgia, fever, depression | V. A. Pt will remain comfortable during therapy | V. A. Assess pt for symptoms during and after treatment |
| | | | B. Premedicate with acetaminophen, antihistamine, or steroids as per MD order |
| | | | C. Evaluate the effectiveness of the symptomatic relief that is prescribed and administered |
| VI. *Alteration in metabolism* A. Hepatotoxicity | VI. A. Drug is metabolized rapidly by the liver | VI. A. Hepatic dysfunction will be identified early | VI. A. 1. Establish a baseline for liver function tests |
| | | | 2. Monitor SGOT, SGPT, LDH, alkaline phosphatase, and bilirubin on a regular basis |
| | | | 3. Notify MD of any elevations |
| | | | 4. Refer to sec. on hepato-toxicity, Chapter 4 |

| | | | |
|---|---|---|---|
| B. Renal toxicity | B. Drug is metabolized rapidly by the kidneys | B. Renal toxicity will be minimal | B. 1. Monitor BUN and creatinine prior to drug dose<br>2. Provide fluid and teach pt the importance of hydration<br>3. See sec. on nephrotoxicity, Chapter 4 |
| VII. *Potential for sexual dysfunction* | VII. A. Drug is mutagenic and teratogenic | VII. A. Pt and significant other will understand need for contraception<br>B. Pt and significant other will identify strategies to cope with sexual dysfunction | VII. A. As appropriate, explore with pt and significant other reproductive patterns and impact chemotherapy will have<br>B. Discuss strategies to preserve sexuality and reproductive health (sperm banking, contraception)<br>C. See sec. on gonadal dysfunction, Chapter 4 |

# Daunorubicin hydrochloride
(Cerubidine, Daunomycin)

*Class:* Anthracycline antibiotic isolated from streptomycin products, in particular the rhodomycin products

## MECHANISM OF ACTION

No clearly defined mechanism. Intercalates DNA, therefore blocking DNA, RNA, and protein synthesis. Binds to DNA and inhibits DNA replication and DNA-dependent RNA synthesis.

## METABOLISM

Site of significant metabolism is in the liver. Doses need to be modified in presence of abnormal liver function. Excreted in urine and bile.

## DOSAGE/RANGE

30–60 mg/m$^2$/day IV for 3 consecutive days

## DRUG PREPARATION

Add sterile water to produce liquid. Drug will form a precipitate when mixed with heparin and is incompatible with dexamethasone.

## DRUG ADMINISTRATION

Give IV push through the sidearm of a freely flowing IV or as a bolus over 1–2 hours or as a continuous infusion over 24 hours. Must be given via a central line if given via bolus or continuous infusion, as drug is a potent vesicant.

## SPECIAL CONSIDERATIONS

Drug is a potent vesicant. Give through running IV to avoid extravasation.

Moderate to severe nausea and vomiting occur in 50% of patients within first 24 hours.

Causes discoloration of urine (pink to red for up to 48 hours after administration).

Cardiac toxicity—dose limit at 550 mg/m$^2$. Patients may exhibit irreversible congestive heart failure. Acute toxicity may be seen within hours after administration. This is unrelated to cumulative dose and may manifest symptoms of pump or conduction function. Rarely, transient EKG abnormalities, CHF, pericardial effusion (whole syndrome referred to as myocarditis-pericarditis syndrome) may occur, which may lead to demise of patient.

## Daunorubicin hydrochloride

| Nursing Diagnosis | Defining Characteristics | Expected Outcomes | Nursing Interventions |
|---|---|---|---|
| I. *Potential for infection and bleeding related to bone marrow depression* | I. A. Leukopenia onset in 7 days; nadir 10–14 days; recovery 21–28 days<br>B. Thrombocytopenia occurs with BMD | I. A. Pt will be without s/s of infection or bleeding<br>B. Early s/s of infection and bleeding will be identified | I. A. Monitor CBC, platelet count prior to drug administration<br>B. Monitor s/s of infection and bleeding<br>C. Instruct pt in self-assessment of s/s of infection and bleeding<br>D. Dose reduction may be necessary<br>E. Transfuse with red cells, platelets per MD order<br>F. Administer growth factors as ordered<br>G. Refer to sec. on bone marrow depression, Chapter 4 |
| II. *Potential for altered cardiac output* | II. A. Acute: 6–30% of pts develop transient EKG changes 1–3 days after dose<br>B. Chronic: cumulative, dose-related cardiomyopathy<br>C. CHF may develop 1–16 months after therapy ceases | II. A. Early s/s of cardiomyopathy will be identified | II. A. Assess for s/s of cardiomyopathy<br>B. Assess quality and regularity of heartbeat<br>C. Baseline EKG<br>D. Instruct pt to report dyspnea, shortness of breath, swelling of extremities, orthopnea<br>E. Chronic cardiomyopathy: monitor gated blood pool scan (GBPS) and ejection fraction, baseline and periodically through treatment as cumulative dosages approach maximum<br>F. See sec. on cardiotoxicity, Chapter 4 |

*(continued)*

## Daunorubicin hydrochloride (continued)

| Nursing Diagnosis | Defining Characteristics | Expected Outcomes | Nursing Interventions |
|---|---|---|---|
| III. *Alteration in nutrition, less than body requirements* | III. A. Mild nausea, vomiting day of therapy (50% incidence) | III. A. Pt will be without nausea and vomiting, or if they | III. A. 1. Premedicate with antiemetic, as ordered, and occur, will be minimal continue prophylactically to prevent nausea and vomiting<br>2. Encourage small, frequent feedings of cool, bland foods and liquids<br>3. Refer to sec. on nausea and vomiting, Chapter 4 |
| | B. Infrequent stomatitis 3–7 days after dose | B. Oral mucous membranes will remain intact | B. 1. Encourage small, frequent feedings of favorite foods, especially high-calorie, high-protein foods<br>2. Encourage use of spices<br>3. Weekly weights<br>4. Assess oral mucous membranes<br>5. Instruct pt in oral assessment and mouth care<br>6. See sec. on stomatitis, Chapter 4 |
| IV. *Potential for impaired skin integrity*<br>A. Extravasation | IV. A. Extravasation of drug can cause tissue necrosis | IV. A. Extravasation, if it occurs, is detected early, with early intervention; skin and underlying tissue damage is minimized | IV. A. 1. Careful technique is used during venipuncture. See sec. on intravenous administration, Chapters 9 and 10<br>2. Administer vesicant through freely flowing IV, constantly monitoring IV site and pt response<br>3. Nurse should be thoroughly familiar with institutional policy and procedure for administration of a vesicant agent<br>4. If vesicant drug is administered as a continuous infusion, drug must be given through a patent central line |

5. If extravasation is suspected:
   a. Stop drug being administered
   b. Aspirate any residual drug and blood from IV tubing, IV catheter/needle, and IV site if possible
   c. *If antidote exists*, instill antidote into area of apparent infiltration as per MD orders and institutional policy and procedure
   d. Apply cold or topical medication as per MD order and institutional policy and procedure
6. Assess site regularly for pain, progression of erythema, induration, and evidence of necrosis
7. When in doubt whether drug is infiltrating, *treat as an infiltration*
8. Teach pt to assess site and notify MD if condition worsens
9. Arrange next clinic visit for assessment of site depending on drug, amount infiltrated, extent of potential injury, and pt variables
10. Document in pts record as per institutional policy and procedure. See sec. on reactions, Chapter 9

*(continued)*

## Daunorubicin hydrochloride (continued)

| Nursing Diagnosis | Defining Characteristics | Expected Outcomes | Nursing Interventions |
|---|---|---|---|
| IV. B. Alopecia | IV. B. Alopecia (complete) 3–4 weeks after treatment begins | IV. B. Pt will verbalize feelings re hair loss and identify strategies to cope with changes in body images | IV. B. 1. Discuss with pt impact of hair loss<br>2. Suggest wig as appropriate prior to actual hair loss<br>3. Explore with pt response to actual hair loss and plan strategies to minimize distress (e.g., wig, scarf, cap)<br>4. Refer to sec. on alopecia, Chapter 4 |
| C. Skin reactions | C. Reactivation of radiation induced lesions (radiation recall); hyperpigmentation, rash; onycholysis (nail loosening from nail bed) | C. Skin discomfort will be minimized and skin will remain intact; pt will verbalize feelings re skin changes | C. 1. This is not an indication to stop the drug<br>2. Discuss with MD symptomatic management<br>3. Reinforce pt teaching on the action and side effects of daunorubicin<br>4. Offer emotional support |
| V. *Potential for sexual dysfunction* | V. A. Drug is mutagenic and teratogenic | V. A. Pt and significant other will understand the need for contraception<br>B. Pt and significant other will identify strategies to cope with sexual dysfunction | V. A. As appropriate, explore with pt and significant other reproductive and sexuality pattern and impact chemotherapy will have<br>B. Discuss strategies to preserve sexuality and reproductive health (e.g., sperm banking, contraception)<br>C. See sec. on gonadal dysfunction, Chapter 4 |
| VI. *Potential for alteration in comfort, i.e., pain* | VI. A. Abdominal pain may occur | VI. A. Pt will be supported during therapy | VI. A. Offer emotional support to pt<br>B. Reinforce information on the action and side effects of daunorubicin hydrochloride<br>C. Discuss with MD medicating for the pain |

# Daunorubicin citrate liposome injection
## (DaunoXome)

*Class:* Anthracycline antibiotic that is isolated from streptomycin products, in particular the rhodomycin products, and encapsulated in a liposome

## MECHANISM OF ACTION

No clearly defined mechanism. Intercalates DNA, therefore blocking DNA, RNA, and protein synthesis. Binds to DNA and inhibits DNA replication and DNA-dependent RNA synthesis. Drug is encapsulated within liposomes (lipid vesicles) and is preferentially delivered to solid tumor sites. The liposomal encapsulated drug is protected from chemical and enzymatic degradation, protein binding, and uptake by normal tissues while circulating in the blood. The exact mechanism for selective targeting of tumor sites is unknown but is believed to be related to increased permeability of the tumor neovasculature. Once delivered to the tumor, the drug is slowly released and exerts its antineoplastic action.

## METABOLISM

Cleared from the plasma at 17 ml/min with a small steady-state volume of distribution. As compared to standard IV daunorubicin, the liposomal encapsulated daunorubicin has higher daunorubicin exposure (plasma area under the curve, ARC). The elimination half-life (4.4 hours) is shorter than standard daunorubicin.

## DOSAGE/RANGE

$40 mg/m^2$/day IV bolus over 60 minutes every 2 weeks

## DRUG PREPARATION

Drug is available as 50 mg of daunorubicin base in a total volume of 25 ml (2 mg/ml).

Visually inspect for particulate matter and discoloration (drug appears as a translucent dispersion of liposomes that scatters light but should not be opaque or have precipitate or foreign matter present).

Withdraw the calculated volume of drug and add to an equal volume of 5% Dextrose to deliver a 1:1, or 1 mg/ml solution.

Administer immediately, or may be stored in the refrigerator at 2–8°C (36–46°F) for 6 hours.

Use ONLY 5% Dextrose, NOT 0.9% sodium chloride or any other solution.

Drug contains no preservatives.

Unopened drug vials should be stored in the refrigerator at 2–8°C (36–46°F), but should not be frozen. Protect from light.

## DRUG ADMINISTRATION

IV bolus over 60 minutes, repeated every 2 weeks.

Do not use an inline filter.

Drug is an irritant, not a vesicant.

Dose should be reduced in patients with renal or hepatic dysfunction.

Hold dose if absolute granulocyte count is $< 750$ cells/mm$^3$.

# Daunorubicin citrate liposome injection
*(continued)*

## *SPECIAL CONSIDERATIONS*

Drug is embryotoxic, so female patients should use contraceptive measures as appropriate.

Back pain, flushing, and chest tightness may occur during the first 5 minutes of drug administration and resolve with cessation of the infusion. Most patients do not experience recurrence when the infusion is restarted at a slower rate.

Drug indicated in the treatment of Kaposi's sarcoma. Activity reported to be equivalent to treatment with ABV (doxorubicin, vincristine, bleomycin) but with less alopecia, cardiotoxicity, and neurotoxicity.

Daunorubicin citrate liposome injection

| Nursing Diagnosis | Defining Characteristics | Expected Outcomes | Nursing Interventions |
|---|---|---|---|
| I. *Potential for infection and bleeding related to bone marrow depression* | I. A. Myelosuppression can be severe and affects the granulocytes primarily<br><br>B. Incidence of neutropenia—36%<br><br>C. Neutropenia with < 500 cells/mm³ occurs in 15% of pts | I. A. Pt will be without s/s of infection or bleeding<br><br>B. Signs of infection and/or bleeding will be identified and reported early | I. A. Monitor Hct, WBC with differential, and platelets prior to drug administration. Discuss any abnormalities with physician (drug should not be given if ANC is < 750 cells/mm³)<br><br>B. Drug dose to be reduced with renal impairment: if creatinine is greater than 3 mg/dl, reduce dose by 50%<br><br>C. Drug dose to be reduced with hepatic dysfunction: 50% reduction if serum bilirubin is greater than 3mg/dl, 25% reduction if serum bilirubin is 1.2–3.0 mg/dl<br><br>D. Assess for s/s infection and bleeding, and instruct pt in self-assessment and to report s/s immediately<br><br>E. Teach pt self-care measures to minimize risk of infection and bleeding, including avoidance of OTC aspirin-containing medications<br><br>F. Refer to section on bone marrow depression, Chapter 4 |

*(continued)*

## Daunorubicin citrate liposome injection (continued)

| Nursing Diagnosis | Defining Characteristics | Expected Outcomes | Nursing Interventions |
|---|---|---|---|
| II. *Alteration in comfort related to back pain, flushing, chest tightness* | II. A. Occurs in 13.8% of pts and is mild to moderate<br>B. The syndrome resolves with cessation of the infusion, and does not usually recur when the infusion is resumed at a slower infusion rate | II. A. Pt will report comfort throughout infusion | II. A. Infuse drug at prescribed rate (over 60 mins); assess for, and teach pt to report, back pain, flushing, and chest tightness<br>B. Stop infusion if any of the above occur; resume infusion at a slower rate once symptoms subside |
| III. *Potential for alteration in skin integrity related to alopecia, changes in skin* | III. A. Mild alopecia occurs in 6% of pts and moderate alopecia in 2% of pts | III. A. Pt's skin will remain intact | III. A. Teach pt about small chance of hair loss, and measures to cope with it, should it occur<br>B. Teach pt that hair loss is uncommon |
| IV. *Potential for alteration in nutrition, less than body requirements, related to nausea and vomiting, anorexia, diarrhea* | IV. A. Mild nausea occurs in 35% of pts, moderate nausea in 16% of pts, and severe nausea in 3% of pts<br>B. Vomiting is less common<br>C. Anorexia may occur (21%) or increased appetite may occur in < 5% of pts<br>D. Diarrhea occurs in 38% of pts. Other GI problems, occurring < 5% of the time, are dysphagia, gastritis, hemorrhoids, hepatomegaly, dry mouth, and tooth caries | IV. A. Pt will be without nausea or vomiting<br>B. Nausea and vomiting, should they occur, will be minimal<br>C. Pt's weight will remain within 5% of baseline | IV. A. Premedicate with antiemetics. Encourage small, frequent feedings of cool, bland foods<br>B. If pt has anorexia, teach patient or caregiver to make foods ahead of time, use spices, and encourage weekly weights<br>C. Encourage pt to report diarrhea, and to use self-management strategies (medications as ordered, diet modifications)<br>D. Instruct patient to report other GI symptoms |

DAUNORUBICIN CITRATE LIPOSOME INJECTION **289**

V. *Potential for alteration in cardiac output related to cardiac changes*

V. A. Daunorubicin may cause cardiotoxicity and CHF, but studies with liposomal daunorubicin show rare clinical cardiotoxicity at cumulative doses > 600 mg/m$^2$

V. A. Pt will maintain baseline cardiac function

V. A. Assess cardiac status prior to chemotherapy administration (esp. in patients with preexisting cardiac disease or prior anthracycline treatment). Tests may include s/s CHF, quality, regularity and rate of heartbeat, results of prior tests of left ventricular ejection fraction (LVEF) or echocardiogram, if performed

B. Instruct pt to report dyspnea, palpitations, swelling in extremities

C. Maintain accurate records of total dose, and expect GBPS to be repeated periodically during treatment

D. Testing of cardiac function should be performed at cumulative doses of 320 mg/m$^2$, 480 mg/m$^2$, and every 240 mg/m$^2$ thereafter

# Dexrazoxane for injection
(Zinecard)

*Class:* Cardioprotector

## MECHANISM OF ACTION

Enters easily through cell membranes, but the exact mechanism of cardiac cell protection is unclear. A possible mechanism is that the drug becomes a chelating agent within the cell and interferes with iron-mediated free-radical formation that otherwise would cause cardiotoxicity from anthracyclines. Drug is a derivative of edetic acid (EDTA).

## METABOLISM

42% of the dose is excreted in the urine. No plasma protein binding of drug.

## DOSAGE/RANGE

10:1 ratio of dexrazoxane to doxorubicin (i.e., 500 mg/m$^2$ of dexrazoxane to 50 mg/m$^2$ of doxorubicin)

## DRUG PREPARATION

Available in 250- or 500-mg vials.

Reconstitute drug with provided diluent.

Drug may be further diluted in 0.9% sodium choride or 5% dextrose to a concentration of 1.3–5 mg/ml.

Stable 6 hours at room temperature or refrigerated.

## DRUG ADMINISTRATION

Give slow IV push or IVB < 30 minutes prior to beginning doxorubicin.

## SPECIAL CONSIDERATIONS

Drug is indicated for reduction of the incidence and severity of cardiomyopathy associated with doxorubicin in women with metastatic breast cancer who have received a cumulative doxorubicin dose of 300 mg/m$^2$ and who would benefit from continuing doxorubicin.

Drug may reduce the response from 5-FU, doxorubicin, cyclophosphamide (FAC) chemotherapy when given concurrently on the first cycle of therapy (48% response rate versus 63% without the drug, and shorter time to disease progression).

## Dexrazoxane for injection

| Nursing Diagnosis | Defining Characteristics | Expected Outcomes | Nursing Interventions |
|---|---|---|---|
| I. *Potential for injury related to bone marrow depression* | I. Drug may increase doxorubicin-induced bone marrow depression | I. Pt will be without s/s of infection or bleeding | I. A. Monitor WBC, hematocrit/hemoglobin, and platelets prior to each dose<br>B. Instruct pt in self-assessment for s/s of infection and bleeding, and how and when to report changes<br>C. Teach pt self-care measure to minimize risk<br>D. Refer to sec. on bone marrow depression, Chapter 4 |
| II. *Potential alteration in metabolism related to hepatic and renal alterations* | II. A. Possible elevations in liver and renal function studies may occur<br>B. Incidence did not differ from pts who received same chemotherapy without the protector | II. A. Liver and renal function tests will remain within normal limits | II. A. Assess hepatic and renal function tests (bili, BUN, creatinine, and alk phos) at baseline and prior to each treatment. Notify physician of any abnormalities |
| III. *Alteration in comfort related to pain at injection site* | III. Pain at the injection site may occur | III. Pt will report comfort throughout infusion | III. A. Assess site during and after infusion<br>B. Instruct pt to notify nurse if discomfort occurs<br>C. Apply local measures to reduce discomfort |

# Dihydro-5-Azacytidine
(DHAC)

*Class:* Antimetabolite (investigational)

## MECHANISM OF ACTION

Decreases synthesis of methylated bases into RNA and proteins by inhibiting methylation of ribosomal. and transfer RNA. Is cell cycle–specific.

## METABOLISM

Extensively metabolized by plasma enzymes

## DOSAGE/RANGE

1500 mg/m$^2$ in a 5-day continuous infusion. Cycle repeats every 21 days.

## DRUG PREPARATION

Reconstitute the 500-mg vial with 9.6 ml of sterile water for injection. Further dilute in D$_5$W, NS, or lactated Ringer's (stable for 48 hours as a diluted solution).

## DRUG ADMINISTRATION

By continuous infusion over 5 days

## SPECIAL CONSIDERATIONS

Patient should be monitored for signs and symptoms of supraventricular tachycardia.

# Dihydro-5-Azacytidine

| Nursing Diagnosis | Defining Characteristics | Expected Outcomes | Nursing Interventions |
|---|---|---|---|
| I. *Potential impaired gas exchange and alteration in comfort* | I. A. Pleurisy has been the dose-limiting toxic effect of DHAC, often accompanied by significant chest pain | I. A. Pt will report breathing pattern/comfort within normal range | I. A. Encourage pt to report discomfort in chest during respiratory cycle<br>B. Administer pain medications as needed (may require morphine)<br>C. Refer to sec. on pulmonary toxicity, Chapter 4 |
| II. *Potential alteration in cardiac output* | II. A. Supraventricular tachycardia and pericardial effusion have been noted with administration of drug | II. A. Pericardial tamponade will be detected early<br>B. Vital signs will remain within normal range | II. A. Monitor vital signs frequently; check for pulsus paradoxus<br>B. Refer to sec. on cardiotoxicity, Chapter 4 |
| III. *Potential alteration in nutrition, less than body requirements* | III. A. Nausea and vomiting moderate and occasionally severe; lasts the duration of treatment<br>B. Stomatitis | III. A. 1. Pt will be without nausea and vomiting<br>2. Nausea and vomiting, if they occur, will be minimal<br>3. Pt will maintain baseline weight ± 5%<br>B. Oral mucous membrane will remain intact and without infection | III. A. 1. Premedicate with antiemetics and continue prophylactically × 24 hrs to prevent nausea and vomiting<br>2. Encourage small, frequent feedings of cool, bland foods and liquids<br>3. Refer to sec. on nausea and vomiting, Chapter 4<br>B. 1. Teach pt oral assessment<br>2. Encourage pt to report early signs of stomatitis<br>3. See sec. on stomatitis/mucositis, Chapter 4 |

# Docetaxel
## (Taxotere)

*Class:* Taxoid, mitotic spindle poison

## MECHANISM OF ACTION

Enhances microtubule assembly and inhibits tubulin depolymerization, thus arresting cell division in metaphase. Cell cycle specific for M-phase.

## METABOLISM

Drug is extensively protein-bound (94–97%). Triphasic elimination when infused over 1–2 hours. Metabolism appears to involve P-450 3A (CYP3A4) isoenzyme system (in vitro testing). Fecal elimination is main route, accounting for excretion of 75% of the drug within 7 days; 80% of the fecal excretion occurred during the first 48 hours. Mild to moderate liver impairment (SGOT+/or SGPT > 1.5 times normal and alk phos > 2.5 times normal) results in delayed metabolism of drug by 27%, resulting in a 38% increase in systemic exposure (AUC).

## DOSAGE/RANGE

Breast cancer: 60–100 mg/m$^2$ IV as a 1-hour infusion 3 weeks

Non-small-cell-lung-cancer: 75 mg/m$^2$ as a 1-hour infusion every 3 weeks

Premedication regime with corticosteroids: e.g., dexamethasone 8 mg bid × 3 days, starting 1 day prior to docetaxel to reduce risk of fluid retention and hypersensitivity reactions.

## DRUG PREPARATION

Vials available as 80 mg/2 ml (40 mg/ml) and 20 mg/0.5 ml, also (40 mg/ml) single-dose vials in blister packs with diluent.

Unopened vials require refrigeration and protection from bright light. Allow to stand at room temperature for 5 minutes prior to reconstitution.

Reconstitute 20-mg and 80-mg vials with accompanying diluent (13% ethanol in water for injection).

Use only glass or polypropylene or polyolefin plastic (bag) IV containers.

Withdraw ordered dose, and further dilute in 250 ml of 5% dextrose or 0.9% sodium Chloride for a final concentration of 0.3–0.9 mg/ml. If the dose exceeds 240 mg of docetaxel, use a larger volume of diluent to achieve a final concentration of < 0.9 mg/ml.

Inspect for any particulate matter or discoloration, and, if found, discard.

Reconstituted vials (premix solution) stable for 8 hours at either room temperature or refrigeration.

## DRUG ADMINISTRATION

Assess patient's ANC, and treat only if ANC > 1500/mm$^3$; assess liver function studies and if abnormality, discuss with physician. See Special Considerations.

Use only glass or polypropylene bottles, or polypropylene or polyolefin plastic bags for drug infusion, and administer infusion ONLY through polyethylene-lined administration sets.

Patient should receive corticosteroid premedication (e.g., dexamethasone 8 mg bid) for 3 days beginning 1 day before drug administration to reduce the incidence and severity of fluid retention and hypersensitivity reactions. Administer drug infusion over 1 hour.

## SPECIAL CONSIDERATIONS

- Indicated for the treatment of 1) locally advanced or metastatic breast cancer after failure of prior chemotherapy, and 2) locally advanced or metastatic non-small-cell lung cancer (NSCLC) after failure of prior platinum-based chemotherapy.

- Contraindicated in patients with history of severe hypersensitivity reactions to docetaxel or to other drugs formulated with polysorbate 80; drug should not be used in patients with neutrophil counts of < 1500 cells/mm$^3$; Drug should not be used in pregnant or breast-feeding women; women of child-bearing age should use effective birth control measures.

- Radiosensitizing effect

- Theoretically, CYP3A4 inhibitors such as ketoconazole, erythromycin, troleandomycin, cyclosporine, terfenadine, and nifedipine can inhibit docetaxel metabolism and result in elevated serum levels of docetaxel; use together with caution or not at all.

- Theoretically, CYP3A4 inducers, such as anticonvulsants and St. John's Wort, may increase metabolism, and decrease serum levels of docetaxel.

- Docetaxel generally should not be administered to patients with bilirubin > upper limit of normal (ULN) or to patients with SGOT and/or SGPT > 1.5 × ULN concomitant with alkaline phosphatase > 2.5 × ULN. Patients treated with elevated bilirubin or abnormal transaminases plus alkaline phosphatase have an increased risk of grade 4 neutropenia, febrile neutropenia, severe stomatitis, infections, severe thrombocytopenia, severe skin toxicity, and toxic death. Serum bilirubin, SGOT or SGPT, and alkaline phosphatase should be obtained and reviewed by the treating physician before each cycle of docetaxel treatment.

- Dose modifications during treatment: 1) Patients with breast cancer dosed initially at 100 mg/m$^2$ who experience either febrile neutropenia, ANC < 500/mm$^3$ for > 1 week, or severe or cumulative cutaneous reactions, should have dose reduced to 75 mg/m$^2$. If reactions continue at the reduced dose, further reduce to 55 mg/m$^2$ or discontinue drug. Patients dosed initially at 60 mg/m$^2$ who do not experience febrile neutropenia. ANC < 500/mm$^3$ for > 1 week, severe cutaneous reactions, or severe peripheral neuropathy during drug therapy may tolerate higher drug doses and may be dose-escalated. Patients who develop > grade 3 peripheral neuropathy should have drug discontinued; 2) Patients with NSCLC dosed initially at 75 mg/m$^2$ who experience either febrile neutropenia, ANC < 500 mg/m$^2$ for > 1 week, severe or cumulative cutaneous reactions, or other non-hematologic toxicity grades 3 or 4 should have treatment withheld until toxicity resolves, and then have dose reduced to 55 mg/m$^2$; patients who develop > grade 3 peripheral neuropathy should discontinue docetaxel chemotherapy.

- Patients should receive 3-day dexamethasone premedication.

## Docetaxel
*(continued)*

Administration of docetaxel in Europe is not subject to United States Federal Drug Administration recommendations—non-PVC containers and tubing are not required.

Incomplete cross-resistance between paclitaxel and docetaxel in many tumor types.

Studies ongoing to determine effectiveness of docetaxel 30–45 mg/m$^2$ weekly in metastatic breast cancer, as drug given in this fashion may act as antiangiogenesis agent, and also provides "dose-dense" therapy, which provides less opportunity for malignant cells to develop resistant clones. Weekly dose schedules being studied are 3 weeks of treatment, one week off or 6 weeks of treatment, and 2 weeks off, with drug being administered as a 30-minute infusion. Most common side effects when drug is given this way are asthenia, anemia, fluid retention, nail toxicity, and hyperlacrimation. Corticosteroid premedication is often dexamethasone 4 or 8 mg po q 12 hours × 3 doses beginning day before treatment.

# Docetaxel

| Nursing Diagnosis | Defining Characteristics | Expected Outcomes | Nursing Interventions |
|---|---|---|---|
| I. *Infection and bleeding related to bone marrow depression* | I. A. Neutropenia is dose-limiting toxicity<br>B. Thrombocytopenia is less frequent | I. A. 1. Pt will be without s/s of infection and bleeding<br>2. Early s/s of infection or bleeding will be identified | I. A. Monitor WBC, platelet count prior to drug administration and periodically after treatment<br>B. Monitor pt for s/s of infection or bleeding and teach pt self-assessment and how to seek medical advice/care<br>C. Drug dose should be reduced or held for low blood values<br>D. Refer to sec. on bone marrow depression, Chapter 4 |
| II. *Potential for injury related to hypersensitivity reactions* | II. A. Hypersensitivity reactions usually occur with initial treatment, if at all | II. A. Early s/s of hyper-sensitivity reactions will be identified | II. A. Review standing orders for management of hyper-sensitivity reactions and identify location of anaphylaxis kit containing epinephrine 1:1000, hydrocortisone sodium succinate (SoluCortef), diphenhydramine HCl (Benadryl), Aminophylline, and other medications<br>B. Prior to drug administration, obtain baseline vital signs and record mental status assessment<br>  1. Premedicate with diphenhydramine and dexamethasone as ordered<br>  2. Assess pt for at least 30 mins after the drug is given for s/s of a reaction<br>  3. Teach pt to report any hypersensitivity reactions or unusual symptoms |

*(continued)*

## Docetaxel (continued)

| Nursing Diagnosis | Defining Characteristics | Expected Outcomes | Nursing Interventions |
|---|---|---|---|
| | | | C. Observe for the following s/s during infusion, usually occurring within first 15 mins of start of infusion: |
| | | | 1. *Subjective* |
| | | |   a. generalized itching |
| | | |   b. nausea |
| | | |   c. chest tightness |
| | | |   d. crampy abdominal pain |
| | | |   e. difficulty speaking |
| | | |   f. anxiety |
| | | |   g. agitation |
| | | |   h. sense of impending doom |
| | | |   i. uneasiness |
| | | |   j. desire to urinate or defecate |
| | | |   k. dizziness |
| | | |   l. chills |
| | | | 2. *Objective* |
| | | |   a. flushed appearance (angioedema of face, lips, neck, eyelids, hands) |
| | | |   b. localized or generalized urticaria |
| | | |   c. respiratory distress ± wheezing |
| | | |   d. hypotension |
| | | |   e. cyanosis |
| | | | D. If reaction occurs, stop infusion and notify MD |
| | | | E. Place pt in supine position to promote perfusion of visceral organs |
| | | | F. Monitor vital signs until stable |
| | | | G. Provide emotional support to patient and family |
| | | | H. Maintain pt airway and have equipment for CPR close by |
| | | | I. Document incident and pt response to treatment |

J. Discuss with MD desensitization and increased premedication for future treatments

III. *Potential impairment of skin integrity related to*

A. Rash

III. A. Maculopapular, violaceous rash may occur

III. A. Pt will verbally report skin rash and describe self-care measures

III. A. 1. Assess skin for any cutaneous changes, such as rash, and any associated symptoms, such as pruritis; discuss with MD
2. Instruct patient in self-care measures
  a. Avoiding abrasive skin products, clothing
  b. Avoiding tight-fitting clothing
  c. Use of skin emollients appropriate for skin alteration
  d. Measures to avoid scratching involved areas

B. Alopecia

B. Alopecia may occur

B. Pt will verbalize feelings re hair loss and strategies to cope with change in body image

B. 1. Discuss potential impact of hair loss prior to drug administration, coping strategies, and plan to minimize body image distortion (e.g., wig, scarf, cap)
2. Assess pt for s/s of hair loss
3. Assess pts response and use of coping strategies
4. Refer to sec. on alopecia, Chapter 4

IV. *Potential alterations in fluid and electrolyte balance*

A. Peripheral edema and pleural effusions may occur

A. Edema or effusions will be identified early

IV. A. Assess baseline skin turgor, especially extremities
B. Assess respiratory status, including breath sounds
C. Teach pt to report any alterations in breathing patterns
D. Discuss abnormal findings with MD

# Doxorubicin hydrochloride
## (Adriamycin, Rubex)

*Class:* Anthracycline antibiotic isolated from streptomycin products, in particular from the rhodomycin products

## MECHANISM OF ACTION

Antitumor antibiotic—no clearly defined mechanism. Binds directly to DNA base pairs (intercalates) and inhibits DNA and DNA-dependent RNA synthesis, as well as protein synthesis. Cell cycle–specific for S phase.

## METABOLISM

Excretion of drug predominates in the liver; renal clearance is minor. Drug excreted through urine and may discolor urine 1–48 hours after administration.

## DOSAGE/RANGE

30–75 mg/m$^2$ IV every 3–4 weeks

20–45 mg/m$^2$ IV for 3 consecutive days

For bladder instillation: 3–60 mg/m$^2$

For intraperitoneal instillation: 40 mg in 2 liters dialysate (no heparin)

Continuous infusion: varies with individual protocol

## DRUG PREPARATION

Drug will form a precipitate if mixed with heparin or 5-fluorouracil. Dilute with sodium chloride (preservative-free) to produce 2 mg/ml concentration.

## DRUG ADMINISTRATION

Give IV push through the sidearm of a freely flowing IV or as a bolus over 1–2 hours or as a continuous infusion over 24 hours. Must be given via a central line if given via bolus or continuous infusion, as drug is a potent vesicant.

## SPECIAL CONSIDERATIONS

Drug is a potent vesicant. Give through running IV to avoid extravasation and tissue necrosis.

Give through central line if drug is to be given by continuous infusion.

Causes discoloration of urine (from pink to red) for up to 48 hours.

Skin changes: may cause "recall phenomenon"—recalls reaction to previously irradiated tissue.

Cardiac toxicity: dose limit at 550 mg/m$^2$. Patients may exhibit irreversible CHF. May see acute toxicity in hours or days after administration. This is unrelated to cumulative dose and may manifest symptoms of pump or conduction function. Rarely, transient EKG abnormalities, CHF, pericardial effusions (whole syndrome referred to as myocarditis-pericarditis syndrome) may occur, which may lead to demise of patient.

Vein discoloration.

Increased pigmentation in black patients.

When given with barbiturates, there is increased plasma clearance of doxorubicin.

When given with cyclophosphamide, there is risk of hemorrhage and cardiotoxicity.

When given with mitomycin, there is increased risk of cardiotoxicity.

There is decreased oral bioavailability of digoxin when given together.

When given with mercaptopurine, there is increased risk of hepatotoxicity.

Abnormalities in liver function require dose modification.

# Doxorubicin hydrochloride

| Nursing Diagnosis | Defining Characteristics | Expected Outcomes | Nursing Interventions |
|---|---|---|---|
| I. Potential for infection and bleeding related to bone marrow depression | I. A. Nadir 10–14 days, with recovery 15–21 days<br>B. Myelosuppression may be severe; overall incidence 60–80%, less common with weekly dosing | I. A. Pt will be without s/s of infection or bleeding<br>B. Early s/s of infection or bleeding will be identified | I. A. 1. Monitor CBC, platelet count prior to drug administration, as well as s/s of infection and bleeding<br>2. Instruct pt in self-assessment of s/s of infection and bleeding<br>3. Dose reduction may be necessary; discuss with MD<br>4. Transfuse with red cells and platelets per MD order<br>5. Administer growth factors as ordered<br>6. Refer to sec. on bone marrow depression, Chapter 4 |
| II. Potential for alteration in nutrition, less than body requirements<br><br>A. Nausea and vomiting | II. A. 1. Moderate to severe; 50% incidence as single agent, with increased incidence in combination with Cytoxan<br>2. Onset 1–3 hrs after drug administration, lasting up to 24 hrs | II. A. 1. Pt will be without nausea and vomiting<br>2. Nausea and vomiting, if they occur, will be minimal | II. A. 1. Premedicate with antiemetics and continue prophylactically × 24 hrs to prevent nausea and vomiting, at least first treatment<br>2. Encourage small, frequent feedings of cool, bland foods and liquids<br>3. Refer to sec. on nausea and vomiting, Chapter 4 |
| B. Anorexia | B. Occurs frequently | B. Pt will maintain baseline weight ± 5% | B. 1. Encourage small, frequent feedings of favorite foods, especially high-calorie, high-protein foods<br>2. Encourage use of spices<br>3. Weekly weights |

*(continued)*

## Doxorubicin hydrochloride (continued)

| Nursing Diagnosis | Defining Characteristics | Expected Outcomes | Nursing Interventions |
|---|---|---|---|
| C. Stomatitis | C. 10% incidence esophagitis | C. Oral mucous membrane will remain intact and without infection | C. 1. Teach pt oral assessment<br>2. Encourage pt to report early signs of stomatitis<br>3. See sec. on stomatitis, mucositis, Chapter 4 |
| III. *Potential for alteration in cardiac output* | III. A. Acute: pericarditis-myocarditis syndrome with nonspecific EKG changes (flat T waves, ST, PVCs) during infusion or immediately after (non-life threatening)<br>B. Cumulative dose cardiomyopathy: risk if dose > 550 mg/m² or > 450 mg/m² when receiving chest XRT or Cytoxan | III. A. Early s/s of cardiomyopathy will be identified | III. A. If pt is receiving cyclophosphamide in addition to doxorubicin, assess for s/s of cardiomyopathy<br>B. Cardiac evaluation on a regular basis<br>C. Discuss gated blood pool scans with MD, baseline and periodically<br>D. Assess pts baseline cardiac function prior to beginning chemotherapy<br>E. Assess quality and regularity of heartbeat<br>F. Instruct pt to report dyspnea, shortness of breath<br>G. See sec. on cardiotoxicity, Chapter 4 |

IV. *Potential for sexual dysfunction*

  A. Drug is teratogenic and mutagenic

IV. A. Pt and significant other will understand need for contraception

  B. Pt and significant other will identify strategies to cope with sexual dysfunction

IV. A. As appropriate, explore with pt and significant other reproductive and sexuality pattern and impact chemotherapy will have

  B. Discuss strategies to preserve sexuality and reproductive health

  C. See sec. on gonadal dysfunction, Chapter 4

V. *Alteration in skin integrity*

  A. Alopecia

    A. Complete hair loss with 60–75 mg/m$^2$ dosing
    1. Occurs 2–5 weeks after therapy begins
    2. Regrowth usually begins a few months after drug is stopped

V. A. Pt will verbalize feelings re hair loss and identify strategies to cope with change in body image

V. A. 1. Assess pt for s/s of hair loss
  2. Discuss with pt impact of hair loss and strategies to minimize distress (e.g., wig, scarf, cap)
  3. See sec. on alopecia, Chapter 4

  B. Changes in nails and skin, radiation recall reaction, flare reaction

    B. 1. Nail beds and dermal creases (especially in black patients) become hyperpigmented
    2. Reactivation of the erythema and skin damage of prior sites of skin irradiation
    3. Erythematous streaking along vein during drug administration, often with urticaria and pruritis; this condition is self-limiting, usually within 30 mins with or without use of antihistamines

  B. Pt will verbalize feelings re changes in nail or skin color or texture and identify strategies to cope with change in body image

  B. 1. Assess pt for changes in skin and nails
  2. Discuss with pt impact of changes and strategies to minimize distress (e.g., wearing nail polish or long sleeves)

*(continued)*

## Doxorubicin hydrochloride (continued)

| Nursing Diagnosis | Defining Characteristics | Expected Outcomes | Nursing Interventions |
|---|---|---|---|
| C. Extravasation | C. Avoid extravasation, as tissue necrosis may occur | C. 1. Extravasation, if it occurs, will be detected early, with early intervention<br>2. Skin and underlying tissue damage will be minimized | C. 1. Careful technique is used during venipuncture; see sec. on intravenous administration, Chapter 10<br>2. Administer vesicant through freely flowing IV, constantly monitoring IV site and patient response<br>3. Nurse should be *thoroughly* familiar with institutional policy and procedure for administration of a vesicant agent<br>4. If vesicant drug is administered as a continuous infusion, drug must be given through a patent central line<br>5. If extravasation is suspected:<br>a. Stop drug being administered<br>b. Aspirate any residual drug and blood from IV tubing, IV catheter/needle, and IV site if possible<br>c. *If antidote exists,* instill antidote into area of apparent infiltration as per MD order and institutional policy and procedure<br>d. Apply cold or topical medication as per MD order and institutional policy and procedure |

2. Assess site regularly for pain, progression of erythema, induration, and evidence of necrosis
3. When in doubt about whether drug is infiltrating, *treat as an infiltration*
4. Teach pt to assess site and notify MD if condition worsens
5. Arrange next clinic visit for assessment of site depending on drug, amount infiltrated, extent of potential injury, and patient variables
6. Document in pts record as per institutional policy and procedure; see sec. on reactions, Chapter 9

# Epirubicin hydrochloride
(Farmorubicin(e), Farmorubicina, Pharmorubicin, Ellence)

*Class:* Antitumor Antibiotic

## MECHANISM OF ACTION

Antitumor antibiotic—no clearly defined mechanism. Binds directly to DNA base pairs (intercalates) and inhibits DNA and DNA-dependent RNA synthesis, as well as protein synthesis. Cell cycle specific for S phase.

## METABOLISM

Rapidly and extensively bound to plasma proteins and distributed into body tissues, undergoes metabolism in the liver, and is predominantly excreted in the bile.

## DOSAGE/RANGE

60–90 mg/m$^2$ as a single dose q 3 weeks: dose may be divided over 2–3 days

120 mg/m$^2$ every 3 weeks, or 45 mg/m$^2$ for 3 consecutive days every 3 weeks

20 mg as a single weekly dose.

Intravesicle: 50 mg weekly as a 0.1% solution for 8 weeks; reduce dose for chemical cystitis.

## DRUG PREPARATION

Dilute in NS or sterile water for injection.

## DRUG ADMINISTRATION

Give IVP through a free-flowing line of NS or D5W over 3–5 minutes, or by bolus over 30 minutes.

## SPECIAL CONSIDERATIONS

Dose reduce with liver dysfunction, bone marrow compromise, or when given with other antineoplastics.

Do not exceed total cumulative dose of 0.9–1 gram/m$^2$ because of risk of cardiotoxicity. Cardiac toxicity may occur at lower cumulative doses, whether or not cardiac risk factors are present.

May cause severe myelosuppression.

Has caused secondary leukemia in a small number of patients.

Drug is a potent vesicant. Give through a running IV to avoid extravasation and tissue necrosis.

Skin changes: may cause "recall phenomenon"—recalls reaction to previously irradiated tissue.

Causes discoloration of urine (from pink to red color) for up to 48 hours.

## Epirubicin hydrochloride

| Nursing Diagnosis | Defining Characteristics | Expected Outcomes | Nursing Interventions |
|---|---|---|---|
| I. *Potential for infection and bleeding related to bone marrow depression* | I. A. Nadir 10–14 days, with recovery 15–21 days<br>B. Myelosuppression may be severe; overall incidence 60–80% | I. A. Pt will be without s/s of infection or bleeding<br>B. Early s/s of infection or bleeding will be identified | I. A. 1. Monitor CBC, platelet count prior to drug administration, as well as s/s of infection and bleeding<br>2. Instruct pt in self-assessment of s/s of infection and bleeding<br>3. Dose reduction may be necessary; discuss with MD<br>4. Transfuse with red cells and platelets per MD order<br>5. Refer to sec. on bone marrow depression, Chapter 4 |
| II. *Potential for alteration in nutrition, less than body requirements*<br>A. Nausea and vomiting | II. A. 1. Moderate to severe; 50% incidence as single agent, with increased incidence in combination with Cytoxan<br>2. Onset 1–3 hrs after drug administration, lasting up to 24 hrs | II. A. 1. Pt will be without nausea and vomiting<br>2. Nausea and vomiting, if they occur, will be minimal | II. A. 1. Premedicate with antiemetics and continue prophylactically × 24 hrs to prevent nausea and vomiting, at least first treatment<br>2. Encourage small, frequent feedings of cool, bland foods and liquids<br>3. Refer to sec. on nausea and vomiting, Chapter 4 |

*(continued)*

## Epirubicin hydrochloride (continued)

| Nursing Diagnosis | Defining Characteristics | Expected Outcomes | Nursing Interventions |
|---|---|---|---|
| B. Anorexia | B. Occurs frequently | B. Pt will maintain baseline weight ± 5% | B. 1. Encourage small, frequent feedings of favorite foods, especially high-calorie, high-protein foods<br>2. Encourage use of spices<br>3. Weekly weights |
| C. Stomatitis | C. 10% incidence esophagitis | C. Oral mucous membrane will remain intact and without infection | C. 1. Teach pt oral assessment<br>2. Encourage pt to report early signs of stomatitis<br>3. See sec. on stomatitis, mucositis, Chapter 4 |
| III. *Potential for alteration in cardiac output* | III. A. Acute: pericarditis-myocarditis syndrome with nonspecific EKG changes (flat T waves, ST, PVCs) during infusion or immediately after (non–life threatening)<br>B. Cumulative dose cardiomyopathy: risk if dose > 1 gm/m²<br>C. Cardiotoxicity and myelotoxicity may be less than with doxorubicin, but is more likely when the cumulative dose exceeds 0.9 to 1 gm/m² body surface area | III. A. Early s/s of cardiomyopathy will be identified | III. A. If pt is receiving cyclophosphamide in addition to doxorubicin, assess for s/s of cardiomyopathy<br>B. Cardiac evaluation on a regular basis<br>C. Discuss gated blood pool scans with MD, baseline and periodically<br>D. Assess pts baseline cardiac function prior to beginning chemotherapy<br>E. Assess quality and regularity of heartbeat<br>F. Instruct pt to report dyspnea, shortness of breath<br>G. See sec. on cardiotoxicity, Chapter 4 |

| Nursing Diagnosis | Defining Characteristics | Expected Outcomes | Nursing Interventions |
|---|---|---|---|
| IV. *Potential for sexual dysfunction* | IV. A. Drug is teratogenic and mutagenic | A. Pt and significant other will understand need for contraception<br>B. Pt and significant other will identify strategies to cope with sexual dysfunction | IV. A. As appropriate, explore with pt and significant other reproductive and sexuality pattern and impact chemotherapy will have<br>B. Discuss strategies to preserve sexuality and reproductive health<br>C. See sec. on gonadal dysfunction, Chapter 4 |
| V. *Alteration in skin integrity*<br>A. Alopecia | V. A. Complete hair loss<br>1. Occurs 2–5 weeks after therapy begins<br>2. Regrowth usually begins a few months after drug is stopped | V. A. Pt will verbalize feelings re hair loss and identify strategies to cope with change in body image | V. A. 1. Assess pt for s/s of hair loss<br>2. Discuss with pt impact of hair loss and strategies to minimize distress (e.g., wig, scarf, cap)<br>3. See sec. on alopecia, Chapter 4 |
| B. Flare reaction | B. 1. Reactivation of the erythema and skin damage of prior sites of skin irradiation<br>2. Erythematous streaking along vein during drug administration, often with urticaria and pruritis; this condition is self-limiting, usually within 30 mins with or without use of antihistamines | B. Skin changes will be identified early | B. 1. Assess patient for changes in skin and nails<br>2. Slow infusion if facial flushing and/or local erythematous streaking along a vein occur |

*(continued)*

## Epirubicin hydrochloride (continued)

| Nursing Diagnosis | Defining Characteristics | Expected Outcomes | Nursing Interventions |
|---|---|---|---|
| C. Extravasation | C. Avoid extravasation, as tissue necrosis may occur | C. 1 Extravasation, if it occurs, will be detected early, with early intervention<br>2. Skin and underlying tissue damage will be minimized | C. 1. Careful technique is used during venipuncture; see sec. on intravenous administration, Chapter 10<br>2. Administer vesicant through freely flowing IV, constantly monitoring IV site and patient response<br>3. Nurse should be *thoroughly* familiar with institutional policy and procedure for administration of a vesicant agent<br>4. If vesicant drug is administered as a continuous infusion, drug must be given through a patent central line<br>5. If extravasation is suspected:<br>  a. Stop drug being administered<br>  b. Aspirate any residual drug and blood from IV tubing, IV catheter/needle, and IV site if possible<br>  c. If antidote exists, instill antidote into area of apparent infiltration as per MD order and institutional policy and procedure<br>  d. Apply cold or topical medication as per MD order and institutional policy and procedure<br>6. Assess site regularly for pain, progression of erythema, induration, and evidence of necrosis |

7. When in doubt about whether drug is infiltrating, treat as an infiltration

8. Teach pt to assess site and notify MD if condition worsens

9. Arrange next clinic visit for assessment of site depending on drug, amount infiltrated, extent of potential injury, and pt variables

10. Document in pt's record as per institutional policy and procedure; see sec. on reactions, Chapter 9

# Estramustine phosphate
## (Estracyte, Emcyt)

*Class:* Alkylating agent

## MECHANISM OF ACTION

At usual therapeutic concentrations, acts as a weak alkylator. A chemical combination of mechlorethamine and estradiol phosphate, estramustine is believed to selectively enter cells with estrogen receptors, where the drug acts as an alkylating agent due to bis-chlorethyl side-chain and liberated estrogens.

## METABOLISM

Well absorbed orally, metabolized in liver, partly excreted in urine. Induces a marked decline in serum calcium and phosphate levels.

## DOSAGE/RANGE

600 mg/m$^2$ (15 mg/kg) orally daily in 3 divided doses (range 10–16 mg/kg/day in most studies, with evaluation after 30–90 days)

## DRUG PREPARATION

Available in 140-mg capsules

## DRUG ADMINISTRATION

Oral

## SPECIAL CONSIDERATIONS

Administer with food or antacids to decrease gastrointestinal side effects.

IV preparation is a *vesicant;* avoid extravasation.

Transient perineal itching and pain after IV administration.

## Estramustine phosphate

| Nursing Diagnosis | Defining Characteristics | Expected Outcomes | Nursing Interventions |
|---|---|---|---|
| I. *Potential for alteration in nutrition, less than body requirements related to* | | | |
| A. Nausea and vomiting | I. A. Occurs at higher dosing<br>1. Pt may develop tolerance<br>2. Dose may need to be reduced or temporarily stopped for moderate to severe nausea and vomiting<br>3. Delayed (6–8 weeks), and intractable nausea and vomiting may occur, requiring discontinuance of therapy | I. A. 1. Nausea and vomiting will be prevented<br>2. Nausea and vomiting, if they occur, will be minimal | I. A. 1. Premedicate with antiemetic and instruct patient in self-administration of antiemetic, especially for high doses<br>2. Refer to sec. on nausea and vomiting, Chapter 4 |
| B. Diarrhea | B. Occurs occasionally | B. Pt will have minimal diarrhea | B. 1. Encourage pt to report onset of diarrhea<br>2. Administer or teach pt to self-administer antidiarrheal medications<br>3. Teach pt diet modifications<br>4. Refer to sec. on diarrhea, Chapter 4 |
| C. Hepatic dysfunction | C. Mild elevations in liver function studies may occur<br>1. LDH, SGOT especially<br>2. Usually are transient and self-limiting<br>3. Jaundice | C. Hepatic dysfunction will be identified early | C. 1. Monitor SGOT, LDH as well as SGPT, alkaline phosphatase, bilirubin periodically during treatment<br>2. Notify MD of any elevations |
| D. ↓ Ca++ and phosphorous levels | D. Serum Ca++ and phosphorus may decrease related to changes in metabolism of bone | D. Abnormalities in Ca++, phosphorous levels will be identified and corrected | D. Monitor Ca++, phosphorous levels; replace per MD orders |
| II. *Body image disturbance related to gynecomastia* | II. A. Occurs less frequently than with DES<br>B. Nipple tenderness may occur initially | II. A. Pt will verbalize feelings re changes in body image<br>B. Pt will identify strategies to cope with changes in body image | II. A. Instruct pt in potential drug side effect of gynecomastia and breast tenderness<br>B. Encourage pt to verbalize feelings re breast enlargement<br>C. Discuss with pt potential coping strategies to deal with these changes |

*(continued)*

**Estramustine phosphate** (*continued*)

| Nursing Diagnosis | Defining Characteristics | Expected Outcomes | Nursing Interventions |
|---|---|---|---|
| III. *Alteration in cardiac output* | III. A. CHF may occur rarely, possibly related to estrogen property of salt retention | III. A. Early CHF or worsening CHF will be detected | III. A. Drug should be used cautiously in patients with history of congestive heart failure or myocardial infarction<br>B. Assess cardiac function (i.e., heart rate and heart sounds—S3, BP, RR, breath sounds) and symptoms of edema, dyspnea, SOB at each visit<br>C. Instruct pt to report any changes in health (i.e., symptoms of dyspnea, SOB, edema) |
| IV. *Altered tissue perfusion* | IV. A. Circulatory changes may occur—thrombophlebitis, thrombosis | IV. A. Early changes in circulation will be detected | IV. A. Drug should be used cautiously in pts with a history of thrombophlebitis, thrombosis, cerebrovascular or coronary artery disease, other thromboembolic states<br>B. Assess circulatory function (pulses, temperature of extremities, etc.) and for s/s of thrombophlebitis, thrombosis<br>C. Instruct pt to report any changes in health (e.g., coolness of extremities, redness/warmth of extremities, leg cramps)<br>D. Instruct pt to avoid crossing legs |
| V. *Potential for alteration in comfort* | V. A. Perineal symptoms, headache, rash, urticaria may occur<br>B. Transient paresthesias of mouth with IV administration | V. A. Pt will be comfortable | V. A. Assess for occurrence of perineal itching and pain after IV administration and for headaches, rash, urticaria; discuss with MD symptomatic treatment<br>B. Use careful IV administration technique, as drug may cause severe thrombophlebitis |

| | | | |
|---|---|---|---|
| VI. *Potential for infection and bleeding related to bone marrow depression* | VI. A. Approximately 5% of pts experience bone marrow depression | VI. A. Pt will be without infection and bleeding<br>B. Early s/s of infection or bleeding will be identified | VI. A. Monitor CBC and platelet count prior to drug administration<br>B. Assess pt for and teach pt self-assessment for s/s of infection and bleeding<br>C. Transfuse with red cells, platelets per MD order<br>D. Drug dosage should be reduced for lower than normal blood values<br>E. See sec. on bone marrow depression, Chapter 4 |
| VII. *Alteration in skin integrity related to extravasation* | VII. A. Estramustine is a potent vesicant<br>B. Vesicant drugs cause erythema, burning, tissue necrosis, and tissue sloughing if extravasated | VII. A. Extravasation, if it occurs, will be detected early, with early intervention<br>B. Skin and underlying tissue damage will be minimized | VII. A. Careful technique is used during venipuncture. See sec. on intravenous administration, Chapter 10<br>B. Administer vesicant through freely flowing IV, constantly monitoring IV site and patient response<br>C. Nurse should be *thoroughly* familiar with institutional policy and procedure for administration of a vesicant agent<br>D. If vesicant drug is administered as a continuous infusion, drug must be given through a patent central line<br>E. If extravasation is suspected:<br>  1. Stop drug being administered<br>  2. Aspirate any residual drug and blood from IV tubing, IV catheter/needle, and IV site if possible<br>  3. *If antidote exists,* instill antidote into area of apparent infiltration as per MD order and institutional policy and procedure |

*(continued)*

## Estramustine phosphate (continued)

| Nursing Diagnosis | Defining Characteristics | Expected Outcomes | Nursing Interventions |
|---|---|---|---|
| | | | 4. Apply cold or topical medication as per MD order and institutional policy and procedure |
| | | | F. Assess site regularly for pain, progression of erythema, induration, and evidence of necrosis |
| | | | G. When in doubt about whether drug is infiltrating, *treat as an infiltration* |
| | | | H. Teach pt to assess site and notify MD if condition worsens |
| | | | I. Arrange next clinic visit for assessment of site depending on drug, amount infiltrated, extent of potential injury, and pt variables |
| | | | J. Document in pts record as per institutional policy and procedure; see sec. on reactions, Chapter 9 |

# Estrogens
Diethylstilbestrol (DES), Diethylstilbestrol diphosphate (Stilphostrol, Stilbestrol diphosphate), Ethinyl estradiol (Estinyl), Conjugated equine estrogen (Premarin), Chlorotrianisene (Tace)

*Class:* Hormones

## MECHANISM OF ACTION

Unknown. Estrogens change the hormonal milieu of the body.

## METABOLISM

Metabolized mainly in the liver. Undergoes enterohepatic recirculation. DES is metabolized more slowly than natural estrogens.

## DOSAGE/RANGE

DES—prostate cancer: 1–3 mg orally daily; breast cancer: 5 mg orally TID

Diethylstilbestrol diphosphate—prostate cancer: 50–200 orally TID, 0.5–1.0 gm IV daily × 5 days, then 250–1000 mg each week

Chlorotrianisene—1–10 orally TID

Ethinyl estradiol—0.5–1.0 mg orally TID

## DRUG PREPARATION

None

## DRUG ADMINISTRATION

Oral

## SPECIAL CONSIDERATIONS

Long-term dosage of DES in males has been associated with cardiovascular deaths. Maximum dose should be 1 mg TID for prostate cancer.

Can cause inaccurate laboratory results (liver, adrenal, thyroid).

Causes rapid rise in serum calcium in patients with bony metastases; watch for symptoms of hypercalcemia.

## Estrogens

| Nursing Diagnosis | Defining Characteristics | Expected Outcomes | Nursing Interventions |
|---|---|---|---|
| I. *Altered nutrition, less than body requirements related to nausea and vomiting* | I. A. Occurs in 25% of pts on estrogens<br>B. Degree of nausea varies depending on the specific drug and is usually dose dependent<br>C. Nausea tends to decrease after a few weeks of therapy | I. A. Pt will be without nausea or vomiting<br>B. Nausea and vomiting, should they occur, will be minimal | I. A. Inform pt that nausea and vomiting can occur; encourage patient to report nausea or vomiting<br>B. Instruct pt to take estrogens at bedtime to decrease nausea<br>C. Consider starting pt at a low dose and increase dose as tolerated<br>D. Refer to sec. on nausea and vomiting, Chapter 4 |
| II. *Potential for injury related to*<br>A. Sodium and water retention | II. A. 1. May occur<br>2. Estrogens should be used with great caution in pts with underlying cardiac, renal, hepatic disease | II. A. 1. Fluid and electrolyte balance will be maintained | II. A. 1. Identify pt with underlying cardiac, hepatic, and renal disease<br>2. Inform pt of potential for sodium and water retention and s/s to watch for; instruct pt to report s/s to MD<br>3. Assess pt for s/s of fluid overload |
| B. Hypercalcemia | B. 1. Occurs in 5–10% of women with breast cancer metastatic to bone<br>2. Particular risk of hypercalcemia in first 2 weeks of therapy<br>3. Renal disease can aggravate hypercalcemia | B. 1. Serum calcium will remain within normal limits<br>2. Hypercalcemia will be identified and treated early | B. 1. Identify pts at risk and monitor serum calcium closely during the first few weeks of treatment<br>2. Teach pt s/s of hypercalcemia (drowsiness, increased thirst, constipation, increased urine output); instruct patient to notify MD if s/s occur |

| | | | |
|---|---|---|---|
| C. Cardiotoxicity | C. 1. Increased incidence of cardiovascular-associated death, especially in men on high-dose estrogens for prostate cancer<br>2. Effects of digitalis are potentiated by estrogens | C. Cardiotoxicity will be avoided | C. 1. Identify pts at risk for cardiotoxicity<br>2. Inform pts of risk, s/s to report<br>3. Monitor cardiac drug levels; alert cardiologist that pt is on estrogen |
| D. Thromboembolic complications | D. Occurrence infrequent but more common with long-term use and high doses | D. Pt will avoid injury related to abnormal blood clotting | D. 1. Teach pt s/s of thromboemboli (i.e., positive Homan's sign, localized swelling, pain, tenderness, erythema, sudden CNS changes, shortness of breath)<br>2. Instruct pt to notify MD if any of above occur |

III. *Potential for sexual dysfunction related to*

| | | | |
|---|---|---|---|
| A. Gynecomastia, loss of libido, impotence, and voice changes | III. A. 1. May occur in men<br>2. Gynecomastia may be prevented by pretreating each breast with radiation therapy<br>3. Feminine characteristics disappear when therapy is stopped | III. A. 1. Pt and significant other will verbalize understanding of changes in sexuality that may occur<br>2. Pt and significant other will identify strategies to cope with sexual dysfunction | III. A. 1. As appropriate, explore with pt and significant other reproductive and sexuality patterns and impact therapy may have on them<br>2. Discuss strategies to preserve sexuality and reproductive health<br>3. See sec. on gonadal dysfunction, Chapter 4 |
| B. Breast tenderness, engorgement in women | B. Engorgement may occur in postmenopausal women | B. Pt will identify strategies to cope with changes in breast physiology | B. 1. As appropriate, explore with pt and significant other reproductive and sexuality patterns and impact therapy may have on them<br>2. Application of heat for local treatment of breast tenderness |

*(continued)*

## Estrogens (continued)

| Nursing Diagnosis | Defining Characteristics | Expected Outcomes | Nursing Interventions |
|---|---|---|---|
| C. Uterine prolapse, exacerbation of preexisting uterine fibroids with possible uterine bleeding | C. May occur | C. Pt will identify the side effects of treatment | C. 1. Discuss with MD symptomatic management<br>2. Reinforce pt teaching on the action and side effects of estrogen therapy<br>3. Offer emotional support |
| D. Urinary incontinence | D. May occur in women | D. Pt will identify strategies to cope with incontinence | D. 1. Reinforce information on the action and side effects of estrogen therapy<br>2. Offer emotional support<br>3. Offer specific suggestions (pads, Attends, exercises, physical therapy, biofeedback) |

# Etoposide
## (VP-16, Vepesid)

*Class:* Plant alkaloid, a derivative of the mandrake plant (mayapple plant)

## MECHANISM OF ACTION

Inhibits DNA synthesis in S and $G_2$ so that cells do not enter mitosis. Causes single-strand breaks in DNA. Cell cycle specific for S and $G_2$ phases.

## METABOLISM

VP-16 is rapidly excreted in the urine and, to a lesser extent, the bile. About 30% of drug is excreted unchanged. Binds to serum albumin (94%), then becomes extensively tissue bound.

## DOSAGE/RANGE

50–100 mg/m² IV qd × 5 (testicular cancer) q 3–4 weeks

75–200 mg/m² IV qd × 3 (small-cell lung cancer) q 3–4 weeks

Oral dose is twice intravenous dose.

## DRUG PREPARATION

Available in 5 cc (100 mg) vials

Oral capsules available in 50-mg and 100-mg capsules

## DRUG ADMINISTRATION

IV infusion: over 30–60 minutes to minimize risk of hypotension and bronchospasm (wheezing). In some instances, a test dose may be infused slowly (0.5 ml in 50 NS) and the remaining drug infused if no untoward reaction after 5 minutes.

Stability: drug must be diluted with either 5% dextrose injection, USP, or 0.9% sodium chloride solution and is stable 96 hours in glass and 48 hours in plastic containers at room temperature (77°F, 25°C) under normal fluorescent light at a concentration of 0.2 mg/ml.

Inspect for clarity of solution prior to administration.

Oral administration: may give as a single dose if ≤ 400 mg; otherwise divide dose.

## SPECIAL CONSIDERATIONS

Reduce drug dose by 50% if bilirubin > 1.5 mg/dl, by 75% if bilirubin > 3.0 mg/dl.

Synergistic drug effect in combination with cisplatin.

Radiation recall may occur when combined therapies are used.

## Etoposide

| Nursing Diagnosis | Defining Characteristics | Expected Outcomes | Nursing Interventions |
|---|---|---|---|
| I. *Potential for injury during drug administration related to* | | | |
| A. Allergic reaction | I. A. Bronchospasm as evidenced by wheezing may occur; may experience fever, chills | I. A. 1. Bronchospasm will be prevented<br>2. Bronchospasm, if it occurs, will be identified early and terminated | I. A. 1. Infuse drug slowly over at least 30–60 mins<br>2. Discontinue drug and notify MD if bronchospasm occurs; have antihistamines ready (e.g., diphenhydramine) |
| B. Hypotension | B. Hypotension may occur during rapid infusion | B. Hypotension will be prevented | B. 1. Monitor BP prior to drug administration and periodically during infusion, at least during first drug administration<br>2. Infuse drug over *at least* 30–60 mins; slow rate of infusion if BP drops |
| C. Anaphylaxis | C. Anaphylaxis may occur but is rare | C. Anaphylaxis, if it occurs, will be managed successfully | C. 1. Monitor pt closely during infusion<br>2. Review standing orders for management of pt in anaphylaxis and identify location of anaphylaxis kit containing epinephrine 1:1000, hydrocortisone sodium succinate (SoluCortef), diphenhydramine HCL (Benadryl), Aminophylline, and others<br>3. Prior to drug administration, obtain baseline vital signs and record mental status |

4. Observe for following s/s during infusion, usually occurring within first 15 mins of start of infusion
   a. *Subjective*
      (1) generalized itching
      (2) nausea
      (3) chest tightness
      (4) crampy abdominal pain
      (5) difficulty speaking
      (6) anxiety
      (7) agitation
      (8) sense of impending doom
      (9) uneasiness
      (10) desire to urinate or defecate
      (11) dizziness
      (12) chills
   b. *Objective*
      (1) flushed appearance (angioedema of face, neck, eyelids, hands, feet)
      (2) localized or generalized urticaria
      (3) respiratory distress ± wheezing
      (4) hypotension
      (5) cyanosis
5. Stop infusion if reaction occurs and notify MD
6. Place pt in supine position to promote perfusion of visceral organs
7. Monitor vital signs until stable

*(continued)*

# Etoposide (continued)

| Nursing Diagnosis | Defining Characteristics | Expected Outcomes | Nursing Interventions |
|---|---|---|---|
| | | | 8. Provide emotional reassurance to pt and family |
| | | | 9. Maintain patent airway and have CPR equipment ready if needed |
| | | | 10. Document incident |
| | | | 11. Discuss with MD desensitization versus drug discontinuance for further dosing |
| | | | 12. See sec. on reactions, Chapter 9 |
| II. *Potential for infection and bleeding related to bone marrow depression* | II. A. Nadir 7–14 days<br>B. Dose-limiting toxicity<br>C. Granulocytopenia can be severe<br>D. Neutropenia, thrombocytopenia, anemia can all occur<br>E. Recovery 20–22 days | II. A. Pt will be without s/s of infection or bleeding<br>B. Early s/s of infection or bleeding will be identified | II. A. Monitor CBC, platelet count prior to drug administration and at time of expected nadir<br>B. Assess for s/s of infection and bleeding<br>C. Instruct pt in self-assessment of s/s of infection and bleeding<br>D. Dose reduction may be necessary with compromised bone marrow function, low nadir counts, or hepatic dysfunction<br>E. Refer to sec. on bone marrow depression, Chapter 4 |
| III. *Altered nutrition, less than body requirements related to* A. Nausea and vomiting | III. A. 1. Usually mild, occurring soon after infusion<br>2. Intensity and frequency increase with oral dosing and may be severe | III. A. 1. Pt will be without nausea and vomiting<br>2. If nausea and vomiting occur, they will be minimal | III. A. 1. Premedicate with antiemetics and continue prophylactically for at least 4–6 hrs after drug administration, at least first treatment<br>2. Encourage small, frequent feedings of cool, bland foods and liquids<br>3. Refer to sec. on nausea and vomiting, Chapter 4 |

B. Anorexia

B. Usually mild but may be severe with oral dosing

B. Pt will maintain weight within ± 5% baseline

B. 1. Encourage small, frequent feedings of favorite foods, especially high-calorie, high-protein foods
   2. Encourage use of spices
   3. Weekly weights in ambulatory setting

IV. *Body image disturbance related to alopecia*

IV. A. Incidence 20–90% depending on dose; regrowth may occur between drug cycles

IV. A. Pt will verbalize feelings re hair loss and identify strategies to cope with change in body image

IV. A. Discuss with pt anticipated impact of hair loss; suggest wig as appropriate prior to actual hair loss
   B. Explore with pt response to hair loss and strategies used to minimize distress (e.g., wig, scarf, cap)
   C. Refer to sec. on alopecia, Chapter 4

V. *Potential for sexual dysfunction*

V. A. Drug is teratogenic and embryocidal in rats
   B. Drug is mutagenic

V. A. Pt and significant other will understand need for contraception
   B. Pt and significant other will identify strategies to cope with sexual dysfunction

V. A. As appropriate, explore with pt and significant other issues of reproductive and sexual patterns and expected impact chemotherapy will have
   B. Discuss strategies to preserve sexuality and reproductive health (e.g., sperm banking, contraception)
   C. See sec. on gonadal dysfunction, Chapter 4

VI. *Altered skin integrity related to*
A. Radiation recall

VI. A. Radiation sensitizer: may reactivate skin reactions from prior radiation therapy

VI. A. Skin surface will remain intact or heal following injury

VI. A. 1. Assess skin in area of prior XRT when combined therapies are given
   2. If radiation recall results in skin breakdown, drug may need to be withheld until skin healing occurs
   3. Wound management based on type of skin reaction

*(continued)*

## Etoposide (continued)

| Nursing Diagnosis | Defining Characteristics | Expected Outcomes | Nursing Interventions |
|---|---|---|---|
| B. Irritation | B. Perivascular irritation may occur if drug extravasates | B. Skin irritation will be minimal | B. 1. Use careful venipuncture techniques and administer drug over 30–60 mins, diluted as directed by manufacturer<br>2. Refer to sec. on reactions, Chapter 9 |
| VII. *Alteration in cardiac output* | VII. A. Rare<br>B. Myocardial infarction has been reported after prior mediastinal XRT and in pts receiving VP-16-containing combination chemotherapy<br>C. Arrhythmias have been reported but are rare | VII. A. Early cardiac dysfunction will be identified | VII. A. Monitor pt closely during treatment, especially with coexisting cardiac dysfunction<br>B. Notify MD of any abnormalities<br>C. Document any irregular cardiac rhythm on EKG<br>D. Refer to sec. on cardiotoxicity, Chapter 4 |
| VIII. *Sensory/perceptual alterations related to neurological toxicities* | VIII. A. Peripheral neuropathies may occur but are rare and mild | VIII. A. Peripheral neuropathies will be identified early<br>B. Pt will verbalize feelings re discomfort and dysfunction related to neuropathies and will identify alternate coping strategies | VIII. A. Assess motor and sensory function prior to therapy<br>B. Encourage pt to verbalize feelings re discomfort and sensory loss if these occur<br>C. Assist pt to discuss alternative coping strategies<br>D. Refer to sec. on neurotoxicity, Chapter 4 |

# Floxuridine
## (FUDR, 5-FUDR, 5-fluoro-2'-deoxyuridine)

*Class:* Antimetabolite

## MECHANISM OF ACTION

Antimetabolite (fluorinated pyrimidine) that is metabolized to 5-fluorouracil when given by IV bolus or metabolized to 5-FUDR-MP when smaller doses are given by continuous infusion intra-arterially. FUDR-MP is four times more effective in inhibiting the enzyme thymidine synthetase than 5-FU, and this prevents the synthesis of thymidine, an essential component of DNA, resulting in interruption of DNA synthesis and cell death. Other FUDR metabolites inhibit RNA synthesis. Drug is cell cycle–specific, with activity during the S phase.

## METABOLISM

When given IV, drug is transformed to 5-FU; 70–90% of drug is extracted by liver on first pass. Metabolites are excreted by kidneys and lungs. Continuous infusion decreases metabolism of drug, with more of the drug being converted to the active metabolite FUDR-MP.

## DOSAGE/RANGE

Intra-arterially by slow infusion pump: 0.3 mg/kg/day (range 0.1–0.6 mg/kg/day)
   *or*
5–20 mg/m$^2$/day every day $\times$ 14–21 days

## DRUG PREPARATION

Reconstitute 500 mg vial of lyophilized powder with sterile water, then dilute with NS.

## DRUG ADMINISTRATION

Usually administered by slow intra-arterial infusion using a surgically placed catheter or percutaneous catheter in a major artery.

## SPECIAL CONSIDERATIONS

Drug usually given for 14 days, then heparinized saline for 14 days to maintain line patency.

Dose reductions or infusion breaks may be necessary depending on toxicity.

FDA approved for intrahepatic arterial infusion only.

## Floxuridine

| Nursing Diagnosis | Defining Characteristics | Expected Outcomes | Nursing Interventions |
|---|---|---|---|
| I. *Altered nutrition, less than body requirements related to* | | | |
| A. Nausea and vomiting | I. A. Occur infrequently and are mild | I. A. 1. Pt will be without nausea and vomiting<br>2. Nausea and vomiting, if they occur, will be mild | I. A. 1. Premedicate with antiemetics and continue prophylactically as needed<br>2. Instruct pt in self-assessment and self-administration of antiemetics at home<br>3. Encourage small, frequent feedings of cool, bland foods and liquids<br>4. If intractable nausea and vomiting occur, stop drug and infuse heparinized saline; *notify MD*<br>5. Refer to sec. on nausea and vomiting, Chapter 4 |
| B. Anorexia | B. Occurs commonly | B. Pt will maintain baseline weight ± 5% | B. 1. Encourage small, frequent feedings of favorite foods, especially high-calorie, high-protein foods<br>2. Encourage use of spices<br>3. Weekly weights |
| C. Stomatitis/esophagopharyngitis | C. 1. Milder than 5-FU-induced stomatitis when drug is given as hepatic artery infusion<br>2. More severe when administered intracarotid (external) arterial infusion | C. Oral mucous membranes will remain intact and without infection | C. 1. Teach pt oral assessment and mouth care<br>2. Assess oral mucosa prior to and during therapy<br>3. Encourage pt to report early stomatitis<br>4. If stomatitis occurs in pt receiving hepatic artery infusion, stop drug, infuse with heparinized saline, and notify MD<br>5. Refer to sec. on stomatitis, mucositis, Chapter 4 |

| | Defining Characteristics | Expected Outcomes | Nursing Interventions |
|---|---|---|---|
| **D. Diarrhea** | D. Occurs occasionally and is mild to moderately severe | D. Pt will have minimal diarrhea | D. 1. Encourage pt to report onset of diarrhea<br>2. Administer or teach pt to administer antidiarrheal medication<br>3. Teach pt diet modifications<br>4. Stop drug and infuse heparinized saline if moderate to severe diarrhea occurs; notify MD<br>5. Refer to sec. on diarrhea, Chapter 4 |
| **E. Gastritis** | E. 1. Epigastric distress (mild to moderately severe) with abdominal pain; cramping may occur<br>2. Moderately severe gastritis may occur<br>3. Incidence greater in pts receiving hepatic artery infusions<br>4. Duodenal ulcer occurs in 10% of pts, may be painless, and may lead to gastric outlet obstruction and vomiting<br>5. Biliary sclerosis may occur | E. 1. Gastric distress and injury will be detected early and minimized<br>2. Gastric complications will be prevented | E. 1. Assess for s/s of abdominal distress, cramping prior to and during infusion<br>2. Discuss with MD use of antacids and antisecretory agents<br>3. Stop drug for moderate to severe symptoms, infuse heparinized saline, and notify MD<br>4. Catheter placement should be verified prior to each infusion cycle, and inadvertent drug infusion into gastric/duodenal-supplying arteries should be investigated |
| **F. Hepatic dysfunction** | F. 1. Chemical hepatitis may be severe, with ↑ alkaline phosphatase, liver enzymes, and finally bilirubin<br>2. Incidence greater in pts receiving hepatic artery infusions<br>3. Drug interruption allows healing of injured hepatocytes | F. 1. Early hepatic dysfunction will be identified<br>2. Injury to liver will be temporary | F. 1. Monitor LFTs prior to drug initiation, during therapy, and at end of 14-day cycle<br>2. Discuss dose modifications if LFTs are elevated and if symptoms occur<br>a. If SGOT/SGPT ↑ by 100% at end of 2-week treatment cycle, dose reduced 25% of original dose at next cycle |

*(continued)*

**Floxuridine (continued)**

| Nursing Diagnosis | Defining Characteristics | Expected Outcomes | Nursing Interventions |
|---|---|---|---|
| | | | b. If AST increases by 3 ×, hold cycle until AST normal |
| | | | 3. Assess for s/s of liver dysfunction: lethargy, weakness, malaise, ↓ appetite, fever, presence of jaundice, icterus |
| | | | 4. If pt becomes jaundiced, discuss with MD ultrasound study to evaluate obstruction versus parenchymal liver injury |
| II. *Infection and bleeding related to bone marrow depression* | II. A. Occurs rarely when FUDR given as single agent by continuous intra-arterial infusion | II. A. Pt will be without s/s of infection or bleeding<br>B. Early s/s of infection or bleeding will be detected | II. A. Monitor CBC, platelet count prior to drug administration; assess for s/s of infection or bleeding<br>B. Instruct pt in self-assessment of s/s of infection or bleeding<br>C. Stop drug if WBC < 3500, platelet count < 100,000; infuse heparinized saline and notify MD<br>D. Refer to sec. on bone marrow depression, Chapter 4 |
| III. *Potential for injury related to intra-arterial catheter* | III. A. Catheter-related problems can occur | III. A. Catheter-related problems will be identified early | III. A. Carefully assess catheter prior to each cycle of therapy: patency, access site of implanted port or pump for s/s of infection or bleeding, and pt comfort during palpation of device and abdomen |

| | | | |
|---|---|---|---|
| | 1. Leakage<br>2. Arterial ischemia or aneurysm<br>3. Catheter occlusion<br>4. Bleeding at catheter site<br>5. Thrombosis or embolism of artery<br>6. Vessel perforation or dislodgement of catheter<br>7. Infection<br>8. Biliary sclerosis | B. Further injury will be prevented | B. Catheter position and patency should be determined prior to each cycle of chemotherapy (radionucleotide scan), as catheter may migrate and develop clot; flow study will evaluate this<br>C. Do not force flush into catheter if unable to infuse drug or flush solution; reaccess, and if still unsuccessful, notify MD and arrange for flow study |
| IV. *Sensory perceptual alterations* | IV. A. Hand and foot syndrome occurs in 30–40% of pts, characterized by numbness, sensory changes in hands and feet | IV. A. Syndrome will be prevented<br>B. If syndrome occurs, pt will identify strategies to minimize distress | IV. A. Discuss with MD use of pyridoxine 50 mg TID to prevent occurrence of this syndrome<br>B. Assess for occurrence of syndrome and impact on pt in performing ADLs and level of comfort |
| V. *Alteration in skin integrity* | V. A. May be manifested as localized erythema, dermatitis, nonspecific skin toxicity, or rash | V. A. Skin will remain intact | V. A. Assess for skin changes<br>B. Assess impact of skin changes on pt: self-image, comfort, ability to perform ADLs<br>C. Treat symptomatically |

# Fludarabine phosphate
(Fludara, FLAMP)

*Class:* Antimetabolite

## MECHANISM OF ACTION

Interferes with DNA synthesis by inhibiting ribonucleotide reductase.

## METABOLISM

Rapidly converted to the active metabolite 2-fluoroara-A (2-FLAA). About 23% of the dose is excreted as 2-FLAA over 5 days.

## DOSAGE/RANGE

20–30 mg/m$^2$ IV over 30 minutes daily for 5 days. Cycle resumes every 28 days except with bone marrow or other toxicity
*or*
20 mg/m$^2$ loading dose (bolus), then 30 mg/m$^2$ continuous infusion for 48 hours

## DRUG PREPARATION

50-mg vial. Reconstitute with 2 ml sterile water. Discard unused solutions after 8 hours, as drug contains no preservative.

## DRUG ADMINISTRATION

Administer as an IV bolus or continuous infusion.

## SPECIAL CONSIDERATIONS

Use drug with caution in patients with advanced age, renal insufficiency, bone marrow impairment, or neurological deficiency.

Severe risk of pulmonary toxicity when fludarabine is given with pentostatin.

May cause tumor lysis syndrome (TLS). Hydrate and use allopurinol to prevent TLS.

Do not use in patients with known hypersensitivity to fludarabine.

# Fludarabine phosphate

| Nursing Diagnosis | Defining Characteristics | Expected Outcomes | Nursing Interventions |
|---|---|---|---|
| I. *Infection and bleeding related to bone marrow depression* | I. A. Anemia, thrombocytopenia, neutropenia occur, with nadir at 13 days<br>B. Bone marrow fibrosis and hemolytic anemia may occur<br>C. Myelosuppression is the dose-limiting toxicity | I. A. Pt will be without s/s of infection or bleeding | I. A. Monitor CBC, platelet count prior to drug administration<br>B. Monitor for s/s of infection and bleeding<br>C. Instruct pt in self-assessment of s/s of infection and bleeding<br>D. Transfuse with RBCs, platelets per MD order<br>E. Refer to sec. on bone marrow depression, Chapter 4 |
| II. *Alteration in nutrition, less than body requirements related to*<br>A. Nausea and vomiting<br><br><br><br><br>B. Stomatitis | II. A. Nausea, vomiting, diarrhea occur in 30% of pts<br><br><br><br><br><br><br>B. Stomatitis and GI bleeding | II. A. 1. Pt will be without nausea and vomiting<br>2. Pt will maintain weight within 5% of baseline<br><br><br><br>B. Mucous membranes of GI tract will remain intact | II. A. 1. Premedicate with antiemetics and continue prophylactically × 24 hrs to prevent nausea and vomiting, at least for first treatment<br>2. Encourage small, frequent feedings of cool, bland foods and liquids<br>3. I&O, daily weights if inpatient (assess for s/s of fluid and electrolyte imbalance)<br>4. Refer to sec. on nausea and vomiting, Chapter 4<br>B. 1. Assess oral cavity every day; teach pt to do own oral assessment and oral hygiene regimen<br>2. Encourage pt to report early stomatitis<br>3. Pain relief measures if indicated<br>4. See sec. on stomatitis, mucositis, Chapter 4 |

*(continued)*

Fludarabine phosphate (continued)

| Nursing Diagnosis | Defining Characteristics | Expected Outcomes | Nursing Interventions |
|---|---|---|---|
| C. Anorexia | C. Anorexia | C. Pt will maintain baseline weight ± 5% | C. 1. Encourage small, frequent feedings of favorite foods, especially high-calorie, high-protein foods<br>2. Encourage use of spices<br>3. Weekly weights<br>4. Dietary consult as needed |
| III. *Potential impaired gas exchange related to pulmonary toxicity* | III. A. Pulmonary toxicity can include dyspnea, cough, fever, hypoxia, interstitial pulmonary infiltrates, effusions<br>B. Onset is 3–28 days after third to fifth cycle | III. A. Early s/s of pulmonary toxicity will be identified | III. A. Discuss with MD the need for pulmonary function tests and CXR prior to beginning therapy<br>B. Assess lung sounds prior to drug administration<br>C. Instruct pt to report cough, dyspnea, shortness of breath<br>D. See sec. on pulmonary toxicity, Chapter 4 |
| IV. *Potential alteration in cardiac output* | IV. A. Pericardial effusion and edema sometimes occur | IV. A. Pt will maintain vital signs within normal limits | IV. A. Monitor vital signs, especially BP; listen for pulsus paradoxus, an indication of possible cardiac tamponade<br>B. Cardiac evaluation as needed<br>C. See sec. on cardiotoxicity, Chapter 4 |
| V. *Potential for sensory/ perceptual alterations related to neurological toxicity* | V. A. CNS neurotoxicity can include weakness, headache, confusion, agitation, visual disturbances, hearing loss, coma<br>B. Peripheral paresthesias | V. A. S/s of neurotoxicity will be identified early | V. A. Monitor for s/s of neurotoxicity before and during each treatment<br>B. Teach pt about possible neurotoxicity and s/s |

# 5-Fluorouracil
(Fluorouracil, Adrucil, 5-FU, Efudex [topical])

*Class:* Pyrimidine antimetabolite

## MECHANISM OF ACTION

Acts as a "false" pyrimidine, inhibiting the formation of an enzyme (thymidine synthetase) necessary for the synthesis of DNA. Also incorporates into RNA, causing abnormal synthesis. Methotrexate given prior to 5-fluorouracil results in synergism and enhanced efficacy.

## METABOLISM

Metabolized by the liver. Most is excreted as respiratory $CO_2$; remainder is excreted by the kidneys. Plasma half-life is 20 minutes.

## DOSAGE/RANGE

12–15 mg/kg IV once a week
  *or*
12 mg/kg IV every day × 5 days every 4 weeks
  *or*
500 mg/m² every week or every week × 5

Hepatic infusion: 22 mg/kg in 100 ml $D_5W$ infused into hepatic artery over 8 hours for 5–21 consecutive days

Head and neck: 1000 mg/m² day as continuous infusion for 4–5 days

## DRUG PREPARATION

No dilution required. Can be added to NS or $D_5W$.

Store at room temperature; protect from light. Solution should be clear. If crystals do not disappear after holding vial under hot water, discard vial.

## DRUG ADMINISTRATION

Given IV push or bolus (slow drip) or as continuous infusion.

Given topically as cream.

## SPECIAL CONSIDERATIONS

Patients who have had adrenalectomy may need higher doses of prednisone while receiving 5-FU, or dose of 5-FU may be reduced in postadrenalectomy patients.

Reduce dose in patients with compromised hepatic, renal, or bone marrow function and malnutrition.

Inspect solution for precipitate prior to continuous infusion.

When given with cimetidine, there are increased pharmacologic effects of fluorouracil.

When given with thiazide diuretics, there is increased risk of myelosuppression.

## 5-Fluorouracil

| Nursing Diagnosis | Defining Characteristics | Expected Outcomes | Nursing Interventions |
|---|---|---|---|
| I. *Altered nutrition, less than body requirements related to* | | | |
| A. Nausea and vomiting | I. A. Occur occasionally, may last 2–3 days, usually preventable with antiemetics | I. A. 1. Pt will be without nausea or vomiting<br>2. Nausea and vomiting, if they occur, will be minimal | I. A. 1. Premedicate with antiemetics and continue prophylactically × 24 hrs to prevent nausea and vomiting, at least with the first treatment<br>2. Encourage small, frequent feedings of cool, bland foods and liquids<br>3. Assess for s/s of fluid and electrolyte imbalance: monitor I&O and daily weights if inpatient<br>4. Refer to sec. on nausea and vomiting, Chapter 4 |
| B. Stomatitis | B. 1. Onset 5–8 days<br>2. May herald severe bone marrow depression<br>3. Indication to interrupt therapy | B. Oral mucous membranes will remain intact and free of infection | B. 1. Assess mouth prior to each dose; stomatitis is sometimes preceded by a beefy, painful tongue or small, shallow ulcers on the inner lip<br>2. Report stomatitis to MD; may need to interrupt therapy<br>3. Teach pt oral assessment and mouth care<br>4. Use pain relief measures<br>5. Refer to sec. on stomatitis, mucositis, Chapter 4 |

C. Diarrhea

C. 1. Indication to interrupt treatment
2. May occur with esophagopharyngitis—sore throat with dysphagia

C. 1. Pt will have minimal diarrhea
2. Early s/s of esophagopharyngitis will be identified and treated

C. 1. Encourage pt to report onset of diarrhea
2. Administer or teach pt to self-administer antidiarrheal medication
3. Guaiac all stools
4. Encourage adequate hydration
5. Refer to sec. on diarrhea, Chapter 4
6. Assess pt for sore throat, dysphagia
7. Treat with topical anesthetics

II. *Infection and bleeding related to bone marrow depression*

II. A. Common
B. Neutropenia, thrombocytopenia are most significant
C. Nadir 7–14 days after first dose

II. A. Pt will be without s/s of infection or bleeding
B. Early s/s of infection or bleeding will be identified

II. A. Monitor CBC, platelet count prior to drug administration, as well as s/s of infection and bleeding
B. Instruct pt in self-assessment of s/s of infection and bleeding
C. Refer to sec. on bone marrow depression, Chapter 4

III. *Alteration in skin integrity related to*

A. Alopecia

III. A. 1. More common with 5-day course of treatment; uncommon with 1-day course
2. Diffuse thinning, loss of eyelashes and eyebrows

III. A. Pt will verbalize feelings re hair loss and identify strategies to cope with change in body image

III. A. 1. Assess pt for s/s of hair loss
2. Discuss with pt impact of hair loss and strategies to minimize distress (e.g., wig, scarf, cap); begin before therapy is initiated
3. Refer to sec. on alopecia, Chapter 4

*(continued)*

## 5-Fluorouracil (continued)

| Nursing Diagnosis | Defining Characteristics | Expected Outcomes | Nursing Interventions |
|---|---|---|---|
| B. Changes in nails and skin | B. 1. Nail loss and brittle cracking of nails may occur<br>2. Photosensitivity/photophobia may occur<br>3. Maculopapular rash sometimes occurs on the extremities and trunk (rarely serious); hyperpigmentation on the palms of hands, face<br>4. Chemical phlebitis may occur during continuous infusions, related to high pH of drug | B. Pt will verbalize feelings re changes in nails and skin and identify strategies to cope with change in body image | B. 1. Assess pt for changes in nails and skin<br>2. Discuss with pt impact of changes and strategies to minimize distress (e.g., wearing nail polish or long sleeves)<br>3. Instruct pt in importance of staying out of sun or wearing sunscreen if sun exposure is unavoidable<br>4. Assess skin for rash or other changes; report changes to MD (pt may need antihistamines or steroids)<br>5. Consider implanted venous access device and discuss with pt and physician |
| IV. *Sensory perceptual alterations* | IV. A. Occasional cerebellar ataxia (reversible when drug is discontinued)<br>B. Somnolence<br>C. Ocular changes: conjunctivitis, increased lacrimation, photophobia, oculomotor dysfunction, blurred vision<br>D. Occasional euphoria | IV. A. Early neurological changes will be identified<br>B. Pt will identify strategies for coping with neurological changes | IV. A. Assess cerebellar function prior to each treatment<br>B. Teach pt safety precautions as needed<br>C. Assess pt for ocular changes; report changes<br>D. Refer to sec. on neurotoxicity, Chapter 4 |

# Flutamide
(Eulexin)

*Class:* Antiandrogen

## MECHANISM OF ACTION

Exerts its effect by inhibiting androgen uptake or by inhibiting nuclear binding of androgen in target tissues or both.

## METABOLISM

Rapidly and completely absorbed. Excreted mainly via urine. Biologically active metabolite reaches maximum plasma levels in approximately 2 hours. Plasma half-life is 6 hours. Largely plasma bound.

## DOSAGE/RANGE

250 mg every 8 hours

## DRUG PREPARATION

Available in 125-mg tablets

## DRUG ADMINISTRATION

Oral

## SPECIAL CONSIDERATIONS

None

# Flutamide

| Nursing Diagnosis | Defining Characteristics | Expected Outcomes | Nursing Interventions |
|---|---|---|---|
| I. *Alteration in comfort* | I. A. Hot flashes occur commonly | I. A. Pt will be without hot flashes<br>B. Discomfort will be identified and treated early | I. A. Inform pt that hot flashes may occur<br>B. Encourage pt to report symptoms early |
| II. *Sexual dysfunction* | II. A. Causes decreased libido and impotence in about a third of pts<br>B. Gynecomastia occurs in about 10% of pts | II. A. Pt and significant other will verbalize understanding of changes in sexuality and body image that may occur | II. A. As appropriate, explore with pt and significant other issues of reproductive and sexuality patterns and the impact chemotherapy may have on them<br>B. Discuss strategies to preserve sexuality and reproductive health<br>C. See sec. on gonadal dysfunction, Chapter 4 |
| III. *Altered nutrition, less than body requirements related to*<br>A. Diarrhea | III. A. Occurs in about 10% of pts | III. A. 1. Pt will have minimal diarrhea | III. A. 1. Encourage pt to report onset of diarrhea<br>2. Administer or teach pt to self-administer antidiarrheals<br>3. Guaiac stools<br>4. Refer to sec. on diarrhea, Chapter 4 |
| B. Nausea and vomiting | B. Occurs in about 10% of pts | B. 1. Pt will be without nausea and vomiting<br>2. Nausea and vomiting, should they occur, will be minimal | B. 1. Inform pt of possibility of nausea and vomiting. Obtain prescription for antiemetic if necessary<br>2. Encourage small, frequent feedings of cool, bland foods<br>3. Refer to sec. on nausea and vomiting, Chapter 4 |

# Ftorafur
## (Tegafur) and Uracil (UFT, Orzel)

*Class:* Pyrimidine antimetabolite (Tegafur) plus uracil (investigational)

## MECHANISM OF ACTION

Acts as a "false" pyrimidine, inhibiting the formation of an enzyme (thymidine sythetase) necessary for the synthesis of DNA. Also incorporates into RNA causing abnormal synthesis and suppression of tumor cell replication. Uracil is thought to inhibit the degradation of 5-FU.

## METABOLISM

Quickly absorbed by the GI tract. Tegafur is metabolized by the liver into 5-FU; most is excreted as respiratory $CO_2$; a small amount is excreted by the kidneys. Uracil is rapidly metabolized and excreted, but enhances the cytotoxic effect of 5-FU by increasing its concentration in tumors and inhibiting its degradation.

## DOSAGE/RANGE

200 mg/m$^2$/da with 5 or 50 mg leukovorin × 28 days per cycle

300–350 mg/m$^2$/da in three divided doses 8 hours apart × 28 days

## DRUG PREPARATION

None

## DRUG ADMINISTRATION

Oral

## DRUG INTERACTIONS

Unknown

## LAB EFFECTS/INTERFERENCE

Decreased CBC
Decreased potassium, magnesium
Increased or decreased calcium
Increased PT
Increased LFTs

## SPECIAL CONSIDERATIONS

Cutaneous side effects occur, e.g., pigmentation changes
Can cause asthenia, paresthesias, and headaches

## Ftorafur

| Nursing Diagnosis | Defining Characteristics | Expected Outcomes | Nursing Interventions |
|---|---|---|---|
| I. *Potential for infection and bleeding related to bone marrow depression* | I. A. Decreased WBC, platelet count usually mild and reversible | I. A. Pt will be without s/s of infection or bleeding | I. A. Monitor CBC, platelet count prior to therapy and periodically during therapy<br>B. Instruct pt in self-assessment of s/s of infection and bleeding<br>C. See section on bone marrow depression, Chapter 4 |
| II. *Alteration in nutrition, less than body requirements related to*<br>A. Nausea and vomiting | II. A. Nausea and vomiting can be severe | II. A. 1. Pt will be without nausea and vomiting<br>2. Nausea and vomiting, should they occur, will be minimal | II. A. 1. Teach pt to self-administer antiemetic one hour prior to dose if nausea and/or vomiting occur; teach pt to report nausea/vomiting that is prevented by antiemetic<br>2. Encourage small, frequent feedings of cool, bland foods and liquids<br>3. Assess for symptoms of fluid and electrolyte imbalance; teach pt to monitor I&O, weekly weights<br>4. See section on nausea and vomiting, Chapter 4 |
| B. Diarrhea | B. Diarrhea can be severe | B. Pt will have minimal diarrhea | B. 1. Assess pt's bowel elimination pattern<br>2. Encourage pt to report onset of diarrhea<br>3. Administer or teach pt to self-administer antidiarrheal medications<br>4. See section on diarrhea, Chapter 4 |

C. Stomatitis

C. Stomatitis can be severe

C. Oral mucous membranes will remain intact and without infection

C.
1. Assess baseline oral mucosa, and use of agents that may damage oral mucosa, such as alcohol containing mouth rinses, increased oral intake of alcohol; teach pt to avoid agents that may damage oral mucosa
2. Teach pt oral assessment and mouth care regimen
3. Encourage pt to report early s/s of stomatitis
4. Provide pain relief measures if needed
5. See section on stomatitis, Chapter 4

D. Anorexia

D. Anorexia may be severe

D. Pt will maintain baseline weight ± 5%

D.
1. Encourage small, frequent feedings of favorite foods, especially high-calorie, high-protein foods
2. Encourage use of spices as tolerated
3. Encourage weekly weights, and to call nurse if continued weight loss

# Gallium nitrate
## (Ganite)

*Class:* Group IIIa heavy metal

## MECHANISM OF ACTION

In hypercalcemia, probably inhibits calcium resorption from bone.

## METABOLISM

65% of drug is excreted in urine within the first 24 hours.

## DOSAGE/RANGE

For hypercalcemia, 200 mg/m$^2$ daily for 5 or fewer days; 100 mg/m$^2$ daily for milder cases.

Has been used as an antitumor agent in phase II trials as a one-time dose of 700 mg/m$^2$ over 30 minutes, with cycles repeating every 2 weeks, or up to 350 mg/m$^2$ per day for 5 days continuous infusion

## DRUG PREPARATION

Dilute in 1 liter NS (or D$_5$W for 24-hour infusions). Stable for 48 hours.

## DRUG ADMINISTRATION

Continuous infusion has been found to be less nephrotoxic than bolus doses. Patient should be well hydrated throughout the time the drug is being administered.

## SPECIAL CONSIDERATIONS

Should not be given to patients with creatinine greater than 2.5 mg/dl.

Avoid the use of nephrotoxic drugs when giving gallium nitrate.

## Gallium nitrate

| Nursing Diagnosis | Defining Characteristics | Expected Outcomes | Nursing Interventions |
|---|---|---|---|
| I. *Potential alteration in fluid/electrolyte balance* | I. A. Hypocalcemia may occur in up to 37% of pts<br>B. Hypophosphatemia, decreased serum bicarbonate, hypomagnesemia | I. A. Pt will maintain serum chemistries within normal limits | I. A. Check calcium, phosphate, magnesium, SMA-7 daily<br>B. Obtain MD order for electrolyte replacement<br>C. Refer to sec. on electrolyte disturbances, Chapter 4 |
| II. *Potential decreased urine output* | II. A. Nephrotoxicity was the dose-limiting toxicity in studies where gallium nitrate was used as an antineoplastic agent | II. A. Pt will maintain urine output greater than 50 ml/hr | II. A. Check I&O every 4 hrs; report urine output of less than 50 ml/hr<br>B. Provide IV hydration<br>C. Check renal function studies daily; discuss delaying drug administration with MD if creatinine is greater than 2.5<br>D. Diuretics as needed to balance I&O |
| III. *Potential for fatigue related to anemia* | III. A. Anemia occurs occasionally | III. A. Pt will maintain hematocrit greater than 25 | III. A. Check hematocrit daily; transfuse pt with RBCs as needed<br>B. Energy conservation measures as indicated<br>C. Refer to sec. on bone marrow depression, Chapter 4 |
| IV. *Potential alteration in nutrition, less than body requirements* | IV. A. Nausea and vomiting occur occasionally<br>B. Metallic taste in mouth has been reported<br>C. Diarrhea occasionally | IV. A. Pt will maintain weight within 5% of baseline | IV. A. Administer antiemetics as needed<br>B. Encourage use of hard candies to counteract metallic taste<br>C. Encourage pt to eat cool, bland foods and liquids<br>D. Monitor pt for diarrhea; administer antidiarrheal medication as needed |

# Gemcitabine
## (difluorodeoxycitidine, dFdC)

*Class:* Antimetabolite

## MECHANISM OF ACTION

Structurally similar to Ara-C. Inhibits DNA synthesis by inhibiting DNA polymerase activity. Cell cycle–specific for S phase, causing cells to accumulate at the G-S boundary.

## METABOLISM

Metabolized by enzymes in tumor cells. Cleared renally.

## DOSAGE/RANGE

Current recommendation for phase II trials is 800–1000 mg/m$^2$ weekly for 3 weeks, with the cycle repeating every 4 weeks

*or*

Given at dose of 3600 mg/m$^2$ every 2 weeks

## DRUG PREPARATION

Reconstitute with 2 ml NS (for 20-mg vial) or 10 ml NS (for 100-mg vial).

Further dilute in NS. Drug dose of 2500 mg/m$^2$ or more must be diluted in at least 1000 ml NS and infused over 4 hours or longer.

## DRUG ADMINISTRATION

Most commonly infused over 30 minutes weekly. Doses over 2500 mg/m$^2$ must be infused over at least 4 hours.

## SPECIAL CONSIDERATIONS

Peripheral (ankle) edema sometimes occurs.

Gemcitabine

| Nursing Diagnosis | Defining Characteristics | Expected Outcomes | Nursing Interventions |
|---|---|---|---|
| I. *Potential for bleeding related to bone marrow depression* | I. A. Thrombocytopenia is dose-limiting toxicity<br>B. Relatively little leukopenia seen, rare anemia<br>C. Myelosuppression resolves rapidly when drug is discontinued | I. A. Pt will remain free of s/s of bleeding<br>B. Hematocrit will be maintained at greater than 25, platelets at greater than 10,000 | I. A. Monitor CBC, platelet count prior to drug administration, as well as s/s of infection and bleeding<br>B. Instruct pt in self-assessment of s/s of infection and bleeding<br>C. Transfuse with red cells, platelets per MD order<br>D. Refer to sec. on bone marrow depression, Chapter 4 |
| II. *Potential alteration in comfort* | II. A. Flu-like symptoms with transient febrile episodes occur in 50% of pts with first dose only<br>B. 1. Skin rash (occasionally) within 2–3 days of starting drug<br>2. Erythematous, pruritic, maculopapular rash of the neck and extremities | II. A. Pt will report absence of flu-like symptoms<br>B. Skin rash will be identified and treated early | II. A. 1. Encourage pt to report flu-like symptoms<br>2. Treat fevers with acetaminophen<br>B. 1. Treat rash with topical corticosteroids<br>2. Discuss with MD possible dose reductions to avoid rash with subsequent administration<br>3. Refer to sec. on reactions, Chapter 9 |
| III. *Potential alteration in nutrition, less than body requirements* | III. A. Nausea and vomiting mild; respond to conventional antiemetics | III. A. Nausea and vomiting will be prevented | III. A. Treat nausea and vomiting with conventional antiemetics<br>B. Premedicate with antiemetics and continue prophylactically × 24 hrs to prevent nausea and vomiting, at least for first treatment<br>C. Encourage small, frequent feedings of cool, bland foods and liquids<br>D. I&O, daily weights if inpt (assess for s/s of fluid and electrolyte imbalance)<br>E. Refer to sec. on nausea and vomiting, Chapter 4 |

# Goserelin acetate
## (Zoladex)

*Class:* Synthetic analogue of luteinizing hormone-releasing hormone (LHRH)

## MECHANISM OF ACTION

Inhibits pituitary gonadotropin, achieving a chemical orchiectomy in 2–4 weeks. Sustained-release medication provides continuous drug diffusion from the depot into subcutaneous tissue. This permits monthly injection instead of daily.

## METABOLISM

Absorbed slowly for first 8 days, then more rapid and constant absorption for remaining 28 days.

## DOSAGE/RANGE

*Adults*
Subcutaneous: 3.6-mg dose into upper abdominal wall, q 28 days

## DRUG PREPARATION/ADMINISTRATION

Inspect package for damage. Open package and inspect drug in translucent chamber.

Select site on upper abdomen.

Prepare site with alcohol swab, cleansing from center outward.

Administer local anesthetic as ordered.

Aseptically, stretch skin at site with nondominant hand, and insert needle into subcutaneous tissue with dominant hand at 45-degree angle.

Redirect needle so it is parallel to the abdominal wall. Advance needle forward until hub touches skin. Withdraw needle 1 cm (approximately 1/2 inch).

Depress plunger fully, expelling depot into prepared site.

Withdraw needle carefully. Apply gentle pressure bandage to site. Confirm that tip of plunger is visible within needle tip.

Document in chart.

## SPECIAL CONSIDERATIONS

Compliance to 28-day injection schedule is important.

Indicated for palliative treatment of advanced prostate cancer.

Initially, there is transient increase in serum testosterone levels, with flare of symptoms.

Well-tolerated treatment.

## Goserelin acetate

| Nursing Diagnosis | Defining Characteristics | Expected Outcomes | Nursing Interventions |
|---|---|---|---|
| I. *Sexual dysfunction related to decreased testosterone levels* | I. Hot flashes, sexual dysfunction, and decreased erections can occur | I. Pt will verbalize understanding of possible changes in sexual function; will identify resources to aid coping | I. A. Inform pt of possible side effects<br>B. Assess baseline sexual pattern<br>C. Refer for counseling as needed |
| II. *Potential alteration in cardiac output related to arrhythmia, cardiovascular dysfunction* | II. A. Arrhythmia, cerebro-vascular accident (CVA), hypertension, myocardial infarction, peripheral vascular disease, chest pain, occurs in 1–5% of pts | II. A. Pt will maintain baseline cardiac function | II. A. Assess heart rate, blood pressure, peripheral pulses<br>B. Teach pt to report palpitations, shortness of breath, chest pain, leg pain<br>C. Evaluate abnormalities with physician |
| III. *Sensory/perceptual alteration related to anxiety, depression, headache* | III. A. Anxiety, depression, headache may occur (< 5%) | III. A. Pt will maintain baseline cognitive functioning and emotional state | III. A. Assess baseline affect, comfort, emotional state<br>B. Instruct pt to report changes in mood, cognitive functioning<br>C. Provide pt with emotional support, referrals as necessary |

*(continued)*

## Goserelin acetate (continued)

| Nursing Diagnosis | Defining Characteristics | Expected Outcomes | Nursing Interventions |
|---|---|---|---|
| IV. Alteration in nutrition, less than body requirements, related to vomiting, hyperglycemia, constipation, diarrhea | IV. A. Vomiting occurs in less than 5% of pts; may experience weight gain, ulcers, hyperglycemia<br>B. Pts may experience constipation or diarrhea (less than 5%) | IV. A. Pt will maintain weight within 5% of baseline | IV. A. Assess baseline weight, diet<br>B. Teach pt about possible side effects, to report changes in digestion and nutrition, and to weigh self weekly<br>C. Teach pt side effect management strategies per MD |
| V. Alteration in urinary elimination related to obstruction or infection | V. A. Urinary obstruction, urinary tract infection, renal insufficiency may occur | V. A. Patient will maintain baseline urinary elimination pattern | V. A. Assess baseline urinary elimination pattern, kidney function tests; monitor throughout therapy<br>B. Instruct pt to report s/s of urinary tract infections (UTI), other changes in urinary function |
| VI. Alteration in comfort related to fever, chills, tenderness | VI. A. Chills, fever, breast swelling, and tenderness<br>B. Discomfort may result from injection, as a 16-gauge needle is used to inject depot | VI. A. Patient will report comfort throughout treatment course | VI. A. Instruct pt to report discomfort<br>B. Discuss strategies to improve comfort<br>C. Administer local anesthetic per MD order prior to injecting medication |

# Hexamethylmelamine
(HXM, Altretamine)

*Class:* Alkylating agent

## MECHANISM OF ACTION

The exact mechanism of action is unknown. May inhibit incorporation of thymidine and uridine into DNA and RNA, respectively. Hexamethylmelamine is felt not to act as an alkylating agent in vitro, but it may be activated to an alkylating agent in the body in vivo. Also may act as an antimetabolite, with activity in the S phase.

## METABOLISM

Well absorbed orally, although bioavailability is variable. Peak plasma concentration in 1 hour. Metabolized extensively in the liver, with majority excreted in the urine. Some of the drug is excreted as respiratory $CO_2$. Half-life of the parent compound 4.7–10.2 hours.

## DOSAGE/RANGE

4–12 mg/kg/day (divided in 3 or 4 doses) × 21–90 days

*or*

240 mg/m$^2$ (6 mg/kg)–320 mg/m$^2$ (8 mg/kg) daily × 21 days, repeated every 6 weeks

## DRUG PREPARATION

Available in 50-mg and 100-mg capsules

## DRUG ADMINISTRATION

Oral

## SPECIAL CONSIDERATIONS

Nausea and vomiting can be minimized if patient takes dose 2 hours after meal and at bedtime.

Vitamin B$_6$ may be administered concurrently to decrease neurological complications.

Nadir 3–4 weeks after treatment.

## Hexamethylmelamine

| Nursing Diagnosis | Defining Characteristics | Expected Outcomes | Nursing Interventions |
|---|---|---|---|
| I. *Infection and bleeding related to bone marrow depression* | I. A. Mild bone marrow depression<br>B. Nadir 21–28 days after beginning treatment<br>C. Rapid recovery within 1 week of drug discontinuance | I. A. Pt will be without s/s of infection or bleeding<br>B. Early s/s of infection or bleeding will be identified | I. A. Monitor CBC, platelet count prior to drug administration, as well as s/s of infection and bleeding<br>B. Instruct pt in self-assessment of s/s of infection and bleeding<br>C. Refer to sec. on bone marrow depression, Chapter 4 |
| II. *Altered nutrition, less than body requirements related to*<br>A. Nausea and vomiting | II. A. 1. Nausea occurs in 50–70% of pts and is dose dependent<br>2. Tolerance may develop, usually after at least 3 weeks | II. A. 1. Pt will be without nausea and vomiting<br>2. Nausea and vomiting, if they occur, will be minimal | II. A. 1. Premedicate with antiemetics and continue throughout therapy as needed (tolerance may develop after 3 weeks); teach pt self-administration<br>2. If nausea occurs, encourage small, frequent feedings of cool, bland foods<br>3. Divide daily dose into 4 parts and give 1–2 hrs pc and at bedtime<br>4. Refer to sec. on nausea and vomiting, Chapter 4 |
| B. Diarrhea and abdominal cramps | B. Gastrointestinal effects often dose limiting | B. 1. Pt will have minimal diarrhea<br>2. Pt will develop strategies to minimize discomfort from cramps | B. 1. Encourage pt to report onset of diarrhea<br>2. Administer or instruct pt in self-administration of antidiarrheal medication<br>3. Refer to sec. on diarrhea, Chapter 4<br>4. Discuss possible strategies to decrease distress from cramping: heat, position change |
| C. Anorexia | C. Anorexia has been noted as a side effect in clinical trials | C. Pt will maintain baseline weight ± 5% | C. 1. Encourage small, frequent feedings of favorite foods, especially high-calorie, high-protein foods<br>2. Encourage use of spices<br>3. Weekly weights |

| Nursing Diagnosis | Defining Characteristics | Expected Outcomes | Nursing Interventions |
|---|---|---|---|
| III. *Sensory/perceptual alterations related to*<br><br>A. Peripheral neuropathies | III. A. 1. Rarely occur, 5% incidence<br>2. Sensory and motor alterations may include paresthesia, hyperesthesia, hyperreflexia, and numbness; reversible with drug discontinuance<br>3. Drug may exacerbate the neurotoxicity caused by other chemotherapeutic agents (e.g., vinca alkaloids) | III. A. Pt will report alterations in sensation, perception | III. A. 1. Instruct pt that these may occur and to report s/s of sensory/perceptual alterations if they occur<br>2. Discuss with physician initiating *pyridoxine* 100 mg TID when hexamethylmelamine is begun to prevent or minimize these side effects<br>3. If these changes occur, discuss drug discontinuance with MD |
| B. CNS effects | B. 1. Agitation, confusion, hallucinations, depression, and Parkinson's-like symptoms may occur and usually resolve after discontinuance of therapy<br>2. More common with continuous (> 3 months) therapy than with pulse-dosing regimens | B. Neurological s/s will be minimized | B. 1. Monitor pt for changes in neurological function<br>2. Notify MD of any changes<br>3. Refer to sec. on neurotoxicity, Chapter 4 |
| IV. *Alteration in skin integrity* | IV. A. Skin rashes, pruritus, eczematous skin lesions may occur but are rare | IV. A. Skin will remain intact<br>B. Early s/s of alterations in skin integrity will be identified | IV. A. Assess for changes in skin color, texture, and integrity<br>B. Teach pt self-assessment of skin and to report these changes<br>C. Assess type of discomfort that exists and develop strategy to provide symptom relief |

# Hydroxyurea
(Hydrea)

*Class:* Miscellaneous/antimetabolite

## MECHANISM OF ACTION

Antimetabolite that prevents conversion of ribonucleotides to deoxyribonucleotides by inhibiting the converting enzyme ribonucleoside diphosphate reductase. DNA synthesis is thus inhibited. Cell cycle phase–specific—S phase. May also sensitize cells to the effects of radiation therapy, although the process is not clearly understood.

## METABOLISM

Rapidly absorbed from gastrointestinal tract.

Peak plasma level reached in 2 hours, with plasma half-life of 3–4 hours. About half the drug is metabolized in the liver, half excreted in urine as urea and unchanged drug. Some of the drug is eliminated as respiratory $CO_2$. Crosses blood-brain barrier.

## DOSAGE/RANGE

20–30 mg/kg/day orally as a continuous dose
50–75 mg/kg/day IV

## DRUG PREPARATION

Available in 500-mg capsules

## DRUG ADMINISTRATION

Oral

## SPECIAL CONSIDERATIONS

Hydroxyurea has a side effect of dramatically lowering WBC in a relatively short period of time (24–48 hours). In leukemia patients endangered by the potential complication of leukostasis, this is the desired effect.

May need to pretreat with allopurinol to protect patient from tumor lysis syndrome.

Dermatologic radiation recall phenomena may occur.

In combination with radiation therapy, mucosal reactions in the radiation field may be severe.

## Hydroxyurea

| Nursing Diagnosis | Defining Characteristics | Expected Outcomes | Nursing Interventions |
|---|---|---|---|
| I. *Infection and bleeding related to bone marrow depression* | I. A. Leukopenia more common than thrombocytopenia<br>B. WBC may start dropping in 24–48 hrs; nadir seen in 10 days, with recovery within 10–30 days<br>C. Severity of leukopenia is dose related | I. A. Pt will be without s/s of infection or bleeding<br>B. Early s/s of infection or bleeding will be identified | I. A. Monitor CBC, platelet count prior to drug administration as well as s/s of infection or bleeding<br>B. Instruct pt in self-assessment of infection or bleeding<br>C. Drug dosage may be titrated for higher or lower than normal blood values<br>D. See sec. on bone marrow depression, Chapter 4 |
| II. *Altered nutrition, less than body requirements related to*<br><br>A. Anorexia | II. A. Mild to moderate | II. A. Pt will maintain baseline weight ± 5% | II. A. 1. Encourage small, frequent feedings of favorite foods, especially high-calorie, high-protein foods<br>2. Encourage use of spices<br>3. Weekly weights |
| B. Stomatitis | B. Uncommon | B. Oral mucous membranes will remain intact and without infection | B. 1. Teach pt oral assessment and mouth care<br>2. Encourage pt to report early stomatitis<br>3. Teach pt oral hygiene<br>4. See sec. on stomatitis mucositis, Chapter 4 |
| C. Diarrhea | C. Uncommon | C. Pt will have minimal diarrhea | C. 1. Encourage pt to report onset of diarrhea<br>2. Administer or teach pt to self-administer antidiarrheal medications<br>3. See sec. on diarrhea, Chapter 4 |
| D. Hepatic dysfunction | D. Hepatitis is rare but may occur; there are also disturbances in liver function studies | D. Hepatic dysfunction will be identified early | D. 1. Monitor SGOT, SGPT, LDH, alkaline phosphatase, and bilirubin periodically during treatment<br>2. Notify MD of any elevations |

(*continued*)

## Hydroxyurea (continued)

| Nursing Diagnosis | Defining Characteristics | Expected Outcomes | Nursing Interventions |
|---|---|---|---|
| III. *Alteration in skin integrity related to* | | | |
| A. Alopecia | III. A. Uncommon, though may be slight to diffuse thinning | III. A. Pt will verbalize feelings re hair loss and identify strategies to cope with change in body image | III. A. 1. Assess pt for s/s of hair loss<br>2. Discuss with pt impact of hair loss and strategies to minimize distress (i.e., wig, scarf, cap); begin before therapy is initiated<br>3. See sec. on alopecia, Chapter 4 |
| B. Dermatitis | B. 1. Dermatitis is uncommon, usually mild and reversible<br>2. Symptoms may include facial erythema, rash pruritus<br>3. Rarely, postirradiation therapy erythema (recall) may occur | B. 1. Skin will remain intact<br>2. Early skin impairment will be identified | B. 1. Assess skin integrity<br>2. If dermatitis severe, discuss drug discontinuance with MD<br>3. Topical medications as appropriate<br>4. Radiation recall occurs when hydroxyurea is administered during or after radiation therapy and may occur weeks or months after therapy |
| IV. *Alteration in renal function related to chemotherapy (rare)* | IV. A. Reversible renal tubular dysfunction evidenced by elevated BUN, creatinine, and uric acid levels | IV. A. Pt will be without renal dysfunction | IV. A. Monitor BUN and creatinine prior to drug dose, as half of drug is excreted unchanged in urine<br>B. Provide or instruct pt in hydration of *at least* 2–3 liters of fluid/day during and for at least 48 hrs after therapy<br>C. Monitor I&O<br>D. Weekly weights<br>E. Refer to sec. on nephrotoxicity, Chapter 4 |

| | | | |
|---|---|---|---|
| V. *Potential for sexual/ reproductive dysfunction* | A. Gonadal function and fertility are affected (may be permanent or transient) <br> B. Reported to be excreted in breast milk reproductive dysfunction | V. A. Pt and significant other will understand need for contraception <br> B. Pt and significant other will identify strategies to cope with sexual and reproductive dysfunction | V. A. As appropriate, explore with pt and significant other issues of reproductive and sexuality pattern and impact chemotherapy will have <br> B. Discuss strategies to preserve sexuality and reproductive health (e.g., contraception, sperm banking) <br> C. See sec. on gonadal dysfunction, Chapter 4 |
| VI. *Sensory/perceptual alterations* | VI. A. S/s may include disorientation, drowsiness, headache, vertigo <br> B. Symptoms usually do not last more than 24 hrs | VI. A. Mental status changes and other disturbances will be identified early | VI. A. Obtain baseline mental status—neurological function <br> B. Assess status changes during chemotherapy <br> C. Encourage pt to report any changes |

# Idarubicin
## (Idamycin, 4-Demethoxydaunorubicin)

*Class:* Antitumor antibiotic

## MECHANISM OF ACTION

Cell cycle phase–specific for S phase. Analogue of daunorubicin. Has a marked inhibitory effect on RNA synthesis.

## METABOLISM

Excreted primarily in the bile and to a lesser extent the urine, with approximately 25% of the IV dose accounted for over 5 days. The half-life of this agent and its metabolite is 18–50 hours.

## DOSAGE/RANGE

12 mg/m$^2$ daily × 3 days by slow IVB (over 10–15 minutes) in combination with Ara-C 100 mg/m$^2$ IV continuous infusion for 7 days

*or*

25 mg/m$^2$ IVB followed by Ara-C 200 mg/m$^2$ continuous infusion daily for 5 days

## DRUG PREPARATION

Available as a red powder. The drug is reconstituted with normal saline injection.

## DRUG ADMINISTRATION

Drug is a vesicant. Administer IV push over 10–15 minutes into the sidearm of a freely running IV.

## SPECIAL CONSIDERATIONS

Vesicant.

Discolored urine (pink to red) may occur up to 48 hours after administration.

Cardiomyopathy is less common and less severe than with doxorubicin and daunorubicin.

Drug is light sensitive.

Incompatible with heparin (precipitate occurs).

Drug dosage should be reduced in patients with hepatic or renal dysfunction.

# Idarubicin

| Nursing Diagnosis | Defining Characteristics | Expected Outcomes | Nursing Interventions |
|---|---|---|---|
| I. *Infection and bleeding related to bone marrow depression* | I. A. Hematologic toxicity is dose limiting<br>B. Leukopenia nadir 10–20 days, with recovery in 1–2 weeks<br>C. Thrombocytopenia usually follows leukopenia and is mild<br>D. BM toxicity is not cumulative | I. A. Pt will be without s/s of infection or bleeding<br>B. Early s/s of infection or bleeding will be identified<br>C. Administer growth factors (esp. GCSF) as ordered | I. A. Monitor CBC, platelet count prior to drug administration as well as s/s of infection or bleeding<br>B. Instruct pt in self-assessment of s/s of infection or bleeding<br>C. Dose modifications often necessary (35–50%) if bone marrow function is compromised<br>D. See sec. on bone marrow depression, Chapter 4 |
| II. *Altered nutrition, less than body requirements related to*<br>A. Nausea and vomiting | II. A. Usually mild to moderate, though nausea and vomiting are seen to some degree in most pts | II. A. 1. Pt will be without nausea and vomiting<br>2. Nausea and vomiting, if they occur, will be minimal | II. A. 1. Premedicate with antiemetics and continue prophylactically × 24 hrs to prevent nausea and vomiting, at least first treatment<br>2. Encourage small, frequent feedings of cool, bland foods and liquids<br>3. Refer to sec. on nausea and vomiting, Chapter 4 |
| B. Anorexia | B. Commonly occurs | B. Pt will maintain baseline weight ± 5% | B. 1. Encourage small, frequent feedings of favorite foods, especially high-calorie, high-protein foods<br>2. Encourage use of spices<br>3. Weekly weights |
| C. Stomatitis | C. Mild | C. Oral mucous membranes will remain intact and without infection | C. 1. Teach pt oral assessment and mouth care<br>2. Encourage pt to report early stomatitis<br>3. Teach pt oral hygiene<br>4. See sec. on stomatitis, Chapter 4 |

*(continued)*

## Idarubicin (continued)

| Nursing Diagnosis | Defining Characteristics | Expected Outcomes | Nursing Interventions |
|---|---|---|---|
| II. D. Diarrhea | II. D. Infrequent and mild | II. D. Pt will have minimal diarrhea | II. D. 1. Encourage pt to report onset of diarrhea<br>2. Administer or teach pt to self-administer antidiarrheal medications<br>3. See sec. on diarrhea, Chapter 4 |
| E. Hepatic dysfunction | E. 1. Hepatitis is rare but may occur<br>2. There are also disturbances in liver function studies | E. Hepatic dysfunction will be identified early | E. 1. Monitor SGOT, SGPT, LDH, alkaline phosphatase, and bilirubin periodically during treatment<br>2. Notify MD of any elevations |
| III. Alteration in skin integrity related to<br>A. Alopecia | III. A. 1. Occurs in about 30% of pts after oral drug and can be partial after IV drug<br>2. Begins after 3 + weeks, and hair may grow back while on therapy<br>3. May be slight to diffuse thinning | III. A. Pt will verbalize feelings re hair loss and identify strategies to cope with change in body image | III. A. 1. Assess pt for s/s of hair loss<br>2. Discuss with pt impact of hair loss and strategies to minimize distress (e.g., wigs, scarf, cap); begin before therapy is initiated<br>3. See sec. on alopecia, Chapter 4 |
| B. Skin changes: darkening of nail beds, skin ulcer/necrosis, sensitivity to sunlight, skin itching at irradiated areas | B. Skin changes seen as hyperpigmentation of nail beds, sensitivity to sunlight, radiation recall, and potential necrosis with extravasation | B. 1. Skin will remain intact<br>2. Early skin impairment will be identified | B. 1. Assess skin for integrity<br>2. If severe, discuss drug discontinuance with MD<br>3. Assess pt for changes in skin, nails<br>4. Discuss with pt impact of changes and strategies to minimize distress (e.g., wearing nail polish, long sleeves)<br>5. Administer according to policies for vesicant drugs<br>  a. Careful technique is used during veni-puncture; see sec. on intravenous administration, Chapters 9 and 10<br>  b. Administer vesicant through freely flowing IV, constantly monitoring IV site and pt response |

c. Nurse should be *thoroughly* familiar with institutional policy and procedure for administration of a vesicant agent

d. If vesicant drug is administered as a continuous infusion, drug must be given through a patent central line

e. If extravasation is suspected:

(1) stop drug being administered

(2) aspirate any residual drug and blood from IV tubing, IV catheter/needle, and IV site if possible

(3) *if antidote exists*, instill antidote into area of apparent infiltration as per MD order and institutional policy and procedure

(4) apply cold or topical medications as per MD order and institutional policy and procedure

f. Assess site regularly for pain, progression of erythema, induration, and evidence of necrosis

g. When in doubt about whether drug is infiltrating, *treat as an infiltration*

h. Teach pt to assess site and notify MD if condition worsens

*(continued)*

## Idarubicin (continued)

| Nursing Diagnosis | Defining Characteristics | Expected Outcomes | Nursing Interventions |
|---|---|---|---|
| | | | i. Arrange next clinic visit for assessment of site depending on drug, amount infiltrated, extent of potential injury, and pt variables<br>j. Document in pts record as per institutional policy and procedure; see sec. on reactions, Chapter 9 |
| IV. *Alteration in cardiac output related to cumulative doses* | IV. A. Cardiac toxicity is similar characteristically but less severe than that seen with daunorubicin and doxorubicin<br>B. CHF due to cardiomyopathy seen after large cumulative doses | IV. A. Early s/s of cardiomyopathy will be identified | IV. A. Assess pt for s/s of cardiomyopathy<br>B. Obtain baseline cardiac functions (EKG changes uncommon)<br>C. Discuss gated blood pool scan or echocardiogram with MD<br>D. Assess quality and regularity of heartbeat<br>E. Instruct pt to report dyspnea, shortness of breath<br>F. Teach pt the potential of irreversible CHF with cumulative doses<br>G. Refer to sec. on cardiotoxicity, Chapter 4 |

# Idoxirene

*Class:* Investigational

## MECHANISM OF ACTION

Overcomes tamoxifen limitations, such as the estrogenic effects that tamoxifen possesses, and maximizes antiestrogen activity (only about 50% of estrogen-positive women with breast cancer respond to tamoxifen, acquired resistance to tamoxifen eventually develops, and it is probable that the estrogen agonist activity of tamoxifen accounts for the increased risk of developing endometrial cancer after tamoxifen therapy). Drug has 2.5–5-fold higher affinity for estrogen receptors than tamoxifen. It is 1.5-fold more effective in inhibiting estrogen-induced growth in tumor cells, and potently inhibits calmodulin activity (important in breast cancer cell growth) (Coombes et al. 1995).

## METABOLISM

Peak plasma levels at 2–8 hours after a single dose, achieving steady state levels with daily dosing in 6–12 weeks, as compared to tamoxifen's 2–6 weeks, and possessing a very long elimination phase (terminal half-life is 23.3 +/− 5 days, about three times longer than tamoxifen).

## DOSAGE/RANGE

Doses studied include 10–60-mg daily dosing for 2 weeks, and then 20-mg maintenance doses.

Refer to study protocol.

## DRUG PREPARATION

None

## DRUG ADMINISTRATION

Oral

## DRUG INTERACTIONS

Unknown, but probably similar to tamoxifen.

## LAB EFFECTS/INTERFERENCE

None known

## SPECIAL CONSIDERATIONS

Possesses ability to reverse multi-anticancer drug resistance mediated by P-glycoprotein (at least as effective as tamoxifen and verapamil).

Probably has partial cross-resistance with tamoxifen so may be effective in tamoxifen-resistant patients.

# Idoxirene

| Nursing Diagnosis | Defining Characteristics | Expected Outcomes | Nursing Interventions |
|---|---|---|---|
| I. *Alteration in nutrition, less than body requirements, related to nausea and vomiting* | I. A. Nausea and vomiting may occur and are transient | I. A. Pt will be without nausea or vomiting<br>B. Nausea/vomiting will be minimized | I. A. Inform pt of possibility of nausea/vomiting, and in self-administration of antiemetics per MD order<br>B. Encourage small, frequent feedings of cool, bland foods and liquids<br>C. Instruct pt in oral self-care measures, and to report nausea/vomiting to health care providers<br>D. Refer to sec. on nausea/vomiting, Chapter 4 |
| II. *Activity intolerance related to fatigue, lethargy, weakness* | II. A. Tiredness, lethargy, weakness may occur; do not appear to be dose related | II. A. Pt will verbalize ways to cope with activity intolerance | II. A. Inform pt about possibility of changes in energy level<br>B. Assess baseline activity level, changes that may have occurred with treatment<br>C. Teach pt energy conservation measures as needed |

# Ifosfamide
(IFEX)

*Class:* Alkylating agent

## MECHANISM OF ACTION

Analogue of cyclophosphamide and is cell cycle phase nonspecific. Destroys DNA throughout the cell cycle by binding to protein and DNA, cross-linking with DNA and causing chain scission as well as inhibition of DNA synthesis. Ifosfamide has been shown to be effective in tumors previously resistant to cyclophosphamide. Activated by microsomes in the liver.

## METABOLISM

Only about 50% of the drug is metabolized, with much of the drug excreted in the urine almost completely unchanged. Half-life is 13.8 hours for high dose versus 3–10 hours for lower doses.

## DOSAGE/RANGE

IV bolus 50 mg/kg/day
  *or*
700–2000 mg/m$^2$/day $\times$ 5 days
  *or*
2400 mg/m$^2$/day $\times$ 3 days
Continuous infusion: 1200 mg/m$^2$/day $\times$ 5 days
Single dose: 5000 mg/m$^2$ q 3–4 weeks
Dose reduce by 25–50% if serum creatinine is 2.1–3.0 mg/dl

## DRUG PREPARATION

Available as a powder and should be reconstituted with sterile water for injection.

Solution is chemically stable for 7 days, but discard after 8 hours due to lack of bacteriostatic preservative of the solution.

May be diluted further in either D$_5$W or normal saline.

## DRUG ADMINISTRATION

IV bolus: administer over 30 minutes.

Continuous infusion: administer IV for 5 days. Mesna should be administered with ifosfamide: it is begun simultaneously with the drug and repeated at 4 and 8 hours after the ifosfamide. (See drug sheet on mesna.) Mesna, ascorbic acid, and Mucomyst have been utilized to protect the bladder. Prehydration and posthydration (150–2000 cc/day) or continuous bladder irrigations are recommended to prevent hemorrhagic cystitis.

## SPECIAL CONSIDERATIONS

Metabolic toxicity is increased by simultaneous administration of barbiturates.

Activity and toxicity of the drug may be altered by allopurinol, chloroquine, phenothiazines, potassium iodide, chloramphenicol, imipramine, vitamin A, corticosteroids, and succinylcholine.

Therapy requires the concomitant administration of a uroprotector such as mesna and prehydration and posthydration; may also require catheterization and constant bladder irrigation, and/or ascorbic acid.

## Ifosfamide

| Nursing Diagnosis | Defining Characteristics | Expected Outcomes | Nursing Interventions |
|---|---|---|---|
| I. *Altered urinary elimination related to* | | | |
| A. Hemorrhagic cystitis | I. A. 1. Symptoms of bladder irritation<br>2. Hemorrhagic cystitis with hematuria, dysuria, urinary frequency<br>3. Preventable with uroprotection and hydration | I. A. 1. Pt will be without hemorrhagic cystitis<br>2. Hemorrhagic cystitis, if it occurs, will be detected early | I. A. 1. Assess presence of RBC in urine prior to successive doses, especially if symptoms are present, as well as BUN and creatinine<br>2. Administer drug with concomitant uroprotector (e.g., mesna)<br>3. Encourage *prehydration*: po intake of 2–3 l/day prior to chemotherapy; *posthydration*: increase po fluids to 2–3 l/day for 2 days after chemotherapy<br>4. If possible, administer drug in morning to minimize drug accumulation in bladder during sleep<br>5. Instruct pt to empty bladder every 2–3 hours, before bedtime, and during night when awake<br>6. Monitor urinary output and total body balance |
| B. Renal toxicity | B. 1. ↑ BUN, ↑ serum creatinine, ↓ urine creatinine clearance (usually reversible)<br>2. Acute tubular necrosis, pyelonephritis, glomerular dysfunction<br>3. Metabolic acidosis | B. Renal dysfunction will be identified early | B. 1. Assess urinary elimination pattern prior to each drug dose<br>2. If rigorous regimen is adhered to, minimal renal toxicity will result<br>3. Monitor BUN and creatinine<br>4. IV hydration as ordered<br>5. Drug dose should be reduced if serum creatinine 2.1–3.0 mg/dl. Hold drug if > 3.0 |

| Nursing Diagnosis | Defining Characteristics | Expected Outcomes | Nursing Interventions |
|---|---|---|---|
| II. *Altered nutrition, less than body requirements*<br><br>A. Nausea and vomiting | II. A. 1. Nausea and vomiting occur in 58% of pts<br>2. Dose and schedule dependent; ↑ severity with higher dose and rapid injection<br>3. Occurs within a few hours of drug administration and may last 3 days | II. A. 1. Pt will be without nausea and vomiting<br>2. Nausea and vomiting, if they occur, will be minimal | II. A. 1. Premedicate with antiemetics and continue prophylactically to *prevent* nausea and vomiting for 24 hrs, at least first treatment<br>2. Encourage small, frequent feedings of cool, bland foods and liquids<br>3. Refer to sec. on nausea and vomiting, Chapter 4 |
| B. Hepatotoxicity | B. 1. Elevations of serum transaminase and alkaline phosphatase may occur<br>2. Usually transient and resolves spontaneously<br>3. No apparent sequelae | B. Early hepatotoxicity will be identified | B. Monitor LFTs during treatment; report elevation to MD |
| III. *Infection and bleeding related to bone marrow depression* | III. A. Leukopenia is mild to moderate<br>B. Thrombocytopenia and anemia are rare<br>C. Bone marrow depression more severe when ifosfamide is combined with other chemotherapy agents<br>D. Pts at risk for BMD: pts with impaired renal function and 0 bone marrow reserve (bone marrow metastases, prior XRT) | III. A. Pt will be without s/s of infection or bleeding<br>B. Early s/s of infection or bleeding will be identified | III. A. Monitor CBC, platelet count prior to drug administration, as well as s/s of infection or bleeding<br>B. Instruct pt in self-assessment of s/s of infection or bleeding<br>C. Dose reduction may be necessary when given in combination with other agents causing BMD<br>D. Refer to sec. on bone marrow depression, Chapter 4 |

*(continued)*

**Ifosfamide** (*continued*)

| Nursing Diagnosis | Defining Characteristics | Expected Outcomes | Nursing Interventions |
|---|---|---|---|
| IV. *Alteration in skin integrity related to*<br>A. Alopecia | IV. A. Incidence 83%, with 50% experiencing severe hair loss in 2–4 weeks | IV. A. Pt will verbalize feelings re hair loss and identify strategies to cope with change in body image | IV. A. 1. Discuss with pt anticipated impact of hair loss; suggest wig, as appropriate, prior to actual hair loss<br>2. Explore with pt response to hair loss and alternative strategies to minimize distress<br>3. See sec. on alopecia, Chapter 4 |
| B. Sterile phlebitis at injection site; irritation with extravasation | B. Drug is not activated until it reaches hepatic microsomes, so drug doesn't cause tissue damage (is not a vesicant); incidence < 2% | B. 1. Skin injury will be prevented<br>2. Early injury will be identified | B. Carefully monitor injection site during drug administration and infusion for s/s of phlebitis, irritation, vein patency |
| C. Skin changes | C. Skin hyperpigmentation, dermatitis, nail ridging may occur | C. 1. Early skin impairment will be identified<br>2. Pt will verbalize feelings re changes in nail or skin color or texture and identify strategies to cope with change in body image | C. 1. Assess skin integrity<br>2. Assess impact of skin changes on body image<br>3. Discuss strategies to minimize distress |
| V. *Sensory/perceptual alterations: confusion, activity intolerance, fatigue* | V. A. Intact drug passes easily into CNS; however, *active* metabolitesdo not<br>B. Lethargy and confusion may be seen with high doses, lasting 1–8 hours; usually spontaneously reversible | V. A. Neurologic alterations will be identified early<br>B. Pt and family will manage distress safely | V. A. Identify pts at risk (↓ renal function) and observe closely<br>B. Assess neurological and mental status prior to and during drug administration and on follow-up<br>C. Instruct pt to report any |

| | | | |
|---|---|---|---|
| | C. CNS side effects occur in about 12% of pts treated, including somnolence, confusion, depressive psychosis, hallucinations<br>D. Less frequent: dizziness, disorientation, cranial nerve dysfunction, seizures<br>E. Incidence of CNS side effects may be higher in pts with compromised renal function, as well as in pts receiving high dose | | C. alterations in behavior, sensation, perception<br>D. If side effects develop, a plan of care with pt and family to manage distress and promote safety |
| VI. *Potential for sexual dysfunction* | VI. A. Drug is carcinogenic, mutagenic, and teratogenic<br>B. Drug is excreted in breast milk | VI. A. Pt and significant other will understand need for contraception<br>B. Pt and significant other will identify strategies to cope with sexual dysfunction | VI. A. As appropriate, explore with pt and significant other issues of reproductive and sexual pattern and impact chemotherapy will have<br>B. Discuss strategies to preserve sexuality and reproductive health (e.g., sperm banking, contraception)<br>C. See sec. on gonadal dysfunction, Chapter 4 |

# Irinotecan
## (Camptosar, Camptothecin-11, CPT-11)

*Class:* Topoisomerase inhibitor

## MECHANISM OF ACTION

Induces protein-linked DNA single-strand breaks and blocks DNA and RNA synthesis in dividing cells, preventing cells from entering mitosis. Prevents DNA repair.

## METABOLISM

Metabolized to active metabolite SN-38 in the liver; 11–20% of drug excreted in urine, and 5–39% in the bile, over a 48-hour period. Mean terminal half-life is 6 hours, while that of SN-38 is 10 hours. Drug is moderately protein-bound (30–68%) while SN-38 is highly protein-bound (95%).

## DOSAGE/RANGE

Starting dose is 125 mg/m$^2$ IV over 90 minutes weekly × 4, followed by 2-week rest period. Repeat 6-week cycle.

If well-tolerated, dose can be increased to 150 mg/m$^2$.

350 mg/m$^2$ IV day/repeated q 3 weeks has same efficacy (300 mg/m$^2$ if age ≥ 70, prior pelvic/abdominal XRT, or performance status of 2).

Drug combined with 5FU and leukovorin is more active than 5FU/leukovorin alone.

## DRUG PREPARATION

Store at room temperature protected from light. Dilute and mix drug in 5% glucose solution.

## DRUG ADMINISTRATION

Administer IV bolus over 90 minutes.

## SPECIAL CONSIDERATIONS

Drug is indicated for treatment of metastatic colon or rectal cancer recurring or progressing after 5FU treatment.

Dose-limiting toxicities are diarrhea and severe myelosuppression.

Drug is synergistic with cisplatin; give irinotecan *after* cisplatin to maximize cell kill.

Drug is teratogenic and contraindicated in pregnant women.

Drug is an irritant; if infiltration occurs, manufacturer recommends flushing IV site with sterile water, and then applying ice.

All patients should receive self-care instruction on management of diarrhea, self-administration of loperamide for delayed diarrhea, and accurate assessment of the patient's ability to purchase and take loperamide if diarrhea develops.

Dose reduce for neutropenia and diarrhea.

Response to therapy usually evaluable after 2 cycles.

Drug active in other solid tumors, including non-small-cell lung cancer.

Irinotecan

| Nursing Diagnosis | Defining Characteristics | Expected Outcomes | Nursing Interventions |
|---|---|---|---|
| I. *Potential for infection, fatigue related to bone marrow depression* | I. A. Leukopenia has been noted in 50–60% of pts on the single-dose schedule<br>B. Anemia reported in 15% of pts | I. A. Pt is without s/s of infection<br>B. Pt reports ability to participate in normal ADLs | I. A. 1. Monitor CBC, platelet count prior to drug administration, as well as s/s of infection and bleeding<br>2. Instruct pt in self-assessment of s/s of infection and bleeding<br>3. Transfuse with platelets per MD order<br>4. Refer to sec. on bone marrow depression, Chapter 4<br>B. 1. Check hematocrit; transfuse with RBCs per MD order<br>2. Instruct pt in energy conservation measures |
| II. *Potential alteration in bowel elimination pattern related to diarrhea* | II. A. Diarrhea common and may occur during or immediately after treatment (cholinergic response). Often associated with diaphoresis, abdominal cramping; preventable by IV atropine 0.25 mg IV<br>B. Delayed diarrhea occurs day 8–13, may be severe and requires compliance to antidiarrheal medicines | II. A. Diarrhea will be prevented<br>B. Diarrhea, if it occurs, will be managed effectively | II. A. Assess normal bowel elimination status, ability to manage self-care and ability to purchase loperamide<br>B. Ensure patient understands required self-administration of loperamide if diarrhea develops<br>C. Teach pt to administer Immodium, 2 tabs after first episode of diarrhea then 1 tab q 2 hrs until no diarrhea × 12 hours (at bedtime, take 2 tabs) (recommended by Camptosar manufacturer)<br>D. Teach pt to modify diet to eliminate fiber, fruits/vegetables that cause diarrhea, to eat small, frequent meals, try BRAT diet, increase po fluids.<br>E. See Chapter 4 |

*(continued)*

## Irinotecan (continued)

| Nursing Diagnosis | Defining Characteristics | Expected Outcomes | Nursing Interventions |
|---|---|---|---|
| III. *Alteration in nutrition related to nausea and vomiting* | III. A. Nausea and vomiting mod-severe<br>B. Occurs in 35–60% of pts<br>C. Preventable using serotonin antagonist antiemetic therapy | III. A. Pt will be without nausea and vomiting<br>B. Pt will maintain weight within 5% of baseline | III. A. Premedicate with antiemetics and continue prophylactically × 24 hrs to prevent nausea and vomiting, at least for first treatment<br>B. Encourage small, frequent feedings of cool, bland foods and liquids<br>C. Monitor I&O, total body balance, electrolyte balance<br>D. Teach pt self-administration of antiemetics at home, and to report if they are ineffective<br>E. Refer to sec. on nausea and vomiting, Chapter 4 |
| IV. *Alteration in skin integrity* | IV. A. Alopecia occurs in 30–40% of pts | IV. A. Pt verbalizes feelings about hair loss and identifies strategies to cope with change in body image | IV. A. Assess pt for hair loss<br>B. Discuss with pt impact of hair loss and strategies to minimize distress (e.g., scarf, cap, wig)<br>C. See section on alopecia, Chapter 4 |
| V. *Potential impaired gas exchange related to pulmonary toxicity* | V. A. Diffuse interstitial infiltrates have occurred in 8% of pts with fever and dyspnea<br>B. Interstitial pneumonitis rare | V. A. Pt will maintain baseline pulmonary function | V. A. Discuss with MD the need for pulmonary function tests and CXR prior to beginning therapy<br>B. Assess lung sounds prior to drug administration<br>C. Instruct pt to report cough, dyspnea, shortness of breath<br>D. Administer glucocorticoids as directed<br>E. See section on pulmonary toxicity, Chapter 4 |

# L-asparaginase
(ELSPAR)

*Class:* Miscellaneous/enzyme

## MECHANISM OF ACTION

Hydrolysis of serum asparagine occurs, which deprives leukemia cells of the required amino acid. Normal cells are spared because they generally have the ability to synthesize their own asparagine.

Cell cycle specific for $G_1$ postmitotic phase.

Some leukemic cells are unable to synthesize asparagine. These cells must obtain asparagine from an exogenous source—the patient's serum. Administration of the enzyme L-asparaginase causes hydrolysis of asparagine to aspartate, resulting in rapid depletion of the asparagine concentration in the patient's serum.

## METABOLISM

Metabolism of L-asparaginase is independent of renal and hepatic function. The drug is not recovered in the urine and does not appear to cross the blood-brain barrier.

## DOSAGE/RANGE

IM or IV, varies with protocol

## DRUG PREPARATION

IV injection: Reconstitute with sterile water for injection or sodium chloride injection (without preservative) and use within 8 hours of reconstitution.

IV infusion: Dilute with sodium chloride injection or 5% dextrose injection and use within 8 hours, only if clear; if gelatinous particles develop, filter through a 5-micron filter.

The lyophilized powder must be stored under refrigeration. The reconstituted solution must also be stored under refrigeration if it is not used immediately. The solution must be discarded within 8 hours after preparation.

## DRUG ADMINISTRATION

Use in a hospital setting. Make preparations to treat anaphylaxis at each administration of the drug.

## SPECIAL CONSIDERATIONS

Potential reduction in antineoplastic effect of methotrexate when given in combination.

Anaphylaxis is associated with the administration of this drug.

Intravenous administration of L-asparaginase concurrently with or immediately before prednisone and vincristine administration may be associated with increased toxicity.

## L-asparaginase

| Nursing Diagnosis | Defining Characteristics | Expected Outcomes | Nursing Interventions |
|---|---|---|---|
| I. *Potential for injury related to hypersensitivity or anaphylactic reaction* | I. A. Occurs in 20–35% of pts<br>B. Increased incidence after several doses administered but may occur with first dose<br>C. Occurs less often with IM route of administration<br>D. May be life-threatening reaction but usually mild<br>  1. Urticardial eruptions<br>  2. Fever (100°–101°F, 37.5°–38°C) seen in half of pts<br>  3. Chills<br>  4. Facial redness<br>  5. Hypotension<br>  6. Shortness of breath<br>  7. Hives<br>  8. Diaphoresis | I. A. Early s/s of hypersensitivity or anaphylactic reactions will be identified | I. A. Teach pt the potential of a hypersensitivity or anaphylaxis reaction and to immediately report any unusual symptoms<br>B. Obtain baseline vital signs and note pts mental status<br>C. Skin testing, prior to administering full dose, is recommended by manufacturer<br>D. Assess pt for at least 30 mins after the drug is given or s/s of a reaction; see sec. on reactions, Chapter 9<br>E. 1. Administer therapy according to MD orders<br>  2. Review standing orders for management of pt in anaphylaxis and identify location of anaphylaxis kit containing epinephrine 1:1000, hydrocortisone sodium succinate (Solucortef), diphenhydramine HCl (Benadryl), Aminophylline, and others<br>  3. Observe for following s/s during infusion, usually occurring within first 15 mins of start of infusion<br>    a. *Subjective*<br>      (1) generalized itching<br>      (2) nausea<br>      (3) chest tightness<br>      (4) crampy abdominal pain<br>      (5) difficulty speaking<br>      (6) anxiety<br>      (7) agitation |

(8) sense of impending doom

(9) uneasiness

(10) desire to urinate/defecate

(11) dizziness

(12) chills

b. *Objective*

(1) flushed appearance (angioedema of face, neck, eyelids, hands, feet)

(2) localized or generalized urticaria

(3) respiratory distress ± wheezing

(4) hypotension

(5) cyanosis

4. If reaction occurs, stop infusion and notify MD

5. Place pt in supine position to promote perfusion of visceral organs

6. Monitor vital signs until stable

7. Provide emotional reassurance to pt and family

8. Maintain patent airway and have CPR equipment ready if needed

9. Document incident

10. Discuss with MD desensitization versus drug discontinuance for further dosing

*(continued)*

**L-asparaginase** (*continued*)

| Nursing Diagnosis | Defining Characteristics | Expected Outcomes | Nursing Interventions |
|---|---|---|---|
| | | | F. *Escherichia coli* preparation of L-asparaginase and *Erwinia carotovora* preparation are non-cross-resistant, so if an anaphylaxis reaction occurs with one, the other preparation may be used |
| II. *Altered nutrition, less than body requirements related to* A. Nausea and vomiting | II. A. 50–60% of pts experience mild to severe nausea and vomiting starting within 4–6 hrs after treatment | II. A. 1. Pt will be without nausea and vomiting 2. Nausea and vomiting if they occur, will be minimal | II. A. 1. Premedicate with antiemetics and continue prophylactically × 24 hrs to *prevent* nausea and vomiting 2. Encourage small, frequent feedings of cool, bland foods and liquids 3. Refer to sec. on nausea and vomiting, Chapter 4 |
| B. Anorexia | B. Commonly occurs | B. Pt will maintain baseline weight ± 5% | B. 1. Encourage small, frequent feedings of favorite foods, especially high-calorie, high-protein foods 2. Encourage use of spices 3. Weekly weights |
| C. Hyperglycemia | C. 1. Transient reaction caused by effects on the pancreas 2. ↓ insulin synthesis 3. Pancreatitis in 5% of pts | C. 1. Pt will be without s/s of hyperglycemia or pancreatitis 2. Early s/s of hyperglycemia or pancreatitis will be identified | C. 1. Teach pt the potential of hyperglycemia and pancreatitis and to report any unusual symptoms (i.e., increased thirst, urination, and appetite) 2. Monitor serum glucose, amylase, and lipase levels periodically during treatment 3. Report any laboratory elevations to MD 4. Treat hyperglycemia issues with diet or insulin as ordered by MD 5. Treat pancreatitis per MD orders |

| Nursing Diagnosis | Defining Characteristics | Expected Outcomes | Nursing Interventions |
|---|---|---|---|
| III. *Hepatic dysfunction or thromboembolic potential* | A. Two-thirds of pts have elevated LFTs starting within first 2 weeks of treatment (i.e., SGOT, bilirubin, alkaline phosphatase)<br>B. Hepatically derived clotting factors may be depressed, resulting in excessive bleeding or blood clotting; relatively uncommon | III. A. Hepatic dysfunction will be identified early | III. A. Monitor SGOT, bilirubin, alkaline phosphatase, albumin, and clotting factors—PT, PTT, fibrinogen<br>B. Teach pt the potential of excessive bleeding or blood clotting and to report any unusual symptoms<br>C. Assess pt for s/s of bleeding or thrombosis |
| IV. *Mental status alteration* | IV. A. 25% of pts experience some changes in mental status—commonly lethargy, drowsiness, and somnolence; rarely coma<br>B. Predominantly seen in adults<br>C. Malaise occurs in most pts and generally gets worse with subsequent doses<br>D. Drug does not cross blood-brain barrier | IV. A. Pt will be without changes in mental status (e.g., depression) | IV. A. Teach pt of the potential of CNS toxicity and to report any unusual symptoms<br>B. Obtain baseline neurologic and mental function<br>C. Assess pt for any neurologic abnormalities and report changes to MD<br>D. Discuss with pt the impact of malaise on his or her general sense of well-being and strategies to minimize distress |
| V. *Alteration in mobility related to soreness at injection site* | V. A. Pt may complain of sore muscle at injection site | V. A. Pt will not complain of altered mobility due to sore muscles | V. A. Rotate injection sites to decrease potential for soreness<br>B. Utilize standard nursing practice for IM injections |
| VI. *Infection, bleeding, and fatigue related to bone marrow depression* | VI. A. Bone marrow depression is not common<br>B. Mild anemia may occur<br>C. Serious leukopenia and thrombocytopenia are rare | VI. A. Pt will be without s/s of infection, bleeding, or anemia<br>B. Early s/s of infection, bleeding, or anemia will be identified | VI. A. Monitor CBC, platelet count prior to drug administration, as well as s/s of infection, bleeding, or anemia<br>B. Instruct pt in self-assessment of s/s of infection, bleeding, or anemia<br>C. Refer to sec. on bone marrow depression, Chapter 4 |
| VII. *Potential for sexual dysfunction* | VII. A. Drug is teratogenic | VII. A. Pt and significant other will understand need for contraception | VII. A. As appropriate, explore with pt and significant other issues of reproductive and sexual pattern<br>B. Discuss strategies to preserve sexuality and reproductive health (e.g., sperm banking, contraception)<br>C. See sec. on gonadal dysfunction, Chapter 4 |

# Leucovorin calcium
## (Folinic acid, Citrovorum factor)

*Class:* Water-soluble vitamin in the folate group (folinic acid)

## MECHANISM OF ACTION

Acts as an antidote for methotrexate and other folic acid antagonists. Circumvents the biochemical block of the enzyme inhibitors (e.g., dihydrofolate reductase [DHFR]) to permit DNA and RNA synthesis. Used as a potentiator of 5-FU, causes 5-FU to bind more tightly to thymidylate synthetase.

## METABOLISM

Metabolized primarily in the liver; 50% of the single dose is excreted in 6 hours in the urine (80–90% of dose) and stool (8% of dose).

## DOSAGE/RANGE

Dose of drug and duration of rescue is dependent on serum methotrexate levels.

| MTX Level | Leucovorin |
|---|---|
| $< 5.0(10)^{-7}$M | 10 mg/m² every 6 hours |
| $5(10)^{-7}$M to $5(10)^{-6}$M | 30–40 mg/m² every 6 hours |
| $> 5(10)^{-6}$M | 100 mg/m² every 3–6 hours |

Drug combinations/dosages are under investigation. The following are sample doses.

5-FU 370 mg/m²/day for 5 days continuous infusion. Leucovorin 500 mg/m²/day continuous infusion starting 24 hours before 5'-FU and continuing until 12 hours after

5-FU 600 mg/m² plus leucovorin 500 mg/m² weekly for 6 weeks

5-FU 350–500 mg/m² IVB over 2 hours with leucovorin 350–500 mg/m² IVP midway during infusion weekly for 6 weeks

5-FU 500 mg/m² qd × 5 plus leucovorin 200 mg/m² qd × 5

## DRUG PREPARATION

Drug is supplied in ampules·or vials. Reconstitute vials with sterile water for injection. Dilute reconstituted vials or ampules further with $D_5W$ or normal saline.

## DRUG ADMINISTRATION

Administer 24 hours after first methotrexate dose is begun. Dose every 6 hours for up to 12 doses.

First dose is given IV: others can be administered orally or IM.

IV doses are given via bolus over 15 minutes.

Doses must be given *exactly on time* in order to rescue normal cells from methotrexate toxicity.

## SPECIAL CONSIDERATIONS

It is imperative that the patient receive the leucovorin on schedule to avoid fatal methotrexate toxicity. Notify the physician if the patient is unable to take the dose orally, as it must then be given IV.

Usually free of side effects but allergic reaction and local pain may occur.

Drug metabolite may accumulate in CSF, thus decreasing effectiveness of intrathecal methotrexate.

## Leucovorin calcium


| Nursing Diagnosis | Defining Characteristics | Expected Outcomes | Nursing Interventions |
|---|---|---|---|
| I. *Potential for injury related to* | | | |
| A. Allergic reaction | I. A. Allergic sensitization has been reported: facial flushing, itching | I. A. 1. Pt will be without an allergic reaction 2. If allergic reaction occurs, it will be minimized | I. A. 1. Monitor pt for s/s of allergic reaction 2. Diphenhydramine is effective for relieving symptoms of allergic reaction |
| B. Drug interaction | B. Leucovorin in large amounts may counteract the antiepileptic effects of phenobarbital, phenytoin, and pyrimidone | B. Pt will maintain baseline neurological status | B. 1. Monitor pt for symptoms of increased seizure activity (if on antiepileptic drugs) 2. Monitor antiepileptic drug levels |
| II. *Altered nutrition, less than body requirements related to nausea and vomiting* | II. A. Oral leucovorin rarely causes nausea or vomiting | II. A. Pt will be without nausea and vomiting | II. A. Administer oral leucovorin with antacids or milk |

# Letrozole
## (Femara)

*Class:* Nonsteroidal aromatase inhibitor

## MECHANISM OF ACTION

Highly selective, potent agent which significantly suppresses (90%) serum estradiol levels within 14 days without interfering with other steroid hormone synthesis. Binds to the heme group of aromatasae, a cytochrome P450 enzyme necessary for the conversion of androgens to estrogens. Aromatase is thus inhibited, leading to a significant reduction in plasma estradiol, estrone, and estrone sulfate. After 6 weeks of therapy, there is 97% suppression of estradiol.

## METABOLISM

Rapidly and completely absorbed after oral administration, with a terminal half-life of 2 days. Metabolized in the liver and excreted in the urine.

## DOSAGE/RANGE

2.5 mg po qd

## PREPARATION/ADMINISTRATION

Oral

## DRUG INTERACTIONS

None known

## LAB EFFECTS/INTERFERENCE

Liver transaminases may be transiently elevated.

## SPECIAL CONSIDERATIONS

Indicated for the treatment of advanced breast cancer in postmenopausal women with disease progression following antiestrogen therapy.

Potent aromatase inhibitor with response rate of 20%.

Drug has not been evaluated in premenopausal women.

Glucocorticoid replacement is not necessary.

About 200 times more potent than aminoglutethamide.

## Letrozole

| Nursing Diagnosis | Defining Characteristics | Expected Outcomes | Nursing Interventions |
|---|---|---|---|
| I. *Alteration in comfort related to pain, fatigue, and hot flushes* | I. A. Most common side effects were musculoskeletal pain (21%: muscle, skeletal, back, arm, leg), arthralgia (8%), headache (9%), fatigue (8%) and chest pain (6%) <br> B. Hot flushes occur in approximately 6% of pts | I. A. Pt will be comfortable | I. A. Assess baseline comfort levels, and teach pt that this discomfort may occur <br> B. Teach pt symptomatic measures, and to report if symptoms are unrelieved |
| II. *Alteration in nutrition, less than body requirements related to nausea* | II. A. Nausea occurs in 13% of pts <br> B. Vomiting and anorexia less frequent | II. A. Pt will be without nausea | II. A. Determine baseline weight, and monitor at each visit <br> B. Teach pt that these side effects may occur, and to report this <br> C. Discuss strategies to minimize nausea, including diet and dosing time |
| III. *Alteration in bowel elimination related to diarrhea and constipation* | III. A. Diarrhea or constipation occur in about 6% of pts | III. A. Pt will have normal bowel elimination | III. A. Assess for change in bowel patterns, and teach pt to report diarrhea or constipation <br> B. Teach pt that diarrhea or constipation are usually relieved by nonprescription medications such as kaopectate for diarrhea, and stool softeners or metamucil for constipation <br> C. Teach pt to report unrelieved diarrhea or constipation |

# Leuprolide acetate
## (Lupron, Viadur)

*Class:* Antihormone

## MECHANISM OF ACTION

Is a luteinizing hormone-releasing hormone (LHRH) analogue that suppresses the secretion of follicle-stimulating hormone (FSH) and luteinizing hormone (LH) from the pituitary gland. The decrease in LH causes the Leydig cells to reduce testosterone production to castrate levels.

## METABOLISM

Metabolism and elimination characteristics of leuprolide in humans have not yet been fully elucidated. Several enzymes in the hypothalamus and anterior pituitary may be responsible for the metabolism of endogenous gonadotropin-releasing hormones and leuprolide may be metabolized in a similar way.

## DOSAGE/RANGE

For palliative treatment of prostate cancer: 1 mg/day subcutaneous (up to 20 mg/day have been used, but without clear clinical advantages)

Lupron depot (7.5 mg active drug)

## DRUG PREPARATION

Daily dose solution: use syringes provided by manufacturer. Solution should be inspected for particulate matter, discoloration. Store solution at room temperature.

Depot: add 1 ml of provided diluent to 7.5-mg vial, forming a milky suspension (stable for 24 hours).

## DRUG ADMINISTRATION

Give daily SQ (1 mg = 0.2 ml) dose.

Give monthly depot (7.5 mg) dose IM.

Give 12-month implant (65 mg) subcutaneously in inner aspect of upper arm.

## SPECIAL CONSIDERATIONS

Patient should be instructed in proper administration techniques and signs and symptoms of infection at site. Sites should be rotated. Daily SQ or monthly IM.

Initially, drug causes increased LH secretion, resulting in increased testosterone secretion and tumor flare. Usually disappears after 2 weeks.

Drug is active in metastatic breast and refractory ovarian cancer.

Viadur implant kit contains implant, implanter, and sterile field/supplies. Sterile gloves must be added.

Procedure is sterile and uses a special implant technology. Kit contains specific directions for insertion of implant, removal, and reinsertion after 1 year.

Leuprolide acetate

| Nursing Diagnosis | Defining Characteristics | Expected Outcomes | Nursing Interventions |
|---|---|---|---|
| I. *Altered nutrition, less than body requirements related to*<br><br>A. Anorexia | I. A. Causes decreased appetite (< 5%)<br><br>B. May occur (< 5%) | I. A. Pt will maintain baseline weight ± 5%<br><br>B. 1. Pt will be without nausea and vomiting<br>2. Nausea and vomiting, should they occur, will be minimal | I. A. 1. Encourage small, frequent feedings of favorite foods, especially high-calorie, high-protein foods<br>2. Encourage use of spices<br>3. Monitor weight weekly<br><br>B. 1. Inform pt of possibility of nausea and vomiting<br>2. Obtain order or prescription for antiemetic if necessary<br>3. Encourage small feedings of cool, bland foods<br>4. Refer to sec. on nausea and vomiting, Chapter 4 |
| | B. Nausea and vomiting | | |
| II. *Alteration in comfort* | II. A. Hot flashes may occur in 50% of men; headache, dizziness may occur<br>B. Tumor "flare" may occur initially in 10% of pts (bone and tumor pain, transient increase in tumor size) due to transient ↑ in testosterone levels<br>C. Breast tenderness has been reported<br>D. Peripheral edema may occur (8%) | II. A. Pt will be without headache, hot flashes, pain<br>B. Discomfort will be identified and treated early | II. A. Inform pt that symptoms may occur and that "flare" reaction will subside after the initial 2 weeks of therapy<br>B. Encourage pt to report symptoms early; administer analgesics as needed |
| III. *Potential for sexual dysfunction* | III. A. In men, frequently causes decreased libido and erectile impotence (2%)<br>B. Gynecomastia may occur (3%)<br>C. In women, amenorrhea occurs after 10 weeks of therapy | III. A. Pt and significant other will verbalize understanding of changes in sexuality that may occur<br>B. Pt and significant other will identify strategies to cope with sexual dysfunction | III. A. As appropriate, explore with pt and significant other issues of reproductive and sexual patterns and impact chemotherapy may have on them<br>B. Discuss strategies to preserve sexuality and reproductive health<br>C. See sec. on gonadal dysfunction, Chapter 4 |

# Levamisole hydrochloride
(Ergamisol)

*Class:* Antihelminthic agent

## MECHANISM OF ACTION

Nonspecific immunomodulating agent that appears to restore immune function; when given in combination with 5-fluorouracil, has antiproliferative activity against small metastatic lesions in the colon.

## METABOLISM

Rapidly absorbed from the GI tract, with an elimination half-life of 3–4 hours. Extensively metabolized by liver, and metabolites are excreted by kidneys (70% by 3 days).

## DOSAGE/RANGE

Adjuvant chemotherapy with 5-fluorouracil (5-FU) for Duke's C colon cancer.

Initial therapy: 50 mg po q 8 hrs × 3 days, starting 7–30 days postop; with 5-FU 450 mg/m$^2$/day IV × 5 days (concomitant with a 3–day course of levamisole, starting 21–34 days postsurgery).

Maintenance therapy: 50 mg po q 8 hrs × 3 days q 2 weeks × 1 year; 5-FU 450 mg/m$^2$ IV q week × 48 weeks, beginning 28 days after initiation of 5-day course.

Dose is held for stomatitis, diarrhea, and leukopenia. Dose is reduced 20% if symptoms are moderate or severe.

## DRUG PREPARATION

Available as 50-mg tablets

## DRUG ADMINISTRATION

Oral

## SPECIAL CONSIDERATIONS

Drug interactions: alcohol can cause disulfiram-like reaction when taken concurrently. When given together with 5-FU, may increase phenytoin serum levels.

5-FU with levamisole in Duke's C colon cancer: reduces risk of recurrence by 41% and risk of death by 33%.

Much of reported toxicity is due to 5-FU.

May cause agranulocytosis.

# Levamisole hydrochloride

| Nursing Diagnosis | Defining Characteristics | Expected Outcomes | Nursing Interventions |
|---|---|---|---|
| I. *Alteration in nutrition, less than body requirements related to* | | | |
| A. Nausea and vomiting | I. A. Usually mild and preventable with antiemetics; incidence 20–65%; nausea more common | I. A. 1. Pt will be without nausea and vomiting<br>2. Nausea and vomiting, if they occur, will be mild<br>3. Pt will maintain weight within 5% of baseline | I. A. 1. Premedicate with antiemetics prior to drug administration and postchemotherapy PRN<br>2. Encourage small, frequent feedings of cool, bland foods and liquids<br>3. Assess for symptoms of fluid/electrolyte imbalance if pt has severe nausea and vomiting<br>4. Monitor I&O, daily weights, lab electrolyte values<br>5. Refer to sec. on nausea and vomiting, Chapter 4 |
| B. Diarrhea | B. Incidence 52%; indication to interrupt or hold therapy; reduce dose if moderate to severe | B. Pt will have minimal diarrhea | B. 1. Encourage pt to report onset of diarrhea<br>2. Administer or teach pt to self-administer antidiarrheal medication<br>3. Refer to sec. on diarrhea, Chapter 4 |
| C. Stomatitis | C. Uncommon but requires interruption of therapy or dose reduction if moderate to severe | C. Oral mucous membranes will remain infection-free | C. 1. Assess baseline oral mucous membranes<br>2. Teach pt oral care and to report any alterations<br>3. Refer to sec. on mucositis, Chapter 4 |
| D. Anorexia | D. Incidence 5% | D. Anorexia will be minimized, pt will maintain weight within 5% of baseline | D. 1. Encourage small, frequent feedings of favorite foods, especially high-calorie, high-protein foods<br>2. Monitor or have pt monitor weekly weights |

*(continued)*

## Levamisole hydrochloride (continued)

| Nursing Diagnosis | Defining Characteristics | Expected Outcomes | Nursing Interventions |
|---|---|---|---|
| II. *Infection and bleeding related to bone marrow depression* | II. A. Bone marrow depression most likely due to 5-FU; uncommon<br><br>B. Agranulocytosis may occur and may be preceded by fever, chills | II. A. Pt will be without s/s of infection or bleeding<br><br>B. Early s/s of infection or bleeding will be identified | II. A. Monitor CBC, platelet count prior to drug administration and postchemotherapy; assess for s/s of infection or bleeding<br><br>B. Teach pt self-assessment of s/s of infection or bleeding and to seek medical advice/care<br><br>C. Teach pt self-care measures to reduce risk of infection and bleeding<br><br>D. Expect the following:<br>1. Hold 5-FU if WBC < 3500/mm$^3$<br>2. Hold 5-FU and levamisole if platelets < 100,000/mm$^3$<br>3. Reduce dose 20% if 5-FU nadir < 2500/mm$^3$<br><br>E. Refer to sec. on bone marrow depression, Chapter 4 |
| III. *Potential impairment of skin integrity related to*<br><br>A. Rash | III. A. Incidence 23% and may be pruritic | III. A. Pt will verbally report skin rash and describe self-care measures | III. A. 1. Assess skin for any cutaneous changes, such as rash, and any associated symptoms, such as pruritis; discuss with MD<br>2. Instruct pt in self-care measures<br>a. Avoiding abrasive skin products, clothing<br>b. Avoiding tight-fitting clothing<br>c. Use of skin emollients appropriate for skin alteration<br>d. Measures to avoid scratching involved areas |

| | | | |
|---|---|---|---|
| B. Alopecia | B. Incidence 22% | B. Pt will verbalize feelings re hair loss and strategies to cope with change in body image | B. 1. Discuss potential impact of hair loss with pt prior to drug administration; include coping strategies and plan to minimize body image change (e.g., wig, scarf, cap)<br>2. Assess pt for s/s of hair loss<br>3. Assess pt's response and use of coping strategies |
| IV. *Potential for sensory/ perceptual alterations related to neurotoxicity* | IV. A. Dizziness, headaches, paresthesias, ataxia, taste perversion, altered sense of smell (4–8%)<br>B. Somnolence, depression, insomnia (2%) | IV. A. Early s/s of neurological toxicity will be identified<br>B. Function will be maintained | IV. A. Assess baseline neurological and mental function and reassess prior to drug infusion<br>B. Teach pt to report any changes in sensation or function<br>C. Discuss alterations with MD<br>D. Identify strategies to promote pt comfort and safety |

# Lomustine
(CCNU, CeeNU)

*Class:* Alkylating agent (nitrosourea)

## MECHANISM OF ACTION

Nitrosourea alkylates DNA with a reactive chloroethyl carbonium ion, producing strand breaks and cross-links that inhibit RNA and DNA synthesis. Interferes with enzymes and histadine utilization. Is cell cycle phase–nonspecific.

## METABOLISM

Completely absorbed from gastrointestinal tract. Metabolized rapidly, partly protein bound. Undergoes hepatic recirculation. Lipid soluble; crosses blood-brain barrier; 75% excreted in urine within 4 days.

## DOSAGE/RANGE

100–300 mg/m$^2$ orally every 6 weeks

## DRUG PREPARATION

Available in 10-mg, 30-mg, and 100-mg capsules

## DRUG ADMINISTRATION

Oral

## SPECIAL CONSIDERATIONS

Give orally at bedtime, on empty stomach.

Consumption of alcohol should be avoided for a short period after taking CCNU.

Absorbed 30–60 minutes after administration. Therefore, vomiting usually does not affect efficacy.

## Lomustine

| Nursing Diagnosis | Defining Characteristics | Expected Outcomes | Nursing Interventions |
|---|---|---|---|
| I. Infection and bleeding related to myelosuppression | I. A. Nadir: platelets— 26–34 days, lasting 6–10 days; WBC—41–46 days, lasting 9–14 days<br>B. Delayed and cumulative bone marrow depression with successive dosing; recovery 6–8 weeks<br>C. Bone marrow depression is dose-limiting toxicity | I. A. Pt will be without infection or bleeding<br>B. Early s/s of infection and bleeding will be identified | I. A. Drug should be administered every 6–8 weeks due to delayed nadir and recovery<br>B. Monitor CBC, platelets prior to drug administration (WBC > 4000/mm$^3$ and platelets > 100,000/mm$^3$)<br>C. Dispense only *one* dose at a time<br>D. See sec. on bone marrow depression, Chapter 4 |
| II. Alteration in nutrition, less than body requirements related to | | | |
| A. Nausea and vomiting | II. A. Onset 2–6 hrs after taking dose; may be severe | II. A. Nausea and vomiting will be minimized or prevented | II. A. 1. Administer drug on an empty stomach at bedtime<br>2. Premedicate with antiemetic and sedative or hypnotic to promote sleep<br>3. Discourage food or fluid intake for 2 hrs after drug administration<br>4. Refer to sec. on nausea and vomiting, Chapter 4 |
| B. Anorexia | B. May last for several days | B. Pt will maintain weight ± 5% of baseline | B. 1. Encourage small, frequent feedings of favorite foods<br>2. Encourage high-calorie, high-protein foods<br>3. Weekly weights |
| C. Diarrhea | C. Occurs infrequently | C. Pt will have minimal diarrhea | C. 1. Encourage pt to report onset of diarrhea<br>2. Administer or teach pt to self-administer antidiarrheal medication<br>3. See sec. on diarrhea, Chapter 4 |

*(continued)*

## Lomustine (continued)

| Nursing Diagnosis | Defining Characteristics | Expected Outcomes | Nursing Interventions |
|---|---|---|---|
| II. D. Stomatitis | II. D. Occurs infrequently | II. D. Oral mucous membranes will remain intact and without infection | II. D. 1. Teach pt oral assessment and mouth care<br>2. Encourage pt to report early stomatitis<br>3. See sec. on stomatitis, mucositis, Chapter 4 |
| E. Hepatic dysfunction | E. Transient reversible elevations in liver function studies may occur | E. Hepatic dysfunction will be identified early | E. Monitor SGOT, SGPT, LDH, alkaline phosphatase, and bilirubin; notify MD of elevations |
| III. Activity intolerance | III. A. Neurologic dysfunction may occur rarely: confusion, lethargy, disorientation, ataxia | III. A. Neurologic dysfunction will be identified early | III. A. Perform neurologic assessment as part of prechemotherapy assessment<br>B. Assess orientation and level of consciousness, gait, activity tolerance |
| IV. Altered urinary elimination | IV. A. After prolonged therapy with high cumulative doses, tubular atrophy, glomerular sclerosis, and interstitial nephritis have occurred, leading to renal failure | IV. A. Early renal dysfunction will be identified | IV. A. Monitor BUN, creatinine prior to dosing, especially in pts receiving prolonged or high cumulative dose therapy<br>B. If abnormalities are noted, a creatinine clearance should be determined |
| V. Sensory/perceptual alterations (visual) | V. A. Ocular damage may occur rarely: optic neuritis, retinopathy, blurred vision | V. A. Visual disturbances will be identified early | V. A. Assess vision during prechemotherapy assessment<br>B. Encourage pt to report any visual changes |
| VI. Potential for sexual dysfunction related to mutagenic and teratogenic qualities of CCNU | VI. A. Drug is teratogenic, mutagenic, and carcinogenic | VI. A. Pt and significant other will understand the need for contraception | VI. A. As appropriate, discuss birth control measures<br>B. See sec. on gonadal dysfunction, Chapter 4 |
| VII. Body image disturbance related to alopecia (rare) | VII. A. Alopecia is rare but may occur | VII. A. Pt will verbalize feelings re hair loss and strategies to cope with change in body image | VII. A. Assess pt for hair loss<br>B. Discuss with pt impact of hair loss and obtaining wig or alternative<br>C. See sec. on alopecia, Chapter 4 |

# Mechlorethamine hydrochloride
(Nitrogen Mustard, Mustargen, HN$_2$)

*Class:* Alkylating agent

## MECHANISM OF ACTION

Produces interstrand and intrastrand cross-linkages in DNA, causing miscoding, breakage, and failures of replication. Is cell cycle phase–nonspecific.

## METABOLISM

Undergoes chemical transformation after injection, with less than 0.01% excreted unchanged in urine. Drug is rapidly inactivated by body fluids; 50% of the inactive metabolites are excreted in the urine within 24 hours.

## DOSAGE/RANGE

IV: 0.4 mg/kg *or* 12–16 mg/m$^2$ IV as single agent; 6 mg/m$^2$ IV days 1 and 8 of 28-day cycle with MOPP regimen

Topical: dilute 10 mg in 60 ml sterile water; apply with rubber gloves

Intracavitary (pleural, peritoneal, pericardial): 0.2–0.4 mg/kg

## DRUG PREPARATION

Add sterile water or NS to each vial.

Drug must be used within 15 minutes of reconstitution.

## DRUG ADMINISTRATION

Intravenous. This drug is a *potent vesicant*. Give through a freely running IV to avoid extravasation, which can lead to ulceration, pain, and necrosis. Check hospital's policy and procedure for administration of a vesicant.

## SPECIAL CONSIDERATIONS

Drug is a *vesicant*. Give through a running IV to avoid extravasation. *Antidote* is sodium thiosulfate (dilute 4 ml sodium thiosulfate injection, USP [10%] with 6 ml sterile water of injection, USP and inject subcutaneously in area of infiltration).

Nadir is 6–8 days after treatment.

Side effects occur in the reproductive system, such as amenorrhea and azoospermia.

Severe nausea and vomiting.

Systemic toxic effects may occur with intracavitary drug administration.

## Mechlorethamine hydrochloride

| Nursing Diagnosis | Defining Characteristics | Expected Outcomes | Nursing Interventions |
|---|---|---|---|
| I. *Altered nutrition, less than body requirements related to* | | | |
| A. Nausea and vomiting | I. A. 1. Occurs in ~100% of pts<br>2. Within 30 mins to 2 hrs of drug administration and up to 8 hrs after<br>3. Can be severe | I. A. 1. Pt will be without nausea and vomiting<br>2. Nausea and vomiting, if they occur, will be minimal | I. A. 1. Premedicate with antiemetics and continue prophylactically<br>2. Antiemetic and sedative may need to be started evening before if pt develops anticipatory nausea and vomiting<br>3. Encourage small, frequent feedings of cool, bland foods, dry toast, crackers<br>4. Monitor I&O to detect fluid volume deficit<br>5. Notify MD for more aggressive antiemetic if vomitus ≥ 750 cc<br>6. Refer to sec. on nausea and vomiting, Chapter 4 |
| B. Anorexia, taste distortion (metallic taste) | B. Taste alterations contribute to the anorexia that pts experience | B. Pt will maintain baseline weight ± 5% | B. 1. Encourage small, frequent feedings of favorite foods, especially high-calorie high-protein foods<br>2. Encourage use of spices<br>3. Weekly weights |
| C. Diarrhea | C. May occur up to several days after drug administration | C. Pt will have minimal diarrhea | C. 1. Encourage pt to report onset of diarrhea<br>2. Administer or teach pt to self-administer antidiarrheal medication<br>3. Diet modifications<br>4. Refer to sec. on diarrhea, Chapter 4 |
| D. Stomatitis | D. Occurs rarely | D. Oral mucous membrane will remain intact and without infection | D. 1. Teach pt oral assessment and mouth care<br>2. Perform oral assessment prior to drug administration<br>3. Encourage pt to report early stomatitis<br>4. See sec. on stomatitis, mucositis, Chapter 4 |

| Nursing Diagnosis | Defining Characteristics | Expected Outcomes | Nursing Interventions |
|---|---|---|---|
| II. *Infection and bleeding related to bone marrow depression* | II. A. Potent myelosuppressant<br>B. Nadir 6–8 days, with recovery in 4 weeks<br>C. Pts at risk for profound BMD are those with previous extensive XRT, previous chemotherapy, or compromised bone marrow function<br>D. Lymphocyte depression occurs within 24 hrs of drug dose | II. A. Pt will be without s/s of infection or bleeding<br>B. Early s/s of infection or bleeding will be identified | II. A. Monitor CBC, platelet count prior to drug administration; assess for s/s of infection or bleeding<br>B. Instruct pt in self-assessment of s/s of infection or bleeding<br>C. Refer to sec. on bone marrow depression, Chapter 4 |
| III. *Impaired skin integrity related to*<br>A. Alopecia | III. A. Usually occurs as diffuse thinning | III. A. Pt will verbalize feelings re hair loss and identify strategies to cope with change in body image | III. A. 1. Discuss with pt anticipated impact of hair loss; suggest wig as appropriate prior to actual hair loss<br>2. Explore with pt response to actual hair loss and plan strategies to minimize distress (e.g., wig, scarf, cap)<br>3. Refer to sec. on alopecia, Chapter 4 |
| B. Extravasation | B. 1. Drug is a *potent vesicant*, causing tissue necrosis and sloughing if extravasation occurs<br>2. Thrombosis or thrombophlebitis may occur despite all precautions, and venous access device may be required | B. 1. Extravasation will not occur<br>2. If extravasation occurs, tissue damage will be minimal | B. 1. Use careful technique during venipuncture; see sec. on intravenous administration, Chapter 10<br>2. Administer vesicant through freely flowing IV, constantly monitoring IV site and pt response<br>3. Nurse should be *thoroughly* familiar with institutional policy and procedure for administration of a vesicant agent |

*(continued)*

## Mechlorethamine hydrochloride (continued)

| Nursing Diagnosis | Defining Characteristics | Expected Outcomes | Nursing Interventions |
|---|---|---|---|
| | | | 4. If extravasation is suspected: |
| | | |   a. Stop drug administered |
| | | |   b. Aspirate any residual drug and blood from IV tubing, IV catheter/needle, and IV site if possible |
| | | |   c. Instill antidote into area of apparent infiltration—sodium thiosulfate (1/6 M)—as per MD order and institutional policy and procedure |
| | | |   d. Apply cold or topical medication as per MD order and institutional policy and procedure |
| | | | 5. Assess site regularly for pain, progression of erythema, induration, and evidence of necrosis |
| | | | 6. When in doubt about whether drug is infiltrating, *treat as an infiltration* |
| | | | 7. Teach pt to assess site and notify MD if condition worsens |
| | | | 8. Arrange next clinic visit for assessment of site depending on drug, amount infiltrated, extent of potential injury, and pt variables |
| | | | 9. Document in pt's record as per institutional policy and procedure; see sec. on reactions, Chapter 9 |
| | | | 10. *Consider* venous access device if peripheral veins are difficult to access |

| | | | |
|---|---|---|---|
| | | | 11. Warm packs may decrease discomfort of phlebitis<br>12. Have standing orders and sodium thiosulfate injection, USP (10%) close by in the event of actual infiltration of drug; dilute sodium thiosulfate with sterile water for injection and inject subcutaneously in area of infiltration |
| C. Skin eruptions | C. Maculopapular rash (rare) | C. Skin discomfort will be minimized, and skin will remain intact | C. 1. This is not an indication to stop the drug<br>2. Discuss with MD symptomatic management |
| D. Delayed cutaneous hypersensitivity | D. Is seen with topical application | D. Skin will be monitored for delayed cutaneous hypersensitivity | D. 1. This is not an indication to stop the drug<br>2. Discuss with MD symptomatic management |
| IV. *Alteration in comfort related to chills, fever, diarrhea* | IV. A. May occur immediately after drug administration<br>B. Also weakness, drowsiness, headache may occur | IV. A. Pt will verbalize discomfort | IV. A. Assess pt for these symptoms during hour following treatment<br>B. Instruct pt to report these symptoms and teach self-management at home if outpatient<br>C. Provide symptomatic management per MD with acetaminophen, antidiarrheal medication |
| V. *Potential for sexual dysfunction* | V. A. Drug is teratogenic, carcinogenic<br>B. Amenorrhea occurs in females<br>C. Impaired spermatogenesis occurs in males<br>D. If administered to pregnant pt, spontaneous abortion or fetal abnormalities may occur | V. A. Pt and significant other will understand need for contraception<br>B. Pt and significant other will identify strategies to cope with sexual dysfunction | V. A. As appropriate, explore with pt and significant other issues of reproductive and sexual pattern, and anticipated impact chemotherapy will have<br>B. Discuss strategies to preserve sexuality and reproductive health (sperm banking, contraception, etc.)<br>C. Refer to sec. on gonadal dysfunction, Chapter 4 |

*(continued)*

## Mechlorethamine hydrochloride *(continued)*

| Nursing Diagnosis | Defining Characteristics | Expected Outcomes | Nursing Interventions |
|---|---|---|---|
| VI. *Sensory/perceptual alterations related to*<br>A. Tinnitus, deafness | VI. A. Tinnitus, deafness, and other signs of eighth cranial nerve damage occur *rarely*, especially with high drug doses or regional perfusion techniques | VI. A. Hearing problems will be identified early | VI. A. 1. Assess hearing ability, presence of tinnitus prior to drug doses<br>2. If high doses of drug are given, or regional perfusion used, schedule pt for periodic audiometry<br>3. Instruct pt to report s/s of hearing loss |
| B. Temporary aphasia and paresis | B. Occur very rarely | B. Sensory and perceptual changes will be identified early | B. Refer to sec. on neurotoxicity, Chapter 4 |
| VII. *Potential for injury related to severe allergic reactions or anaphylaxis* | VII. A. Occur rarely | VII. A. Allergic reaction or anaphylaxis will be detected early<br>B. Airway will remain patent<br>C. Systolic BP will remain within 20 mmHg of baseline | VII. A. Review standing orders for management of pt in anaphylaxis and identify location of anaphylaxis kit containing epinephrine 1:1000, hydrocortisone sodium succinate (SoluCortef) diphenhydramine HCI (Benadryl), Aminophylline, and others<br>B. Prior to drug administration, obtain baseline vital signs and record mental status<br>C. Observe for following s/s during infusion, usually occurring within first 15 mins of start of infusion:<br>1. *Subjective*<br>a. generalized itching<br>b. nausea<br>c. chest tightness<br>d. crampy abdominal pain<br>e. difficulty speaking<br>f. anxiety<br>g. agitation<br>h. sense of impending doom<br>i. uneasiness<br>j. desire to urinate or defecate |

k. dizziness

l. chills

2. *Objective*

a. flushed appearance (angioedema of face, neck, eyelids, hands, feet)

b. localized or generalized urticaria

c. respiratory distress ± wheezing

d. hypotension

e. cyanosis

D. Stop infusion and notify MD

E. Place pt in supine position to promote perfusion of visceral organs

F. Monitor vital signs until stable

G. Provide emotional reassurance to pt and family

H. Maintain patent airway and have CPR equipment ready if needed

I. Document incident

J. Discuss with MD desensitization versus drug discontinuance for further dosing

# Melphalan
## (Alkeran, L-PAM, Phenylalanine Mustard, L-sarcolysin)

*Class:* Alkylating agent

## MECHANISM OF ACTION

Prevents cell replication by causing breaks and cross-linkages in DNA strands, with subsequent miscoding and breakage. Is cell cycle phase nonspecific. Drug is derivative of nitrogen mustard.

## METABOLISM

Variable bioavailability after oral administration, especially if taken with food. Therefore, dose is titrated to WBC count; 20–50% of drug is excreted in feces over 6 days, 50% excreted in urine within 24 hours. After IV administration, parent compound disappears from plasma, with a half-life of about 2 hours.

## DOSAGE/RANGE

6 mg/m² orally daily × 5 days every 6 weeks for myeloma
*or*
0.1 mg/kg orally × 2–3 weeks, then maintenance of 2–4 mg daily when bone marrow has recovered
8 mg/m² IV daily × 5 days (experimental)

## DRUG PREPARATION

Oral: available in 2-mg tablets.
IV: dilute reconstituted vial in D₅W. Administer over 30–45 minutes.

## DRUG ADMINISTRATION

Serious hypersensitivity reactions reported with IV.
Take oral preparation on an empty stomach.
IV infusion should be given in 100–150 ml of D₅W or NS over 15–30 minutes.

## SPECIAL CONSIDERATIONS

Nadir 14–21 days after treatment.
Increased risk of nephrotoxicity when given with cyclosporine.
Doses used in bone marrow transplant are 140–200 mg/m².
Drug is used experimentally in regional perfusion.
Drug dose reduction recommended in patients with renal compromise.
Drug activity enhanced with concurrent administration of misonidazol (investigational).

# Melphalan

| Nursing Diagnosis | Defining Characteristics | Expected Outcomes | Nursing Interventions |
|---|---|---|---|
| I. *Infection and bleeding related to bone marrow depression* | I. A. Bone marrow depression may be pronounced<br>B. Leukopenia and thrombocytopenia 14–21 days after intermittent dosing schedules<br>C. May be delayed in onset and cumulative, with nadir extended to 5–6 weeks<br>D. Combined immunosuppression from disease (i.e., multiple myeloma) and drug may prolong vulnerability to infection<br>E. Thrombocytopenia may be persistent | I. A. Pt will be without s/s of infection or bleeding<br>B. Early s/s of infection or bleeding will be identified early | I. A. Monitor CBC, platelets prior to drug administration, and assess for s/s of infection or bleeding<br>B. Hold drug if WBC $< 3000/mm^3$ or platelet count $< 100,000/mm^3$; discuss with MD<br>C. Teach pt self-assessment techniques and self-care measures to minimize risk of infection and bleeding<br>D. Refer to sec. on bone marrow depression, Chapter 4 |
| II. *Altered nutrition, less than body requirements related to*<br>A. Nausea and vomiting | II. A. Mild at low, continuous dosing; severe following high doses | II. A. 1. Pt will be without nausea and vomiting<br>2. Nausea and vomiting, if they occur, will be minimal | II. A. 1. Administer drug (oral) on empty stomach<br>2. Premedicate with antiemetic (oral) 1 hr before oral dose<br>3. Use aggressive antiemetic regimen for IV Alkeran<br>4. Refer to sec. on nausea and vomiting, Chapter 4 |
| B. Anorexia | B. Occurs rarely | B. Pt will maintain baseline weight ± 5% | B. 1. Encourage small, frequent feedings of favorite foods, especially high-calorie, high-protein foods<br>2. Encourage use of spices<br>3. Weekly weights |
| C. Stomatitis | C. Infrequent occurrence (rare) | C. Oral mucous membrane will remain intact and without infection | C. 1. Teach pt oral assessment<br>2. Assess oral mucosa prior to drug administration<br>3. Encourage pt to report (early) stomatitis<br>4. Refer to sec. on stomatitis, Chapter 4 |

*(continued)*

## Melphalan (continued)

| Nursing Diagnosis | Defining Characteristics | Expected Outcomes | Nursing Interventions |
|---|---|---|---|
| III. *Impaired skin integrity related to alopecia, maculopapular rash, urticaria* | III. A. Alopecia is minimal, if it occurs at all<br>B. Maculopapular rash and urticaria are infrequent | III. A. Pt will develop strategy to manage distress associated with skin side effects | III. A. Assess skin integrity and presence of rash, urticaria, alopecia prior to dosing<br>B. Assess impact of these alterations on pt and develop plan to manage symptom distress |
| IV. *Potential for impaired gas exchange related to pulmonary toxicity* | IV. A. Rare but may occur, especially with continued chronic dosing<br>B. Bronchopulmonary dysplasia and pulmonary fibrosis | IV. A. Early s/s of pulmonary toxicity will be identified | IV. A. Assess pulmonary status for s/s of pulmonary dysfunction<br>B. Assess lung sounds prior to dosing<br>C. Instruct pt to report cough or dyspnea<br>D. Discuss pulmonary function studies to be performed periodically with MD |
| V. *Potential for injury related to*<br>A. Second malignancy | V. A. 1. Acute myelogenous and myelomonocytic leukemias may occur after continuous long-term dosing<br>2. Especially in pts with ovarian cancer and multiple myeloma<br>3. Heralded by preleukemic pancytopenia of several weeks' duration<br>4. Chromosomal abnormalities characteristic of acute leukemia | V. A. Malignancy, if it occurs, will be identified early | V. A. Pts receiving prolonged continuous therapy should be closely followed during and after treatment |
| B. Drug infiltration when given IV | B. Painful burning can occur | B. Drug infiltration will not occur | B. Drug administration technique should be meticulous; refer to sec. on intravenous administration, Chapter 10 |

C. Anaphylaxis and hypersensitivity reactions

C. Severe hypersensitivity reactions can occur with IV administration, including diaphoresis, hypotension, and cardiac arrest

C. 1. Hypersensitivity reactions will be detected early
2. Airway will be patent
3. BP will remain within 20 mmHg of baseline
4. Anaphylaxis, if it occurs, will be detected early

C. 1. Review standing orders for management of pt in anaphylaxis and identify location of anaphylaxis kit containing epinephrine 1:1000, hydrocortisone sodium succinate (SoluCortef), diphenhydramine HCl (Benadryl), Aminophylline, and others
2. Prior to drug administration, obtain baseline vital signs and record mental status
3. Administer drug slowly, diluted as per MD order
4. Observe for following s/s, usually occurring within first 15 mins of infusion
   a. *Subjective*
      (1) generalized itching
      (2) nausea
      (3) chest tightness
      (4) crampy abdominal pain
      (5) difficulty speaking
      (6) anxiety
      (7) agitation
      (8) sense of impending doom
      (9) uneasiness
      (10) desire to urinate/defecate
      (11) dizziness
      (12) chills

*(continued)*

## Melphalan (continued)

| Nursing Diagnosis | Defining Characteristics | Expected Outcomes | Nursing Interventions |
|---|---|---|---|
| | | | b. *Objective*<br>  (1) flushed appearance (angioedema of face, neck, eyelids, hands, feet)<br>  (2) localized or generalized urticaria<br>  (3) respiratory distress ± wheezing<br>  (4) hypotension<br>  (5) cyanosis<br>5. For generalized allergic reaction, stop infusion and notify MD<br>6. Place pt in supine position to promote perfusion of visceral organs<br>7. Monitor vital signs<br>8. Provide emotional reassurance to pt and family<br>9. Maintain patent airway and have CPR equipment ready if needed<br>10. Document incident<br>11. Discuss with MD desensitization versus drug discontinuance for further dosing |
| VI. *Potential for sexual dysfunction* | VI. A. Potentially mutagenic and teratogenic | VI. A. Pt and significant other will understand potential sexual dysfunction | VI. A. Encourage pt to verbalize goals re family and discuss options, such as sperm banking<br>B. As appropriate, discuss or refer for counseling re birth control measures during therapy<br>C. Refer to sec. on gonadal dysfunction, Chapter 4 |

# 6-Mercaptopurine
(Purinethol, 6-MP)

*Class:* Antimetabolite

## MECHANISM OF ACTION

One of two thiopurine antimetabolites (with 6-TG) that are converted to monophosphate nucleotides and inhibit de novo purine synthesis. The nucleotides are also incorporated into DNA. Cell cycle phase specific (S phase).

## METABOLISM

Metabolized by the enzyme xanthine oxidase in the kidney and liver. Because xanthine oxidase is inhibited by allopurinol, concurrent use of the latter necessitates a dose reduction of 6-MP to one-fourth the normal dose. Fifty percent of the drug is excreted in the urine. Plasma half-life: 20–40 minutes.

## DOSAGE/RANGE

100 mg/m$^2$ orally daily × 5 days

Children: 70 mg/m$^2$ daily for induction, then 40 mg/m$^2$ daily for maintenance

IV use is investigational.

## DRUG PREPARATION

Oral: available in 50-mg tablets.

IV: reconstitute 500 mg vial with sterile water for concentration of 10 mg/ml.

Store IV solution at room temperature; discard after 8 hours.

## DRUG ADMINISTRATION

IV use is investigational; consult protocol.

## SPECIAL CONSIDERATIONS

Elevated serum glucose levels and elevated serum uric acid levels could be related to the effects of medication.

Patients receiving allopurinol concurrently may require dosage reduction due to xanthine oxidase inhibition.

When given with nondepolarizing muscle relaxants, there is decreased neuromuscular blockade.

When given with warfarin, there is a decreased hypothrombinemic effect.

Reduce dose in cases of hepatic or renal dysfunction.

## 6-Mercaptopurine

| Nursing Diagnosis | Defining Characteristics | Expected Outcomes | Nursing Interventions |
|---|---|---|---|
| I. *Altered nutrition, less than body requirements related to* | | | I. A. |
| A. Nausea and vomiting | I. A. Uncommon; mild when they occur | I. A. 1. Pt will be without nausea and vomiting<br>2. Nausea and vomiting, if they occur, will be minimal | 1. Consider premedicating with antiemetics for first dose<br>2. Encourage small, frequent feedings of cool, bland foods and liquids<br>3. Assess for symptoms of fluid/electrolyte imbalance if pt's vomiting is significant<br>4. Monitor I&O, daily weights; check lab results<br>5. Refer to sec. on nausea and vomiting, Chapter 4 |
| B. Anorexia | B. Infrequent; mild | B. Pt will maintain baseline weight ± 5% | B. 1. Encourage small, frequent feedings of favorite foods, especially high-calorie, high-protein foods<br>2. Encourage use of spices |
| C. Stomatitis | C. Uncommon; appears as white patchy areas similar to thrush | C. Oral mucous membranes will remain intact and without infection | C. 1. Teach oral assessment and mouth care regimen<br>2. Encourage pt to report early stomatitis<br>3. Provide pain relief measures if indicated<br>4. Refer to sec. on stomatitis, Chapter 4 |
| D. Diarrhea | D. Occurs occasionally; mild | D. Pt will have minimal diarrhea | D. 1. Encourage pt to report onset of diarrhea<br>2. Administer or teach pt to self-administer antidiarrheal medication<br>3. Guaiac all stools<br>4. If diarrhea is protracted, ensure adequate hydration, monitor I&O and electrolytes, and teach hygiene to pt<br>5. Refer to sec. on diarrhea, Chapter 4 |

| Nursing Diagnosis | | Expected Outcomes | Interventions |
|---|---|---|---|
| E. Hepatotoxicity | E. <br> 1. Reversible cholestatic jaundice may develop after 2–5 months of treatment <br> 2. Hepatic necrosis may develop | E. Early hepatotoxicity will be identified | E. <br> 1. Monitor SGOT, SGPT, LDH, alkaline phosphatase, and bilirubin periodically during treatment <br> 2. Notify MD of any elevations <br> 3. Hepatotoxicity may be an indication for discontinuing treatment |
| II. *Potential for infection and bleeding related to bone marrow depression* | II. <br> A. Nadir varies from 5 days to 6 weeks after treatment <br> B. Leukopenia more prominent than thrombocytopenia <br> C. Blood counts may continue to fall after therapy is stopped | II. <br> A. Pt will be without s/s of infection or bleeding <br> B. Early s/s of infection or bleeding will be identified | II. <br> A. Monitor CBC, platelet count prior to drug administration, as well as s/s of infection or bleeding <br> B. Instruct in self-assessment of s/s of infection or bleeding <br> C. Refer to sec. on bone marrow depression, Chapter 4 |
| III. *Potential for impaired skin integrity* | III. <br> A. Skin eruptions, rash may occur | III. <br> A. Distress related to alterations in skin condition will be minimized | III. <br> A. Advise pt these changes may occur <br> B. Instruct pt in symptomatic care if distress related to skin reactions occurs |

# Mesna

*Class:* Sulfhydryl

## MECHANISM OF ACTION

Used to prevent ifosfamide- or cyclophosphamide-induced hemorrhagic cystitis. Drug is rapidly metabolized to the metabolite dimesna. In the kidney, dimesna is reduced to mesna, which binds to the urotoxic metabolites resulting in detoxification.

## METABOLISM

Drug is rapidly metabolized, remains in the vascular compartment, and is then rapidly eliminated via the kidneys. The majority of the dose is excreted within 4 hours.

## DOSAGE/RANGE

240 mg/m$^2$ IV bolus 15 minutes before ifosfamide, 4 hours after ifosfamide, and 8 hours after ifosfamide. Mesna dose is 20% of ifosfamide dose.

Continuous ifosfamide infusions: loading mesna dose, followed by mesna dose equal to ifosfamide dose added to ifosfamide in same infusion bag, followed by 24-hour mesna infusion alone (dosage same as daily ifosfamide dose).

Oral mesna: dose is 40% of ifosfamide dose (not recommended for initial dose if the patient experiences nausea and vomiting).

## DRUG PREPARATION

Further dilute mesna with 5% dextrose, D$_5$NS, or 0.9% sodium chloride to create desired final concentration. Diluted solution is stable for 24 hours at room temperature.

## DRUG ADMINISTRATION

Administer as IV bolus or IV continuous infusion based on method of ifosfamide administration.

## SPECIAL CONSIDERATIONS

Can cause false positive result on urinalysis for ketones.

# Mesna

| Nursing Diagnosis | Defining Characteristics | Expected Outcomes | Nursing Interventions |
|---|---|---|---|
| I. *Alteration in nutrition, less than body requirements related to* | | | |
| A. Nausea and vomiting | I. A. Minor incidence and severity | I. A. 1. Pt will be without nausea and vomiting<br>2. Nausea and vomiting, if they occur, will be mild<br>3. Pt will maintain weight within 5% of baseline | I. A. 1. Assess baseline nutritional status<br>2. Usual premedication for ifosfamide provides protection from mesna-induced nausea and vomiting<br>3. Encourage small, frequent feedings of cool, bland foods and liquids; avoid greasy, spicy foods<br>4. Teach pt to report nausea and vomiting post-chemotherapy<br>5. Monitor I&O, daily weights, lab electrolyte values |
| B. Diarrhea | B. Mild | B. Pt will have minimal diarrhea | B. 1. Encourage pt to report onset of diarrhea<br>2. Administer or teach pt to self-administer antidiarrheal medication<br>3. See sec. on mucositis, diarrhea, Chapter 4 |

# Methotrexate
(Amethopterin, Mexate, Folex)

*Class:* Antimetabolite (folic acid antagonist)

## MECHANISM OF ACTION

Blocks the enzyme dihydrofolate reductase (DHFR), which inhibits the conversion of folic acid to tetrahydrofolic acid, resulting in an inhibition of the key precursors of DNA, RNA, and cellular proteins. May synchronize malignant cells in the S phase. At high plasma levels, passive entry of the drug into tumor cells can potentially overcome drug resistance.

## METABOLISM

Bound to serum albumin; concurrent use of drugs that displace methotrexate from serum albumin should be avoided. Salicylates, sulfonamides, dilantin, some antibacterials (including tetracycline, chloramphenicol, paraminobenzoic acid), and alcohol should be avoided, as they will delay excretion. Drug is absorbed from gastrointestinal tract and peaks in 1 hour. Plasma half-life is 2 hours; 50–100% of dose is excreted into the systemic circulation, with peak concentration 3–12 hours after administration.

## DOSAGE/RANGE

IV:  Low, 10–50 mg/m$^2$
     Medium, 100–500 mg/m$^2$
     High, 500 mg/m$^2$ and above, with leucovorin rescue
IT:  10–15 mg/m$^2$
IM:  25 mg/m$^2$

## DRUG PREPARATION

Five-mg, 50-mg, 100-mg, and 200-mg vials are available already reconstituted.

Powder is available in vials without preservative for IT and high-dose administration (reconstitute with preservative-free NS).

## DRUG ADMINISTRATION

5–149 mg: slow IVP
150–499 mg: IV drip over 20 minutes
500–1500 mg: infusion per protocol, with leucovorin rescue

## SPECIAL CONSIDERATIONS

High doses cross the blood-brain barrier: reconstitute with preservative-free NS.

With high doses (1–7.5 gm/m$^2$), urine should be alkalinized both before and after administration, as the drug is a weak acid and can crystallize in the kidneys at an acid pH. Alkalinize with bicarbonate and add to prehydration and posthydration. High doses should be given only under the direction of a qualified oncologist at an institution that can provide rapid serum methotrexate level readings.

Leucovorin rescue must be given *on time* per orders to prevent excessive toxicity and to achieve maximum therapeutic response (see leucovorin calcium table).

Avoid folic acid and its derivatives during methotrexate therapy.

Kidney function must be adequate to excrete drug and avoid excessive toxicity. Check BUN and creatinine before each dose.

# Methotrexate

| Nursing Diagnosis | Defining Characteristics | Expected Outcomes | Nursing Interventions |
|---|---|---|---|
| I. *Altered nutrition, less than body requirements related to* | | | |
| A. Nausea and vomiting | I. A. 1. Nausea and vomiting uncommon with low dose; more common (39%) with high dose 2. May occur during drug administration and last 24–72 hours | I. A. 1. Pt will be without nausea and vomiting 2. Nausea and vomiting, should they occur, will be minimal | I. A. 1. Premedicate with antiemetics if giving high-dose methotrexate; continue prophylactically for 24 hrs (at least) to *prevent* nausea and vomiting 2. Encourage small, frequent feedings of cool, bland foods and liquids 3. Assess for symptoms of fluid and electrolyte imbalance: monitor I&O, daily weights if inpt 4. See sec. on nausea and vomiting, Chapter 4 |
| B. Stomatitis | B. 1. Common; indication for interruption of therapy 2. Occurs in 3–5 days with high dose, 3–4 weeks with low dose 3. Appears initially at corners of mouth | B. Oral mucous membranes will remain intact and without infection | B. 1. Assess oral cavity every day 2. Teach pt oral assessment and mouth care regimens 3. Encourage pt to report early stomatitis 4. Provide pain relief measures if indicated 5. See sec. on stomatitis, Chapter 4 6. Explore pt compliance to rescue; discuss ↑ rescue dose |
| C. Diarrhea | C. 1. Common; indication for interruption of therapy, as enteritis and intestinal perforation may occur 2. Melena, hematemesis may occur | C. Pt will have minimal diarrhea | C. 1. Assess pt for diarrhea; guaiac all stools 2. Encourage pt to report onset of diarrhea 3. Administer or teach pt to self-administer antidiarrheal medications 4. See sec. on diarrhea, Chapter 4 |
| D. Hepatotoxicity | D. 1. Usually subclinical and reversible but can lead to cirrhosis | D. Early hepatotoxicity will be identified | D. 1. Monitor LFTs prior to drug dose, especially with high-dose methotrexate |

*(continued)*

**Methotrexate** (*continued*)

| Nursing Diagnosis | Defining Characteristics | Expected Outcomes | Nursing Interventions |
|---|---|---|---|
| | 2. Increased risk of hepatotoxicity when given with other hepatotoxic agents, like alcohol<br>3. Transient increase in LFTs with high dose 1–10 days after treatment; pt may become jaundiced | | 2. Assess pt prior to and during treatment for s/s of hepatotoxicity |
| E. Anorexia | E. Mild | E. Pt will maintain baseline weight ±5% | E. 1. Encourage small, frequent feedings of favorite foods, especially high-calorie, high-protein foods<br>2. Encourage use of spices<br>3. Daily weights |
| II. *Potential for infection and bleeding related to bone marrow depression* | II. A. Nadir seen 7–9 days after drug administration<br>B. Nadir range: WBC, 4–7 days; platelets, 5–12 days<br>C. Bone marrow depression of pts | II. A. Pt will be without s/s of infection or bleeding<br>B. S/s of infection or bleeding will be identified early | II. A. Monitor CBC, platelet count prior to drug administration, as well as s/s of infection or bleeding<br>B. Instruct in self-assessment of s/s of infection or bleeding<br>C. Administer leucovorin calcium as ordered<br>D. See care plan for leucovorin calcium |
| III. *Potential for altered urinary elimination related to renal toxicity* | III. A. As an organic acid, methotrexate is insoluble in acid urine<br>B. At doses greater than 1 gm/m² (i.e., high dose), drug may precipitate in renal tubules, causing acute tubular necrosis (ATN) | III. A. Pt will maintain normal patterns of urinary elimination<br>B. Renal toxicity will be avoided | III. A. Prehydrate pt with alkaline solution for several hours prior to drug administration<br>B. Maintain high urine output with a urine pH of greater than 7 (hydration fluid may need further alkalinization); dipstick each void<br>C. Record I&O |

| Nursing Diagnosis | Defining Characteristics | Expected Outcomes | Nursing Interventions |
|---|---|---|---|
| | | | D. Monitor BUN and serum creatinine before, during, and after drug administration; increases in these values may require methotrexate dose reductions or leucovorin dose increases |
| IV. Potential for impaired gas exchange related to pulmonary toxicity | IV. A. Pneumothorax (high dose) rare; occurs within first 48 hours after drug administration in pts with pulmonary metastasis. B. Allergic pneumonitis (high dose) rare but accompanied by eosinophilia, patchy pulmonary infiltrates, fever, cough, shortness of breath; occurs 1–5 months after initiation of treatment. C. Pneumonitis (low dose) symptoms usually disappear within a week, with or without use of steroids; interstitial pneumonitis may be a fatal complication | IV. A. Early s/s of pulmonary toxicity will be identified | IV. A. Assess for s/s of pulmonary dysfunction before each dose and between doses (see "Defining Characteristics"). B. Discuss pulmonary function studies to be performed periodically with MD. C. Assess lung sounds prior to drug administration. D. Instruct pt to report cough or dyspnea |
| V. Potential for alteration in skin integrity | V. A. Alopecia and dermatitis are uncommon. B. Pruritis and urticaria may occur. C. Photosensitivity and sunburn-like rash 1–5 days after treatment; also radiation recall reaction | V. A. Pt will verbalize feelings about potential change in body image and identify strategies to cope with them. B. Pt will identify strategies to minimize, avoid, or treat body image change | V. A. Assess pt for s/s of hair loss. B. Discuss with pt impact of hair loss and strategies to minimize distress. C. See sec. on alopecia, Chapter 4. D. Instruct pt to avoid sun if possible, to stay covered or wear sunscreen if sun exposure is unavoidable |

*(continued)*

**Methotrexate** *(continued)*

| Nursing Diagnosis | Defining Characteristics | Expected Outcomes | Nursing Interventions |
|---|---|---|---|
| VI. *Potential for sensory and perceptual alterations* | VI. A. CNS effects: dizziness, malaise, blurred vision<br>B. IT administration may increase CSF pressure<br>C. Brain XRT followed by IV MTX may cause neurological changes | VI. A. Early s/s of neurological toxicity will be identified | VI. A. Monitor for CNS effects of drug: dizziness, blurred vision, malaise<br>B. Monitor for symptoms of increased CSF pressure: seizures, paresis, headache, nausea and vomiting, brain atrophy, fever<br>C. If IV methotrexate follows brain XRT, monitor for symptoms of increased CSF pressure |
| VII. *Potential for alterations in comfort* | VII. A. Sometimes causes back pain during administration | VII. A. Pt will report comfort throughout drug administration | VII. A. Monitor pt for back and flank pain; slow infusion rate if it occurs<br>B. Administer analgesics if pain occurs (must avoid ASA-containing products, as they displace methotrexate from serum albumin) |

# Methyl-CCNU
## (Semustine, MeCCNU, Methyl Lomustine)

*Class:* Alkylating agent (nitrosourea); investigational

## MECHANISM OF ACTION

Alkylation and carbamoylation by semustine metabolites interfere with the synthesis and function of DNA, RNA, and proteins. Also inhibits DNA repair. Semustine is lipid soluble and easily enters the brain. Is cell cycle phase nonspecific.

## METABOLISM

Ten to 20 percent of the drug is excreted in the urine.

## DOSAGE/RANGE

150–200 mg/m$^2$ po once every 6–10 weeks

## DRUG PREPARATION

Available in 10-mg, 50-mg, and 100-mg capsules.

## DRUG ADMINISTRATION

Administer po at bedtime on an empty stomach or 3–4 hours after a meal to minimize nausea and vomiting.

## SPECIAL CONSIDERATIONS

Dose reduction necessary if patient has liver impairment.

Dispense one dose of semustine at a time.

Bone marrow recovery should occur prior to administration: WBC > 4000/mm$^3$ and platelets > 100,000/mm$^3$.

## Methyl-CCNU

| Nursing Diagnosis | Defining Characteristics | Expected Outcomes | Nursing Interventions |
|---|---|---|---|
| I. *Potential for infection and bleeding related to myelosuppression* | I. A. Nadir: platelets 4 weeks but may be delayed to 8 weeks, with recovery 4–10 weeks later; WBC occurs later than platelets <br><br> B. Cumulative bone marrow suppression with subsequent dosing may occur; 2nd or 3rd drug dose may be reduced 25–50% <br><br> C. Persistent thrombo-cytopenia may occur | I. A. Pt will be without infection or bleeding <br> B. Early s/s of infection and bleeding will be identified | I. A. Monitor WBC, platelets prior to drug administration (see "Special Considerations") WBC > 4000/mm$^3$ and platelets > 100,000/mm$^3$ <br> B. Dispense only one drug dose at a time <br> C. Do not administer more often than once every 6 weeks <br> D. Reduce dose with bone marrow or liver impairment <br> E. Refer to sec. on bone marrow depression, Chapter 4 |
| II. *Alteration in nutrition, less than body requirements related to* <br> A. Nausea and vomiting | II. A. Onset 4–6 hrs after drug dosing and may be severe | II. A. Nausea and vomiting will be minimized or prevented | II. A. 1. Premedicate with antiemetic and sedative or hypnotic <br> 2. Administer at night on empty stomach <br> 3. Discourage food or fluid for 6 hrs after drug dose <br> 4. Refer to sec. on nausea and vomiting, Chapter 4 |
| B. Anorexia | B. Occurs rarely | B. Pt will maintain baseline weight ± 5% | B. 1. Encourage favorite foods especially high-calorie high-protein foods <br> 2. Encourage small, frequent feedings |
| C. Stomatitis | C. Occurs rarely | C. Oral mucous membranes will remain intact and without infection | C. 1. Inspect oral mucosa prior to dosing <br> 2. Teach pt oral exam, mouth care pc and hs <br> 3. Refer to sec. on stomatitis, mucositis, Chapter 4 |
| D. Hepatic dysfunction | D. Delayed hepatocullular damage may occur *rarely* | D. Hepatic dysfunction will be identified early | D. 1. Monitor SGOT, LDH, alkaline phosphatase, bilirubin <br> 2. Notify MD of elevations and discuss prior to administering subsequent drug dose |

| | | | |
|---|---|---|---|
| III. *Activity intolerance* | III. A. Neurologic dysfunction may occur *rarely*, including disorientation, lethargy, ataxia | II. A. Neurologic dysfunction will be identified early | III. A. Perform neurologic assessment as part of prechemotherapy assessment<br>B. Assess orientation and level of consciousness, gait, activity tolerance |
| IV. *Sensory/perceptual alterations (visual)* | IV. A. Ocular damage may occur *rarely*, including optic neuritis, retinopathy, blurred vision | IV. A. Visual disturbances will be identified early | IV. A. Assess vision during prechemotherapy assessment<br>B. Encourage pt to report any visual changes |
| V. *Altered urinary elimination* | V. A. Renal dysfunction infrequent but may occur late in treatment<br>B. Tubular atrophy and glomerular sclerosis, ultimately renal failure | V. A. Early renal dysfunction will be identified | V. A. Monitor BUN, creatinine prior to dosing, especially in pts receiving prolonged or high cumulative doses<br>B. If abnormalities are noted, determine renal creatinine clearance |
| VI. *Potential for sexual dysfunction* | VI. A. Drug is teratogenic and mutagenic | VI. A. Pt and significant other will understand need for contraception | VI. A. As appropriate, discuss birth control measures<br>B. See sec. on gonadal dysfunction, Chapter 4 |
| VII. *Body image disturbance* | VII. A. Alopecia infrequent | VII. A. Pt will verbalize feelings re hair loss and strategies to cope with change in body image | VII. A. Assess pt for hair loss<br>B. Discuss with pt impact of hair loss and obtaining wig or alternative head cover<br>C. See sec. on alopecia, Chapter 4 |
| VIII. *Impaired gas exchange related to pulmonary fibrosis* | VIII. A. Pulmonary fibrosis occurs rarely | VIII. A. Early pulmonary fibrosis/dysfunction will be identified | VIII. A. Assess pts at risk (i.e., those with preexisting lung disease, high cumulative doses)<br>B. Monitor pulmonary function studies periodically for pulmonary dysfunction |

# Misonidazole
## (NSC-261037)

*Class:* Nitroimidazole (investigational)

## MECHANISM OF ACTION

When combined with melphalan, enhances DNA cross-linking, causing cell arrest.

## METABOLISM

Unknown

## DOSAGE/RANGE

By protocol; for example, misonidazole 4 gm/m$^2$ plus melphalan 0.6 mg/kg

## DRUG PREPARATION

Available as 500 mg for injection in 30-ml vial.

Drug may crystallize, requiring warming or further dilution to 20 mg/ml.

Reconstituted vials stable for at least 14 days at room temperature or mixed 1 gm/L 5% dextrose injection, USP. Vials are single use, and should be discarded within 8 hours of opening.

## DRUG ADMINISTRATION

IV

## SPECIAL CONSIDERATIONS

Drug is a radiosensitizer.

Potentiates lomustine activity in vitro.

# Misonidazole

| Nursing Diagnosis | Defining Characteristics | Expected Outcomes | Nursing Interventions |
|---|---|---|---|
| I. *Infection and bleeding related to bone marrow depression* | I. A. Dose-limiting side effect caused by melphalan | I. A. Pt will be without s/s of infection or bleeding | I. A. Monitor CBC, platelet count prior to drug administration<br>B. Monitor for s/s of infection and bleeding<br>C. Instruct pt in self-assessment of s/s of infection and bleeding and to call MD or go to emergency room<br>D. Transfuse platelets per MD order<br>E. Refer to sec. on bone marrow depression, Chapter 4 |
| II. *Sensory/perceptual alterations related to peripheral neuropathy* | II. A. Usually mild | II. A. Early s/s of neurological toxicity will be identified<br>B. Function will be maintained | II. A. Assess baseline neuromuscular function and reassess prior to drug infusion, especially presence of paresthesias<br>B. Teach pt to report any changes in sensation or function<br>C. Discuss alterations with MD<br>D. Identify strategies to promote comfort and safety<br>E. Refer to sec. on neurotoxicity, Chapter 4 |

# Mitoguazone dihydrochloride
(methyl-GAG, methyl-G)

*Class:* Investigational

## MECHANISM OF ACTION

Methyl-GAG interferes with protein synthesis by inhibiting specific enzyme products. This process ultimately inhibits DNA synthesis. There are also theories that it may bind directly to DNA and act as a mitochondrial poison. The exact mechanism of action is not clearly understood. Is cell cycle nonspecific.

## METABOLISM

Methyl-GAG is administered by intravenous infusion or by deep intramuscular injection. There is a prolonged retention of methyl-GAG, with an associated delay in excretion; 60% of drug dose is excreted intact in urine, with < 20% being excreted in feces. At 72 hours postinfusion, only 14% of drug dose is excreted in urine. The remainder of the drug is slowly excreted over at least the next 2 weeks. The mean half-life is 136–224 hours.

## DOSAGE/RANGE

Currently methyl-GAG is given in doses of 260–800 mg/m$^2$ IV weekly, or 3–4 mg/kg deep IM injection weekly. Clinical trials with methyl-GAG have been under way since the 1960s, but the optimal dosing schedule has yet to be determined. It is clear that schedules of administering it every 10–14 days offer less toxicity.

## DRUG PREPARATION

Methyl-GAG is available as a lyophilized powder in 30-ml vials of 1 gm of drug. The drug is supplied by the National Cancer Institute.

Each 30-ml vial is reconstituted with 9.3 ml of sodium chloride injection. This solution is chemically stable for 48 hours at room temperature or refrigerated, but as it lacks bacteriostatic preservatives, the solution should be discarded after 8 hours. The reconstituted solution may be further diluted in 500 ml D$_5$W or NS.

## DRUG ADMINISTRATION

Methyl-GAG IV infusions should be administered over 30–45 minutes. IV push administration may cause orthostatic hypotension and thus is not recommended. This drug may also be administered by deep IM injection. The total volume of drug per each injection site should not exceed 7.5 ml.

## SPECIAL CONSIDERATIONS

Irritant.

Administered by IV infusion or deep IM injection.

Reports of rare occurrences of hypotension and bronchospasm during infusion.

Toxicities somewhat unpredictable. Seem to be cumulative rather than dose related (may be due to rate of excretion).

Majority of patients experience facial flushing (may involve whole body) and warmth halfway into infusion, which resolve completely within 15 minutes after infusion. This problem can be decreased by decreasing the rate of infusion.

Dose-limiting toxicities include muscle weakness, malaise, myopathies, GI mucositis, and hypoglycemia.

Mucositis may represent toxicity from drug accumulation.

Anorexia and weight loss have been noted in clinical trials.

# Mitoguazone dihydrochloride

| Nursing Diagnosis | Defining Characteristics | Expected Outcomes | Nursing Interventions |
|---|---|---|---|
| I. *Potential for injury related to hypersensitivity reactions* | I. A. Almost all pts experience some hypersensitivity reactions, usually facial flushing and numbness but may involve entire body; bronchospasm occurs in 4% of pts<br><br>B. Especially seen with IM injections<br><br>C. Starts 5–15 mins after injection<br><br>D. Hypotension may occur, especially with rapid infusions<br><br>E. Dizziness and bronchospasm rarely occur<br><br>F. Usually responds to or steroids, epinephrine, antihistamines | I. A. Early s/s of hypersensitivity reactions will be identified | I. A. Review standing orders for management of pt in anaphylaxis and identify location of anaphylaxis kit containing epinephrine 1:1000, hydrocortisone sodium succinate (SoluCortef), diphenhydramine HCl (Benadryl), Aminophylline, and others<br><br>B. 1. Prior to drug administration, obtain baseline vital signs and record mental status<br>2. Assess pt for at least 30 mins after the drug is given for s/s of a reaction<br>3. Teach pt about the potential for hypersensitivity reactions and to report any unusual symptoms<br><br>C. Observe for following s/s during infusion, usually occurring within first 15 mins of start of infusion:<br>1. *Subjective*<br>a. generalized itching<br>b. nausea<br>c. chest tightness<br>d. crampy abdominal pain<br>e. difficulty speaking<br>f. anxiety<br>g. agitation<br>h. sense of impending doom<br>i. uneasiness<br>j. desire to urinate or defecate<br>k. dizziness<br>l. chills |

(continued)

## Mitoguazone dihydrochloride (continued)

| Nursing Diagnosis | Defining Characteristics | Expected Outcomes | Nursing Interventions |
|---|---|---|---|
| | | | C. 2. *Objective*<br>a. flushed appearance (angioedema of face, neck, eyelids, hands, feet)<br>b. localized or generalized urticaria<br>c. respiratory distress ± wheezing<br>d. hypotension<br>e. cyanosis<br>D. If reaction occurs, stop infusion and notify MD<br>E. Place pt in supine position to promote perfusion of visceral organs<br>F. Monitor vital signs until stable<br>G. Provide emotional reassurance to pt and family<br>H. Maintain patent airway and have CPR equipment ready if needed<br>I. Document incident<br>J. Discuss with MD desensitization versus drug discontinuance for further dosing |
| II. *Potential for infection and bleeding related to bone marrow depression* | II. A. Dose related, occurring in 13% of pts; profound with daily dosing; rare with intermittent dosing<br>B. Leukopenia is more common than thrombocytopenia<br>C. Thrombocytopenia is mild to moderate | II. A. Pt will be without s/s of infection or bleeding<br>B. Early s/s of infection or bleeding will be identified | II. A. Monitor CBC, platelet count prior to drug administration, as well as s/s of infection or bleeding<br>B. Instruct pt in self-assessment of s/s of infection or bleeding<br>C. Dose reduction may be necessary in setting of compromised bone marrow function<br>D. See sec. on bone marrow depression, Chapter 4 |

III. *Altered nutrition, less than body requirements related to*

A. Nausea and vomiting

III. A. 1. Nausea is more common than vomiting
2. Rarely, an unclear reaction occurs, resulting in prolonged vomiting
3. Nausea usually limited to first 24 hrs after therapy

III. A. 1. Pt will be without nausea and vomiting
2. Nausea and vomiting, if they occur, will be minimal

III. A. 1. Premedicate with antiemetics and continue prophylactically × 24 hrs to prevent nausea and vomiting, at least for first treatment
2. Encourage small, frequent feedings of cool, bland foods and liquids
3. See sec. on nausea and vomiting, Chapter 4

B. Mucositis

B. 1. May be severe and dose limiting
2. May progress from stomatitis to ulcerative mucositis with bloody diarrhea in 24% of pts
3. S/s start 7–14 days after administration
4. S/s may include inflammation or ulceration of any mucosal membrane, anorexia, weight loss, abdominal pain, diarrhea
5. Occurs in 20% of pts and may represent drug accumulation

B. 1. Mucous membranes will remain intact without infection
2. Pt will maintain baseline weight ± 5%
3. Pt will have minimal diarrhea

B. 1. Teach pt oral assessment
2. Encourage pt to report onset of mucositis, diarrhea
3. Teach pt oral hygiene
4. Encourage small, frequent feedings of favorite foods, especially high-calorie, high-protein foods
5. Encourage use of spices
6. Weekly weights
7. Administer or teach pt to self-administer antidiarrheal medications
8. See sec. on stomatitis, mucositis, Chapter 4

C. Hypoglycemia

C. 1. Rare and delayed reaction, more common with daily dosing than intermittent dosing
2. S/s include muscle weakness, lethargy, flushing, confusion, restlessness, numbness, malaise

C. 1. Pt will be without s/s of hypoglycemia
2. Early s/s of hypoglycemia will be identified

C. 1. Teach pt about the potential for hypoglycemia and to report any unusual symptoms (i.e., mental status changes, muscle weakness, palpitations)
2. Monitor serum glucose levels
3. Report any laboratory abnormalities to MD
4. Treat hypoglycemia with diet or medication as ordered by MD

*(continued)*

## Mitoguazone dihydrochloride (continued)

| Nursing Diagnosis | Defining Characteristics | Expected Outcomes | Nursing Interventions |
|---|---|---|---|
| IV. *Impaired skin integrity related to*<br>A. Alopecia | IV. A. Uncommon; may be slight to diffuse thinning | IV. A. Pt will verbalize feelings regarding hair loss and identify strategies to cope with change in body image | IV. A. 1. Assess pt for s/s of hair loss<br>2. Discuss with pt impact of hair loss and strategies to minimize distress (e.g., wigs, scarf, cap); begin before therapy initiated<br>3. See sec. on alopecia, Chapter 4 |
| B. Changes in skin | B. 1. May be inflammatory reactions on hands, feet, lower extremities<br>2. S/s may include erythema, edema, pain, dermatitis, ulcers, vasculitis<br>3. Subcutaneous nodules may for at injection site<br>4. Chemical thrombophlebitis and cellulitis occur | B. Pt. will verbalize feelings regarding skin changes and identify strategies to cope with change in body image | B. 1. Assess pt for inflammatory skin reactions or formation of subcutaneous nodules at injection sites<br>2. Discuss with pt impact of changes and strategies to minimize distress (e.g., wearing nonirritating socks, cotton gloves, long pants)<br>3. Rotate injection sites<br>4. Warm soaks for nodules as appropriate<br>5. Administer corticosteroids as ordered |
| V. *Potential for injury related to myopathy and peripheral neuropathies* | V. A. 24% of pts experience myopathy syndrome; may be quite severe, necessitating narcotic analgesia; reversible when treatment is held<br>B. Peripheral neuropathies are rare | V. A. Early s/s of myopathy and peripheral neuropathies will be identified<br>B. Pt will not experience injuries as a result of skeletal or neurological changes | V. A. Teach pt about the potential for myopathy or peripheral neuropathies and to report any unusual symptoms (i.e., muscle weakness and wasting, numbness)<br>B. Obtain baseline physical; assess muscular and neurological function<br>C. Dose decrease or rescheduling of dose administration may be necessary |

# Mitomycin
## (Mitomycin C, Mutamycin)

*Class:* Antitumor antibiotic

## MECHANISM OF ACTION

Drug acts as alkylating agent and inhibits DNA synthesis by cross-linking of DNA. Alkylating and cross-linking mitomycin metabolites interfere with structure and function of DNA.

## METABOLISM

Drug is rapidly cleared by the liver. May need to modify dose in presence of liver abnormalities. Ten percent of drug is excreted unchanged.

## DOSAGE/RANGE

2 mg/m$^2$ IV every day × 5 days
15–20 mg/m$^2$ IV every 6–8 weeks
Bladder instillations 20–60 mg (1 mg/ml)

## DRUG PREPARATION

Depending on vial size, dilute with sterile water to obtain concentration of 0.5 mg/ml.

## DRUG ADMINISTRATION

This drug is a potent vesicant. Give through the sidearm of a running IV to avoid extravasation, which can lead to ulceration, pain, and necrosis. Check individual hospital policy for administration of a vesicant.

## SPECIAL CONSIDERATIONS

Drug is a potent vesicant. Give through running IV to avoid extravasation.

Interstitial pneumonitis.

Special investigational applications include administration via intra-arterial, intra-peritoneal, and intrapleural routes.

## Mitomycin

| Nursing Diagnosis | Defining Characteristics | Expected Outcomes | Nursing Interventions |
|---|---|---|---|
| I. *Altered nutrition, less than body requirements related to* A. Nausea and vomiting | I. A. Mild to moderate nausea and vomiting occur within 1–2 hrs, lasting up to 3 days | I. A. 1. Pt will be without nausea and vomiting 2. Nausea and vomiting, if they occur, will be minimal | I. A. 1. Premedicate with antiemetics and continue prophylactically × 24 hrs to prevent nausea and vomiting, at least for first treatment 2. Encourage small, frequent feedings of cool, bland foods and liquids 3. See sec. on nausea and vomiting, Chapter 4 |
| B. Stomatitis | B. Mucocutaneous toxicity | B. Oral mucous membrane will remain intact and without infection | B. 1. Teach pt oral assessment and oral hygiene regimen 2. Encourage pt to report early stomatitis 3. See sec. on stomatitis, Chapter 4 |
| II. *Potential for infection related to myelosuppression* | II. A. Myelosuppression is the dose-limiting toxicity; toxicity is delayed and cumulative B. Initial nadir occurs at approximately 4–6 weeks C. Usually by the third course, 50% drug modifications are necessary | II. A. Pt will be without infection B. Early s/s of infection will be identified | II. A. Monitor WBC, hematocrit, platelets prior to drug administration B. Monitor pts for s/s of infection; teach pt self-assessment C. Drug dosage should be reduced or held for lower-than-normal blood values D. See sec. on bone marrow depression, Chapter 4 |
| III. *Potential for alteration in comfort related to fever* | III. A. Fever with malaise in almost all pts is related to length and duration of drug schedule | III. A. Pt will remain comfortable during therapy | III. A. Assess pt for symptoms during treatment; discuss with MD B. Premedicate with prescribed medication C. Evaluate the effectiveness of the symptomatic relief prescribed and administered D. Monitor the quantity of cumulative dose |

IV. *Potential for impaired skin integrity related to*

A. Extravasation

IV. A. Extravasation of drug can cause severe tissue necrosis, erythema, burning, tissue sloughing

IV. A. 1. Extravasation will be prevented or treated appropriately if it occurs

2. Skin and underlying tissue damage will be minimized

IV. A. 1. Careful technique is used during venipuncture; see sec. on intravenous administration, Chapter 10

2. Administer vesicant through freely flowing IV, constantly monitoring IV site and pt response

3. Nurse should be *thoroughly* familiar with institutional policy and procedure for administration of a vesicant agent

4. If vesicant drug is administered as a continuous infusion, drug must be given through a patent central line

5. If extravasation is suspected:

  a. Stop drug administered

  b. Aspirate any residual drug and blood from IV tubing, IV catheter/ needle, and IV site if possible

  c. *If antidote exists,* instill antidote into area of apparent infiltration as per MD order and institutional policy and procedure

  d. Apply cold or topical medication as per MD order and institutional policy and procedure

6. Assess site regularly for pain, progression of erythema, induration, and evidence of necrosis

7. When in doubt about whether drug is infiltrating, *treat as an infiltration*

8. Teach pt to assess site and notify MD if condition worsens

*(continued)*

## Mitomycin (continued)

| Nursing Diagnosis | Defining Characteristics | Expected Outcomes | Nursing Interventions |
|---|---|---|---|
| | | | 9. Arrange next clinic visit for assessment of site depending on drug, amount infiltrated, extent of potential injury, and pt variables |
| | | | 10. Document in pt's record as per institutional policy and procedure; see sec. on reactions, Chapter 9 |
| B. Alopecia | B. Alopecia has been reported | B. Pt will verbalize feelings re hair loss and identify strategies to cope with change in body image | B. 1. Discuss with pt impact of hair loss |
| | | | 2. Suggest wig as appropriate prior to actual hair loss |
| | | | 3. Explore with pt response to actual hair loss and plan strategies to minimize distress (e.g., wig, scarf, cap) |
| | | | 4. See sec. on alopecia, Chapter 4 |
| C. Skin reactions | C. Discoloration of fingernails; usually dark half circles | C. 1. Skin discomfort will be minimized, and skin will remain intact | C. 1. Discuss with pt feelings about skin changes |
| | | 2. Pt will verbalize feelings re skin changes | 2. Reinforce pt teaching on the action and side effects of mitomycin |
| | | | 3. Offer emotional support |
| V. *Potential for injury related to hemolytic uremic syndrome* | V. A. Pts (2%) may experience significant increase in creatinine unrelated to total dose or duration of therapy | V. A. Alterations in renal function will be identified early | V. A. Monitor renal function, hematocrit, platelets prior to each drug dose; hold dose if serum creatinine is > 1.7 mg/dl |
| | B. Hold drug for creatinine >1.7 mg/dl | | B. If renal failure occurs, hemofiltration or dialysis may be necessary |
| | C. Thrombotic microangiopathy may occur with anemia, thrombocytopenia | | C. Discuss risks and benefits with MD and pt if renal insufficiency is present and blood transfusion is required |
| | D. Blood transfusions may exacerbate condition | | |
| | E. Often fatal | | |

# Mitotane
(o,p'-DDD; Lysodren)

*Class:* Antihormone

## MECHANISM OF ACTION

Adrenocortical suppressant with direct cytotoxic effect on mitochondria of adrenal cortical cells. Forces a drop in steroid secretion and alters the peripheral metabolism of steroids.

## METABOLISM

34–45% of oral dose is absorbed from the gastrointestinal tract. Metabolized partly in the liver and kidneys to a water-soluble metabolite that is then excreted in the bile and urine. Small amount of drug passes into the CSF.

## DOSAGE/RANGE

2–16 gm/day orally
Usual doses 2–10 gm/day
Treatment usually begins with low doses (2 gm/day) and gradually increases.
Daily dose is divided into 3–4 doses.

## DRUG PREPARATION

Available as 500-mg tablets

## DRUG ADMINISTRATION

Oral

## SPECIAL CONSIDERATIONS

Hypersensitivity reactions are rare but have occurred.
Indicated for the palliation of inoperable carcinoma of the adrenal cortex.

## Mitotane

| Nursing Diagnosis | Defining Characteristics | Expected Outcomes | Nursing Interventions |
|---|---|---|---|
| I. *Altered nutrition, less than body requirements related to*<br>A. Nausea and vomiting | I. A. 1. Occurs in 75% of pts and may be dose-limiting toxicity<br>2. Anorexia may also occur | I. A. 1. Pt will be without nausea and vomiting<br>2. Nausea or vomiting, should they occur, will be treated early | I. A. 1. Nausea and vomiting may be reduced by beginning therapy with a low dose and increasing it as tolerated<br>2. Premedicate with antiemetics to prevent nausea and vomiting; continue as needed<br>3. Encourage small, frequent feedings of cool, bland foods and liquids<br>4. Inform pt that nausea and vomiting can occur; encourage pt to report onset<br>5. See sec. on nausea and vomiting, Chapter 4 |
| B. Diarrhea | B. Occurs in 20% of pts | B. Pt will have minimal diarrhea | B. 1. Encourage pt to report onset of diarrhea<br>2. Administer or teach administration of antidiarrheal medication<br>3. If diarrhea is protracted, ensure adequate hydration, monitor I&O and electrolytes, teach perineal hygiene<br>4. See sec. on diarrhea, Chapter 4 |
| II. *Potential for injury related to neurological toxicity* | II. A. Lethargy and somnolence most common; resolve with discontinuation of therapy<br>B. Dizziness, vertigo occur in about 15% of pts<br>C. Other CNS manifestations are depression, vertigo, muscle tremors, confusion, headache | II. A. Pt will maintain baseline cognitive function<br>B. Pt will report onset of cognitive changes | II. A. Teach the pt and family about possible neurological toxicity; assess safety of planned activities (i.e., pt should avoid activities that require alertness)<br>B. Encourage pt and family to report onset of symptoms, as they may necessitate discontinuing therapy |

*III. Potential for impaired skin integrity*

III.
A. Skin irritation or rash occurs in about 15% of pts
B. Sometimes resolves during treatment

III.
A. Skin will remain intact
B. Early signs of skin impairment will be identified

III.
A. Inform pt that rash is expected and will resolve when treatment is finished
B. Assess skin for integrity; recommend measures to decrease irritation if indicated

# Mitoxantrone
(Novantrone)

*Class:* Anthracenediones; antitumor antibiotic

## MECHANISM OF ACTION

Inhibits both DNA and RNA synthesis regardless of the phase of cell division. Intercalates between base pairs, thus distorting DNA structure. DNA-dependent RNA synthesis and protein synthesis are also inhibited.

## METABOLISM

Excreted in both the bile and urine for 24–36 hours as virtually unchanged drug. Mean half-life is 5.8 hours. Peak levels achieved immediately. FDA approved for acute non-lymphocytic leukemia in adults.

## DOSAGE/RANGE

10–14 mg/m² daily for 1–3 days

10–24 mg/m²/day (clinical trials; see specific protocol)

## DRUG PREPARATION

Available as dark blue solution.

May be diluted in $D_5W$, NS, or $D_5NS$.

Solution is chemically stable at room temperature for at least 48 hours.

Intact vials should be stored at room temperature. If refrigerated, a precipitate may form. This precipitate can be redissolved when vial is warmed to room temperature.

## DRUG ADMINISTRATION

IV push over 3 minutes through the arm of a freely running infusion.

IV bolus over 5–30 minutes.

## SPECIAL CONSIDERATIONS

Nonvesicant. There have been rare reports of tissue necrosis after drug infiltration.

Incompatible with admixtures containing heparin.

Patient may experience blue-green urine for 24 hours after drug administration.

# Mitoxantrone

| Nursing Diagnosis | Defining Characteristics | Expected Outcomes | Nursing Interventions |
|---|---|---|---|
| I. *Potential for injury related to* | | | |
| A. Infection | I. A. 1. Significant bone marrow depression; nadir 9–10 days<br>2. Granulocytopenia is usually the dose-limiting toxicity<br>3. Toxicity may be cumulative | I. A. 1. Pt will be without infection<br>2. Early s/s of infection and bleeding will be identified | I. A. 1. Monitor WBC, hematocrit, platelets prior to drug administration<br>2. Drug dosage should be reduced or held for lower-than-normal blood values<br>3. Instruct pt in self-assessment of s/s of infection<br>4. See sec. on bone marrow depression, Chapter 4 |
| B. Bleeding | B. Thrombocytopenia uncommon but can be severe when it occurs | B. 1. Pt will be without s/s of bleeding<br>2. Bleeding, if it occurs, will be identified and treated early | B. Instruct pt in self-assessment of s/s of bleeding |
| C. Allergic reactions | C. 1. Hypersensitivity has been reported occasionally<br>2. Hypotension<br>3. Urticaria<br>4. Dyspnea<br>5. Rashes | C. Allergic reactions will be detected early | C. 1. Prior to drug administration, obtain baseline vital signs<br>2. Observe for s/s of allergic reaction<br>3. Subjective s/s: generalized itching, dizziness<br>4. Objective s/s: flushed appearance (angioedema of face, neck, eyelids, hands, feet), localized or generalized urticaria<br>5. Document incident<br>6. Discuss with MD desensitization for future dose versus drug discontinuance |
| II. *Nutrition alteration, less than body requirements related to*<br>A. Nausea and vomiting | II. A. 1. Typically not severe<br>2. Occurs in 30% of pts | II. A. 1. Pt will be without nausea and vomiting<br>2. Nausea and vomiting, if they occur, will be minimal | II. A. 1. Premedicate with antiemetic and continue prophylactically × 24 hrs to prevent nausea and vomiting, at least for first treatment |

(continued)

## Mitoxantrone (continued)

| Nursing Diagnosis | Defining Characteristics | Expected Outcomes | Nursing Interventions |
|---|---|---|---|
| | | | 2. Encourage small, frequent feedings of cool, bland foods and liquids<br>3. Refer to sec. on nausea and vomiting, Chapter 4 |
| B. Mucositis | B. 1. More common with prolonged dosing<br>2. Occurs in 5% of pts<br>3. Usually within 1 week of therapy | B. Oral mucous membranes will remain intact and without infection | B. 1. Teach pt oral assessment and oral hygiene regimen<br>2. Encourage pt to report early stomatitis<br>3. See sec. on stomatitis, Chapter 4 |
| III. *Potential for impaired skin integrity related to*<br>A. Alopecia | III. A. 1. Mild to moderate<br>2. Occurs in 20% of pts | III. A. 1. Pt will verbalize feelings regarding hair loss<br>2. Pt will identify strategies to cope with change in body image | III. A. 1. Discuss with pt impact of hair loss<br>2. Suggest wig as appropriate prior to actual hair loss<br>3. Explore with pt response to actual hair loss and plan strategies to minimize distress, (e.g., wig, scarf, cap)<br>4. Refer to sec. on alopecia, Chapter 4 |
| B. Extravasation | B. 1. Not a vesicant<br>2. Stains skin blue, without ulcers<br>3. Rare reports of tissue necrosis following extravasation | B. 1. Skin discomfort will be minimized<br>2. Skin will remain intact<br>3. Pt will verbalize feelings re skin changes | B. 1. Careful technique is used during venipuncture; see sec. on intravenous administration, Chapter 10<br>2. Administer drug through freely flowing IV, constantly monitoring IV site and pt response<br>3. Teach pt to assess site and notify provider if condition worsens<br>4. Arrange next clinic visit for assessment of site depending on drug, amount infiltrated, extent of potenial injury, and pt variables<br>5. Document in pt's record as per institutional policy and procedure; see sec. on reactions, Chapter 9 |

| Nursing Diagnosis | Defining Characteristics | Expected Outcomes | Nursing Interventions |
|---|---|---|---|
| IV. *Potential for alteration in cardiac output* | A. CHF<br>B. Decreased left ventricular ejection fraction occurs in about 3% of pts<br>C. Increased cardiotoxicity with cumulative dose greater than 180 mg/m$^2$<br>D. Cumulative lifetime dose must be reduced if pt has had previous anthracycline therapy | IV. A. Early s/s of cardiomyopathy will be identified | IV. A. Assess for s/s of cardiomyopathy<br>B. Assess quality and regularity of heartbeat<br>C. Baseline EKG<br>D. Instruct pt to report dyspnea, shortness of breath, swelling of extremities, orthopnea<br>E. Discuss frequency of gated blood pool scan with MD |
| V. *Alteration in metabolic pattern* | A. In leukemia pts, rapid tumor lysis may occur, with resultant hyperuricemia | V. A. Hyperuricemia will be identified early | V. A. Hydrate pt<br>B. Alkalinize urine<br>C. Administer allopurinol as per MD order<br>D. Evaluate the effects of allopurinol by monitoring uric acid levels<br>E. Monitor blood values of electrolytes, BUN, and creatinine |
| VI. *Potential for anxiety* | A. Urine will be green/blue for 24 hrs<br>B. Sclera may become discolored blue | VI. A. Pt will verbalize understanding of physiological changes expected with treatment | VI. A. Explain to pt changes that may occur with therapy and that they are only temporary |
| VII. *Potential for sexual dysfunction* | A. Drug is mutagenic and teratogenic | VII. A. Pt and significant other will understand the need for contraception | VII. A. As appropriate, explore with pt and significant other issues of reproductive and sexuality pattern and impact chemotherapy may have<br>B. Discuss strategies to preserve sexual and reproductive health (e.g., sperm banking, contraception)<br>C. See sec. on gonadal dysfunction, Chapter 4 |

# Oxaliplatin

*Class:* Alkylating agent

## MECHANISM OF ACTION

Blocks DNA replication and transcription into RNA by causing intrastrand and interstrand cross-links in DNA strands.

## METABOLISM

Heavily bound to plasma proteins; about 50% of the platinum found in the bloodstream is bound to RBCs. Concentrates most significantly in the kidney and spleen. Renally excreted as platinum-containing metabolites.

## DOSAGE/RANGE

135 mg/m$^2$ every 3 weeks
In phase II trials with 5-FU and leucovorin, dose of 25–35 mg/m$^2$ per day for 5 days (continuous infusion) is used (125 mg/m$^2$ total).

## DRUG PREPARATION

Reconstitute 50-mg and 100-mg vials with 25 ml and 50 ml of sterile water, respectively, then dilute in D$_5$W up to a volume of 500 ml. *Unstable in chloride-containing solutions.*

## DRUG ADMINISTRATION

Administer by IV bolus (500 ml) or continuous infusion over 5 days.

## SPECIAL CONSIDERATIONS

Avoid use of aluminum needles and infusion sets containing aluminum.

Oxaliplatin

| Nursing Diagnosis | Defining Characteristics | Expected Outcomes | Nursing Interventions |
|---|---|---|---|
| I. *Potential alteration in nutrition, less than body requirements* | I. A. Nausea and vomiting moderate to severe<br>B. Emesis may last 2–3 days | I. A. Nausea and vomiting will be prevented | I. A. Premedicate with antiemetics and continue prophylactically × 24 hrs to prevent nausea and vomiting, at least for first treatment. Serotonin antagonist effective<br>B. Encourage small, frequent feedings of cool, bland foods and liquids<br>C. I&O, daily weights if inpatient (assess for s/s of fluid and electrolyte imbalance)<br>D. Refer to sec. on nausea and vomiting, Chapter 4 |
| II. *Potential sensory/perceptual alterations related to neurotoxicity* | II. A. Peripheral neuropathy is dose-related<br>B. Dysesthesia appears to be precipitated by exposure to cold. Laryngo-pharyngeal dysesthesia may occur, characterized by sensation of difficulty breathing or swallowing. This is self-limiting but requires emotional support and close monitoring<br>C. Characterized by paresthesias of hands, feet, and occasionally lips and throat<br>D. Symptom intensity increases with repeated courses of drugs, and may progress from sensory only to fine-motor dysfunction<br>E. Symptoms of neurotoxicity usually resolve within 1 week of stopping therapy (no permanent effects) | II. A. Neurotoxicity will be identified early<br>B. Function will be maintained<br>C. Laryngopharyngeal dysesthesia, if it occurs, will be managed | II. A. Assess neurological function baseline and before each drug dose<br>B. Teach pt cold may cause dysesthesias, and to avoid exposure (avoid drinking cold beverages, eating ice cream, avoid exposing hand to cold [e.g., wear gloves when going outside or getting food from refrigerator/freezer])<br>C. Assess fine-motor movement baseline and before each treatment (writing name, picking up coin from flat surface)<br>D. Assess risk for injury and develop strategies to prevent injury. Refer to sec. on neurotoxicity, Chapter 4 |

*(continued)*

## Oxaliplatin (continued)

| Nursing Diagnosis | Defining Characteristics | Expected Outcomes | Nursing Interventions |
|---|---|---|---|
| III. *Potential for infection and bleeding related to bone marrow depression* | III. A. Mild leukopenia; mild to moderate thrombocytopenia | III. A. Pt will be free of s/s of infection and bleeding | III. A. Monitor CBC, platelet count prior to drug administration, as well as s/s of infection and bleeding<br>B. Instruct pt in self-assessment of s/s of infection and bleeding<br>C. Transfuse with red cells, platelets per MD order<br>D. Refer to sec. on bone marrow depression, Chapter 4 |

# Paclitaxel
(Taxol)

*Class:* Mitotic inhibitor (spindle poison)

## MECHANISM OF ACTION

Promotes early microtubule assembly; prevents depolymerization, bringing about cell arrest.

## METABOLISM

Extensively protein bound, resulting in an initial sharp decline in serum levels; metabolized by the liver. Metabolites excreted in bile.

## DOSAGE/RANGE

Previously untreated ovarian cancer: 135 mg/m$^2$ IV over 24 hours, followed by cisplatin 75 mg/m$^2$ every 3 weeks.

Previously treated ovarian cancer: 135–175 mg/m$^2$ IV over 3 hours every 3 weeks.

Adjuvant node positive breast cancer: 175 mg/m$^2$ IV over 3 hours, every 3 weeks, for 4 courses administered sequentially to doxorubicin-containing combination chemotherapy.

Metastatic breast cancer overexpressing HER2 protein: 175 mg/m$^2$ IV over 3 hours, every 3 weeks in combination with trastuzumab.

Metastatic breast cancer, after failure of initial therapy or relapse within 6 months of adjuvant therapy: 175 mg/m$^2$ IV over 3 hours every 3 weeks.

Non-small-cell lung cancer (NSCLC), not candidate for potentially curative surgery and/or XRT: 135 mg/m$^2$ IV over 24 hours, followed by cisplatin 75 mg/m$^2$ repeated every 3 weeks.

Second line AIDS-related Kaposi's Sarcoma: 135 mg/m$^2$ IV over 3 hours, repeated every 3 weeks or 100 mg/m$^2$ IV over 3 hours, repeated every 2 weeks (dose intensity of 45–50 mg/m$^2$ per week).

Other regimes used/being studied/reported: Advanced or metastatic NSCLC Phase II study of weekly paclitaxel 50 mg/m$^2$ IV over 1 hour in combination with carboplatin AUC 2 with concurrent XRT, and after completion of XRT, paclitaxel 200 mg/m$^2$ and carboplatin AUC 6 q 3 weeks × 2 cycles; studies in other tumor types (bladder, small cell lung, head and neck cancers).

## DRUG PREPARATION

Taxol is poorly soluble in water, so it is formulated using Cremaphor EL (polyoxyethylated castor oil) and dehydrated alcohol. Dilute in 5% dextrose or 0.9% sodium chloride.

## DRUG ADMINISTRATION

IV as 3-hour infusion or 24-hour continuous infusion, repeated every 21 days.

Glass or polyolefin containers and polyethylene-lined nitroglycerine tubing *must be used. Do not use* polyvinyl chloride plastic, as diethyl-hexlphthalate leaches into drug solution.

Use 0.22-micron in-line filter.

### Paclitaxel (Taxol) *(continued)*

#### *SPECIAL CONSIDERATIONS*

Premedicate with steroid, $H_2$ blocker, diphenhydramine to prevent hypersensitivity reaction.

Reversal of multidrug resistance experimentally successful with quinidine, cyclosporin A, quinine, or verapamil.

Has radiosensitizing effects.

Hypersensitivity reactions occur in 10% of patients, and cardiac arrythmias can occur; keep resuscitation equipment nearby.

Monitor vital signs every 15 minutes for 1 hour and then every hour if no adverse effects occur.

*Do not give drug* as a bolus, as it may cause bronchospasm and hypotension.

Phlebitis may occur rarely.

Drug is embryofetal toxic; benefit should outweigh risk if drug is used during pregnancy.

Breast-feeding should be avoided, as drug may be excreted in breast milk.

Contraindicated in patients with hypersensitivity to paclitaxel or other drugs formulated in Cremaphor EL. However, there are reports of rechallenge following multiple high doses of corticosteroids.

Contraindicated in patients with baseline absolute neutrophil count < 1500 cells/mm$^3$, and < 1000 cells/mm$^3$ in AIDS-related Kaposi's Sarcoma patients.

Drug may interact with ketoconazole, resulting in decreased paclitaxel metabolism; monitor patient closely.

If severe neuropathy develops, drug dose should be reduced 20%.

# Paclitaxel

| Nursing Diagnosis | Defining Characteristics | Expected Outcomes | Nursing Interventions |
|---|---|---|---|
| I. *Potential for injury related to hypersensitivity reactions* | I. A. 10% of pts experience anaphylaxis<br>B. S/s include tachycardia, wheezing, hypotension, facial edema, supraventricular tachycardia with hypotension and chest pain (1–2%) | I. A. Early s/s of hypersensitivity reactions will be identified | I. A. Review standing orders for management of hypersensitivity reactions and identify location of anaphylaxis kit containing epinephrine 1:1000, hydrocortisone sodium succinate (SoluCortef), diphenhydramine HC1 (Benadryl), Aminophylline, and other medications<br>B. Prior to drug administration, obtain baseline vital signs and record mental status assessment<br>C. Administer or teach pt to self-administer (as ordered) the following:<br>  1. Dexamethasone 20-mg IV or po 12–14 hrs and 6–7 hrs prior to paclitaxel administration<br>  2. Diphenhydramine 50-mg IV 30 mins prior to chemotherapy<br>  3. Ranitidine 50-mg IV or cimetidine 300 mg IV or other $H_2$ blocker 30 mins prior to chemotherapy<br>D. Assess pt for at least 30 mins after drug is given for s/s of a reaction<br>E. Teach pt to report any hypersensitivity reactions or unusual symptoms<br>F. Observe for the following s/s during infusion, usually occurring within first 15 mins of start of infusion:<br>  1. *Subjective*<br>    a. generalized itching<br>    b. nausea |

*(continued)*

**Paclitaxel** (*continued*)

| Nursing Diagnosis | Defining Characteristics | Expected Outcomes | Nursing Interventions |
|---|---|---|---|
| | | | c. chest tightness<br>d. crampy abdominal pain<br>e. difficulty speaking<br>f. anxiety<br>g. agitation<br>h. sense of impending doom<br>i. uneasiness<br>j. desire to urinate or defecate<br>k. dizziness<br>l. chills<br>2. *Objective*<br>a. flushed appearance (angioedema of face, lips, neck, eyelids, hands)<br>b. localized or generalized urticaria<br>c. respiratory distress ± wheezing<br>d. hypotension<br>e. cyanosis<br>G. If reaction occurs, stop infusion and notify MD<br>H. Place pt in supine position to promote perfusion of visceral organs<br>I. Monitor vital signs until stable<br>J. Provide emotional support to pt and family<br>K. Maintain patent airway and have equipment for CPR close by<br>L. Document incident and pt response to treatment<br>M. Discuss with MD desensitization and increased premedication for future treatments |

| Nursing Diagnosis | Defining Characteristics | Expected Outcomes | Nursing Interventions |
|---|---|---|---|
| II. *Potential alteration in cardiac output* | II. A. Sinus bradycardia occurs in 29% of pts up to 8 hrs after drug infusion<br>B. Ventricular tachycardia rare | II. A. Cardiac arrhythmias will be identified early<br>B. BP will remain within normal limits | II. A. Assess baseline cardiac status, including apical pulse, and note rate and rhythm; repeat every 15 mins for 1 hr then every hour if stable<br>B. Notify MD if abnormalities occur, and prepare to stabilize pt<br>C. Teach pt to report any discomfort, dizziness, weakness, chest pain |
| III. *Infection and bleeding related to bone marrow depression* | III. A. Neutropenia may be severe; nadir 7–10 days after dose, with recovery in 1 week<br>B. Neutropenia is dose dependent, with severe neutropenia (ANC < 500 cells/mm$^3$) occurring in 47–67% of pts<br>C. Pts with prior XRT are at risk<br>D. Anemia occurs frequently, but thrombocytopenia is uncommon | III. A. Pt will be without s/s of infection or bleeding<br>B. Early s/s of infection or bleeding will be identified | III. A. Monitor CBC, platelet count prior to drug administration and postchemotherapy; assess for s/s of infection or bleeding<br>B. Teach pt self-assessment of s/s of infection or bleeding and how to seek medical advice/care<br>C. Teach pt self-administration of granulocyte colony-stimulating factor (G-CSF) as ordered<br>D. Refer to sec. on bone marrow, Chapter 4 |
| IV. *Potential for sensory/ perceptual alterations* | IV. A. Peripheral neuropathy may occur within 24 hrs of high-dose therapy (burning pain in feet, hyperesthesias, numbness, periorbital numbness, decreased deep tendon reflexes); severity is dose dependent<br>B. Mild paresthesias most common (62%)<br>C. Symptoms improve within months of drug discontinuance | IV. A. Early s/s of neurological toxicity will be identified<br>B. Function will be maintained | IV. A. Assess baseline neuromuscular function and, prior to drug infusion, especially presence of paresthesias<br>B. Teach pt to report any changes in sensation or function<br>C. Discuss alterations with MD<br>D. Identify strategies to promote comfort and safety |

*(continued)*

**Paclitaxel** (continued)

| Nursing Diagnosis | Defining Characteristics | Expected Outcomes | Nursing Interventions |
|---|---|---|---|
| V. *Alteration in skin integrity related to alopecia*<br><br>A. Nausea and vomiting | V. A. Complete alopecia occurs in most pts<br>B. Reversible | V. A. Pt will verbalize feelings re hair loss and strategies to cope with change in body image | V. A. 1. Discuss potential impact of hair loss prior to drug administration, coping strategies, and plan to minimize body image distortion (e.g., wig, scarf, cap)<br>2. Assess pt for s/s of hair loss<br>3. Assess pt's response and use of coping strategies |
| VI. *Alteration in nutrition, less than body requirements related to*<br><br>A. Nausea and vomiting | VI. A. Nausea and vomiting are usually mild and preventable with antiemetics; incidence is 59% | VI. A. 1. Pt will be without nausea and vomiting<br>2. Nausea and vomiting, if they occur, will be mild<br>3. Pt will maintain weight within 5% of baseline | VI. A. 1. Premedicate with antiemetics prior to drug administration and postchemotherapy<br>2. Encourage small, frequent feedings of cool, bland foods and liquids<br>3. Assess for symptoms of fluid/electrolyte imbalance if pt has severe nausea and vomiting<br>4. Monitor I&O, daily weights, lab electrolyte values<br>5. Refer to sec. on nausea and vomiting, Chapter 4 |
| B. Diarrhea | B. Mild, with 43% incidence | B. Pt will have minimal diarrhea | B. 1. Encourage pt to report onset of diarrhea<br>2. Administer or teach pt to self-administer antidiarrheal medication<br>3. See sec. on diarrhea, Chapter 4 |
| C. Mucositis | C. Mild, with 39% incidence | C. Oral mucous membranes will remain infection-free | C. 1. Assess baseline oral mucous membranes<br>2. Teach pt oral assessment and mouth care and to report any alterations<br>3. See sec. on mucositis, Chapter 4 |

| | | |
|---|---|---|
| D. Dysgeusia | D. Occurs rarely | D. Taste distortions will be minimized | D. 1. Assess presence of taste distortions and ask pt to identify abnormal taste responses to specific foods<br>2. Discuss alternative foods that do not cause dysgeusia<br>3. Discuss use of condiments that may minimize dysgeusia (e.g., Crazy Jane salt and pepper)<br>4. Refer to nutritionist/ dietitian as appropriate |
| E. Hepatotoxicity | E. Mild increase in liver function studies may occur | E. Hepatic dysfunction will be identified early | E. 1. Assess liver function studies prior to drug administration and periodically during treatment<br>2. Dose modification necessary for severe hepatic dysfunction (see "Special Considerations") |
| VII. *Alteration in comfort related to flu-like syndrome* | VII. A. Occurs rarely and may include arthralgias, myalgias, fever, rash, headache, and fatigue | VII. A. Pt will report early s/s of flu-like syndrome | VII. A. Teach pt about the potential for flu-like syndrome and how to distinguish from actual infection<br>B. Instruct pt to report symptoms<br>C. Teach pt self-care measures to minimize symptoms |

# Pala

(NSC-224131, N-phosphonoacetyl-
disodium L-aspartic acid)

*Class:* Antimetabolite (investigational)

## MECHANISM OF ACTION

Blocks pyrimidine synthesis.

## METABOLISM

Excreted by kidneys (70% in 24 hours). Crosses
blood-brain barrier; excreted in tears.

## DOSAGE/RANGE

Varies with protocol; schedules commonly found
are 2.5 gm/day IV × 2 days, repeated every
2 weeks

## DRUG PREPARATION

Available as 100 mg/ml in 10-ml ampules from
the National Cancer Institute. Dilute to a
final concentration of 1 mg/ml in 0.9%
sodium chloride or 5% dextrose.

## DRUG ADMINISTRATION

Under investigation; usually administered as IV
infusion over 1 hour.

## SPECIAL CONSIDERATIONS

Synergistic with 5-fluorouracil.

Pala

| Nursing Diagnosis | Defining Characteristics | Expected Outcomes | Nursing Interventions |
|---|---|---|---|
| I. *Alteration in nutrition, less than body requirements related to* | | | |
| A. Mucositis | I. A. Mucositis is a dose-limiting toxicity | I. A. Oral mucous membranes will remain infection-free | I. A. 1. Assess baseline oral mucous membranes<br>2. Teach pt oral assessment and mouth care and to report any alterations<br>3. See sec. on mucositis, Chapter 4 |
| B. Diarrhea | B. Diarrhea is a dose-limiting toxicity | B. Pt will have minimal diarrhea | B. 1. Encourage pt to report onset of diarrhea<br>2. Administer or teach pt to self-administer antidiarrheal medication<br>3. See sec. on mucositis, diarrhea, Chapter 4 |
| C. Nausea and vomiting | C. Nausea and vomiting are mild and can be controlled | C. 1. Pt will be without nausea and vomiting<br>2. Nausea and vomiting, if they occur, will be mild<br>3. Pt will maintain weight within 5% of baseline | C. 1. Premedicate with antiemetics prior to drug administration and postchemotherapy<br>2. Encourage small, frequent feedings of cool, bland foods and liquids<br>3. Assess for symptoms of fluid/electrolyte imbalance if pt has severe nausea and vomiting<br>4. Monitor I&O, daily weights, and lab electrolyte values<br>5. Refer to sec. on nausea and vomiting, Chapter 4 |
| II. *Potential alteration in skin integrity* | II. A. Rash can be a dose-limiting side effect<br>B. Begins as erythema and progresses to desquamation of hands and feet | II. A. Rash will be identified | II. A. Assess baseline skin integrity and condition<br>B. Teach pt to report skin rash<br>C. Teach pt measures to protect skin integrity<br>D. Discuss drug discontinuance with MD |

(continued)

## Pala (continued)

| Nursing Diagnosis | Defining Characteristics | Expected Outcomes | Nursing Interventions |
|---|---|---|---|
| III. Infection and bleeding related to bone marrow depression | III. A. Usually mild | III. A. Pt will be without s/s of infection or bleeding<br>B. Early s/s of infection or bleeding will be identified | III. A. Monitor CBC, platelet count prior to drug administration and post-chemotherapy; assess for s/s of infection or bleeding<br>B. Teach pt self-assessment of s/s of infection or bleeding and how to seek medical advise/care<br>C. Refer to sec. on bone marrow depression, Chapter 4 |
| IV. Potential for sensory/perceptual alterations | IV. A. Paresthesias, rare seizures, headache, lethargy, and confusion can occur rarely<br>B. Ataxia may occur with 24-hr drug infusion | IV. A. Early s/s of neurological toxicity will be identified | IV. A. Assess baseline neuromuscular function and mental status<br>B. Teach pt to report any changes in sensation or function<br>C. Discuss alterations with MD<br>D. Identify strategies to promote comfort and safety |

# Pentostatin
## (2'-deoxycofomycin, DCF)

*Class:* Antitumor antibiotic
(investigational)

## MECHANISM OF ACTION

Cell cycle phase–nonspecific. A potent inhibitor of adenosine deaminase. Interferes with DNA replication and disrupts RNA processing. It has potent lymphocytotoxic properties. The major mechanism of action is not yet clearly understood.

## METABOLISM

The majority of pentostatin is excreted from the body via urine as unchanged drug. The mean halflife is 4.9–6.2 hours.

Clinical trials have shown a relationship between pentostatin's complete excretion and the patient's renal function. Patients with creatinine clearance $\leq$ 50 ml/min should *not* receive this agent.

## DOSAGE/RANGE

Drug is undergoing clinical trials; consult individual protocol for specific dosages.

## DRUG PREPARATION

This drug is supplied by the National Cancer Institute.

Available as a white powder.

Reconstitute with sodium chloride injection.

This solution is chemically stable at room temperature for at least 72 hours, but since it lacks bacteriostatic preservatives, discard the solution after 8 hours.

## DRUG ADMINISTRATION

Drug is a vesicant. Administer IV push over 5 minutes through the sidearm of a freely running IV.

## SPECIAL CONSIDERATIONS

Drug is a vesicant.

Dose-limiting toxicities involve renal and neurotoxicities.

Requires adequate renal function.

Enhanced toxicity when allopurinol is administered concurrently. *Avoid concurrent use.*

Severe, potentially fatal pulmonary toxicity when drug is administered with fludarabine. *Avoid concurrent use.*

**Pentostatin**

| Nursing Diagnosis | Defining Characteristics | Expected Outcomes | Nursing Interventions |
|---|---|---|---|
| I. *Potential for infection and bleeding related to bone marrow depression* | I. A. Severe/profound leukopenia and thrombocytopenia<br>B. Mild anemia | I. A. Pt will be without s/s of infection or bleeding<br>B. Early s/s of infection or bleeding will be identified | I. A. Monitor CBC, platelet count prior to drug administration, as well as s/s of infection or bleeding<br>B. Instruct pt in self-assessment of s/s of infection or bleeding<br>C. Dose reduction often necessary (35–50%) with compromised bone marrow function<br>D. Transfuse with platelets, red cells per MD order<br>E. Refer to sec. on bone marrow depression, Chapter 4 |
| II. *Potential for altered urinary elimination related to nephrotoxicity* | II. A. Renal insufficiency—mild, increased BUN and creatinine common—reversible<br>B. May include hyperuricemia if hydration, allopurinol are inadequate or if tumor lysis is acute | II. A. Pt will be without s/s of nephrotoxicity | II. A. Monitor BUN and creatinine prior to drug dose, as drug is excreted in urine<br>B. Provide or instruct pt in hydration of at least 3 liters of fluid/day<br>C. Monitor I&O<br>D. Hold drug if renal functions are elevated<br>E. Refer to sec. on nephrotoxicity, Chapter 4 |
| III. *Altered nutrition, less than body requirements related to*<br>A. Nausea and vomiting | III. A. Nausea and vomiting may be mild to severe and seen in at least two-thirds of pts | III. A. 1. Pt will be without nausea and vomiting<br>2. Nausea and vomiting, if they occur, will be minimal | III. A. 1. Premedicate with antiemetics and continue prophylactically × 24 hrs to prevent nausea and vomiting<br>2. Encourage small, frequent feedings of cool, bland foods and liquids<br>3. Refer to sec. on nausea and vomiting, Chapter 4 |
| B. Hepatic dysfunction | B. Hepatitis is rare but may occur; disturbances in liver functions, (i.e., mild SGOT) | B. Hepatic dysfunction will be identified early | B. 1. Monitor LFTs, especially SGOT<br>2. Notify MD of any elevations<br>3. Refer to sec. on hepatotoxicity, Chapter 4 |

| Nursing Diagnosis | Expected Outcomes | Defining Characteristics | Nursing Interventions |
|---|---|---|---|
| IV. *Potential for mental status changes* | IV. A. Neurotoxicity will be identified early | IV. A. Neurotoxicity varies from lethargy to somnolence to coma<br>B. Occurs in 60% of cases<br>C. Begins several days after pentostatin infusion and may last for up to 3 weeks | IV. A. Teach pt about the potential for neurological reactions and to report any unusual symptoms<br>B. Obtain baseline neurological and mental function<br>C. Assess pt for any neurological abnormalities and report changes to MD<br>D. Concomitant psychotropic drugs may exacerbate s/s<br>E. Refer to sec. on neurotoxicity, Chapter 4 |
| V. *Potential for impaired gas exchange related to pulmonary toxicity* | V. A. Early s/s of pulmonary toxicity will be identified | V. A. Infiltrates and nodules may occur in pts with prior history of receiving bleomycin or lung irradiation | V. A. Obtain baseline pulmonary function<br>B. Assess for s/s of pulmonary dysfunction (i.e., lung sounds)<br>C. Discuss with MD pulmonary function studies to be performed periodically<br>D. Instruct pt to report cough or dyspnea<br>E. Refer to sec. on pulmonary toxicity, Chapter 4 |
| VI. *Potential for sensory/ perceptual alterations* | VI. A. Conjunctivitis will be prevented (or at least identified early) | VI. A. Severe yet reversible conjunctivitis<br>B. Responds to steroid eyedrops | VI. A. Obtain baseline ophthalmic assessment<br>B. Teach pt of the potential of ophthalmic reactions and to report any unusual symptoms<br>C. Administer steroid eyedrops during drug administration |
| VII. *Alteration in skin integrity related to extravasation* | VII. A. Extravasation, if it occurs, is detected early, with early intervention<br>B. Skin and underlying tissue damage is minimized | VII. A. Pentostatin is a potent vesicant<br>B. Vesicants cause erythema, burning, tissue necrosis, tissue sloughing | VII. A. Careful technique is used during venipuncture; see sec. on intravenous administration, Chapter 9<br>B. Administer vesicant through freely flowing IV, constantly monitoring IV site and pt response |

*(continued)*

## Pentostatin (continued)

| Nursing Diagnosis | Defining Characteristics | Expected Outcomes | Nursing Interventions |
|---|---|---|---|
| | | | C. Nurse should be *thoroughly* familiar with institutional policy and procedure for administration of a vesicant agent |
| | | | D. If vesicant drug is administered as a continuous infusion, drug must be given through a patent central line |
| | | | E. If extravasation is suspected: |
| | | |   1. Stop drug being administered |
| | | |   2. Aspirate any residual drug and blood from IV tubing, IV catheter/needle, and IV site if possible |
| | | |   3. *If antidote exists*, instill antidote into area of apparent infiltration as per MD order and institutional policy and procedure |
| | | |   4. Apply cold or topical medication as per MD order and institutional policy and procedure |
| | | | F. Assess site regularly for pain, progression of erythema, induration, and evidence of necrosis |
| | | | G. When in doubt about whether drug is infiltrating, *treat as an infiltration* |
| | | | H. Teach pt to assess site and notify MD if condition worsens |
| | | | I. Arrange next clinic visit for assessment of site depending on drug, amount infiltrated, extent of potential injury, and pt variables |
| | | | J. Document in pt's record as per institutional policy and procedure; see sec. on reactions, Chapter 9 |

# Plicamycin
(mithramycin, Mithracin)

*Class:* Antibiotic; isolated from *Streptomyces plicatus*

## MECHANISM OF ACTION

In the presence of magnesium ions, the drug binds with guanine bases of DNA and inhibits DNA-directed RNA synthesis. Cell cycle–specific for S phase.

## METABOLISM

Metabolism is not clearly understood. About half of the drug is excreted within 18–24 hours. Crosses blood-brain barrier and concentration of drug in CSF equals blood concentration 4–6 hours after administration.

## DOSAGE/RANGE

Testicular cancer: 25–30 µg/kg IV alternating days until toxicity occurs

Hypercalcemia: 25 µg/kg IV × 1

## DRUG PREPARATION

For each 2.5-mg vial, add sterile water to obtain concentration of 500 µg/ml.

## DRUG ADMINISTRATION

IV. Drug is an irritant; avoid extravasation. Administer over 4–6 hours to minimize nausea and vomiting.

## SPECIAL CONSIDERATIONS

Alternate-day therapy greatly reduces the incidence and severity of stomatitis, hemorrhage, and facial flushing and swelling.

Do not administer to patient with a coagulation disorder or impaired bone marrow function because of the risk of hemorrhagic diathesis.

Crosses the blood-brain barrier.

Metallic taste with administration.

## Plicamycin

I. *Altered nutrition, less than body requirements related to*

| Nursing Diagnosis | Defining Characteristics | Expected Outcomes | Nursing Interventions |
|---|---|---|---|
| A. Nausea and vomiting | I. A. Severe nausea and vomiting begin 6 + hrs after dose and may last 24 hrs (at therapeutic doses) | I. A. 1. Pt will be without nausea and vomiting 2. Nausea and vomiting, if they occur, will be minimal | I. A. 1. Premedicate with antiemetics and continue prophylactically to *prevent* nausea and vomiting, at least for first treatment 2. Encourage small, frequent feedings of cool, bland foods and liquids 3. See sec. on nausea and vomiting, Chapter 4 |
| B. Anorexia | B. Commonly occurs | B. Pt will maintain baseline weight ±5% | B. 1. Encourage small, frequent feedings of favorite foods, especially high-calorie, high-protein foods 2. Encourage use of spices 3. Weekly weights |
| C. Stomatitis | C. Alternate-day therapy greatly reduces the incidence and severity of stomatitis | C. Oral mucous membranes will remain intact and without infection | C. 1. Teach pt oral assessment and oral hygiene regimens 2. Encourage pt to report early stomatitis 3. Pain relief measures if needed 4. See sec. on stomatitis, Chapter 4 |
| D. Potential for taste alterations | D. Taste alterations can occur | D. Pt will eat adequate calories, proteins, minerals | D. 1. Suggest increased use of spices as tolerated 2. Help pt and significant other develop menus based on past favorite foods 3. Dietary consultation as needed 4. Discuss dietary supplements of zinc and selenium |

| Nursing Diagnosis | Assessment Data | Expected Outcomes | Interventions |
|---|---|---|---|
| II. *Potential for infection and bleeding related to bone marrow depression* | II. A. Leukopenia nadir 7–14 days, with recovery by 1–2 weeks<br>B. Less frequent thrombocytopenia, but one-third of pts develop a coagulopathy; alternate-day dosing reduces bleeding<br>C. Mild anemia<br>D. Potent immunosuppressant | II. A. Pt will be without s/s of infection or bleeding<br>B. Early s/s of infection or bleeding will be identified | II. A. Monitor CBC, platelet count prior to drug administration, as well as s/s of infection or bleeding<br>B. Instruct pt in self-assessment of s/s of infection or bleeding<br>C. Dose reduction often necessary (35–50%) if compromised bone marrow function<br>D. See sec. on bone marrow depression, Chapter 4 |
| III. *Potential for impaired skin integrity related to*<br><br>A. Alopecia | III. A. 1. Occurs in 30–50% of pts, especially with IV dosing<br>2. Some degree of hair loss expected in all pts<br>3. Begins after 3 + weeks, and hair may grow back during therapy<br>4. May be slight to diffuse thinning | III. A. Pt will verbalize feelings re hair loss and identify strategies to cope with change in body image | III. A. 1. Assess pt for s/s of hair loss<br>2. Discuss with pt impact of hair loss and strategies to minimize distress (e.g., wig, scarf, cap); begin before therapy initiated<br>3. See sec. on alopecia, Chapter 4 |
| B. Changes in nails, skin | B. Hyperpigmentation of nails and skin, transverse ridging of nails ("banding") may occur | B. Pt will verbalize feelings re changes in nail or skin color or texture and identify strategies to cope with change in body image | B. 1. Assess pt for changes in skin, nails<br>2. Discuss with pt impact of changes and strategies to minimize distress (e.g., wearing nail polish, long sleeves) |

*(continued)*

**Plicamycin** *(continued)*

| Nursing Diagnosis | Defining Characteristics | Expected Outcomes | Nursing Interventions |
|---|---|---|---|
| IV. *Potential for sexual dysfunction* | IV. A. Drug is mutagenic and teratogenic<br>B. Testicular atrophy sometimes with reversible oligospermia and azoospermia<br>C. Amenorrhea often occurs in females<br>D. Drug is excreted in breast milk | IV. A. Pt and significant other will understand need for contraception<br>B. Pt and significant other will identify strategies to cope with sexual dysfunction | IV. A. As appropriate, explore with pt and significant other issues of reproductive and sexuality pattern and impact chemotherapy will have<br>B. Discuss strategies to preserve sexual and reproductive health (e.g., sperm banking, contraception)<br>C. See sec. on gonadal dysfunction, Chapter 4 |
| V. *Alteration in metabolism* | V. A. Drug may decrease calcium and lead to hypocalcemia; monitor for muscle stiffness, twitching<br>B. In some cases when calcium is abnormally high (as in hypercalcemia from breast cancer), this drug may be used to decrease calcium level | V. A. Hypocalcemia will be identified and treated early | V. A. Monitor blood calcium levels<br>B. Instruct pt about s/s of neuromuscular involvement, such as muscle stiffness, weakness, or twitching<br>C. Instruct pt about CNS manifestations of hypocalcemia; weakness, drowsiness, lethargy, irritability, headache, confusion, depression |

# Polifeprosan 20 with carmustine (BCNU) implant (Gliadel™)

*Class:* Alkylating agent

## MECHANISM OF ACTION

Wafer (copolymer) containing carmustine is implanted in the surgical cavity created when brain tumor is resected. In water, the anhydride bonds of the wafer are hydrolyzed, releasing the carmustine into the surgical cavity. The carmustine diffuses into the surrounding brain tissue, reaching any residual tumor cells, and causing cell death by alkylating DNA and RNA.

## METABOLISM

Unknown. Wafer is biogradable in brain tissue, with a variable rate. More than 70% of the copolymer degrades by 3 weeks. In some patients, wafer fragments remained up to 232 days after implantation, with almost all drug gone.

## DOSAGE/RANGE

Each wafer contains 7.7 mg of carmustine, and the recommended dose is 8 wafers, or a total dose of 61.6 mg of carmustine.

## DRUG PREPARATION

Drug must be stored at or below −20° C (−4° F) until time of use. Unopened foil packages can stay at room temperature for a maximum of 6 hours at a time. The manufacturer recommends that the treatment box be removed from the freezer and taken to the operating room just prior to surgery. The box and pouches should be opened just before the surgeon is ready to implant the wafers. Open the sealed treatment box and remove double foil packages, handling the unsterile outer foil packet by the crimped edge VERY CAREFULLY to prevent damage to the wafers. See product information for opening the inner foil pouch and removing the wafer with sterile technique. Chemotherapy precautions should be used to limit exposure to the chemotherapy: surgical instruments used to remove and implant the wafers should be kept separate from other instruments and sterile fields, and should be cleaned after the procedure according to hospital chemotherapy procedure; all personnel handling the inner foil pouches containing the wafers, or the wafers, should wear double gloves, which, along with unused wafers or fragments, inner foil packages, opened outer foil package, and gloves, should be disposed of as chemotherapeutic waste.

## DRUG ADMINISTRATION

Neurosurgeon places 8 wafers into surgical resection cavity if size and shape appropriate; wafers are placed contiguously or with slight overlapping. Wafer may be broken into 2 pieces *only* if needed.

## DRUG INTERACTIONS

Unknown but unlikely as drug is probably not systemically absorbed.

## LAB EFFECTS/INTERFERENCE

Unknown, but unlikely.

# Polifeprosan 20 *(continued)*

## SPECIAL CONSIDERATIONS

Indicated for use as an adjunct to surgery to prolong survival in patients with recurrent glioblastoma multiforme for whom surgical resection is indicated.

Manufacturer reports that in a study of 222 patients with recurrent glioma who failed initial surgery and radiotherapy, 6-month survival rate after surgery increased from 47% (placebo) to 60%, and in patients with glioblastoma multiforme. Six-month survival for patients receiving placebo was 36% vs. 56% for patients receiving polifeprosan 20 with carmustine implant.

Patients require close monitoring for complications of craniotomy, as intracerebral mass effect has occurred that does not respond to corticosteroid treatment, and in one case, resulted in brain herniation.

Studies have not been conducted during pregnancy or in nursing mothers. Carmustine is a known teratogen, and is embryotoxic. Use during pregnancy should be avoided, and mothers should stop nursing during use of the drug.

## Polifeprosan 20 with carmustine (BCNU) implant (Gliadel™)

| Nursing Diagnosis | Defining Characteristics | Expected Outcomes | Nursing Interventions |
|---|---|---|---|
| I. *Potential sensory/perceptual alterations related to seizures, brain edema, mental status changes* | I. A. Incidence of new or worsened seizures was 19% in both the group receiving the implant and those receiving the placebo. Seizures were mild to moderate in severity. In pts with new or worsened seizures postoperatively, the group receiving the implant had a 56% incidence, with median time to first new or worsened seizure of 3.5 days, versus placebo incidence of 9%, and median time to first new or worsened seizure of 61 days. Incidence of brain edema was 4%, and there were cases of intracerebral mass effect that did not respond to corticosteroids<br><br>B. Other nervous system effects: hydrocephalus (3%), depression (3%), abnormal thinking (2%), ataxia (2%), dizziness (2%), insomnia (2%), visual field defect (2%), eye pain (1%), monoplegia (2%), coma (1%), amnesia (1%), diplopia (1%), and paranoid reaction (1%)<br><br>C. Rarely (< 1%), cerebral infarct or hemorrhage may occur | I. A. Early s/s of increased ICP or CNS changes will be defected, and managed | I. A. Monitor neurovital signs closely postoperatively, and notify MD of any abnormalities<br><br>B. Expect pt to be taken to surgery for removal of the wafer or remnants if increased ICP, or a mass effect is suspected that is unresponsive to corticosteroids<br><br>C. Assess baseline mental status and regularly postoperatively; validate any changes with family members, report any changes immediately to MD, and continue to monitor neurovital signs closely |

*(continued)*

## Polifeprosan 20 with carmustine (BCNU) implant (Gliadel™) (continued)

| Nursing Diagnosis | Defining Characteristics | Expected Outcomes | Nursing Interventions |
|---|---|---|---|
| II. Potential for infection related to healing abnormalities | II. A. 1. Most abnormalities were mild to moderate, occurred in 14% of pts, and included: cerebrospinal leaks, subdural fluid collections, subgaleal or wound effusions, and breakdown<br>2. The incidence of intracranial infection (e.g., meningitis or abscess) was 4%<br>B. Incidence of deep wound infection was 6% (same as placebo) and included infection of subgaleal space, bone, meninges, and brain tissue | II. A. Pt will be without s/s of infection<br>B. If infection develops, s/s will be identified early and managed | II. A. Using aseptic technique, assess postoperative wound dressing immediately after surgery, and regularly thereafter<br>B. Assess systematically for s/s of infection or wound breakdown;<br>C. If s/s of infection or wound breakdown, discuss management and antimicrobial therapy with MD |
| III. Alteration in nutrition, less than body requirements related to GI side effects, electrolyte abnormalities | III. A. Rarely, GI disturbances occurred: diarrhea (2%), constipation (2%), dysphagia (1%), gastrointestinal hemorrhage (1%), fecal incontinence (1%)<br>B. Hyponatremia (3%), hypokalemia (1%), and hyperglycemia (3%) also occurred | III. A. Pt will maintain weight within 5% of baseline<br>B. Pt's electrolyte balance will be WNL | III. A. Assess baseline nutritional status, including electrolytes<br>B. Assess bowel elimination status and monitor nutritional and elimination status closely postoperatively<br>C. Discuss management strategies with MD |

| Nursing Diagnosis | Data | Expected Outcomes | Nursing Interventions |
|---|---|---|---|
| IV. *Alteration in circulation, potential, related to changes in blood pressure* | IV. A. Hypertension occurred in 3% of pts, and hypotension (1%) | IV. A. Changes in BP will be detected early | IV. A. Assess baseline vital signs, and monitor closely during postoperative phase<br>B. Discuss any abnormalities with MD |
| V. *Alteration in comfort related to edema, pain, asthenia* | V. A. The following occur rarely: peripheral edema (2%), neck pain (2%), rash (2%), back pain (1%), asthenia (1%), chest pain (1%) | V. A. Pt will be comfortable | V. A. Assess baseline comfort level, and monitor closely during postoperative course<br>B. Provide physical and mental comfort measures<br>C. If ineffective, discuss alternative strategies with MD for symptom management |

# Procarbazine hydrochlorozide
(Natulanar, Matulane)

*Class:* Miscellaneous agent

## MECHANISM OF ACTION

Uncertain, but appears to affect preformed DNA, RNA, and protein. It is a methylhydrazine derivative.

## METABOLISM

Most of the drug is excreted in urine. Procarbazine crosses the blood-brain barrier. Rapidly absorbed from the gastrointestinal tract, metabolized by the liver.

## DOSAGE/RANGE

100–300 mg daily po for 7–14 days every 4 weeks; given in combination with other drugs

## DRUG PREPARATION

Available in 50-mg capsules.

## DRUG ADMINISTRATION

Oral

## SPECIAL CONSIDERATIONS

Procarbazine is synergistic with CNS depressants. Barbiturates, antihistamines, narcotics, hypotensive agents, or phenothiazine antiemetics should be used with caution.

Antabuse-like reaction may result if the patient consumes ETOH. Symptoms include headache, respiratory difficulties, nausea and vomiting, chest pain, hypotension, and mental status changes.

Exhibits weak MOA (monoamine oxidase) inhibitor activity. Foods containing high amounts of tyramine should be avoided: beer, wine, cheese, brewer's yeast, chicken livers, bananas. Consumption of foods high in tyramine in combination with procarbazine may lead to intracranial hemorrhage or hypertensive crisis.

When taken in combination with digoxin, there is a decreased bioavailability of digoxin.

## Procarbazine hydrochlorozide

| Nursing Diagnosis | Defining Characteristics | Expected Outcomes | Nursing Interventions |
|---|---|---|---|
| I. *Potential for infection and bleeding related to bone marrow depression* | I. A. Major dose-limiting toxicity<br>B. Thrombocytopenia occurs in 50% of pts, evidenced by a delayed onset (28 days after treatment) and lasting 2–3 weeks<br>C. Leukopenia seen in two-thirds of pts, with nadir occurring after initial thrombocytopenia<br>D. Anemias may be due to BMD or hemolysis | I. A. Pt will be without s/s of infection or bleeding<br>B. Early s/s of infection or bleeding will be identified | I. A. Monitor CBC, platelet count prior to drug administration, as well as s/s of infection, bleeding, and anemia<br>B. Instruct pt in self-assessment of s/s of infection, bleeding, and anemia<br>C. Dose reduction often necessary (35–50%) if compromised bone marrow function<br>D. Platelet and red cell transfusions per MD order<br>E. Refer to sec. on bone marrow depression, Chapter 4 |
| II. *Altered nutrition, less than body requirements related to*<br>A. Nausea and vomiting | II. A. Nausea and vomiting occur in 70% of pts and may be a dose-limiting toxicity | II. A. 1. Pt will be without nausea and vomiting<br>2. Nausea and vomiting, if they occur, will be minimal | II. A. 1. Premedicate with antiemetics and continue prophylactically × 24 hrs to *prevent* nausea and vomiting<br>2. Encourage small, frequent feedings of cool, bland foods and liquids<br>3. Minimize nausea and vomiting by dividing the total daily dosage into 3–4 doses; taking pills at bedtime may decrease nausea<br>4. May administer nonphenothiazine antiemetics<br>5. Refer to sec. on nausea and vomiting, Chapter 4 |

*(continued)*

## Procarbazine hydrochlorozide (continued)

| Nursing Diagnosis | Defining Characteristics | Expected Outcomes | Nursing Interventions |
|---|---|---|---|
| B. Diarrhea | B. Uncommon, but rarely may be protracted and thus would be an indication for dose reduction | B. Pt will have minimal diarrhea | B. 1. Encourage pt to report onset of diarrhea<br>2. Administer or teach pt to self-administer antidiarrheal medications<br>3. Teach pt perineal hygiene routine<br>4. See sec. on diarrhea, Chapter 4 |
| C. Stomatitis | C. Rare | C. Oral mucous membranes will remain intact and without infection | C. 1. Teach pt oral assessment<br>2. Encourage pt to report early stomatitis<br>3. Teach pt oral hygiene regimen<br>4. See sec. on stomatitis, Chapter 4 |
| D. Anorexia | D. Rare | D. Pt will maintain baseline weight ± 5% | D. 1. Encourage small, frequent feedings of favorite foods, especially high-calorie, high-protein foods<br>2. Encourage use of spices<br>3. Weekly weights |
| III. *Potential for sensory/ perceptual alterations* <br> A. Neurotoxicity | III. A. 1. Symptoms occur in 10–30% of pts; lethargy, depression, frequent nightmares, insomnia, nervousness, hallucinations<br>2. Tremors, coma, convulsions are less common<br>3. Symptoms usually disappear when drug is discontinued<br>4. Crosses into CSF | III. A. Early s/s of neurotoxicity will be identified | III. A. 1. Teach pt the potential of neurotoxicity and provide early counseling about these effects<br>2. Assess pts for any symptoms of neurotoxicity<br>3. Discuss strategies with pt to preserve general sense of well-being<br>4. Obtain baseline neurological and motor function<br>5. CNS toxicity may be manifested as reactions to other drugs (e.g., barbiturates, narcotics, phenothiazine antiemetics) |

| Nursing Diagnosis | Defining Characteristics | Expected Outcomes | Nursing Interventions |
|---|---|---|---|
| B. Peripheral neuropathy | B. 1. 10% of pts exhibit paresthesias, decrease in deep tendon reflexes 2. Foot drop and ataxia occasionally reported 3. Reversible when drug discontinued | B. Pt will be without s/s of peripheral neuropathy | B. 1. Obtain baseline neurological and motor function 2. Assess pt for any changes in motor function (e.g., picking up pencil, buttoning buttons) |
| C. Flu-like syndrome | C. Commonly occurs: fever, chills, sweating, lethargy, myalgias, arthralgias | C. Pt will report early s/s of flu-like syndrome | C. 1. Teach pt the potential for flu-like syndrome and how to distinguish from actual infection 2. Instruct pt to report any changes in condition |
| IV. *Potential for impaired skin integrity related to rare dermatitis reactions* | IV. A. Rarely occurs as alopecia, pruritis, rash, hyperpigmentation | IV. A. Pt will verbalize feelings regarding changes in hair loss, skin color, or integrity and will identify strategies to cope with change in body image | IV. A. Assess pt for changes in skin, nails, and hair loss B. Discuss with pt impact of changes and strategies to minimize distress (e.g., wearing nail polish, long sleeves, wigs, scarves, caps) |
| V. *Potential for sexual dysfunction* | V. A. Drug is teratogenic B. Causes azoospermia C. Cessation of menses, though may be reversible | V. A. Pt and significant other will understand need for contraception B. Pt and significant other will identify strategies to cope with sexual dysfunction | V. A. As appropriate, explore with pt and significant other issues of reproductive and sexuality pattern and impact chemotherapy may have B. Discuss strategies to preserve sexual and reproductive health (e.g., sperm banking, contraception) C. See sec. on gonadal dysfunction, Chapter 4 |
| VI. *Potential for injury related to secondary malignancy, leukemia* | VI. A. Prolonged therapy may cause leukemia (related to drug's carcinogenic properties) | VI. A. Malignancy, if it occurs, will be identified early | VI. A. If receiving prolonged therapy, pt should be screened periodically B. Educate pt on the potential for secondary malignancies |

# Progestational agents
medroxyprogesterone acetate (Provera, Depo-Provera), megestrol acetate (Megace, Pallace)

*Class:* Hormones

## MECHANISM OF ACTION

Unclear, but progestational agents compete for androgen and progestational receptor sites on the cell. Has potent antiestrogenic properties that disturb estrogen receptor cycle. Also increases synthesis of RNA by interacting with DNA.

## METABOLISM

Rapidly absorbed from gastrointestinal tract. Metabolized in the liver. Excreted in the urine. Peak plasma levels reached in 1–3 hours; biological half-life, 3.5 days.

## DOSAGE/RANGE

*Medroxyprogesterone acetate*
Provera: 20–80 mg orally daily
Depo-Provera: 400–800 mg IM every month; 100 mg IM 3 times weekly; 1000–1500 mg daily (high dose)
*Megestrol acetate (Megace, Pallace)*
Breast cancer: 40 mg orally qid
Endometrial cancer: 80 mg orally qid

## DRUG PREPARATION

IM preparation is ready to use; shake vial well before drawing up medication.

## DRUG ADMINISTRATION

Give via deep IM injection.

## SPECIAL CONSIDERATIONS

Patients may become sensitive to oil carrier (oil in which drug is mixed).

Small risk of hypersensitivity reaction.

Megestrol acetate is indicated for malnutrition related to anorexia and cancer cachexia. Optimal dose is 800 mg qid.

## Progestational agents

| Nursing Diagnosis | Defining Characteristics | Expected Outcomes | Nursing Interventions |
|---|---|---|---|
| I. *Potential for injury related to* | | | |
| A. Fluid retention | I. A. May occur | I. A. Fluid balance will be maintained | I. A. 1. Inform pt of potential for fluid retention and s/s to watch for and to report to nurse or MD<br>2. Assess pt for s/s of fluid overload |
| B. Thromboembolic complications | B. Thromboembolic complications may occur | B. Pt will avoid injury related to abnormal blood clotting | B. 1. Teach pt and family s/s of thromboembolic events: positive Homan's sign, localized pain, tenderness, erythema, sudden CNS changes, shortness of breath<br>2. Instruct pt to notify nurse or MD if any of the above occur |
| C. Sterile abscess | C. May occur with IM administration | C. Pt will avoid injury related to abscess formation | C. 1. Give drug via deep IM injection; apply pressure to injection site after administering<br>2. Inspect used sites; rotate sites systematically |
| II. *Altered nutrition, less than body requirements related to nausea* | II. A. Occurs infrequently | II. A. Pt will be without nausea | II. A. Inform pt that nausea can occur and to report nausea<br>B. Encourage small, frequent feedings of cool, bland liquids and foods<br>C. Refer to sec. on nausea and vomiting, Chapter 4 |

# Raloxifene hydrochloride
(Evista™)

*Class:* Selective Estrogen Receptor Modulator (SERM)

## MECHANISM OF ACTION

Selectively modulates estrogen receptors by binding to them. This binding causes expression of multiple estrogen regulated genes in different tissues; acts as an antagonist by inhibiting breast epithelial and uterine/endometrial proliferation; acts as an agonist (like estrogen) in bone. To preserve bone mineral density, and on lipid metabolism to lower low-density lipids and total cholesterol, while not affecting high-density lipids or triglycerides.

## METABOLISM

Primarily metabolized in the liver, with rapid systemic clearance.

## DOSAGE/RANGE

60 mg qd

## DRUG PREPARATION

None. Oral, available in 60-mg tablets.

## DRUG ADMINISTRATION

Take orally, without regard to food or meals.

## DRUG INTERACTIONS

Cholestyramine: causes 60% reduction in absorption of raloxifene; do not give concurrently.

Warfarin: 10% decrease in PT has been noted; monitor prothrombin closely if drugs given concurrently.

Highly protein-bound drugs: raloxifene is > 95% protein bound. Use together cautiously with the following drugs, and monitor closely for underdosing or toxicity: clofibrate, indomethacin, naproxen, ibuprofen, diazepam, diazoxide.

## LAB EFFECTS/INTERFERENCE

Unknown

## SPECIAL CONSIDERATIONS

Indicated for the prevention of osteoporosis in postmenopausal women, at doses of 30–150 mg/day, together with calcium replacement.

Multiple Outcomes of Raloxifene study showed raloxifene used to treat osteoporosis in postmenopausal women reduced risk of invasive breast cancer by 76% (1999). Thus, drug is currently being tested against tamoxifen in the prevention of breast cancer [National Surgical Adjuvant Breast and Bowel Project (NSABP) Study of Tamoxifen and Raloxifene (STAR)], Prevention Trial 2.

As compared to tamoxifen, raloxifene has 3 times the risk of causing thromboembolic disease, but does not significantly increase the risk of endometrial cancer.

Contraindicated in individuals who are hypersensitive to the drug, have or have had thromboembolic disorders, pregnant women, and women who may become pregnant.

When used to preserve bone density in postmenopausal women, drug should be combined with supplemental calcium, Vitamin D, weight-bearing exercises, lifestyle changes such as cessation of smoking and reduction in alcohol intake.

## Raloxifene hydrochloride

| Nursing Diagnosis | Defining Characteristics | Expected Outcomes | Nursing Interventions |
|---|---|---|---|
| I. *Alteration in circulation, potential, related to thromboembolic event* | I. A. Deep vein thrombosis, pulmonary embolism, and retinal vein thromboses may occur<br>B. Greatest risk is in first 4 months of treatment<br>C. Rarely, pts may experience chest pain | I. A. Pt will report thrombotic events immediately<br>B. Injury from thrombotic events will be minimal | I. A. Assess baseline risk (e.g., malignancy)<br>B. Teach pt to report pain in the legs, especially the calves, any redness or swelling of the legs, sudden onset shortness of breath, chest pain<br>C. If pt complains of leg pain, assess Homan's sign; if positive, discuss diagnostic ultrasound to r/o thromboembolism or thrombophlebitis<br>D. If pulmonary embolism is suspected, assess pulmonary status, discuss VQ scan with physician<br>E. Drug should be discontinued at least 72 hrs prior to and during prolonged bed rest (e.g., postoperative care), and resumed when pt ambulatory<br>F. Teach pt to walk/move around frequently, to avoid prolonged sitting while traveling |
| II. *Alteration in nutrition related to gastrointestinal symptoms* | II. A. Nausea, vomiting, dyspepsia, flatulence, gastroenteritis, and weight gain have been reported > 2% of the time | II. A. Pt will manage gastro-intestinal symptoms should they arise<br>B. Pt will maintain weight within 5% of baseline | II. A. Assess baseline nutritional status, including weight, and occurrence management of these symptoms<br>B. Teach pt that these symptoms may occur and to report them<br>C. Teach pt symptom management strategies<br>D. If symptoms are refractory or unacceptable, discuss pharmacologic symptom management, and if unsuccessful, drug discontinuance with MD |

*(continued)*

## Raloxifene hydrochloride (continued)

| Nursing Diagnosis | Defining Characteristics | Expected Outcomes | Nursing Interventions |
|---|---|---|---|
| III. Alteration in comfort related to headache, insomnia, depression, fever | III. A. Migraine headaches, depression, insomnia, and fever have all been reported as occurring in > 2% of pts | III. A. Pt will be comfortable | III. A. Assess baseline neurological status, including affect and sleeping pattern<br>B. Teach pt that these symptoms may occur, and to report them<br>C. Teach symptomatic management<br>D. If symptoms do not resolve, or become severe, discuss with MD pharmacologic symptom management and possible discontinuance of drug |
| IV. Alteration in comfort related to hot flashes, arthralgias, myalgias, cough, rash | IV. A. Hot flashes (25%), arthralgias (11%), myalgias (8%), leg cramps (6%), arthritis (4%), rash (6%), and flu syndrome (15%) have all been described<br>B. Hot flashes usually occur during first 6 months of treatment | IV. A. Pt will manage symptoms<br>B. Pt will be comfortable | IV. A. Assess baseline comfort level, and history of muscle and joint aches or pains<br>B. Assess skin integrity, and respiratory status<br>C. Teach pt that these symptoms may occur, and to report them, especially rash<br>D. Teach symptomatic management<br>E. If symptoms persist or become severe, discuss drug discontinuation with MD |
| V. Alteration in sexuality related to vaginitis, leukorrhea | V. A. Vaginitis, urinary tract infections (UTIs), cystitis, and leukorrhea have been reported to occur in at least 2% of pts | V. A. Pt will manage vaginal changes | V. A. Assess baseline gynecologic status, and history of UTIs and cystitis<br>B. Teach pt that these problems may occur, and to report them<br>C. Teach pt symptomatic management, and if these are ineffective, discuss other strategies with MD |

# Streptozocin
## (Streptozotocin, Zanosar)

*Class:* Alkylating agent (nitrosourea)

## MECHANISM OF ACTION

A weak alkylating agent (nitrosourea) that causes interstrand cross-linking in DNA (is cell cycle phase nonspecific). Appears to have some specificity for neoplastic pancreatic endocrine cells. Glucose attached to nitrosourea appears to diminish myelotoxicity.

## METABOLISM

60–70% of total dose and 10–20% of parent drug appears in urine. Drug is rapidly eliminated from serum in 4 hours, with major concentrations occurring in liver and kidneys.

## DOSAGE/RANGE

500 mg/m$^2$ IV every day $\times$ 5 days, repeat every 3–4 weeks

*or*

1500 mg/m$^2$ IV every week

## DRUG PREPARATION

Add sterile water or NS to vial.

If powder or solution contacts skin, wash immediately with soap and water.

Solution is stable 48 hours at room temperature, 96 hours if refrigerated.

## DRUG ADMINISTRATION

Administer via volutrol over 1 hour.

Has been given as continuous infusion or continuous arterial infusion into the hepatic artery.

If local pain or burning occurs, slow infusion and apply cool packs above injection site.

Irritant; avoid extravasation.

Administer with 1–2 liters of hydration to prevent nephrotoxicity.

## SPECIAL CONSIDERATIONS

Increased risk of nephrotoxicity if given with other potentially nephrotoxic drugs.

Renal function must be monitored closely.

Drug is an irritant. Give through the sidearm of a running IV.

## Streptozocin

| Nursing Diagnosis | Defining Characteristics | Expected Outcomes | Nursing Interventions |
|---|---|---|---|
| I. *Potential for altered urinary elimination* | I. A. 60% of pts experience renal dysfunction<br>B. Usually transient proteinuria and azotemia but may progress to permanent renal failure, especially if other nephrotoxic drugs are given concurrently<br>C. S/s include: proteinuria, increased BUN, hypophosphatemia, glycosuria, renal tubular acidosis, decreased creatinine clearance<br>D. Hypophosphatemia is probably earliest sign of renal dysfunction | I. A. Early renal dysfunction will be identified<br>B. Permanent renal failure will be prevented | I. A. Closely monitor BUN, creatinine, phosphorus, urine protein, 24-hr creatinine clearance prior to each treatment, and BUN, creatinine, pH of urine, glucose/protein of urine every shift during therapy<br>B. If creatinine clearance is < 25 ml/min, dose should be reduced by 50–75%<br>C. Strictly monitor I&O during therapy<br>D. Hydration per MD, but usually 2–3 l/day<br>E. Refer to sec. on nephrotoxicity, Chapter 4 |
| II. *Altered nutrition, less than body requirements related to*<br>A. Nausea and vomiting | II. A. 1. Nausea and vomiting occur in up to 90% of pts, beginning 1–4 hrs after drug dose<br>2. Significantly reduced when drug is given as continuous infusion<br>3. Nausea and vomiting may worsen during 5-consecutive-day therapy<br>4. Increased severity with doses > 500 mg/m$^2$ | II. A. 1. Pt will be without nausea and vomiting<br>2. Nausea and vomiting, if they occur, will be minimal | II. A. 1. Premedicate with antiemetics and continue prophylactically × 24 hrs; use aggressive antiemetics when drug is given IV over 1 hour<br>2. Encourage small, frequent feedings of cool, bland foods and liquids<br>3. If pt has emesis > 250 cc in 8 hrs, discuss with MD more aggressive antiemetics<br>4. Monitor I&O closely and replace fluids<br>5. Refer to sec. on nausea and vomiting, Chapter 4 |

| | | | |
|---|---|---|---|
| B. Diarrhea | B. 10% of pts experience diarrhea with abdominal cramping | B. Pt will have minimal diarrhea | B. 1. Encourage pt to report onset of diarrhea<br>2. Administer or teach pt to self-administer antidiarrheal medications<br>3. Teach pt dietary modifications<br>4. Instruct pt in perineal hygiene routines<br>5. Refer to sec. on diarrhea, Chapter 4 |
| C. Alterations in glucose metabolism | C. 1. Appears that damage to pancreatic beta cells causes sudden release of insulin, with resulting hypoglycemia in about 20% of pts<br>2. Hyperglycemia may occur in pts with insulinomas and decreased glucose tolerance; increased fasting or postprandial blood levels may occur | C. 1. Hypoglycemia will be identified and corrected<br>2. Hyperglycemia will be identified and corrected | C. 1. Monitor serum glucose levels every day or more frequently as needed; check urine glucose<br>2. Assess for and instruct pt to report following s/s of hypoglycemia:<br>  a. muscle weakness and lethargy<br>  b. perspiration<br>  c. flushed feeling<br>  d. restlessness<br>  e. headache<br>  f. confusion<br>  g. trembling<br>  h. epigastric hunger pains<br>3. If s/s of hyperglycemia are found, encourage pt to eat or drink high-glucose foods and juices and notify MD<br>4. Hypoglycemia can be prevented with nicotinamide<br>5. Assess for s/s of hyperglycemia in pt with insulinomas and instruct pt in self-assessment |

*(continued)*

**Streptozocin** (*continued*)

| Nursing Diagnosis | Defining Characteristics | Expected Outcomes | Nursing Interventions |
|---|---|---|---|
| II. D. Hepatic dysfunction | II. D. 1. Liver function studies may be elevated but will normalize with time <br> 2. Hepatotoxicity occurs in ~50% of pts <br> 3. Liver enzymes increase 2–3 weeks after therapy <br> 4. Albumin decreases <br> 5. Symptoms rarely occur <br> 6. Painless jaundice may occur | II. D. Early hepatotoxicity will be identified | II. D. 1. Monitor LFTs (liver function tests) prior to each treatment (alkaline phosphatase, SGOT, SGPT, albumin) <br> 2. Assess for s/s of hepatic dysfunction: jaundice, yellowing of skin; sclera, orange-colored urine; white or clay-colored stools; itchy skin |
| III. *Potential for infection and bleeding related to bone marrow depression* | III. A. BMD occurs in about 9–20% of pts <br> B. Nadir 1–2 weeks after administration <br> C. Occasionally, severe leukopenia and thrombocytopenia occur <br> D. Mild anemia may occur | III. A. Pt will be without s/s of infection or bleeding <br> B. Early s/s of infection or bleeding will be identified | III. A. Monitor CBC, platelets prior to drug administration, as well as assess for s/s of infection or bleeding <br> B. Instruct pt in self-assessment of s/s of infection or bleeding <br> C. Refer to sec. on bone marrow depression, Chapter 4 |
| IV. *Potential for injury related to secondary malignancies* | IV. A. Drug is carcinogenic; secondary malignancies are well described | IV. A. Malignancy, if it occurs, will be identified early | IV. A. Pts receiving prolonged therapy should be screened periodically |

# Suramin sodium
## (Antrypol, Germanin, Naganol)

*Class:* Antiparasitic agent (trypanosomiasis); investigational

## MECHANISM OF ACTION

Inactivates many normal cellular enzymes, inhibits mitochondrial function, and causes cell death. Binds to some growth factors, thus depriving tumor of hormonal stimulation, and cells do not divide. Inhibits angiogenesis, thus depriving tumor of new capillaries and blood supply. Also is a potent inhibitor of viral reverse transcriptase and anti-HIV activity.

## METABOLISM

98% protein bound; small urinary excretion. Drug does not pass the blood-brain barrier. Has a long terminal half-life and narrow therapeutic range (250–300 µg/ml serum concentration).

## DOSAGE/RANGE

Varies per protocol, but commonly:

*Loading dose*

350 mg/m$^2$/day continuous IV infusion to achieve plasma level of 280–300 µg/ml.

*Maintenance*

2-month break, then q 2 monthly treatments

## DRUG PREPARATION

Reconstitute with 10 ml sterile water for injection, USP (100 mg/ml). Further dilute to 10 mg/ml with 0.9% NS or D$_5$W. Stable for 2 weeks at room temperature.

## DRUG ADMINISTRATION

Continuous IV infusion.

## SPECIAL CONSIDERATIONS

Incompatible with basic drugs such as pentamidine.

Investigationally used as antiretroviral agent in treatment of AIDS (6 weekly injections, each IV over 20 minutes).

Rare incidence of circulatory collapse.

May displace other highly protein-bound drugs.

May require vitamin K and glucocorticoid supplementation.

Increased risk of adrenal insufficiency, so patient should receive hydrocortisone (40 mg po qd) and may require lifelong therapy. Patient also should receive vitamin K 10 mg sc weekly to prevent coagulopathy.

Drug has shown activity against prostate cancer.

## Suramin sodium

| Nursing Diagnosis | Defining Characteristics | Expected Outcomes | Nursing Interventions |
|---|---|---|---|
| I. *Alteration in comfort related to malaise, fatigue, lethargy* | I. A. Most common dose-limiting toxicity<br>B. Generally occurs in third month of therapy and is reversible | I. A. Pt will report comfort | I. A. Assess pt for malaise, fatigue, and lethargy during visits<br>B. Teach pt self-assessment and measures to maximize rest between periods of activity |
| II. *Sensory/perceptual alterations related to neurotoxicity* | II. A. Sensory neuropathy with paresthesia of upper and lower extremities in pts with high serum levels (> 300 µg/dl); reversible within a few days<br>B. Motor weakness has occurred 3–6 months after drug discontinuance, consistent with axonal degeneration<br>  1. Aggressive physical therapy reduced disability<br>  2. All pts studied had residual deficits<br>C. Vortex keratopathy with photophobia, tearing, and blurred vision may occur<br>D. Guillain-Barré–like syndrome rare | II. A. Early s/s of neurological toxicity will be identified<br>B. Function will be maintained | II. A. Assess baseline neuromuscular function and reassess prior to drug infusion, especially presence of alterations in sensation in extremities<br>B. Teach pt to report any changes in sensation or function, tearing of eyes, or visual disturbances<br>C. Discuss alterations with MD<br>D. Identify strategies to promote comfort and safety<br>E. Refer to sec. on neurotoxicity, Chapter 4 |
| III. *Potential for alteration in skin integrity related to rash* | III. A. Diffuse morbilliform rash develops in 89% of pts at some time during therapy | III. A. Pt will report changes in skin and describe self-care measures | III. A. Assess skin for any cutaneous changes, such as rash, and any associated symptoms, such as pruritis; discuss with MD |

| Nursing Diagnosis | Defining Characteristics | Expected Outcomes | Nursing Interventions |
|---|---|---|---|
| | B. Resolves within 5–7 days without interruption of therapy | | B. Instruct pt in self-care measures<br>1. Avoiding abrasive skin products, clothing<br>2. Avoiding tight-fitting clothing<br>3. Use of skin emollients appropriate for skin alteration<br>4. Measures to avoid scratching involved areas |
| IV. *Infection and bleeding related to*<br>A. Bone marrow depression | IV. A. 33% incidence of bone marrow suppression | IV. A. Pt will be without s/s of infection or bleeding | IV. A. 1. Monitor CBC, platelet count prior to drug administration<br>2. Monitor for s/s of infection and bleeding<br>3. Instruct pt in self-assessment of s/s of infection and bleeding and to call physician or go to emergency room<br>4. Refer to sec. on bone marrow depression, Chapter 4 |
| B. Coagulopathy | B. 60% incidence with increased thrombin time (PT, PTT) | B. Pt will be without bleeding | B. 1. Assess nonprescription drugs pt is taking and teach pt to avoid aspirin-containing drugs and nonsteroidals<br>2. Monitor PT, PTT, thrombin time |
| V. *Alteration in urinary elimination related to renal toxicity* | V. A. High incidence of proteinuria (2 gm/day) and increased serum creatinine (60% incidence) | V. A. Renal dysfunction will be identified early | V. A. Assess serum BUN, creatinine, and urine for protein prior to and between treatments<br>B. Discuss abnormalities with MD |

*(continued)*

## Suramin sodium (continued)

| Nursing Diagnosis | Defining Characteristics | Expected Outcomes | Nursing Interventions |
|---|---|---|---|
| VI. *Alteration in nutrition related to liver function abnormalities* | VI. A. SGOT, SGPT elevated in 40% of pts | VI. A. Liver function abnormalities will be identified early | VI. A. Assess liver function tests prior to chemotherapy and between treatments<br>B. Discuss abnormalities with MD |
| VII. *Potential for injury related to hypersensitivity reaction and/or atrial arrhythmias* | VII. A. Rarely, acute complications of nausea and vomiting with circulatory collapse; atrial fibrillation with rapid ventricular response | VII. A. Early s/s of hypersensitivity or cardiac irritability will be identified | VII. A. Prior to drug administration, obtain baseline vital signs and monitor during infusion<br>B. Administer test dose if ordered by MD prior to full dose administration<br>C. Assess pt for at least 30 mins after the drug is given for s/s of a reaction<br>D. Teach pt to report any unusual symptoms, such as rapid heartbeat, light-headedness |

# Tamoxifen citrate
(Nolvadex)

*Class:* Antiestrogen

## MECHANISM OF ACTION

Nonsteroidal antiestrogen that binds to estrogen receptors, forming an abnormal complex that migrates to the cell nucleus and inhibits DNA synthesis.

## METABOLISM

Well absorbed from gastrointestinal tract and metabolized by liver. Undergoes enterohepatic circulation, prolonging blood levels. Excreted in feces. Elimination half-life is 7 days.

## DOSAGE/RANGE

20–80 mg orally daily (most often, 20-mg BID)

## DRUG PREPARATION

Available in 10-mg tablets

## DRUG ADMINISTRATION

Oral

## SPECIAL CONSIDERATIONS

Measurement of estrogen receptors in tumor may be important in predicting tumor response and should be performed at same time as biopsy and before antiestrogen treatment is started.

Avoid antacids within 2 hours of taking enteric-coated tablets.

A "flare" reaction with bony pain and hypercalcemia may occur. Such reactions are short-lived and usually result in a tumor response if therapy is continued.

## Tamoxifen citrate

| Nursing Diagnosis | Defining Characteristics | Expected Outcomes | Nursing Interventions |
|---|---|---|---|
| I. *Potential for sexual dysfunction* | I. A. May cause menstrual irregularity, hot flashes, milk production in breasts, vaginal discharge and bleeding<br><br>B. Symptoms occur in about 10% of pts and are usually not severe enough to discontinue therapy | I. A. Pt and significant other will identify strategies for coping with sexual dysfunction | I. A. As appropriate, explore with pt and significant other issues of reproductive and sexuality pattern and impact drug may have<br><br>B. Discuss strategies to preserve sexual and reproductive health<br><br>C. Refer to sec. on gonadal dysfunction, Chapter 4 |
| II. *Potential for alteration in comfort* | II. A. May cause "flare" reaction initially (bone and tumor pain, transient increase in tumor size)<br><br>B. Nausea and vomiting and anorexia may occur | II. A. Pt will identify s/s of "flare" reaction and strategies to cope with it<br><br>B. Pt will avoid nausea and vomiting and anorexia<br><br>C. Nausea and vomiting and anorexia, should they occur, will be minimal | II. A. Inform pt of possibility of "flare" reactions and s/s to be aware of; encourage pt to report any s/s<br><br>B. Inform pt of possibility of nausea and vomiting and anorexia<br><br>C. Encourage small, frequent feedings of high-calorie, high-protein foods |
| III. *Potential for sensory/perceptual alteration* | III. A. Retinopathy has been reported with high doses<br><br>B. Corneal changes (infrequent), decreased visual acuity, and blurred vision have occurred<br><br>C. Headache, dizziness, and light-headedness are rare | III. A. Visual disturbance and CNS symptoms will be identified early | III. A. Obtain visual assessment prior to starting therapy<br><br>B. Encourage pt to report any visual changes<br><br>C. Instruct pt to report headache, dizziness, light-headedness |
| IV. *Potential for infection and bleeding related to bone marrow depression* | IV. A. Mild transient leukopenia and thrombocytopenia occur rarely | IV. A. Pt will be without s/s of infection or bleeding | IV. A. Monitor CBC, platelet count prior to therapy and after therapy has begun<br><br>B. Instruct pt in self-assessment of s/s of infection or bleeding<br><br>C. See sec. on bone marrow depression, Chapter 4 |

| | | | |
|---|---|---|---|
| V. *Potential for skin integrity impairment* | V. A. Skin rash, alopecia, and peripheral edema are rare | V. A. Skin integrity will be maintained | V. A. Assess pt for s/s of hair loss, edema, and skin rash<br>B. Instruct pt to report any of these symptoms<br>C. Discuss with pt the impact of skin changes |
| VI. *Potential for injury related to hypercalcemia* | VI. A. Hypercalcemia uncommon | VI. A. Serum calcium will remain within normal limits | VI. A. Obtain serum calcium levels prior to therapy and at regular intervals during therapy<br>B. Instruct pt in s/s of hypercalcemia: nausea, vomiting, weakness, constipation, loss of muscle tone, malaise, decreased urine output |

# Temozolomide
(Temodar™)

*Class:* Alkylating agent

## MECHANISM OF ACTION

Drug is a member of the imidazotetrazine class, and related to dacarbazine. Drug is a prodrug, forming the active metabolite monomethyl triazenoimidazole carboxamide (MTIC) when chemically degraded. Drug can pass through blood-brain barrier, where it has been shown to be effective against some brain tumors, possibly because of the alkaline pH. MTIC causes alkylation of DNA and RNA strands.

## METABOLISM

Well absorbed from the GI tract following oral dose, with peak concentrations in 1–2 hours. The elimination half-life is 1.8 hours. The drug is degraded into MTIC plasma and tissues. 15% of the drug is excreted unchanged in the urine. Differs from dacarbazine in that formation of MTIC does not require liver metabolism.

## DOSAGE/RANGE

Initial dose is 150 mg/m$^2$/day × 5 days, repeated every 28 days.

Dosage for subsequent cycles is based on nadir neutrophil and platelet counts.

Day 29 (day 1 of subsequent cycle) dose may be increased to 200 mg/m$^2$/day × 5 days if BOTH nadir of prior cycle, as well as labs on day 1 of dosing are: ANC ≥ 1500/µl and platelets ≥ 100,000/µl.

Assess nadir CBC on day 22 of cycle, and weekly until ANC ≥ 1500/µl and platelets ≥ 100,000/µl.

Dose Modifications (Schering/Oncology/Biotherapy [1999] Temodar™ Package Insert. Kenilworth NJ: Schering Corp, 8/99).

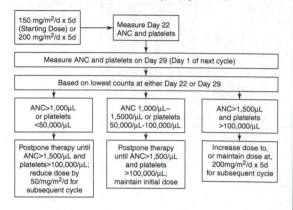

## DRUG PREPARATION

None. Round dose off to nearest 5 mg. Capsules available in 250-mg, 100-mg, 20-mg, and 5-mg strengths. Available in 5-count and 20-count packages. Store at room temperature, protected from light and moisture.

## DRUG ADMINISTRATION

Give orally on an empty stomach, 1 hour before eating or at bedtime. Do not crush, chew or dissolve capsule contents. Drug is given for up to maximum of 2 years or until disease progression, or unacceptable side effects.

## DRUG INTERACTIONS

Valproic acid decreases oral clearance of temozolomide by 5% with unclear clinical implications.

## *Temozolomide (continued)*

### *LAB EFFECTS/INTERFERENCE*

Elevated liver function tests (ALT, AST in up to 40% of patients; alkaline phosphatase); decreased white and red blood cell and platelet counts; hyperglycemia; elevated renal function tests.

### SPECIAL CONSIDERATIONS

Drug causes severe myelosuppression, and thrombocytopenia is the dose limiting factor.

Indicated in the treatment of adult patients with refractory anaplastic astrocytoma who have failed a regime containing a nitrosurea and procarbazine.

Active in high-grade malignant gliomas (glioblastoma multiforme, anaplastic astrocytoma) and malignant melanoma.

Use with caution, if at all, in the following groups of patients: hypersensitive to dacarbazine, myelosuppressed, having bacterial or viral infection, having renal dysfunction, having received prior chemotherapy or radiation therapy, women who are pregnant or breast-feeding.

One percent of patients may develop hypercalcemia.

PET (positive emission tomography) scanning has been used to demonstrate response as there is reduced uptake of fluorodeoxyglucose (FDG) in patients who responded in one study, as compared to those who did not respond and showed increased FDG uptake.

Overall response rates in some studies of patients who have recurred or progressed after surgery and radiation therapy was 15–25%, and 30% in newly diagnosed patients prior to radiotherapy.

## Temozolomide

| Nursing Diagnosis | Defining Characteristics | Expected Outcomes | Nursing Interventions |
|---|---|---|---|
| I. *Potential for infection, bleeding and fatigue related to bone marrow depression* | I. A. 1. Thrombocytopenia and leukopenia are dose-limiting factors, and occur in grade 2 or higher 40% of the time<br><br>2. This does not usually require administration of G-CSF<br><br>3. Nadir at 21–22 days, unless using 5-day treatment schedule where nadir is day 29<br><br>4. Recovery for platelets is 7–42 days, and white blood count in shorter time | I. A. Pt will be without s/s of infection or bleeding<br><br>B. S/s of infection or bleeding will be identified early | I. A. Monitor CBC, platelet count prior to drug administration, as well as s/s of infection or bleeding<br><br>B. Instruct pt in self-assessment of s/s of infection or bleeding<br><br>C. Refer to sec on bone marrow depression, Chapter 4 |
| II. *Fatigue related to anemia, potential* | II. A. Anemia may occur, and is mild | II. A. Pt will manage fatigue | II. A. Monitor hemoglobin and hematocrit and transfuse per MD order or administer erythropoietin per MD order<br><br>B. Teach pt to alternate rest and activity<br><br>C. Teach diet<br><br>D. Teach stress reduction/relaxation techniques<br><br>E. Exercise may improve energy level<br><br>F. Refer to sec. on bone marrow depression, Chapter 4 |

III. *Altered nutrition, less than body requirements related to*

| Nursing Diagnosis | Occurrence | Goal | Interventions |
|---|---|---|---|
| III. A. Nausea and vomiting | A. 1. Nausea and vomiting occur in 75% of pts, especially on day 1<br>2. In one trial using a 5-day regime, 21% had grade 3 nausea, and 23% had grade 4 | III. A. 1. Pt will be without nausea and vomiting<br>2. Nausea and vomiting, should they occur, will be minimal | III. A. 1. Premedicate with antiemetics (serotonin antagonist effective) to *prevent* nausea and vomiting<br>2. Encourage small, frequent feedings of cool, bland foods and liquids<br>3. Assess for symptoms of fluid and electrolyte imbalance; monitor I&O, daily weights if inpatient<br>4. See sec. on nausea and vomiting, Chapter 4 |
| B. Stomatitis | B. May occur in up to 20% of pts | B. Oral mucous membranes will remain intact and without infection | B. 1. Assess oral cavity every day<br>2. Teach pt oral assessment and mouth care regimens<br>3. Encourage pt to report early stomatitis<br>4. Provide pain relief measures if indicated<br>5. See sec. on stomatitis, Chapter 4 |
| C. Constipation | C. May occur in up to 33% of pts | C. Pt will have minimal constipation | C. 1. Assess pt for constipation, bowel elimination patterns<br>2. Encourage pt to report onset of constipation<br>3. Administer or teach pt to self-administer anti-constipation medications<br>4. See sec. on constipation, Chapter 4 |
| D. Anorexia | D. Mild but may occur in 40% of pts | D. Pt will maintain baseline weight ± 5% | D. 1. Encourage small, frequent feedings of favorite foods, especially high-calorie, high-protein foods<br>2. Encourage use of spices<br>3. Daily weights |

*(continued)*

## Temozolomide (continued)

| Nursing Diagnosis | Defining Characteristics | Expected Outcomes | Nursing Interventions |
|---|---|---|---|
| IV. *Alteration in skin integrity/comfort related to rash, pruritis, alopecia* | IV. A. Skin rash, itching, and mild alopecia may occur, and are mild | IV. A. Pt will have intact skin<br>B. Pt will be comfortable | IV. A. Teach pt about the possibility of these side effects, and to notify the nurse if any develop<br>B. Discuss rash with physician if moderate or severe<br>C. Teach pt local symptom management strategies for itch<br>D. Reassure pt that hair loss is usually thinning with mild hair loss, and will grow back |
| V. *Activity intolerance, potential related to central nervous system effects* | V. A. Lethargy (up to 40% in pts with malignant glioma), fatigue, headache, ataxia, and dizziness may occur<br>B. Unclear if due to neurological disease (i.e., malignant glioma), concurrent other drug therapy, or temozolomide | V. A. Pt will be able to do desired activities | V. A. Assess baseline energy and activity level<br>B. Teach pts that these side effects may occur, especially if the primary diagnosis is malignant glioma<br>C. Teach pt to report them<br>D. Teach pt to alternate rest and activity periods, to use supportive device such as cane if ataxia or dizziness occur, and other measures to maximize activity tolerance, and to prevent injury |

# Teniposide
## (Vumon, VM-26)

*Class:* Plant alkaloid, a derivative of the mandrake plant (*Mandragora officinarum*); investigational

## MECHANISM OF ACTION

Cell cycle–specific in late S phase, early $G_2$ phase, causing arrest of cell division in mitosis. Inhibits uptake of thymidine into DNA, so DNA synthesis is impaired.

## METABOLISM

Drug binds extensively to serum protein. Metabolized by the liver and excreted in bile and urine.

## DOSAGE/RANGE

100 mg/m$^2$ weekly for 6–8 weeks

50 mg/m$^2$ twice a week × 4

## DRUG PREPARATION

Available investigationally in 10-mg/ml 5-ml ampules. Add desired NS for injection, or 5% dextrose in water, to reach final concentration of 0.1–0.4 mg/ml (stable for 24 hours) or 1 mg/ml (stable for 4 hours).

## DRUG ADMINISTRATION

Do not administer the solution if a precipitate is noted.

Use only non-DEHP containers such as glass or polyolefin plastic bags or containers.

*Do not use* polyvinyl chloride IV bags, as the DEHP will leach into the solution.

Administer over at least 30–60 minutes.

## SPECIAL CONSIDERATIONS

Rapid infusion, less than 30 minutes, may cause hypotension and sudden death.

Chemical phlebitis may occur if drug is not properly diluted or if it is infused too rapidly.

Severe myelosuppression may occur.

Hypersensitivity reactions, including anaphylaxis-like symptoms, may occur with initial or repeated doses.

Drug is prepared by the manufacturer with polyoxyethylated castor oil and dehydrated alcohol, which may stimulate hypersensitivity.

Reduce doses of tolbutamide, sodium salicylate, or sulfamethizole if given concurrently.

Heparin causes precipitate.

## Teniposide

| Nursing Diagnosis | Defining Characteristics | Expected Outcomes | Nursing Interventions |
|---|---|---|---|
| I. *Potential for injury during drug administration related to* | | | |
| A. Hypotension | I. A. Hypotension may occur during rapid infusion | I. A. Hypotension will be prevented | I. A. 1. Monitor BP prior to drug administration and periodically during infusion at least during first drug administration<br>2. Infuse over at least 30–60 mins |
| B. Anaphylaxis | B. 1. Rarely occurs; may be characterized by fever, dyspnea, lumbar pain, progressive hypotension<br>2. May respond to drug discontinuance and IV hydrocortisone | B. Anaphylaxis, if it occurs, will be managed successfully | B. 1. Have anaphylaxis tray with corticosteroids, antihistamines, epinephrine nearby when chemotherapy is administered<br>2. Monitor pt closely during infusion<br>3. Review standing orders for management of allergic reactions (hypersensitivity and anaphylaxis) as per institutional policy and procedure<br>4. Prior to drug administration, obtain baseline vital signs and record mental status<br>5. Observe for following s/s, usually occurring within the first 15 mins of infusion:<br>  a. *Subjective*<br>    (1) generalized itching<br>    (2) nausea<br>    (3) chest tightness<br>    (4) crampy abdominal pain<br>    (5) agitation<br>    (6) anxiety<br>    (7) sense of impending doom<br>    (8) wheeziness<br>    (9) desire to urinate or defecate<br>    (10) dizziness<br>    (11) chills |

b. *Objective*

  (1) flushed appearance (angioedema of the face, neck, eyelids, hands, feet)

  (2) localized or generalized urticaria

  (3) respiratory distress ± wheezing

  (4) hypotension

  (5) cyanosis

6. For generalized allergic response, stop infusion and notify MD

7. Place pt in supine position to promote perfusion of visceral organs

8. Monitor vital signs

9. Provide emotional reassurance to pt and family

10. Maintain patent airway and have equipment ready for CPR if needed

11. Document incident

12. Discuss with MD desensitization versus drug discontinuance for further dose

*(continued)*

## Teniposide (continued)

| Nursing Diagnosis | Defining Characteristics | Expected Outcomes | Nursing Interventions |
|---|---|---|---|
| II. *Potential for infection and bleeding related to bone marrow depression* | II. A. Dose-limiting toxicity<br>B. Leukopenia; thrombocytopenia may also occur<br>C. Nadir 3–14 days (~7 days)<br>D. Dose reduction indicated for pts heavily pretreated with radiation or chemotherapy | II. A. Pt will be without s/s of infection or bleeding<br>B. Early s/s of infection or bleeding will be identified | II. A. Monitor platelet count prior to drug administration, assess for s/s of infection or bleeding; assess nadir counts<br>B. Instruct pt in self-assessment techniques for infection or bleeding<br>C. Dose reduction may be necessary based on nadir counts, history of previous XRT/chemotherapy, altered hepatic function<br>D. Transfuse with red cells, platelets per MD order |
| III. *Altered nutrition, less than body requirements related to*<br>A. Nausea and vomiting | III. A. May occur, but are usually mild | III. A. Pt will be without nausea and vomiting | III. A. 1. Premedicate with antiemetic and continue prophylactically × 24 hrs to prevent nausea and vomiting, at least for first treatment<br>2. Encourage small, frequent feedings of cool, bland foods and liquids |
| B. Hepatic dysfunction | B. Mild elevation of liver function tests may occur | B. Hepatic dysfunction will be identified early | B. 1. Monitor SGOT, SGPT, LDH, alkaline phosphatase, and bilirubin prior to drug administration<br>2. Notify MD of any elevations |

| | | | |
|---|---|---|---|
| IV. Potential for impaired skin integrity related to<br>A. Alopecia | IV. A. Occurs uncommonly (9–30%) and is reversible | IV. A. 1. Pt will verbalize feelings re hair loss<br>2. Pt will identify strategies to cope with changes in body image | IV. A. 1. Discuss with pt impact of hair loss<br>2. Suggest wig as appropriate prior to actual hair loss<br>3. Explore with pt response to actual hair loss and plan strategies to minimize distress (e.g., wig, scarf, cap) |
| B. Irritation | B. Phlebitis or perivascular irritation may occur if drug is too concentrated or is infused too rapidly | B. Phlebitis, irritation will be minimal | B. Use careful venipuncture technique and administer drug over 30–60 mins, diluted to at least 5 volumes as per manufacturer's specifications |
| V. Potential for alteration in cardiac output | V. A. Rarely, palpitations may occur | V. A. Early cardiac rhythm abnormalities will be identified | V. A. Monitor heart rate, noting rhythm, when administering drug<br>B. Notify MD of any irregularity<br>C. EKG to identify irregular rhythm |
| VI. Potential for sensory/perceptual alterations related to neurological toxicity | VI. A. Peripheral neuropathies may occur and are mild | VI. A. Peripheral neuropathy will be identified early<br>B. Pt will verbalize feelings re discomfort and dysfunction related to neuropathy and identify alternative coping strategies | VI. A. Assess motor and sensory function prior to therapy<br>B. Encourage pt to verbalize feelings re discomfort and sensory loss if these occur<br>C. Assist pt to discuss alternative coping strategies |

# 6-Thioguanine
(Thioguanine, Tabloid, 6-TG)

*Class:* Thiopurine antimetabolite

## MECHANISM OF ACTION

Converts to monophosphate nucleotides and inhibits de novo purine synthesis. The nucleotides are also incorporated into DNA. Cell cycle phase specific (S phase).

Thioguanine interferes with nucleic acid biosynthesis, resulting in sequential blockage of the synthesis and utilization of the purine nucleotides.

## METABOLISM

Absorption is incomplete and variable orally. Is metabolized in the liver by deamination and methylation. Metabolites are excreted in the urine and feces. Plasma half-life is 80–90 minutes.

## DOSAGE/RANGE

Children and adults: 100 mg/m$^2$ orally every 12 hours for 5–10 days, usually in combination with cytarabine

100 mg/m$^2$ IV daily × 5 days

1–3 mg/kg orally daily

## DRUG PREPARATION

Available in 40-mg tablets.
Reconstitute 100-mg vial in 15 ml NS.

## DRUG ADMINISTRATION

IV bolus

## SPECIAL CONSIDERATIONS

Oral dose to be given on empty stomach to facilitate complete absorption.

Dose is titrated to avoid excessive stomatitis and diarrhea.

6-thioguanine can be used in full doses with allopurinol.

## 6–Thioguanine

| Nursing Diagnosis | Defining Characteristics | Expected Outcomes | Nursing Interventions |
|---|---|---|---|
| I. *Altered nutrition, less than body requirements related to* A. Nausea and vomiting | I. A. Nausea and vomiting occur uncommonly, especially in children, but are dose related | I. A. 1. Pt will be without nausea and vomiting 2. Nausea and vomiting, should they occur, will be minimal | I. A. 1. Treat symptomatically with antiemetics 2. Encourage small, frequent feedings of cool, bland foods and liquids 3. If vomiting occurs, assess for fluid and electrolyte imbalance; monitor I&O and daily weights if pt is hospitalized |
| B. Anorexia | B. Rare | B. Pt will maintain baseline weight ± 5% | B. 1. Encourage small, frequent feedings of favorite foods, especially high-calorie, high-protein foods 2. Encourage use of spices 3. Weekly weights |
| C. Stomatitis | C. Rare, but most common with high doses | C. Oral mucous membranes will remain intact and without infection | C. 1. Teach oral assessment and oral hygiene regimen 2. Encourage pt to report early stomatitis 3. Provide pain relief measures if indicated 4. See sec. on stomatitis, Chapter 4 |
| D. Hepatotoxicity | D. Rare, but may be associated with hepatic veno-occlusive disease or jaundice | D. Hepatotoxicity will be identified early | D. 1. Monitor LFTs prior to drug dose 2. Assess pt prior to and during treatment for s/s of hepatotoxicity |
| II. *Potential for infection and bleeding related to bone marrow depression* | II. A. Bone marrow depression occurs 1–4 weeks after treatment B. Leukopenia and thrombocytopenia are most common C. Drug may have prolonged or delayed nadir | II. A. Pt will be without s/s of infection or bleeding B. Early s/s of infection or bleeding will be identified | II. A. Monitor CBC, platelet count prior to drug administration, as well as s/s of infection or bleeding B. Instruct pt in self-assessment of s/s of infection or bleeding C. Administer platelet, red cell transfusions per MD order D. Refer to sec. on bone marrow depression, Chapter 4 |

*(continued)*

## 6–Thioguanine (continued)

| Nursing Diagnosis | Defining Characteristics | Expected Outcomes | Nursing Intervention |
|---|---|---|---|
| III. *Potential for sensory/ perceptual alterations* | III. A. Loss of vibratory sensation, unsteady gait may occur | III. A. Neurological toxicity will be identified early | III. A. Assess vibratory sensation, gait before each dose and between treatments<br>B. Report changes to MD<br>C. Encourage pt to report any changes |

# Thiotepa
## (Triethylene Thiophosphoramide)

*Class:* Alkylating agent

## MECHANISM OF ACTION

Selectively reacts with DNA phosphate groups to produce chromosome cross-linkage with blocking of nucleoprotein synthesis. Acts as a polyfunctional alkylating agent. Cell cycle phase nonspecific. Mimics radiation-induced injury.

## METABOLISM

Rapidly cleared following IV administration; 60% of dose is eliminated in urine within 24–72 hours. Slow onset of action, slowly bound to tissues, extensively metabolized.

## DOSAGE/RANGE

*Intravenous*

$8 \text{ mg/m}^2$ (0.2 mg/kg) IV every day × 5 days, repeated every 3–4 weeks

30–60 mg IV, IM, or SQ once a week, depending on WBC

*Intracavitary*

Bladder: 60 mg in 60 ml sterile water once a week for 3–4 weeks

## DRUG PREPARATION

Add sterile water to vial of lyophilized powder.

Further dilute with NS or $D_5W$.

Do not use solution unless it is clear.

Refrigerate vial until use (reconstituted solution is stable for 5 days).

## DRUG ADMINISTRATION

IV, IM; intracavitary; intratumor; intra-arterial

## SPECIAL CONSIDERATIONS

Hypersensitivity reactions have occurred with this drug.

Is an irritant; should be given via a sidearm of a running IV.

Increased neuromuscular blockage when given with nondepolarizing muscle relaxants.

## Thiotepa

| Nursing Diagnosis | Defining Characteristics | Expected Outcomes | Nursing Interventions |
|---|---|---|---|
| I. *Potential for infection and bleeding related to bone marrow depression* | I. A. Nadir is 5–30 days after drug administration<br>B. Thrombocytopenia and leukopenia may occur<br>C. Anemia may occur with prolonged use<br>D. May be cumulative toxicity, with recovery of bone marrow in 40–50 days<br>E. Thrombocytopenia is dose limiting | I. A. Pt will be without s/s of infection or bleeding<br>B. Early s/s of infection or bleeding will be detected | I. A. Monitor CBC, platelet count prior to drug administration; monitor for s/s of infection or bleeding<br>B. Instruct pt in self-assessment of s/s of infection or bleeding<br>C. Administer red cell and platelet transfusions per MD order<br>D. Refer to sec. on bone marrow depression, Chapter 4 |
| II. *Altered nutrition, less than body requirements related to*<br>A. Nausea and vomiting | II. A. 1. Nausea and vomiting occur in 10–15% of pts<br>2. Dose dependent<br>3. Occur 6–12 hrs after drug dose | II. A. 1. Pt will be without nausea and vomiting<br>2. Nausea and vomiting, if they occur, will be minimal | II. A. 1. Premedicate with antiemetics, especially with parenteral high dose; continue antiemetics at least 12 hrs after drug is given<br>2. Encourage small, frequent feedings of cool, bland, dry foods<br>3. Refer to sec. on nausea and vomiting, Chapter 4 |
| B. Anorexia | B. Occurs occasionally | B. Pt will maintain baseline weight ± 5% | B. 1. Encourage small, frequent feedings of favorite foods, especially high-calorie, high-protein foods<br>2. Encourage use of spices<br>3. Weekly weights |
| III. *Sexual dysfunction* | III. A. Drug is mutagenic<br>B. Sterility may be reversible and incomplete<br>C. Amenorrhea often reverses in 6–8 months | III. A. Pt and significant other will identify coping strategies to deal with sexual dysfunction | III. A. As appropriate, explore with pt and significant other issues of reproductive and sexuality pattern and anticipated impact chemotherapy will have<br>B. Discuss strategies to preserve sexuality and reproductive health (e.g., sperm banking)<br>C. Refer to sec. on gonadal dysfunction, Chapter 4 |

**IV. Potential for injury related to**

| | | | |
|---|---|---|---|
| A. Allergic reaction | IV. A. Allergic responses may occur rarely: hives, bronchospasm, skin rash (dermatitis) | IV. A. Allergic responses will be detected early and treated | IV. A. 1. Assess for s/s of allergic response during drug administration<br>2. Stop drug if bronchospasm occurs and notify MD<br>3. Discuss symptomatic treatment with MD |
| B. Secondary malignancies | B. Secondary malignancies may occur with prolonged therapy | B. Secondary malignancy, if it occurs, will be detected early | B. Instruct pt receiving prolonged therapy in importance of regular health maintenance examinations during and after therapy by primary care provider and oncologist |
| **V. Alteration in comfort** | V. A. Dizziness, headache, fever, and local pain may occur | V. A. Distress will be minimal | V. A. Assess for alterations in comfort<br>B. Treat symptomatically |

# Tretinoin
## (Vesanoid™ All Trans Retinoic Acid/ATRA)

*Class:* Retinoid

## MECHANISM OF ACTION

Induces maturation of acute promyelocytic leukemia cells, thus decreasing proliferation. In patients who achieve a complete response to this therapy, there is an initial maturation of primitive leukemic cells, and then cells in both the bone marrow and peripheral blood are normal, polyclonal blood cells. The exact mechanism is unknown.

## METABOLISM

This drug is well absorbed orally into the systemic circulation with peak concentrations in 1–2 hours. Drug is > 95% protein bound, primarily to albumin. Oxidative metabolism occurs via the Cytochrome P450 enzyme system in the liver. Drug is excreted in the urine (63% in 72 hours) and feces (31% in 6 days).

## DOSAGE/RANGE

45 mg/m$^2$/day

## DRUG PREPARATION

None—oral. Available as 10-mg capsules. Protect from light.

## DRUG ADMINISTRATION

Drug is to be used for induction remission only. Administer in evenly divided doses until complete remission (CR) is achieved, then for an additional 30 days, or after 90 days of treatment, whichever comes first.

## DRUG INTERACTIONS

Drugs which either inhibit or induce the Cytochrome P450 hepatic enzyme system potentially will interact with this drug, but there is no data to suggest that these drugs either increase or decrease tretinoin activity. Drugs that induce the enzyme system: rifampin, glucocorticoids, phenobarbitol, pentobarbitol; drugs that inhibit the enzyme system: ketoconazole, cimetidine, erythromycin, verapamil, diltiazem, cyclosporin.

## LAB EFFECTS/INTERFERENCE

Increased cholesterol and triglyceride levels (60% of patients) and elevated LFTs (50–60% of patients).

## SPECIAL CONSIDERATIONS

Indicated for the induction remission of patients with acute promyelocytic leukemia (FAB-M3) characterized by the presence of the t(15:17) translocation and/or presence of the PML/RARα gene.

Absorption is enhanced when taken with food.

Monitor cbc, platelets, coagulation studies, liver function tests, and triglyceride and cholesterol levels frequently during therapy.

# Tretinoin

| Nursing Diagnosis | Defining Characteristics | Expected Outcomes | Nursing Interventions |
|---|---|---|---|
| I. *Alteration in oxygenation, potential, related to retinoic acid-APL syndrome* | I. A. Syndrome occurs in approximately 25% of pts, and varies in severity, but has resulted in death<br>B. Syndrome is characterized by fever, dyspnea, weight gain, pulmonary infiltrates on X-ray, and pleural and/or pericardial effusions<br>C. May also be accompanied by impaired myocardial contractility, hypotension, ± leukocytosis, and because of progressive hypoxemia and multisystem organ failure, some pts have died<br>D. Usually occurs during first month of treatment, but may follow initial drug dose | I. A. Early s/s of syndrome will be detected early<br>B. Injury will be minimized/prevented | I. A. Assess vital signs, pulmonary exam, and weight at each visit<br>B. Teach pt to do daily weights, and to report any SOB, fever, weight gain<br>C. If this occurs, notify physician and discuss obtaining CXR, and focused exam<br>D. Discuss chest X-ray findings with physician<br>E. Be prepared to give high-dose steroids at the first sign of the syndrome, e.g., Dexamethasone 10 mg IV q 12 hrs × 3 days, or until symptom resolution (necessary in 60% of pts)<br>F. Provide pulmonary and hemodynamic support as necessary<br>G. Discuss whether drug should be discontinued based on severity and pt's response to high-dose steroids |

*(continued)*

## Tretinoin (continued)

| Nursing Diagnosis | Defining Characteristics | Expected Outcomes | Nursing Interventions |
|---|---|---|---|
| II. *Alteration in comfort related to Vitamin A toxicity* | II. A. Almost all pts experience some toxicity, but they do not usually have to discontinue the drug<br>B. Toxicity of high dose Vitamin A includes headache (86%) starting the first week of treatment, but fading after that; fever (83%); skin/mucous membrane dryness (77%); bone pain (77%); nausea/vomiting (57%); rash (54%); mucositis (26%); pruritis (20%); increased sweating (20%); visual disturbances (17%); ocular disorders (17%); alopecia (14%); skin changes (17%); changed visual acuity (6%); visual field defects (3%) | II. A. S/s of vitamin toxicity will be detected early | II. A. Teach pt about possible side effects of high-dose Vitamin A as above, and to report them if they occur<br>B. Teach pt symptom management<br>C. Assess severity of symptom(s) and discuss with physician symptom management of fever, headache unresponsive to acetaminophen, nausea/vomiting<br>D. If headache is severe in a child, have child evaluated for pseudotumor cerebri |
| III. *Potential for injury related to pseudotumor cerebri* | III. A. Benign intracranial hypertension has occurred in children treated with retinoids<br>B. Early signs and symptoms are papilledema, headache, nausea and vomiting, and visual disturbances | III. A. S/s of benign intracranial hypertension will be detected early | III. A. Teach pt/parents to report symptoms<br>B. Assess pt for symptomatology on regular basis<br>C. If headache is severe, discuss with physician analgesics and therapeutic lumbar puncture |

| IV. *Potential disturbance in circulation* | IV. A. The following disturbances may occur: arrythmia (23%), flushing (23%), hypotension (14%), hypertension (11%), phlebitis (11%), cardiac failure (6%), while 3% of pts studied developed cardiac arrest, myocardial infarction, enlarged heart, heart, murmur ischemia, stroke, and other serious disturbances | IV. A. Alterations in circulation will be detected early | IV. A. Assess cardiac status baseline and presence of risk factors (e.g., hypertension) <br> B. Assess vital signs at each visit, and teach pt in a manner not to induce anxiety to report any symptoms such as chest pain, SOB, heart palpitations, or any changes that occur |
| V. *Alteration in nutrition, less than body requirements related to gastrointestinal (GI) dysfunction* | V. A. Some problems are related to APL, and together with drug, may emerge, such as GI bleeding/hemorrhage, which may occur in up to 34% of pts <br> B. Other GI problems include abdominal pain (31%), diarrhea (23%), constipation (17%), dyspepsia (14%), abdominal distention (11%), hepatosplenomegaly (11%), hepatitis (3%), and ulcer (3%) | V. A. Pt will maintain weight within 5% of baseline <br> B. Alterations will be detected early and managed effectively | V. A. Assess GI status, and presence of GI dysfunction baseline <br> B. Teach pt to report any GI disturbances, or changes in bowel status <br> C. If these occur, assess severity and need for symptom management, or discussion/intervention with physician <br> D. Monitor liver function studies frequently during therapy |

*(continued)*

**Tretinoin (continued)**

| Nursing Diagnosis | Defining Characteristics | Expected Outcomes | Nursing Interventions |
|---|---|---|---|
| VI. Sensory/perceptual alterations related to changes in ear sensation/hearing | VI. A. 23% of pts report earache or fullness in ears. Other ear problems that may occur are reversible hearing loss (5%) of pts, and irreversible hearing loss (1%) | VI. A. Early dysfunction will be detected | VI. A. Teach pt that this may occur, and to report it if it occurs<br><br>B. Assess severity, and need for intervention |
| VII. Potential for injury related to CNS, peripheral nervous system changes, and affect changes | VII. A. Changes that may occur include dizziness (20%), paresthesias (17%), anxiety (17%), insomnia (14%), depression (14%), confusion (11%), cerebral hemorrhage (9%), agitation (9%), and hallucinations (6%)<br><br>B. Rarely, the following may occur: forgetfulness, gait disturbances, convulsions, coma, facial paralysis, tremor, leg weakness, somnolence, slow speech, aphasia, and other CNS changes | VII. A. Pt will be free of central and peripheral nervous system changes and affect, or if changes occur, they will be detected early | VII. A. Teach pt to report any changes in affect, sensorium, or functional ability (e.g., to walk, speak) in a manner that does not cause anxiety<br><br>B. Assess severity of symptom(s) if they arise, and potential for injury<br><br>C. If severe, modify pt's environment to minimize risk of injury and discuss medical intervention with physician |
| VIII. Altered urinary elimination, potential related to renal changes | VIII. A. Uncommonly, renal insufficiency may occur (11%), dysuria (9%), acute renal failure (3%), urinary frequency (3%), renal tubular necrosis (3%) and enlarged prostate (3%) | VIII. A. Renal dysfunction will be identified early | VIII. A. Assess baseline urinary elimination pattern<br><br>B. Teach pt to report any changes<br><br>C. Monitor BUN/creatinine periodically during therapy and discuss any abnormalities with physician |

# Topotecan hydrochloride for injection (Hycamptin)

*Class:* Topoisomerase inhibitor

## MECHANISM ACTION

Causes single-strand breaks in DNA to permit relaxation of the DNA helix of before DNA replication. Topotecan binds to the topoisomerase I-DNA complex, thus preventing repair of the breaks, and ultimately DNA synthesis, and leads to cell death.

## METABOLISM

Thirty percent of the drug is excreted in the urine. Moderate renal impairment leads to a 34% decrease in plasma clearance of the drug so a dose reduction is necessary. Minor metabolism occurs in the liver.

## DOSAGE/RANGE

1.5 mg/m$^2$ IV qd × 5, repeated q 21 days

## DRUG PREPARATION

Reconstitute 4-mg-vial with 4 ml sterile water for injection. Further dilute in 0.9% sodium chloride or 5% Dextrose, and use immediately.

## DRUG ADMINISTRATION

Infuse over 30 minutes. Baseline ANC for initial course must be ≥ 1500/mm$^3$ and platelet count ≥ 100,000/mm$^3$, and for subsequent courses, ANC ≥ 1000/mm$^3$, platelets ≥ 100,000/mm$^3$, and hemoglobin ≥ 9 mg/dl.

## LAB EFFECTS/INTERFERENCE

Decrease in CBC; increase in LFTs, RFTs

## DRUG INTERACTIONS

None known

## SPECIAL CONSIDERATIONS

G-CSF (Neupogen) may be required in neutropenia develops first cycle.

Dose modifications recommended by manufacturer:

Renal impairment: mild = creatinine clearance (cr cl) 40–60 ml/min, dose is 0.75 mg/m$^2$; moderate = cr cl 29–39 ml/min, consider drug discontinuance.

Hematologic toxicity: severe neutropenia, dose reduce by 0.25 mg/m$^2$ for subsequent doses or use G-CSF beginning on day 6 (24 hours after last dose of drug).

Minimum of 4 courses needed, as clinical responses occur 9–12 weeks after beginning of therapy.

Indicated for the treatment of relapsed or refractory metastatic ovarian cancer, but has activity in many solid tumors.

## Topotecan hydrochloride for injection

| Nursing Diagnosis | Defining Characteristics | Expected Outcomes | Nursing Interventions |
|---|---|---|---|
| I. *Infection and bleeding related to bone marrow depression* | I. A. Dose limiting toxicity seen during first course in 60% of pts. Febrile neutropenia or sepsis may occur in 26% of pts<br>B. Grade 4 neutropenia<br>C. Nadir occurs on day 11<br>D. Grade 4 thrombocytopenia occurs in 26% of pts (platelet count <25,000/mm$^3$)<br>E. Platelet nadir occurs on day 15 | I. A. Pt will be without s/s of infection or bleeding | I. A. Monitor CBC, platelet count prior to drug administration, as well as start of infection and bleeding. Assess baseline renal function and prior to each cycle<br>B. Teach s/s of infection and bleeding, pt self-assessment, and to call or come to EDR if T > 100.5 or per institutional policy, and s/s of bleeding. Teach pt to avoid aspirin or aspirin containing OTC medicines, NSAIDs, and other medicines without talking to RN or MD first<br>C. Teach pt/family rationale for G-CSF and how to prepare and administer medicine if ordered to prevent febrile neutropenia<br>D. Refer to section on bone marrow depression, Chapter 4 |
| II. *Potential for activity intolerance related to anemia-induced fatigue* | II. A. Severe anemia (Hgb < 8 gm/dl) occurs in 40% of pts<br>B. 56% of pts require transfusions | II. A. Pt will be able to do desired activities<br>B. Early fatigue related to anemia will resolve | II. A. Monitor hemoglobin, hematocrit<br>B. Teach pt/family rationale for EPO, and how to prepare and administer injection if ordered<br>C. Transfuse per MD for hematocrit < 25, s/s of severe anemia<br>D. Teach pt diet high in iron, folic acid; teach self-administration of folic acid, iron medications as ordered<br>E. Teach pt to alternate rest and activity periods<br>F. Refer to sec. on bone marrow depression, Chapter 4 |

| Nursing Diagnosis | | Desired Outcomes | Interventions |
|---|---|---|---|
| III. Alteration in nutrition, less than body requirements related to | | | |
| A. Nausea and vomiting | A. 1. Nausea occurs in 77% of pts and vomiting in 58% of pts without premedication<br>2. Abdominal pain occurs in 33% of pts | III. A. 1. Pt will be without nausea and vomiting<br>2. Nausea and vomiting, should they occur, will be minimal | III. A. 1. Premedicate with antiemetics, such as a serotonin-antagonist to prevent nausea and vomiting<br>2. Encourage small, frequent feedings of cool, bland foods and liquids<br>3. Assess for symptoms of fluid and electrolyte imbalance; monitor daily weights for 5-day course<br>4. See sec. on nausea and vomiting, Chapter 4 |
| B. Diarrhea | B. Diarrhea occurs in 39% of pts | B. Pt will have minimal diarrhea | B. 1. Assess pt's bowel elimination pattern; guaiac all stools<br>2. Encourage pt to report onset of diarrhea<br>3. Administer or teach pt to self-administer antidiarrheal medications<br>4. See sec. on diarrhea, Chapter 4 |
| C. Elevated LFTs | C. Elevated LFTs occur in 5% of pts (AST [SGOT], ALT [SGPT]) | C. Changes in LFTs will be identified early | C. 1. Assess baseline LFTs and monitor periodically during therapy<br>2. Discuss any elevations with physician |
| IV. Potential for hepatotoxicity related preexisting hepatic insufficiency | IV. A. There may be increased drug toxicity in pts with low serum protein and hepatic dysfunction | IV. A. Evidence of hepatotoxicity will be identified early | IV. A. Assess baseline serum albumin, LFTs prior to first dose, and during treatment<br>B. If hepatotoxicity develops, assess for increased drug toxicity and discuss dose reduction with physician |

# Toremifene citrate
## (Fareston)

*Class:* Synthetic tamoxifen analogue

## MECHANISM OF ACTION

Estrogen antagonist

## METABOLISM

Extensively metabolized in the liver by the P-450 enzyme system. Peak serum level after single dose is 3 hours, with terminal half-life of 6.2 days. Increased terminal half-life (decreased clearance) in patients with hepatic dysfunction to 10.9 days and 21 days for the principal metabolite. Only slightly protein bound (0.3%). Clearance not significantly changed with renal impairment.

## DOSAGE/RANGE

60 mg po qd

## DRUG PREPARATION

None—oral

## DRUG ADMINISTRATION

Administer orally qd without regard to meals.

## DRUG INTERACTIONS

Metabolism is inhibited by testosterone and cyclosporin.

Appears to enhance the inhibition of multi-drug resistant cell lines by vinblastine.

Appears to be cross-resistant with tamoxifen.

## LAB EFFECTS/INTERFERENCE

Decreased WBC and platelets (mild)

## SPECIAL CONSIDERATIONS

Activity, side effects, toxicity in postmenopausal women or women with unknown receptor status similar.

## Toremifene citrate

| Nursing Diagnosis | Defining Characteristics | Expected Outcomes | Nursing Interventions |
|---|---|---|---|
| I. *Potential for sexual dysfunction related to menstrual irregularities, hot flashes* | I. A. Similar to tamoxifen toxicity profile<br>B. May cause menstrual irregularity, hot flashes (most common), milk production in breast, and vaginal discharge and bleeding<br>C. Symptoms are usually not severe enough to necessitate drug discontinuance | I. A. Pt and significant other will identify strategies for coping with sexual dysfunction | I. A. As appropriate, explore with pt and significant other issues of reproductive and sexual pattern and impact drug may have<br>B. Discuss strategies to preserve sexual and reproductive health<br>C. Refer to sec. on gonadal dysfunction, Chapter 4 |
| II. *Potential for alteration in comfort* | II. A. May cause "flare" reaction initially (bone and tumor pain, transient increase in tumor size)<br>B. Nausea, vomiting, anorexia rarely occur | II. A. Pt will identify s/s of "flare" reaction and strategies to cope with it<br>B. Pt will be without nausea, vomiting, anorexia<br>C. Nausea, vomiting, anorexia, if they occur, will be minimal | II. A. Inform pt of possibility of "flare" reaction and s/s to assess for; encourage pt to report any s/s<br>B. Inform pt of possibility of nausea, vomiting, and anorexia<br>C. Encourage small, frequent feedings of high-calorie, high-protein food |
| III. *Potential for infection and bleeding related to bone marrow depression* | III. A. Mild transient leukopenia and thrombocytopenia rarely occur | III. A. Pt will be without s/s of infection or bleeding | III. A. Monitor CBC, platelet count prior to therapy and periodically during therapy<br>B. Instruct pt in self-assessment of s/s of infection and bleeding<br>C. See sec. on bone marrow depression, Chapter 4 |
| IV. *Potential for alteration in skin integrity* | IV. A. Skin rash, alopecia, and peripheral edema are rare | IV. A. Skin integrity will be maintained | IV. A. Assess pt for s/s of hair loss, edema, and skin rash<br>B. Teach pt that these may occur, and to report any symptoms<br>C. Explore with pt potential impact of alopecia, skin changes |

# Trimetrexate
## Glucuronate (Neutrexin; Trimexate)

*Class:* Antimetabolite

## MECHANISM OF ACTION

Nonclassical folate antagonist; potent inhibitor of dihydrofolate reductase. May be able to overcome mechanism(s) of methotrexate resistance, as drug reaches higher concentration within tumor cells. Also, inhibits growth of parasitic infective agents (causing pneumocystis carinii, toxoplasmosis) in patients with immunodeficiency or myelodysplastic disorders.

## METABOLISM

Significant percentage of drug is protein bound. Metabolized by liver; 10–20% of dose is excreted by kidneys in 24 hours.

## DOSAGE/RANGE

6–16 mg/m$^2$ IV daily × 5, repeat every 21–28 days

150–200 mg/m$^2$ every 2 weeks

When used to treat pneumocystis carinii:

Oral: 60 mg/m$^2$/day

IV: 90–220mg/m$^2$ q 1–3 weeks
   30 mg/m$^2$/d qd × 21 days
   45 mg/m$^2$ q 6 hours × 21 days

Leucovorin: Oral/IV: 20 mg/m$^2$ q 6 hours during and × 72 hours after last dose of trimetrexate

## DRUG PREPARATION

Stable 24 hours at room temperature or refrigerated.

## DRUG ADMINISTRATION

IV bolus over 5 minutes.

Can be given as an IV infusion.

Incompatible with chloride solutions.

Leucovorin is administered during, and for 72 hours after therapy.

## SPECIAL CONSIDERATIONS

Increased toxicity is seen in patients with low protein (drug is highly protein bound) and hepatic dysfunction. Dose reduction indicated.

Leukopenia is a dose-limiting toxicity first seen at dose of 1.6 mg/m$^2$.

Other side effects are nausea and vomiting, rash, mucositis, diarrhea, SGOT elevations, thrombocytopenia.

Contraindicated during pregnancy and, as drug is excreted in breast milk, nursing mothers should not nurse while receiving drug. Premenopausal women should have a pregnancy test.

Contraindicated in patients hypersensitive to drug methotrexate, or any component, or in patients with preexisting bone marrow suppression.

## Trimetrexate

| Nursing Diagnosis | Defining Characteristics | Expected Outcomes | Nursing Interventions |
|---|---|---|---|
| I. *Infection and bleeding related to bone marrow depression* | I. A. Leukopenia is a dose-limiting toxicity seen at doses of 1.6 mg/m² and higher<br>B. Thrombocytopenia also occurs commonly | I. A. Pt will be without s/s of infection or bleeding<br>B. Early s/s of infection or bleeding will be identified | I. A. Monitor CBC, platelet count prior to drug administration, as well as s/s of infection or bleeding<br>B. Instruct pt in self-assessment of s/s of infection or bleeding<br>C. Administer red cell, platelet transfusions per MD order<br>D. Ensure that leucovorin is administered exactly on time<br>E. Refer to sec. on bone marrow depression, Chapter 4 |
| II. *Altered nutrition, less than body requirements related to*<br>A. Nausea and vomiting | II. A. Nausea and vomiting reported in clinical trials | II, A. 1. Pt will be without nausea and vomiting<br>2. Nausea and vomiting, if they occur, will be minimal | II. A. 1. Premedicate with antiemetics and continue prophylactically × 24 hrs to prevent nausea and vomiting, at least for the first treatment<br>2. Encourage small, frequent feedings of cool, bland foods and liquids<br>3. Assess for symptoms of fluids and electrolyte imbalance; monitor I&O, daily weights if inpatient<br>4. Refer to sec. on nausea and vomiting, Chapter 4 |
| B. Stomatitis | B. Has been reported to cause stomatitis | B. Oral mucous membranes will remain intact and without infection | B. 1. Teach pt oral assessment and oral hygiene regimens<br>2. Encourage pt to report early stomatitis<br>3. Provide pain relief measures if indicated (e.g., topical anesthetics)<br>4. See sec. on stomatitis, mucositis, Chapter 4 |

*(continued)*

# Trimetrexate (continued)

| Nursing Diagnosis | Defining Characteristics | Expected Outcomes | Nursing Interventions |
|---|---|---|---|
| II. C. Diarrhea | II. C. Documented during clinical trials | II. C. Pt will have minimal diarrhea | II. C. 1. Encourage pt to report onset of diarrhea<br>2. Administer or teach pt to self-administer antidiarrheal medication<br>3. Teach pt about perineal hygiene routines<br>4. Ensure adequate hydration, monitor I&O<br>5. See sec. on diarrhea, Chapter 4 |
| III. *Potential for hepatotoxicity* | III. A. Evidenced in SGOT elevations<br>B. Increased drug toxicity in pts with low protein and hepatic dysfunction; dose reductions may be necessary | III. A. Early hepatotoxicity will be identified | III. A. Monitor LFTs prior to drug dose<br>B. Assess pt prior to and during treatment for s/s of hepatotoxicity<br>C. See sec. on hepatotoxicity, Chapter 4 |

# Vinblastine
(Velban)

*Class:* Plant alkaloid extracted from the periwinkle plant (*Vinca rosea*)

## MECHANISM OF ACTION

Drug binds to microtubular proteins, thus arresting mitosis during metaphase; may inhibit RNA, DNA, and protein synthesis. Active in S and M phases (cell cycle phase–specific).

## METABOLISM

About 10% of drug is excreted in feces. Vinblastine is partially metabolized by the liver. Minimal amount of the drug is excreted in urine and bile. Dose modification may be necessary in the presence of hepatic failure.

## DOSAGE/RANGE

0.1 mg/kg or 6 mg/m$^2$ IV weekly: continuous infusion 1.4–1.8 mg/day × 5 days

## DRUG PREPARATION

Available in 10-mg vials. Store in refrigerator until use.

## DRUG ADMINISTRATION

IV push or by continuous infusion. When given as a continuous infusion, must be given via central line, as drug is a potent vesicant.

## SPECIAL CONSIDERATIONS

Drug is a *vesicant*. Give through a running IV to avoid *extravasation*.

Dose modification may be necessary in the presence of hepatic failure.

Decreased pharmacologic effects of phenytoin when given with this drug.

Increases cellular uptake of methotrexate by certain malignant cells when administered sequentially, but less so than vincristine.

## Vinblastine

| Nursing Diagnosis | Defining Characteristics | Expected Outcomes | Nursing Interventions |
|---|---|---|---|
| I. *Potential for infection and bleeding related to bone marrow depression* | I. A. May cause severe BMD<br>B. Nadir 4–10 days<br>C. Neutrophils greatly affected<br>D. In pts with prior XRT or chemotherapy, thrombocytopenia may be severe | I. A. Pt will be without s/s of infection or bleeding<br>B. Early s/s of infection or bleeding will be identified | I. A. Monitor CBC, platelet count prior to drug administration<br>B. Assess for s/s of infection or bleeding<br>C. Instruct pt in self-assessment of s/s of infection or bleeding<br>D. Dose reduction if hepatic dysfunction: 50% if bilirubin > 1.5 mg/dl; 75% if bilirubin > 3.0 mg/dl<br>E. Administer red cell, platelet transfusions as ordered<br>F. Refer to sec. on bone marrow depression, Chapter 4 |
| II. *Potential for sensory/perceptual alterations* | II. A. Occur less frequently than with vincristine<br>B. Occur in pts receiving prolonged or high-dose therapy<br>C. Symptoms: paresthesias, peripheral neuropathy, depression, headache, malaise, jaw pain, urinary retention, tachycardia, orthostatic hypotension, seizures<br>D. Rare ocular changes: diplopia, ptosis, photophobia, oculomotor dysfunction, optic neuropathy | II. A. Sensory/perceptual changes will be identified early<br>B. Dysfunction will be minimized<br>C. Discomfort will be minimized | II. A. Assess sensory/perceptual changes prior to each drug dose, especially if dose is high (> 10 mg) or pt is receiving prolonged therapy<br>B. Notify MD of alterations<br>C. Discuss with pt impact changes have had and strategies to minimize dysfunction and decrease distress<br>D. Refer to sec. on neurotoxicity, Chapter 4 |
| III. *Potential for constipation* | III. A. Constipation results from neurotoxicity (central) and is less common than with vincristine<br>B. Risk factors: high dose (> 20 mg) | III. A. Constipation will be prevented<br>B. Early s/s of adynamic ileus will be identified | III. A. Assess bowel elimination pattern after each drug dose, especially if dose > 20 mg<br>B. Teach pt to promote bowel evacuation by fluids (3 l/day), high-fiber, bulky foods, exercise, stool softeners |

| Nursing Diagnosis | Assessment | Desired Outcomes | Nursing Interventions |
|---|---|---|---|
| | C. May lead to adynamic ileus, abdominal pain | | C. Suggest laxative if unable to move bowels at least once a day<br>D. Instruct pt to report abdominal pain |
| IV. *Altered nutrition, less than body requirements related to*<br>A. Nausea and vomiting | IV. A. Rarely occur | IV. A. 1. Pt will be without nausea and vomiting<br>2. Nausea and vomiting, if they occur, will be minimal | IV. A. 1. Premedicate with antiemetics and continue prophylactically × 24 hrs to prevent nausea and vomiting, at least for the first treatment<br>2. Encourage small, frequent feedings of cool, bland foods and liquids<br>3. Assess for symptoms of fluid and electrolyte imbalance; monitor I&O, daily weights if inpatient<br>4. Refer to sec. on nausea and vomiting, Chapter 4 |
| B. Stomatitis | B. Occurs occasionally; may be severe | B. Oral mucous membranes will remain intact and without infection | B. 1. Teach pt oral assessment<br>2. Teach, reinforce teaching, re oral hygiene regimens<br>3. Encourage pt to report early stomatitis<br>4. Provide pain relief measures if indicated (e.g., topical anesthetics)<br>5. See sec. on stomatitis, mucositis, Chapter 4 |
| C. Diarrhea | C. Occasional, infrequent, and mild | C. Pt will have minimal diarrhea | C. 1. Encourage pt to report onset of diarrhea<br>2. Administer or teach pt to self-administer antidiarrheal medication<br>3. Suggest diet modification<br>4. See sec. on diarrhea, Chapter 4 |

*(continued)*

## Vinblastine (continued)

| Nursing Diagnosis | Defining Characteristics | Expected Outcomes | Nursing Interventions |
|---|---|---|---|
| V. *Potential for impaired skin integrity related to*<br>A. Alopecia | V. A. 1. Reversible and mild<br>2. Occurs in 45–50% of pts receiving drug | V. A. 1. Pt will verbalize feelings re hair loss<br>2. Pt will identify strategies to cope with changes in body image | V. A. 1. Discuss with pt impact of hair loss<br>2. Suggest wig as appropriate prior to actual hair loss<br>3. Explore with pt response to actual hair loss and plan strategies to minimize distress (i.e., wig, scarf, cap)<br>4. Refer to sec. on alopecia, Chapter 4 |
| B. Extravasation | B. Drug is a potent vesicant and can cause irritation and necrosis if infiltrated | B. 1. Extravasation will be avoided<br>2. Skin will heal completely if extravasation occurs | B. 1. For safe administration of vesicant, refer to sec. on reactions, Chapter 9<br>2. Careful technique is used during venipuncture; see sec. on intravenous administration, Chapter 10<br>3. Administer vesicant through freely flowing IV, constantly monitoring IV site and pt response<br>4. Nurse should be *thoroughly* familiar with institutional policy and procedure for administration of a vesicant agent<br>5. If vesicant drug is administered as a continuous infusion, drug must be given through a patent central line<br>6. If extravasation is suspected:<br>  a. Stop drug administered<br>  b. Aspirate any residual drug and blood from IV tubing, IV catheter/needle, and IV site if possible |

c. If drug infiltration is suspected, manufacturer suggests the following after withdrawing any remaining drug from IV: local installation of hyaluronidase, apply moderate heat

7. Assess site regularly for pain, progression of erythema, induration, and evidence of necrosis

8. When in doubt about whether drug is infiltrating, *treat as an infiltration*

9. Teach pt to assess site and notify MD if condition worsens

10. Arrange next clinic visit for assessment of site depending on drug, amount infiltrated, extent of potential injury, and pt variables

11. Document in pt's record as per institutional policy and procedure; see sec. on reactions, Chapter 9

C. Rash

C. Uncommon

C. Pt will identify strategies to cope with rash

C. Assess impact of rash on pt (body image, comfort) and treat symptomatically

VI. *Potential for sexual dysfunction*

VI. A. Drug is possibly teratogenic
B. Likely to cause azoospermia in men

A. Pt and significant other will identify strategies to cope with sexual dysfunction

VI. A. As appropriate, explore with pt and significant other issues of reproductive and sexuality pattern and anticipated impact chemotherapy will have

B. Discuss strategies to preserve reproductive health (e.g., sperm banking)

C. Refer to sec. on gonadal dysfunction, Chapter 4

# Vincristine
## (Oncovin)

*Class:* Plant alkaloid extracted from the peri-winkle plant (*Vinca rosea*)

## MECHANISM OF ACTION

Drug binds to microtubular proteins, thus arrest-ing mitosis during metaphase. Cell cycle phase specific in M and S phases.

## METABOLISM

The primary route for excretion is via the liver, with about 70% of the drug being excreted in feces and bile. These metabolites are a result of hepatic metabolism and biliary excretion. A small amount is excreted in the urine. Dose modification may be necessary in the presence of hepatic failure.

## DOSAGE/RANGE

0.4–1.4 mg/m$^2$ weekly (initially limited to 2 mg per dose)

## DRUG PREPARATION

Supplied in 1-mg, 2-mg, and 5-mg vials. Refrigerate vials until use.

## DRUG ADMINISTRATION

IV push or as a continuous infusion over 24 hours. When given as a continuous infu-sion should be administered through a cen-tral line, as drug is a potent vesicant.

## SPECIAL CONSIDERATIONS

Drug is a *vesicant*. Give through a running IV to avoid *extravasation*.

Dose modification may be necessary in the pres-ence of hepatic failure.

Decreased bioavailability of digoxin when given with this drug.

Increased cellular uptake of methotrexate by some malignant cells when given sequentially.

# Vincristine

| Nursing Diagnosis | Defining Characteristics | Expected Outcomes | Nursing Interventions |
|---|---|---|---|
| I. *Potential for sensory/perceptual alterations related to* | | | |
| A. Peripheral neuropathies | I. A. 1. Peripheral neuropathies occur as a result of toxicity to nerve fibers<br>2. Absent deep tension reflexes<br>3. Numbness, weakness, myalgias, cramping<br>4. Late severe motor difficulties<br>5. Reversal or discontinuance of therapy necessary<br>6. Increased risk in elderly | I. A. 1. Sensory and perceptual changes will be identified early<br>2. Dysfunction will be minimized<br>3. Discomfort will be minimized | I. A. 1. Assess sensory and perceptual changes prior to each drug dose (i.e., presence of numbness or tingling of fingertips or toes)<br>2. Assess for loss of deep tendon reflexes: foot drop, slapping gait<br>3. Assess for motor difficulties: clumsiness of hands, difficulty climbing stairs (buttoning shirt, walking on heels)<br>4. Notify MD of alterations: discuss holding drug if loss of deep tendon reflexes occurs<br>5. Discuss with pt impact alterations have had and strategies to minimize dysfunction and decrease distress<br>6. Discuss with pt type of alteration: memory, sensory/perceptual, temporary and reversible when drug stopped<br>7. See sec. on neurotoxicity, Chapter 4 |
| B. Cranial nerve damage and other nerve involvement | B. 1. Cranial nerve dysfunction may occur (rare)<br>2. Jaw pain (trigeminal neuralgia)<br>3. Diplopia<br>4. Vocal cord paresis<br>5. Mental depression<br>6. Metallic taste | B. Symptoms of nerve dysfunction will be identified early | B. 1. Assess pt for s/s of nerve dysfunction before each dose<br>2. Notify MD of any changes |

*(continued)*

## Vincristine (continued)

| Nursing Diagnosis | Defining Characteristics | Expected Outcomes | Nursing Interventions |
|---|---|---|---|
| C. Constipation | C. 1. Autonomic neuropathy may lead to constipation and paralytic ileus<br>2. A concurrent use of vinblastine, narcotic analgesics, or cholinergic medication may increase risk of constipation | C. 1. Constipation will be prevented<br>2. Early s/s of paralytic ileus will be identified | C. 1. Assess bowel elimination pattern prior to each chemotherapy administration<br>2. Teach pt to include bulky and high-fiber foods in diet, increase fluids to 3 l/day, and exercise moderately to promote elimination<br>3. Suggest stool softeners if needed<br>4. Teach pt to use laxative if unable to move bowels at least once every 2 days<br>5. Instruct pt to report abdominal pain |
| II. Potential for impaired skin integrity related to<br><br>A. Alopecia and subsequent body image disturbance | II. A. 1. Complete hair loss occurs in 12–45% of pts<br>2. Both men and women are at risk for body image disturbance<br>3. Hair will grow back | II. A. Pt will verbalize feelings about hair loss and identify strategies to cope with change in body image | II. A. 1. Discuss with pt anticipated impact of hair loss; suggest wig or toupee as appropriate prior to actual hair loss<br>2. Explore with pt response to hair loss, if it occurs, and strategies to minimize distress (i.e., wig, scarf, cap)<br>3. See sec. on alopecia, Chapter 4 |
| B. Dermatitis | B. Uncommon | B. Pt will identify coping strategies | B. 1. Assess impact on pt: body image, comfort<br>2. Discuss strategies to minimize distress |
| C. Extravasation | C. Drug is potent vesicant, causing irritation and necrosis if infiltrated | C. 1. Extravasation will be avoided<br>2. Skin will heal completely if drug is extravasated | C. 1. Careful technique is used during venipuncture; see sec. on intravenous administration, Chapter 10<br>2. Administer vesicant through freely flowing IV, constantly monitoring IV site and pt response |

3. Nurse should be *thoroughly* familiar with institutional policy and procedure for administration of a vesicant agent

4. If vesicant drug is administered as a continuous infusion, drug must be given through a patent central line

5. If extravasation is suspected:
   a. Stop drug being administered
   b. Aspirate any residual drug and blood from IV tubing, IV catheter/needle and IV site if possible
   c. If drug infiltration is suspected, manufacturer suggests the following after withdrawing any remaining drug from tubing: local injection of hyaluronidase, apply moderate heat

6. Assess site regularly for pain, progression of erythema, induration, and evidence of necrosis

7. When in doubt about whether drug is infiltrating, *treat as an infiltration*

8. Teach pt to assess site and notify MD if condition worsens

9. Arrange next clinic visit for assessment of site depending on drug, amount infiltrated, extent of potential injury, and pt variables

10. Document in pt's record as per institutional policy and procedure; see sec. on reactions, Chapter 9

*(continued)*

## Vincristine (continued)

| Nursing Diagnosis | Defining Characteristics | Expected Outcomes | Nursing Interventions |
|---|---|---|---|
| III. *Potential for infection and bleeding related to bone marrow depression* | III. A. Rare myelosuppression; mild when it occurs <br> B. May have cumulative bone marrow depression over time, requiring transfusion <br> C. Nadir 10–14 days after treatment begins | III. A. Pt will be without bleeding or infection <br> B. Early s/s of bleeding or infection will be detected | III. A. Monitor WBC, hematocrit, platelets prior to drug administration <br> B. Dose reduction if hepatic dysfunction: 50% reduction if bilirubin > 1.5 mg/dl; 75% reduction if bilirubin > 3.0 mg/dl <br> C. See sec. on bone marrow depression, Chapter 4 |
| IV. *Potential for sexual dysfunction* | IV. A. Impotence may occur related to neurotoxicity | IV. A. Pt and significant other will identify strategies to cope with sexual dysfunction | IV. A. As appropriate, explore with pt and significant other issues of reproductive and sexuality pattern and impact chemotherapy may have <br> B. Discuss strategies to preserve sexual health (i.e., alternative expressions of sexuality) <br> C. Reassure pt that impotency, if it occurs, is usually temporary and reversible after drug discontinuance <br> D. Refer to sec. on gonadal dysfunction, Chapter 4 |

# Vindesine
## (Eldisine, Desacetylvinblastine)

*Class:* Synthetic derivative of vinblastine; synthetic vinca alkaloid

## MECHANISM OF ACTION

Inhibits microtubule formation, causing metaphase arrest during M phase and causes some cell death during S phase. Cell cycle phase–specific.

## METABOLISM

Short plasma half-life (probably binds to tissue). Prolonged elimination, suggesting drug may accumulate with repeated dosing. Excreted primarily by bile.

## DOSAGE/RANGE

3–4 mg/m$^2$ q 1–2 weeks

1–1.3 mg/m$^2$/day $\times$ 5–7 days, repeated every 3 weeks

1.5–2 mg/m$^2$ twice a week

## DRUG PREPARATION

A 10-mg vial of lyophilized powder is reconstituted with provided diluent or normal saline. Solution is stable for 2 weeks if refrigerated.

## DRUG ADMINISTRATION

Vesicant precautions. Administer slowly as intravenous push through sidearm of freely running IV. Also may be given as continuous infusion.

## SPECIAL CONSIDERATIONS

Do not give with other vinca alkaloids, such as vincristine or vinblastine, as there is a potential for cumulative neurotoxicity.

Dose reduction may be necessary in patients with abnormal liver function or if patient has received maximal doses of other vinca alkaloids.

## Vindesine

| Nursing Diagnosis | Defining Characteristics | Expected Outcomes | Nursing Interventions |
|---|---|---|---|
| I. *Potential for infection and bleeding related to bone marrow depression* | I. A. Dose-limiting side effect <br> B. Nadir 5–10 days <br> C. Neutropenia mild to moderate <br> D. Thrombocytopenia mild, rare (may increase on treatment) | I. A. Pt will be without s/s of infection or bleeding <br> B. Early s/s of infection or bleeding will be identified | I. A. Monitor CBC, platelet count prior to drug administration, as well as s/s of infection or bleeding <br> B. Instruct pt in self-assessment of s/s of infection or bleeding <br> C. Dose reduction often necessary (35–50%) with compromised bone marrow function <br> D. Refer to sec. on bone marrow depression, Chapter 4 |
| II. *Potential for sensory/perceptual alteration related to* <br><br> A. Peripheral neuropathy, cranial nerve damage, other nerve involvement | II. A. 1. Neurotoxicity similar to vincristine <br> 2. Cumulative toxicity, mild <br> 3. Begins with distal paresthesias, proximal muscle weakness, loss of deep tendon reflexes <br> 4. Hoarseness, jaw pain (severe and transient may occur) | II. A. 1. Sensory/perceptual changes will be identified early <br> 2. Dysfunction will be minimized <br> 3. Discomfort will be minimized | II. A. 1. Obtain visual assessment prior to starting therapy <br> 2. Encourage pt to report any visual changes <br> 3. Instruct pt to report headache, dizziness, light-headedness <br> 4. Refer to sec. on neurotoxicity, Chapter 4 |
| B. Constipation | B. Autonomic neuropathy may lead to abdominal cramping, constipation, and paralytic ileus | B. 1. Constipation will be prevented <br> 2. Early s/s of paralytic ileus will be identified | B. 1. Assess bowel elimination pattern prior to each chemotherapy administration <br> 2. Teach pt to include bulky and high-fiber foods in diet, increase fluids to 3 L/day, exercise moderately to promote elimination <br> 3. Suggest stool softeners if needed <br> 4. Teach pt to use laxative if unable to move bowels at least once every 2 days <br> 5. Instruct pt to report abdominal pain |

III. *Potential for impaired skin integrity related to*

| | Defining Characteristics | Expected Outcomes | Nursing Interventions |
|---|---|---|---|
| **A. Alopecia, with subsequent image disturbance** | III. A. 1. Affects 80–90% of pts with 25–50% experiencing total hair loss<br>2. Alopecia may be progressive<br>3. Both men and women at risk for body image disturbance<br>4. Hair will grow back<br>5. Scalp tourniquet may be helpful if not contraindicated | III. A. 1. Pt will verbalize feelings re hair loss<br>2. Pt will identify strategies to cope with changes in body image | III. A. 1. Discuss with pt impact of hair loss<br>2. Suggest wig as appropriate prior to actual hair loss<br>3. Explore with pt response to actual hair loss and plan strategies to minimize distress (e.g., wig, scarf, cap)<br>4. Refer to sec. on alopecia, Chapter 4 |
| **B. Rash** | B. Uncommon | B. Pt will identify coping strategies | B. Assess impact of rash on pt (body image, comfort) treat symptomatically |
| **C. Extravasation** | C. 1. Inapparent or obvious infiltrations can occur<br>2. Presentation delayed; pain, phlebitis, blister formation occurs; may progress to ulceration and necrosis<br>3. Management similar to vincristine extravasation | C. 1. Extravasation will be avoided<br>2. Skin will heal completely if extravasation occurs | C. 1. Careful technique is used during venipuncture; see sec. on intravenous administration, Chapter 10<br>2. Administer vesicant through freely flowing IV, constantly monitoring IV site and pt response<br>3. Nurse should be *thoroughly* familiar with institutional policy and procedure for administration of a vesicant agent<br>4. If vesicant drug is administered as a continuous infusion, drug must be given through a patent central line |

*(continued)*

## Vindesine (continued)

| Nursing Diagnosis | Defining Characteristics | Expected Outcomes | Nursing Interventions |
|---|---|---|---|
| | | | 5. If extravasation is suspected:<br>a. Stop drug administered<br>b. Aspirate any residual drug and blood from IV tubing, IV catheter/needle and IV site if possible<br>c. If drug infiltration is suspected, manufacturer suggests the following after withdrawing any remaining drug from IV: local installation of hyaluronidase, apply moderate heat |
| | | | 6. Assess site regularly for pain, progression of erythema, induration, and evidence of necrosis |
| | | | 7. When in doubt about whether drug is infiltrating, *treat as an infiltration* |
| | | | 8. Teach pt to assess site and notify MD if condition worsens |
| | | | 9. Arrange next clinic visit for assessment of site depending on drug, amount infiltrated, extent of potential injury, and pt variables |
| | | | 10. Document in pt's record as per institutional policy and procedure; see sec. on reactions, Chapter 9 |
| IV. *Altered nutrition, less than body requirements related to*<br>A. Nausea and vomiting | IV. A. 1. Typically not severe<br>2. Occur in 30% of pts | IV. A. 1. Pt will be without nausea and vomiting<br>2. Nausea and vomiting, if they occur, will be minimal | IV. A. 1. Premedicate with antiemetic and continue prophylactically × 24 hrs to prevent nausea and vomiting, at least for first treatment |

2. Encourage small, frequent feedings of cool, bland foods and liquids
3. Refer to sec. on nausea and vomiting, Chapter 4

| | | | |
|---|---|---|---|
| B. Diarrhea | B. Uncommon, but rarely may be protracted and thus would be an indication for dose reduction | B. Pt will have minimal diarrhea | B. 1. Encourage pt to report onset of diarrhea<br>2. Administer or teach pt to self-administer anti-diarrheal medications<br>3. See sec. on diarrhea, Chapter 4 |
| C. Stomatitis | C. Rare | C. Oral mucous membranes will remain intact and without infection | C. 1. Teach pt oral assessment<br>2. Encourage pt to report early stomatitis<br>3. Teach pt oral hygiene<br>4. See sec. on stomatitis, mucositis, Chapter 4 |
| D. Anorexia | D. Rare | D. Pt will maintain baseline weight ± 5% | D. 1. Encourage small, frequent feedings of favorite foods, especially high-calorie, high-protein foods<br>2. Encourage use of spices<br>3. Weekly weights |

# Vinorelbine
(Navelbine)

*Class:* Semisynthetic vinca alkaloid derived from vinblastine

## MECHANISM OF ACTION

Inhibits mitosis at metaphase by interfering with microtubule assembly. Also appears to interfere with some aspects of cellular metabolism, including cellular respiration and nucleic acid biosynthesis. Cell cycle–specific.

## METABOLISM

Slow elimination; extensive tissue binding (80% bound to plasma proteins); metabolized by the liver. Terminal half-life is 27–43 hours. Excreted in feces (46%) and urine (18%).

## DOSAGE/RANGE

30 mg/m$^2$ IV weekly or in combination with 120 mg/m$^2$ cisplatin given on days 1 and 29, then every 6 weeks. Investigationally, 80 mg/m$^2$ po weekly.

## DRUG PREPARATION

Available as 10-mg/ml solution in 1-ml or 5-ml vials. Further dilute in 75–250 ml 0.9% sodium chloride or 5% dextrose in water. Final concentration should be 1.5–3 mg/ml for syringe and 0.5–2 mg/ml for IV bolus administration. Stable for 24 hours at room temperature. Oral preparation available as 40-mg gelatin capsules.

## DRUG ADMINISTRATION

Drug is a vesicant. It is administered IV over 6–10 minutes by slow IV push via syringe into the sidearm closest to the IV bag of a freely flowing IV, followed by a 75–125 ml flush or by IV bolus infusion via a central line. Refer to individual hospital policy and procedure for vesicant administration.

Oral capsule should be taken on an empty stomach at bedtime.

## SPECIAL CONSIDERATIONS

There has been a 33% response rate in non-small-cell lung cancer when used as single agent and a 65% response in combination with cisplatin, 5-fluorouracil, and leucovorin.

Overall response rate in metastatic breast cancer was 45%, with 20% complete responses.

Increased nausea, vomiting, and diarrhea with oral administration of capsules.

Drug is a vesicant, and as with other vinca alkaloids, hyaluronidase should be administered if extravasation is suspected.

Drug is embryotoxic and mutagenic, so female patients of childbearing age should use contraception.

Administer cautiously in patients with hepatic insufficiency.

Dose modification is necessary in the presence of hepatic dysfunction: total bilirubin 2.1–3.0 mg/dl, use 50% dose reduction (i.e., 15 mg/m$^2$); total bilirubin > 3.0 mg/dl, use 75% dose reduction (i.e., 7.5 mg/m$^2$).

Contraindicated if absolute granulocyte count (AGC) is < 1000 cells/mm$^3$.

Dose modification necessary for hematologic toxicity. If AGC on the day of treatment is 1000–1499 cells/m$^3$, use 50% dose reduction (i.e., 15 mg/m$^2$); drug should be held if AGC is < 1000 cells/m$^3$. If drug is held for 3 consecutive weeks due to AGC < 1000 cells/m$^3$, discontinue drug.

## Vinorelbine *(continued)*

If patient develops granulocytopenic fever or sepsis or drug is held for granulocytopenia for 2 consecutive doses, drug dose should be reduced 25% (i.e., 22.5 mg/m$^2$) if AGC is > 1500 cells/mm$^3$; if AGC is 1000–1499 cells/mm$^3$, drug dose should be decreased to 11.25 mg/m$^2$ as per package insert.

Rarely, acute pulmonary reactions have been reported when drug is administered in combination with Mitomycin C.

# Vinorelbine

| Nursing Diagnosis | Defining Characteristics | Expected Outcomes | Nursing Interventions |
|---|---|---|---|
| I. *Infection and bleeding related to bone marrow depression* | I. A. Leukopenia is dose-limiting toxicity; bone marrow depression noncumulative and short-lived (< 7 days), with nadir 7–10 days<br>B. Use with caution in pts with history of prior radiotherapy or chemotherapy<br>C. Severe thrombocytopenia and anemia uncommon | I. A. Pt will be without s/s of infection or bleeding<br>B. Early s/s of infection or bleeding will be identified | I. A. Monitor CBC, platelet count prior to drug administration and postchemotherapy; assess for s/s of infection or bleeding<br>B. Teach pt self-assessment of s/s of infection or bleeding and how to seek medical advice/care<br>C. Dose may be held until full bone marrow recovery, then reduced 25%; see "Special Considerations"<br>D. See "Special Considerations" for dose reduction with hepatic dysfunction<br>E. Administer growth factor (i.e., G-CSF) > 24 hrs after drug administration, as ordered |
| II. *Potential for sensory/perceptual alterations related to neurological toxicity* | II. A. Incidence of mild to moderate neuropathy is 25%<br>B. Paresthesias occurs in 2–10% of pts, but incidence is increased if pt has received prior chemotherapy with vinca alkaloids or abdominal XRT<br>C. Decreased deep tendon reflexes (6–29%)<br>D. Constipation may occur in 29% of pts<br>E. Reversible neuropathy | II. A. Early s/s of neurological toxicity will be identified<br>B. Function will be maintained | II. A. Assess baseline neuromuscular function and reassess prior to drug infusion, especially presence of paresthesias; risk is increased if drug is given concurrently with cisplatin<br>B. Teach pt to report any changes in sensation or function<br>C. Discuss alterations with MD<br>D. Identify strategies to promote comfort and safety |

III. *Alteration in nutrition, less than body requirements related to*

| | Defining Characteristics | Expected Outcomes | Nursing Interventions |
|---|---|---|---|
| A. Nausea and vomiting | III. A. Incidence increases with oral dosing; mild in IV dosing, with 44% incidence; vomiting occurs in approximately 20% of pts | III. A. 1. Pt will be without nausea and vomiting 2. Nausea and vomiting, if they occur, will be mild 3. Pt will maintain weight within 5% of baseline | III. A. 1. Premedicate with antiemetics prior to drug administration, at least for first treatment 2. Encourage small, frequent feedings of cool, bland foods and liquids 3. Assess for symptoms of fluid/electrolyte imbalance if pt has severe nausea and vomiting 4. Monitor I&O, daily weights, lab electrolyte values |
| B. Diarrhea | B. Increased incidence with oral dosing (17%) | B. Pt will have minimal diarrhea | B. 1. Encourage pt to report onset of diarrhea 2. Administer or teach pt to self-administer antidiarrheal medication |
| C. Stomatitis | C. Usually mild to moderate, with < 20% incidence | C. Oral mucous membranes will remain intact and without infection | C. 1. Teach pt oral self-assessment 2. Teach, reinforce teaching re oral hygiene regimen 3. Encourage pt to report early stomatitis 4. Provide pain relief measures if indicated (i.e., topical anesthetics) |
| D. Hepatotoxicity | D. Transient increase in liver function studies (SGOT) occurs in 67% of pts, without clinical significance | D. Hepatic dysfunction will be identified early | D. 1. Assess liver function studies prior to drug administration and periodically during treatment 2. Dose modification necessary for severe hepatic dysfunction (see "Special Considerations") |

*(continued)*

## Vinorelbine (continued)

| Nursing Diagnosis | Defining Characteristics | Expected Outcomes | Nursing Interventions |
|---|---|---|---|
| IV. Potential for alteration in skin integrity related to<br><br>A. Alopecia | IV. A. Incidence is 12%; reversible and mild | IV. A. Pt will verbalize feelings re hair loss and strategies to cope with change in body image | IV. A. 1. Discuss potential impact of hair loss prior to drug administration, coping strategies, and plan to minimize body image distortion (e.g., wig, scarf, cap)<br>2. Assess pt for s/s of hair loss<br>3. Assess pt's response and use of coping strategies |
| B. Extravasation | B. Drug is a vesicant similar to other vinca alkaloids and can cause irritation and necrosis if drug extravasates | B. 1. Extravasation will be avoided<br>2. Skin will heal completely if extravasation occurs | B. 1. Careful technique is used during venipuncture<br>2. Administer vesicant through freely flowing IV, constantly monitoring IV site and pt response<br>3. Nurse should be *thoroughly* familiar with institutional policy and procedure for administration of a vesicant agent<br>4. If vesicant drug is administered as a continuous infusion, drug must be given through a patent central line<br>5. If extravasation is suspected:<br>  a. Stop drug administered<br>  b. Aspirate any residual drug and blood from IV tubing, IV catheter/ needle, and IV site if possible<br>  c. If drug infiltration is suspected, manufacturer suggests the following after withdrawing any remaining drug from IV: local installation of hyaluronidase, apply moderate heat |

| | | |
|---|---|---|
| C. Injection site reactions | C. Erythema and pain at injection site, vein discoloration (33%), mostly mild or moderate; chemical phlebitis proximal to injection site may occur in 10% of pts | 6. Assess site regularly for pain, progression of erythema, induration, and evidence of necrosis<br>7. When in doubt whether drug is infiltrating, *treat as an infiltration*<br>8. Teach pt to assess site and notify MD if condition worsens<br>9. Arrange next clinic visit for assessment of site depending on drug, amount infiltrated, extent of potential injury, and pt variables<br>10. Document in pt's record as per institutional policy and procedure |
| | C. 1. Skin changes will be identified early<br>2. Skin changes will be minimal | C. 1. Select vein carefully and alternate venipuncture sites<br>2. Consider central access (i.e., VAD) early if pt has limited venous access<br>3. Flush vein after drug administration with at least 75–125 ml of IV solution |
| V. *Potential for sexual/ reproductive dysfunction* | V. A. Drug is teratogenic and fetotoxic | V. A. Pt and significiant other will identify strategies to cope with altered sexual and reproductive pattern |
| | V. A. Pt and significiant other will identify strategies to cope with altered sexual and reproductive pattern | V. A. As appropriate, explore with pt and significant other issues of reproductive and sexuality pattern and anticipated impact chemotherapy may have<br>B. Counsel female pts of childbearing age in contraceptive options |

# BIBLIOGRAPHY

Abratt, R.P., Bezwoda, W.R., Falkson, G., Goedhals, L., Hacking, D., and Rugg, T.A. (1994). Efficacy and safety profile of gemcitabine in non-small cell lung cancer: a phase II study. *Journal of Clinical Oncology* 12(8): 1535–1540.

Agarwal, R. (1980). Deoxycoformycin toxicity in mice after long-term treatment. *Cancer Chemotherapy and Pharmacology* 5(2): 83–87.

Alza Corporation. (2000). VIADUR (leuprolide acetate implant) Healthcare Professional Product Information. Mountain View, Cal.: Alza Corporation: 1–10.

Amrein, P.C., Davis, R.B., Mayer, R.J., and Schiffer, C.A. (1990). Treatment of relapsed and refractory acute myeloid leukemia with diaziquone and mitoxantrone: A CALGB phase I study. *American Journal of Hematology* 35(2): 80–83.

Anderson, H., Lund, B., Bach, F., Thatcher, N., Walling, J., and Hansen, H.H. (1994). Single-agent activity of weekly gemcitabine in advanced non-small cell lung cancer: A phase II study. *Journal of Clinical Oncology* 12(9): 1821–1826.

*Annual Report to the FDA.* (1985). CBDCA (NSC #241-240). Washington, D.C.: Government Printing Office.

Beck, S., and Yasko, J.M. (1984). *A Guideline for Oral Care.* Sage Products.

Becker, T. (1981). *Cancer Chemotherapy: A Manual for Nurses.* Boston: Little, Brown.

Brager, B.L., and Yasko, J.M. (1984). *Care of the Client Receiving Chemotherapy.* Reston, Vir.: Reston Publishing Co.

Cadman, E.D., Ignoffo, R.J., and Stagg, R.J. (1985). *Leucovorin: Uses with Methotrexate, Sequential Methotrexate and 5-Fluorouracil, and with 5-Fluorouracil.* Wayne, N.J.: Lederle Laboratories.

Calvert, A.H., Harland, J.J., Newell, D.R., et al. (1985). Phase 1 studies with carboplatin at the Royal Marsden Hospital. *Cancer Treatment Review* 12 (suppl A): 54.

Canetta, R., Franks, C., Smaldone, L., et al. (1987). Clinical status of carboplatin. *Oncology* (July): 61–69.

Carella, A.M., Santini, G., Martinengo, M., Giordano, D., Nati, S., Congiu, A., Cerri, R., Risso, M., Damasio, E., and Rossi, E. (1985). 4-demethoxy-daunorubicin (Idarubicin) in refractory or relapsed acute leukemia: A pilot study. *Cancer* 55(7): 1452.

Carter, S.K., Canetta, R., and Roxencweig, M. (1985). Carboplatin: future directions. *Cancer Treatment Review* 12 (suppl A): 145.

Chabner, B.A., and Myers, C.E. (1985). Clinical pharmacology of cancer chemotherapy. In V.T. DeVita, Jr., S. Hellman, and S.A. Rosenberg (eds.): *Cancer: Principles and Practice of Oncology.* 2nd ed. Philadelphia: Lippincott.

Daghestani, A.N., et al. (1985). Phase 1–2 clinical and pharmacological study of 4-demethoxy-daunorubicin (DMDR) in adult patients with acute leukemia. *Cancer Research* 45(3): 1408–1412.

Doria, M.I., Shepart, K.V., Lerin, B., and Riddell, R.H. (1986). Liver pathology following hepatic arterial infusion chemotherapy: hepatic toxicity with FUDR. *Cancer* 58(4): 855–861.

Dorr, R.T. (1989). *MESNEX (Mesna) Injection Dosing and Administration Guide—Rationale and Guidelines for Dosing and Administration.* Evansville, Ind.: Bristol-Myers.

Dorr, R.T., and Fritz, W. (1980). *Cancer Chemotherapy Handbook.* New York: Elsevier.

Dorr, R.T., and Von Hoff, D.D. (1994). *Cancer Chemotherapy Handbook.* 2nd ed. Norwalk, Conn.: Appleton and Lange.

Eisenhower, E.A., Zee, B.C., Pater, J.L., et al. (1988). Trimetrexate: Predictors of severe or life-threatening toxic effects. *Journal of the National Cancer Institute* 80(16): 1318–1322.

Fischer, D.S., and Knobf, M.T. (1989). *The Cancer Chemotherapy Handbook.* 3rd ed. Chicago: Yearbook Medical Publishers.

Forastiere, A.A., Natale, R.B., Takasugi, B.J., Goren, M.P., Vogel, W.C., and Kudla-Hatch, V. (1987). A phase I–II trial of carboplatin and 5-fluorouracil combination chemotherapy in advanced carcinoma of the head and neck. *Journal of Clinical Oncology* 5(2): 191.

Foster, B.J., Clagett-Carr, K., Leyland-Jones, B., et al. (1985). Results of NCI sponsored phase I trials with carboplatin. *Cancer Treatment Review* 12 (suppl A): 43.

Goodman, M. (1988). Concepts of hormonal manipulation in the treatment of cancer. *Oncology Nursing Forum* 15(5): 639–647.

———. (1987). Management of nausea and vomiting induced by outpatient cisplatin therapy. *Seminars in Oncology Nursing* 3 (suppl 1): 23–35.

Govani, L.E., and Hayes, J.E. (1982). *Drugs and Nursing Implications*. Norwalk, Conn.: Appleton-Century-Crofts.

Grem, J.L., Ellenberg, S.S, King, S.A., et al. (1989). Correlates of severe or life-threatening toxic effects from trimetrexate. *Journal of the National Cancer Institute* 80(16): 1313–1318.

Grever, M.R., Malspers, L., Balcerzak, S., et al. (1982). 2'-deoxycoformycin: A phase I clinical-pharmacokinetic investigation. *AACR Proceedings* 23(533): 36.

Grever, M.R., Siaw, M.F., Jacob, W.F., Neidhart, J.A., Miser, J.S., Coleman, M.S., Hutton, J.J., and Balcerzak, S.P. (1981). The biochemical and clinical consequences of 2'-deoxycoformycin in refractory lymphoproliferative malignancies. *Blood* 57(2): 406–417.

Grochow, L.B., Noe, D.A., Dole, G.B., and Yarbro, C.H. (1989). Phase I trial of trimetrexate gluconate on a five-day bolus schedule: Clinical pharmacology and pharmacodynamics. *Journal of the National Cancer Institute* 81: 124–130.

Groenwald, S.L., Frogge, M.H., Goodman, M., and Yarbro, C.H. (1990). *Cancer Nursing Principles and Practice*. 2nd ed. Boston: Jones & Bartlett.

Harris, J.R., Hellman, S., Canellos, G.P., et al. (1985). Cancer of the breast. In V.T. DeVita, Jr., S. Hellman, and S.A. Rosenberg (eds.): *Cancer: Principles and Practice of Oncology*. 2nd ed. Philadelphia: Lippincott.

Holmes, F.A., Hwee-Yong, Y.A.P., Esparza, L., Buzdar, A.U., Blumenchein, G.R., Hug, V., and Hortobagyi, G.N. (1987). Mitoxantrone, cyclophosphamide, and fluorouracil in metastatic breast cancer unresponsive to hormonal therapy. *Cancer* 59(12): 1992–1999.

Hubbard, S.M., and Seipp, C. (1985). Administration of cancer treatments: practical guide for physicians and oncology nurses. In V.T. DeVita, Jr., S. Hellman, and S.A. Rosenberg (eds.): *Cancer: Principles and Practice of Oncology*. 2nd ed. Philadelphia: Lippincott.

Hudes, G.R., and Comis, R.L. (1988). Phase I and II studies of trimetrexate administered in combination with fluorouracil to patients with metastatic cancer. *Seminars in Oncology* 15 (suppl 2): 41–45.

Johnson, B.L., and Gross, J. (1985). *Handbook of Oncology Nursing*. New York: John Wiley and Sons.

Kemeny, N., Daly, J., Reichman, B., Geller, N., Botet, J., and Odermany, P. (1987). Intrahepatic or systemic infusion of fluorodeoxyuridine in patients with liver metastases from colorectal carcinoma. *Annals of Internal Medicine* 107(4): 459–465.

Knight, W.A. III, Livingston, R.B., Fabian, C., and Costanzi, J. (1979). Phase I–II trial of methyl-GAG: A SWOG pilot. *Cancer Treatment Report* 63(11-12): 1933.

Knobf, M.K.T., Fischer, D.S., and Welch-McCaffrey, D. (1984). *Cancer Chemotherapy: Treatment and Care*. 2nd ed. Boston: G.K. Hall Medical Publishers.

Koeller, J.M., Earhart, R.H., Davis, T.E., et al. (1983). Phase I trial of CBDCA (NSC #241-240) by bolus intravenous injection. *AACR Proceedings* 24(642): 162 (abstract).

Kris, M.G., D'Acquisto, R.W., Gralla, R.J., Burke, M.T., Marks, L.D., Fanucci, M.P., and Heelan, R.T. (1989). Phase II trial of trimetrexate in patients with stage III and IV non-small cell lung cancer. *American Journal of Clinical Oncology* 12(1): 24–26.

Kufe, D., Major, P., Agarwal, R., et al. (1980). Phase I–II trial of deoxycoformycin (DCF) in T-cell malignancies. *AACR Proceedings* 21: 328.

Lambertenghi-Deleliers, G., Pogliani, E., Maiolo, A.T., et al. (1983). Therapeutic activity of 4-demethoxydaunorubicin (DMDR) in adult leukemia. *TUMORI* 69: 515–519.

Lasley, K., and Ignoffo, R.J. (1981). *Manual of Oncology Therapeutics*. St. Louis: Mosby.

Lederle Laboratories. (1988). *Novantrone Formulary Brochure*. Wayne, N.J.

Lee, E.J., Paciucci, A., Amrein, P., et al. (1990). A randomized phase II trial of 3 regimens in the treatment of relapsed or refractory acute myeloid leukemia (AML) in adults: A CALGB study. *ASH Abstracts* 294a.

Lee, E.J., Van Echo, D.A., Egorin, M.J., Nayar, M.S., Schulman, P., and Schiffer, C.A. (1986). Diaziquone given as a continuous infusion is an active agent for relapsed adult acute nonlymphocytic leukemia. *Blood* 67(1): 182–187.

Ligha, S.S., Gutterman, J.V., Hall, S.W., et al. (1978). Phase I clinical investigation of 4'-(9-acidinyl-amino) methanesulfon-m-aniside (NSC-249992), a new acridine derivative. *Cancer Research* 38(11): 3712–3716.

Lu, K., Savaraj, J., Kavanaugh, J., et al. (1984). Clinical pharmacology of 4-demethoxydauno-rubicin. *ASCO Proceedings* 3(C-147): 88 (abstract).

MacElveen-Hoehn, P. (1985). Sexual assessment and counselling. *Seminars in Oncology Nursing* 1(1): 69–75.

Major, P.P., Agarwal, R.P., and Kufe, D.W. (1981). Clinical pharmacology of deoxycoformycin. *Blood* 58(1): 91–96.

Malspers, L., Weinrib, A.B., Staubus, A.E., et al. (1984). Clinical pharmacokinetics of 2'-deoxyco-formycin. *Cancer Treatment Symposium* 2: 7–15.

Marsh, K.C., Liesman, J., Patton, T.F., Fabian, C.J., and Sternson, L.A. (1981). Plasma levels and uri-nary excretion of methyl-GAG following IV infu-sion in man. *Cancer Treatment Reports* 65(3-4): 253.

Mead Johnson Oncology Products. (1989). *The Introduction of Ifex and Mesna.* Evansville, Ind.

Melmon, K.L., and Morelli, H.F. (1978). *Clinical Pharmacology: Basic Principles in Therapeutics.* 2nd ed. New York: Macmillan.

Micetrick, K.C., Barnes, D., and Erickson, L.C. (1985). A comparison of the cytotoxicity and DNA damaging effects of carboplatin and cisplatin (II). *AACR Proceedings* 26(1036): 263 (abstract).

Micromedex (2000). Epirubicin hydrochloride. Web reference: Martindale/Micromedex.

Moertel, R.J. (1990). Does adjuvant therapy work in colon cancer? *New England Journal of Medicine* 322: 399–401.

Moore, J.O., Schiffer, C.A., Amrein, P., et al. (1992). G-CSF reduces the duration of both granulo-cytopenia and thrombocytopenia after AZQ/mitox-antrone consolidation in acute myelogenous leukemia—CALGB 9022. *ASH Abstracts* 291a.

*National Cancer Institute Investigational Drugs— Pharmaceutical Data 1988.* U.S. Department of Health and Human Services, NIH Publication 89-2141.

Nichols, C., Williams, S., Tricot, G., et al. (1988). Phase I study of high dose etoposide plus carboplatin with autologous bone marrow rescue (ABMT) in refractory germ cell cancer. *ASCO Proceedings* 7(454): 118 (abstract).

Orphan Medical, Inc. (1999). Busulfex (busulfan) injection: Product monograph. Minnetonka, Minn.: Orphan Medical, Inc.

Paciarini, A., et al. (1983). Pharmacokinetic studies of IV and oral 4-demethoxydaunorubicin in man. *13th International Congress of Chemotherapy.* Vienna, Austria.

Patt, Y.Z., Boddie, A.W., Charnsangavej, C., Ajani, J.A., Wallace, S., Soski, M., Claghorn, L., and Mavligit, G.M. (1986). Hepatic arterial infusion with floxuridine and cisplatin: Overriding impor-tance of antitumor effect vs. degree of tumor bur-den as determinants of survival among patients with colorectal cancer. *Journal of Clinical Oncology* 4(9): 1356–1364.

Pazdur, R., Coia, L.R., Hoskins, W.J., et al. (2000). *Cancer Management: A Multidisciplinary Approach.* 4th ed. Melville, N.Y.: PRR.

Perry, M.C., and Yarbro, J.W. (1984). *Toxicity of Chemotherapy.* New York: Grune and Stratton.

Peters, F.T.M., Beijnen, J.H., and ten Bokkel Huinink, W.W. (1987). Mitoxantrone extravasation injury. *Cancer Treatment Reports* 71(10): 992–993.

Physician's Desk Reference. (1986). *Physician's Desk Reference.* 40th ed. Oradell, N.J.: Medical Economics Company, Inc.

———. (2000). 54th ed. (Montvale, N.J.: Medical Economics Company, Inc.

Pratt, W.B., and Ruddon, R.W. (1979). *The Anticancer Drugs.* New York: Oxford University Press.

Rodrigues, V., Cabanillas, F., Bodey, G.P., et al. (1982). Studies with ifosfamide in patients with malignant lymphoma. *Seminars in Oncology* 9 (suppl 1): 87.

Schiffer, C.A., Davis, R.B., Mayer, R.J., Peterson, B.A., and Lee, E.J. (1987). Combination chemotherapy with diaziquone and amsacrine in relapsed and refractory acute nonlymphocyt-ic leukemia: A CALGB study. *Cancer Treatment Reports* 71(9): 879–880.

Silver, R.T., Lauper, R.D., and Jarowski, C.I. (1987). *A Synopsis of Cancer Chemotherapy.* 2nd ed. New York: Yorke Medical Books.

Skeel, R.T., (ed.). (1982). *Manual of Cancer Chemotherapy.* Boston: Little, Brown.

Skidmore-Roth, L. (1989). *Mosby's 1989 Nursing Drug Reference.* St. Louis: Mosby.

Smith, I.E., Evans, B.D., Gore, M.E., et al. (1987). Carboplatin (Paraplatin, JMB) and etoposide (VP-16) as first line combination therapy for small cell lung cancer. *Journal of Clinical Oncology* 5(2): 186.

Solimando, D.A., Bressler, L.R., Kintzel, P.E., and Geraci, M.C. (2000). *Drug Information Handbook for Oncology*. 2nd ed. Cleveland: Lexi-Comp, Inc.

Stewart, J.A., McCormack, J.J., Tong, W., Low, J.B., Roberts, J.D., Blow, A., Whitfield, L.R., Haugh, L.D., Grove, W.R., and Lopez, A.J. (1988). Phase I clinical and pharmacokinetic study of trimetrexate using a daily × 5 schedule. *Cancer Research* 48(17): 5029–5035.

Tamassia, V., Goldaniga, R., Moroma, A., et al. (1983). Pharmacokinetic studies on three new anthracyclines: Epirubicin, DMDR, esorubicin. In *Fourth NCI-EORTC Symposium in New Drugs in Cancer Therapy*. December 14–17: 16 (abstract).

Tenebaum, L. (1989). *Cancer Chemotherapy: A Reference Guide*. Philadelphia: W.B. Saunders.

Trissel, L.A., Xu, Q., Kwan, J., and Martinez, J.F. (1994). Compatibility of paclitaxel injection vehicle with IV administration and extension sets. *Am J Hosp Pharm* 51(24): 2809–2810

von Hoff, D.D. (1987). Whether carboplatin? A replacement for or an alternative to cisplatin. *Journal of Clinical Oncology* 5(2): 169.

Warrell, R.P., and Burchenal, J.H. (1983). Methyl glyoxal-bis-(Guanylhydrazone) (methyl-GAG): Current status and future prospects. *Journal of Clinical Oncology* 1(2): 54.

Warrell, R.P., Lee, B.J., Kempin, S.J., Lacher, M.J., Straus, D.J., and Young, C.W. (1981a). Effectiveness of methyl-GAG (methyl glyoxal-bis-[guanylhydrazone]) in patients with advanced malignant lymphoma. *Blood* 57(6): 1011.

———. (1981b). Clinical evaluation of methyl-GAG (methyl glyoxal-bis-[guanylhydrazone]) alone and in combination with VM-26 (Teniposide), in advanced malignant lymphoma. *AACR and ASCO Proceedings* 22: 521.

Whitacre, M.Y., and Finley, R.S. (1989). *Paraplatin Administration Guide*. Evansville, Ind: Bristol-Myers Co.

Wilkes, G.M., Ingwersen, K., and Barton-Burke, M. (1993). *Oncology Nursing Drug Reference*. Boston: Jones & Bartlett.

Wilkes, G.M., Ingwersen, K., and Barton-Burke, M. (2000). *2000 Oncology Nursing Drug Handbook*. Sudbury, Mass.: Jones & Bartlett.

Yarbro, C.H. (1989). Carboplatin: A clinical review. *Seminars in Oncology Nursing* 5 (suppl 1): 63–69.

# Chapter 6

# Drug Interactions in the Cancer Chemotherapy Patient

Reginald S. King, PHARMD

## INTRODUCTION

Pharmacologic management of the patient with a malignancy is often quite complex. This is true especially with regard to those cancer patients receiving high-dose or marrow ablative chemotherapy and being rescued with either bone marrow or peripheral stem cell transplants. The frequent occurrence of polypharmacy, or treatment with more than one type of medicine, in this patient population clearly increases the risk of drug interactions. In addition, patients may have concomitant illnesses that are being treated or are likely to be receiving drug therapy to manage the numerous toxicities of their antineoplastic therapy. Given the highly variable nature of potential drug interactions, it is crucial to take into consideration each patient's clinical condition when assessing the likelihood or clinical significance of such interactions. The influence of multiple other factors, such as age and kidney or liver function, also cannot be overlooked. One of the most important concepts to remember with regard to any drug interaction is that an interaction commonly occurs when a potentially interacting agent is added to or discontinued from established therapy.

For example, when a patient's anticoagulant therapy with warfarin has been stabilized and a therapeutic international normalized ratio (INR)

has been achieved, subsequent treatment with cimetidine for a duodenal ulcer may affect warfarin's potency. Cimetidine has been demonstrated to gradually inhibit the hepatic metabolism of warfarin, likely resulting in increased blood levels of the drug and an increased risk of bleeding. This interaction would necessitate a decrease in the dosage of warfarin, with careful monitoring of the patient's INR until stabilized. If therapy with both agents continues and eventually cimetidine is discontinued secondary to healing of the patient's ulcer, the inhibition of warfarin's metabolism that had been taking place will gradually cease as cimetidine is completely eliminated from the patient's body. At this point, normal hepatic metabolism of warfarin will resume, excluding any other interfering factors, and an increase in the patient's warfarin dose to what he or she was receiving prior to cimetidine therapy will most likely be initiated.

As more chemotherapy regimens are administered in the outpatient setting, the management of potential drug interactions becomes more difficult, since patients are more responsible for their own care. In addition, patients who receive peripheral blood stem cell transplants are being discharged from the hospital sooner, secondary to more rapid hematologic recovery, thereby becoming part of the expanding pool of outpatients in the hematology and oncology settings. To minimize the extent of polypharmacy, patients should be encouraged to avoid visiting multiple health care providers, especially if those providers are not in communication with one another. Patients should also inform all their providers about the medications they are currently taking or recently stopped taking, including prescription and nonprescription, or over-the-counter (OTC), medications. OTC medications such as analgesics and cough and cold products are commonly used by patients to self-medicate for numerous ailments.

This chapter focuses on drug-drug interactions in the cancer chemotherapy patient. These interactions may involve a cancer chemotherapy agent and their mechanism is either pharmacokinetic or pharmacodynamic. Pharmacokinetic drug interactions involve the alteration of absorption, distribution, metabolism, or elimination of one drug by another. Pharmacodynamic drug interactions can involve two drugs with antagonistic pharmacologic effects, synergistic or additive therapeutic or adverse effects, and indirect effects on one drug's actions by the pharmacologic effects of another. Pharmacokinetic and pharmacodynamic interactions are not necessarily mutually exclusive. The previously described cimetidine-warfarin interaction is an example of a pharmacokinetic drug interaction.

## PHARMACOKINETIC INTERACTIONS

### Absorption (Including Drug-Food) Interactions

The small intestine is the primary site of absorption for the majority of orally administered drugs. Absorption interactions are those that cause an increase or decrease in the amount of drug absorbed. The relative rate at which drugs are absorbed can be affected as well. These interactions may also occur between drugs and food. Clinically significant absorption interactions typically involve decreases in the total amount of drug absorbed, such as that of digoxin and phenytoin, and can be found in Table 6.1.

In general, the absorption of oral digoxin may be substantially decreased in patients receiving certain antineoplastic agents. The mechanism thought to be responsible for this interaction is the transient damage to the intestinal mucosa caused by some cancer chemotherapy, reported in patients receiving bleomycin, carmustine, cyclophosphamide, cytarabine, doxorubicin, methotrexate, procarbazine, and vincristine (Tatro 1990). Thus, serum levels of digoxin need to be monitored and dosing regimens of digoxin adjusted accordingly. Most important, each patient should be assessed for a suboptimal response to digoxin, such as worsening congestive heart failure. To minimize the potential for decreased absorption of oral tablets in these patients, the use of digoxin oral elixir or liquid-filled capsules may help, since the drug from these dosage forms is usually rapidly and extensively absorbed.

In a similar fashion, the absorption of phenytoin may be decreased in patients receiving certain antineoplastic agents, such as bleomycin, carboplatin, carmustine, cisplatin, methotrexate, and vinblastine (Tatro 1991). Increased metabolism of phenytoin may be another mechanism by which this interaction occurs. Decreased absorption of phenytoin would be a concern in patients receiving the drug for the prevention or management of seizures, where a therapeutic concentration of the drug needs to be achieved. In these patients, serum levels of phenytoin must be monitored and doses adjusted accordingly. The use of parenteral phenytoin may be helpful in minimizing this potential interaction because systemic concentrations can be achieved without the need for absorption from the gastrointestinal (GI) tract.

**Table 6.1** Pharmacokinetic Drug Interactions

| Medication | Pharmacokinetic Interactions | Practice Implications |
|---|---|---|
| oral digoxin (Lanoxin) | Absorption may be decreased possibly due to transient damage to intestinal mucosa caused by chemotherapy (i.e., bleomycin, carmustine, cyclophosphamide, cytarabine, doxorubicin, MTX, procarbazine, and vincristine) | 1. Give digoxin as an oral elixir or in liquid-filled capsules instead of tablets<br>2. Monitor heart rate, rhythm, and status of cardiac output<br>3. Monitor digoxin levels in blood |
| phenytoin (Dilantin) | Absorption may be decreased in patients receiving certain chemotherapy (i.e., bleomycin, carboplatin, carmustine, cisplatin, MTX, and vinblastine) | 1. Use parenteral phenytoin to maintain systemic concentrations of phenytoin<br>2. Monitor phenytoin levels in blood<br>3. Monitor patient for seizure activity |
| estramustine (Emcyt) | Decreased bioavailability and peak serum concentrations have been reported with ingestion of milk or food | 1. Administer on empty stomach unless gastrointestinal side effects are present<br>2. Do not give with milk, milk products, or calcium-rich foods or drugs |
| melphalan (Alkeran) | Decreased bioavailability when given with food | 1. Administer on empty stomach |
| aminoglutethimide (Cytadren) | Long-term administration increases drug metabolism in the liver (e.g., aminoglutethimide appears to increase metabolism of tamoxifen and its metabolites, theophylline, and warfarin | 1. If possible, do not administer in combination with tamoxifen<br>2. If possible, do not administer in combination with theophylline<br>3. Monitor respiratory status, including breath sounds and pulmonary function tests<br>4. Monitor blood theophylline levels<br>5. Warfarin dose may need to be increased; monitor international normalized ratio to ensure adequate anticoagulation<br>6. Warfarin dose may need to be decreased after aminoglutethimide is stopped |
| carmustine (BiCNU) | Myelosuppressive effects reported to be enhanced by cimetidine by inhibition of usual metabolism or by additive effects of both agents on bone marrow | 1. Concomitant administration with cimetidine should be avoided<br>2. Monitor blood values: complete blood counts |
| 6-MP (Purinethol) | Simultaneous use of 6-MP and allopurinol has the potential to increase antineoplastic as well as side effects of 6-MP; results from allopurinol's inhibition of xanthine oxidase, the enzyme responsible for metabolism of 6-MP to inactive metabolite | 1. Avoid concomitant administration with allopurinol<br>2. If both drugs must be used, reduce 6-MP to 25-33% of usual dose |
| MTX | Renal clearance affected when given with NSAIDs and large doses of penicillins because these drugs may interfere with active renal tubular secretion of MTX<br>Salicylates may delay renal excretion, possibly through competition for elimination because salicylates and MTX are both weak acids<br>Administration with protein-bound drugs (i.e., salicylates, sulfonamides, sulfonylureas, phenytoin) can cause displacement of MTX from protein-binding sites, resulting in increased amounts of active MTX available. | 1. Avoid concomitant administration with protein-bound drugs, NSAIDs, and large doses of penicillins<br>2. Monitor for MTX side effects: neutropenia, thrombocytopenia, and mucositis |

MTX = methotrexate; 6-MP = 6-mercaptopurine; NSAIDs = nonsteroidal anti-inflammatory drugs.
*Source:* King, R. (1995). Drug interactions with cancer chemotherapy. *Cancer Practice* 3(1): 58–59. Reprinted with permission.

## Drug-Food Interactions

*Estramustine (Emcyt).* The bioavailability and peak serum concentrations of estramustine were reported to be decreased by approximately 65% following concomitant milk ingestion in six patients with prostate cancer (Gunnarsson et al. 1990). A 40% reduction in bioavailability was reported when estramustine was administered with food (Gunnarsson et al. 1990). To ensure that anticancer therapy is optimal, the potential for the reduced efficacy of estramustine needs to be considered. Whenever possible, it should be administered on an empty stomach unless GI side effects, such as nausea, vomiting, and diarrhea, are intolerable for the patient. Products to try to avoid coadministering with estramustine include milk, milk products, and calcium-rich foods or drugs.

*Melphalan (Alkeran).* In patients receiving oral or IV melphalan, the simultaneous administration with food resulted in reductions in bioavailability from approximately 90% to about 55% (Bosanquet and Gilby 1984; Reece et al. 1986). If GI side effects are tolerable, melphalan should be administered on an empty stomach to avoid decreased bioavailability and, possibly, decreased efficacy.

*Itraconazole (Sporanox).* In the oncology population, especially those patients with acute leukemia or receiving a bone marrow transplant (BMT), systemic fungal infections often can be fatal in the setting of a compromised immune system. Itraconazole is a triazole antifungal that is indicated in the management of oropharyngeal and esophageal candidiasis as well as serious systemic infections caused by *Aspergillus* and other fungi. BMT patients with presumed or documented *Aspergillus* infections commonly receive a course of amphotericin B that may be followed by therapy with itraconazole. This is likely to be continued for an extended period of time, especially in allogeneic BMT patients receiving immunosuppressants for prevention or treatment of GVHD.

Clearly, optimal absorption of any oral antifungal agent would be ideal in order to achieve therapeutic systemic concentrations. Itraconazole is available in both capsule and solution formulations. As with ketoconazole, itraconazole in capsule form requires an acidic environment for optimal absorption. This can be extremely problematic in patients who are taking liquid antacids, $H_2$-blockers (cimetidine, ranitidine, nizatidine), or proton pump inhibitors (omeprazole, lansoprazole). Further complicating variable absorption issues may be the patient with mucositis or GVHD of the gut that may involve malabsorption. Because food intake increases the bioavailability of itraconazole capsules, the recommended method of administration should be with food. In patients whose antacid therapy is unavoidable, such therapy should be administered at a minimum of 2 hours following itraconazole. Because measuring of serum itraconazole levels is not routinely performed, close monitoring of the patient for improvement of radiographic and clinical signs and symptoms of infection is the best indicator of itraconazole's efficacy. An empiric increase in itraconazole dose may be warranted if therapeutic failure is suspected.

The development of itraconazole solution is a marked improvement over the capsule formulation. Due to its increased water solubility and dissolution properties, itraconazole solution has greater bioavailability than its capsule form by approximately one-third. In the fasted state, the solution's bioavailability has been demonstrated to increase by another one-third (Stevens 1999). In addition, an acidic environment does not appear to be necessary for optimal absorption of itraconazole solution. In summary, taking itraconazole solution without food seems to be the most prudent method of administration, especially in a patient population that is likely to be receiving or initiated on some form of antacid therapy.

## Induction or Inhibition of Metabolism

Numerous drugs are metabolized by the cytochrome P450 system, a group of enzymes in the liver and small intestine. These enzymes are commonly induced or inhibited by certain drugs, resulting in increases or decreases, respectively, in the metabolic rate of the drugs that are affected. Hepatic enzyme inducers include barbiturates such as phenobarbital, other anticonvulsants such as phenytoin and carbamazepine, and the antimicrobial rifampin. Cimetidine, a histamine-2 ($H_2$) receptor blocker, has inhibitory effects on hepatic enzymes. Metabolism interactions can be unpredictable, depending on the presence of other factors that may influence metabolism. All of these factors need to be taken into consideration when assessing the possibility of a drug interaction.

*Aminoglutethimide (Cytadren).* Aminoglutethimide increases the activity of certain liver enzymes that metabolize drugs. In theory, the plasma clearance of all drugs metabolized by these enzymes would be expected to increase with long-term administration of aminoglutethimide.

Aminoglutethimide appears to increase the metabolism of tamoxifen and its metabolites. This was demonstrated in six women with breast cancer who received the combination of tamoxifen and aminoglutethimide for 6 weeks (Lien, Anker, Lonning, Solheim, Veland 1990). If possible, these two agents should not be administered together, since the response of breast cancer patients to tamoxifen may be compromised. In all likelihood, the concomitant administration of tamoxifen and aminoglutethimide will not occur, since aminoglutethimide is typically reserved for use as a second-line agent for the palliative therapy of metastatic breast cancer.

Aminoglutethimide also appears to partly increase the metabolism of theophylline. In three patients with metastatic breast cancer who were receiving sustained-release theophylline 200 mg twice daily with aminoglutethimide 250 mg four times daily, the clearance of theophylline increased by a mean of approximately 30% following 2–12 weeks of aminoglutethimide administration (Lonning, Kvinnsland, and Bakke 1984). This increase in clearance may result in a serum level of theophylline that is approximately 70% of that expected. Therapy with both of these agents would be likely in a woman with metastatic breast cancer and a history of asthma. Serum theophylline concentrations should be monitored for several weeks after the initiation or discontinuation of aminoglutethimide, since dose adjustment may be necessary to compensate for the increased or decreased clearance of theophylline, respectively, that would be expected to occur. Most important, the patient's clinical condition, as demonstrated by control of her asthmatic symptoms, should be used to judge whether a change in theophylline therapy is warranted.

Finally, a dose-dependent induction of warfarin metabolism by aminoglutethimide in breast cancer patients has been reported. Two patients receiving both of these agents experienced diminished anticoagulant effects of warfarin secondary to a threefold to fivefold increase in warfarin clearance (Lonning, Kvinnsland, and Jahren 1984). Therefore, careful monitoring of INR is necessary to ensure adequate anticoagulation. Increased doses of warfarin may be indicated following initiation of aminoglutethimide therapy.

Similarly, warfarin doses may need to be decreased after discontinuation of aminoglutethimide administration.

*Carmustine (BiCNU).* Cimetidine has been reported to enhance the myelosuppressive effects of carmustine, either by inhibiting the usual metabolism of carmustine, resulting in increased levels of the drug, or through additive effects of the two agents on the bone marrow. Given the typical delayed hematologic toxicity of carmustine (white blood cell count nadir at 3–4 weeks), concomitant administration of the drug with cimetidine should be avoided if possible to decrease the potential for greater myelosuppression. Since therapy with $H_2$ blockers is often necessary in cancer patients for stress or peptic ulcer prophylaxis or treatment and management of stress-related mucosal bleeding, alternative agents that may be tried include ranitidine, famotidine, and nizatidine. In general, these other $H_2$ blockers have not been shown to interact with drugs to the same extent that cimetidine does. To optimally decrease the potential of a drug-drug interaction with carmustine, therapy with either omeprazole or sucralfate can be initiated. Omeprazole's effects on liver enzymes involved in the metabolism of drugs are different from those of cimetidine, and sucralfate is not absorbed to any great extent, since it acts locally rather than systemically.

*6-Mercaptopurine (6-MP, Purinethol).* Allopurinol works by inhibiting the enzyme xanthine oxidase, which is responsible for the production of uric acid. Started prior to and continued throughout the administration of chemotherapy, allopurinol is frequently used to prevent uric acid nephropathy in patients with bulky tumors undergoing tumor lysis. Interestingly, xanthine oxidase is also responsible for the metabolism of 6-MP to an inactive metabolite. Therefore, the simultaneous use of allopurinol and 6-MP has the potential to increase the antineoplastic effects, as well as the adverse effects, of oral 6-MP. When used as maintenance therapy for acute lymphocytic leukemia (ALL), 6-MP can have adverse effects primarily involving the GI tract (anorexia, nausea, vomiting) and usually including mild myelosuppression (leukopenia and thrombocytopenia). These adverse effects may be expected to increase in severity if normal metabolism of 6-MP to an inactive metabolite is interfered with by the addition of allopurinol. If concomitant administration of the two agents cannot be avoided, the recommendation is to reduce the 6-MP dose to 25–33% of the usual dose (McEvoy 1994). One situation where this might occur would be in an adult patient receiving remission maintenance therapy for ALL with 6-MP who is admitted for treatment of an acute gouty attack and is sent home on prophylactic allopurinol therapy. In any patient receiving allopurinol for prophylaxis of uric acid nephropathy, it is important to remember to discontinue its administration when the risk of tumor lysis is over, usually several days after chemotherapy is completed. In an ALL patient, if allopurinol is inadvertently allowed to continue indefinitely, the chance of concomitant therapy with 6-MP when remission maintenance therapy is initiated is increased greatly.

*Warfarin.* When using warfarin therapy in the setting of cancer chemotherapy, there is always an inherent bleeding risk that may cause anemia and/or thrombocytopenia. Depending on the indication for anticoagulation, warfarin often cannot be discontinued. Reports of potential drug interactions between warfarin and individual or combination chemotherapy regimens are often anecdotal. The clinical significance of such reports also can be difficult to conclude. However, since numerous malignancies are treated with scheduled cycles of chemotherapy, sometimes up to six or more, any potentially problematic interactions that may recur with each cycle should be identified and appropriate interventions put in place.

The concomitant use of 5-fluorouracil (5-FU) and warfarin appears to be a clinically significant problem. One case report described multisite mucous membrane bleeding in a patient with metastatic colon cancer who was receiving chronic anticoagulation therapy and was initiated on a chemotherapy regimen with 5-FU and leucovorin (Brown 1997). 5-fluorouracil was administered as a bolus weekly for 4 weeks. Prothrombin time (PT) and INR were elevated. This patient was restarted on a lower dose of warfarin. The author postulated that 5-FU may inhibit the synthesis of cytochrome P450 enzymes responsible for the metabolism of warfarin.

Five patients at another institution were reported to have a similar interaction between 5-FU and warfarin (Kolesar, Johnson, Freeberg, Berlin, Schiller 1999). These patients had either metastatic colon or breast cancer and were treated with 5-FU-containing regimens. 5-FU appears to have been administered as a bolus in the majority of cases. All patients had been receiving chronic anticoagulation prior to initiation of chemotherapy. Prolonged PT and increased INR dictated warfarin dose reductions in all patients. One patient had a major bleeding event. These authors also postulated that 5-FU may have suppressed those cytochrome P450 enzymes involved in warfarin's metabolism.

***Capecitabine (Xeloda)*** is an oral prodrug of 5-FU indicated for the treatment of metastatic breast cancer. There have also been reports of altered coagulation parameters and/or bleeding in patients receiving warfarin and Xeloda concomitantly (Xeloda, Capecitabine Product Information 1999).

Clearly, more intensive monitoring of PT/INR is warranted in patients receiving warfarin and 5-FU or capecitabine. Bleeding risk may be increased and dose reduction of warfarin necessary.

***Cyclosporine (Sandimmune, Neoral)/ Tacrolimus (Prograf, FK506).*** Cyclosporine (CSA) and tacrolimus (FK506) are immunosuppressant agents frequently used to prevent graft versus host disease (GVHD) in patients receiving allogeneic BMT. Both of these medications are metabolized by hepatic cytochrome P450. The triazole antifungals can inhibit the metabolism of CSA and FK506, leading to increased blood levels. At therapeutic doses of these immunosuppressants, toxicities may include hepatotoxicity, neurotoxicity, and nephrotoxicity associated with or without hypertension. Since the concurrent use of a triazole antifungal with either CSA or FK506 is often necessary and not an absolute contraindication, close monitoring for clinical signs and symptoms of increased toxicity is warranted. Although CSA and FK506 blood levels may be obtained, these do not always correlate with toxicity as they may with efficacy. Close observation of a patient for excessive tremors, increases in blood pressure, serum creatinine, or liver function tests are examples of better ways to assess increased toxicity.

With respect to CSA- or FK506-induced hypertension, calcium channel blockers (CCBs) are often effective in managing this drug-induced toxicity. Although not contraindicated, the negative inotropic CCBs diltiazem and verapamil can inhibit metabolism of CSA and FK506, leading to increased blood levels. A better choice of CCB to use would be from the dihydropyridine class that includes nifedipine, amlodipine, and isradipine, which are not likely to interact with CSA or FK506.

Grapefruit juice also has been demonstrated to inhibit the intestinal metabolism of orally administered CSA and FK506, leading to increased blood levels. Patients who drink grapefruit juice regularly should be made aware of the potential interaction and monitored closely for signs of increased toxicity. This type of drug-food as well as inhibition of metabolism interaction is highly variable and requires further investigation to determine its clinical significance.

The antibacterial *Synercid (quinupristin/ dalfopristin)* is being used with increasing frequency for the treatment of vancomycin-resistant *Enterococcus faecium* (VREF) and other complicated skin and skin structure infections. VREF infection in an immunocompromised host, such as an allogeneic BMT patient, can be fatal. Synercid has been demonstrated *in vitro* to significantly inhibit cytochrome P450 metabolism of cyclosporine (CSA) (Synercid I.V. (quinopristin and dalfopristin) Product Information 1999). The metabolism of FK506 would be expected to be inhibited as well, although this has not been investigated. If Synercid and either immunosuppressive agent are used concomitantly, monitoring of CSA or FK506 blood levels and signs and symptoms of toxicity should be performed. Dose reduction of CSA or FK506 may be warranted while Synercid therapy is ongoing.

Equally as important, classic inducers of cytochrome P450 such as rifampin, phenytoin, carbamazepine, and phenobarbital have the potential to decrease CSA and FK506 levels. Patients may be placed at risk for subtherapeutic immunosuppressant levels if these interacting agents are used together. Since three of the mentioned inducers are used for seizure prophylaxis or treatment, they are not likely to be discontinued to avoid the possibility of a drug interaction. One obvious alternative may be to switch to a newer medication indicated for seizure

prophylaxis or treatment that is not an inducer of cytochrome P450. However, if the use of an inducer with CSA or FK506 cannot be avoided, trough concentrations of CSA or FK506 should be monitored closely. More importantly, these patients need to be assessed for adequate immunosuppressive response.

## Distribution and/or Elimination Interactions

Distribution interactions typically involve the displacement of one highly protein-bound drug by another. Only the unbound, or free, fraction of a drug is active. Therefore, competition for protein binding sites by two drugs can increase the free fraction, or availability, of one drug over the other. Increased availability of the free drug most likely will lead to an extension of its usual pharmacologic effects as well as its side effects.

Since the kidneys are major sites of drug elimination or excretion, they are involved in most elimination interactions. Normal elimination can be impaired if changes in glomerular filtration rate, tubular secretion, or urine pH occur. These changes often result from the administration of other drugs.

*Methotrexate (MTX).* Potentially significant drug interactions with MTX, especially if it is given in high doses for osteosarcoma or ALL, include nonsteroidal anti-inflammatory drugs (NSAIDs) such as ibuprofen (Motrin, Advil), diclofenac (Voltaren), flurbiprofen (Ansaid), indomethacin (Indocin), ketoprofen (Orudis), naproxen (Anaprox, Naprosyn, Alleve), and others; penicillins; and salicylates (aspirin-containing products). Nonsteroidal anti-inflammatory drugs and large doses of penicillins may interfere with the active renal tubular secretion of MTX, thus reducing renal clearance of the antineoplastic agent. The mechanism of this interaction is thought to be a decrease in renal perfusion secondary to NSAID inhibition of renal prostaglandin synthesis (McEvoy 1994). Competition with MTX for renal elimination is a second postulated mechanism (McEvoy 1994). Salicylates are weak acids that may delay the renal excretion of MTX, possibly through competition for elimination, since MTX is also a weak acid (McEvoy 1994). An increase in the amount of MTX available potentially can augment MTX's antineoplastic activity as well as its adverse effects, primarily neutropenia and thrombocytopenia, and mucositis, manifested most often as stomatitis.

It is also usually recommended to avoid the concomitant administration of MTX and proteinbound drugs such as salicylates, sulfonamides (sulfamethoxazole-containing products such as Septra and Bactrim), sulfonylureas (tolbutamide, tolazamide, chlorpropamide, glyburide, glipizide), and phenytoin. Displacement of MTX from protein-binding sites would be expected to result in an increased amount of active MTX available, thus increasing the likelihood of greater myelosuppression and/or GI toxicity. The extent to which toxicity may be enhanced is not well defined and varies depending on the presence of other confounding factors that may also worsen expected adverse effects.

The potentially interfering drugs discussed above are all likely to be part of various regimens patients are taking prior to admission for different ailments. A complete medication history, including all OTC drugs, needs to be solicited on admission. Drugs identified to be potentially interfering should not be given prior to initiation of infusions of high-dose MTX and need to be restarted when serum MTX levels have returned to a nontoxic level, usually considered to be a level less than 0.05 micromolar.

If a potentially interfering drug cannot be discontinued, such as phenytoin, needed for the management or prophylaxis of seizures, the patient receiving this drug needs to be monitored carefully.

In the specific case of phenytoin-MTX, not only is displacement of MTX from protein-binding sites by phenytoin possible, but MTX also may cause increased metabolism of phenytoin. As determined by phenytoin serum level monitoring, a patient may require an increase in phenytoin dosage during MTX therapy. At the same time, an increase in phenytoin may be more likely to compete with MTX for protein-binding sites. This is an ideal example of the complexity of some potential drug interactions.

The use of high-dose MTX results in concentrations of metabolites in the renal tubules that are greater than the solubility of MTX, increasing the risk of crystallization of MTX in the renal tubules and damage to the tubules. Typical measures used to aid in the elimination of MTX include vigorous hydration with sodium bicarbonate–containing solutions and/or oral sodium bicarbonate for urinary alkalinization. Alkalinization of urine aims to increase the solubility of MTX metabolites. Leucovorin rescue is also started immediately following high-dose MTX infusions to aid in the prevention of severe mucositis and myelosuppression.

## PHARMACODYNAMIC INTERACTIONS

### Additive Toxicity

In the oncology and bone marrow transplant (BMT) populations, additive toxicities can become very problematic, given the similar side effect profiles of many of the agents that are administered. In some cases, concomitant administration of some of these agents is unavoidable. For example, cancer chemotherapy regimens often contain more than one agent that has myelosuppression or mucositis as a dose-limiting toxicity. Since chemotherapy regimens have been designed for the antineoplastic effects of their agents when given in combination, changes in these regimens are uncommon except for dosage modifications or discontinuation of certain agents that have previously resulted in unacceptable toxicity. Table 6.2 summarizes the pharmacodynamic interactions known to date. When alternative therapy is available, it should be pursued. Fortunately, the supportive care that patients receive following chemotherapy or BMT does allow for choices among agents that have varying

adverse effects, such as antimicrobials, antiemetics, and analgesics. Whenever possible, efforts should be made to select agents that are not likely to compound toxicity already caused by chemotherapy.

***Cisplatin (Platinol).*** Cisplatin possesses the potential to cause both nephrotoxicity and ototoxicity. Both of these adverse effects may be potentiated by the use of additional agents that also have the potential to cause nephrotoxicity and/or ototoxicity. These include the aminoglycoside antibiotics (gentamicin, tobramycin, amikacin), vancomycin, amphotericin B, cyclosporine, the loop diuretics (ethacrynic

**Table 6.2** Pharmacodynamic Drug Interactions

| Medication | Pharmacodynamic Interactions | Practice Implications |
|---|---|---|
| cisplatin (Platinol) | Nephrotoxicity and ototoxicity side effects may be potentiated when used with aminoglycoside antibiotics, vancomycin, amphotericin B, cyclosporine, loop diuretics, and possibly acyclovir, trimethoprim/sulfamethoxazole, erythromycin | 1. Avoid drug combinations that potentiate nephrotoxicity and ototoxicity 2. Monitor for ototoxicity, c/o tinnitus and auditory discomfort 3. Monitor for nephrotoxicity: BUN and creatinine; hydrate vigorously |
| L-asparaginase (Elspar) | Associated with impaired pancreatic function resulting in decreased insulin synthesis; *if* used with prednisone, there is potential for decreased glucose tolerance resulting in hyperglycemia | 1. Monitor blood glucose levels, including baseline 2. Dipstick urine for glucose 3. Sliding-scale insulin therapy may need to be initiated |
| paclitaxel (Taxol) | When administered in combination with cisplatin, drug sequence should be paclitaxel followed by cisplatin; more severe myelosuppression has been demonstrated when cisplatin is followed by paclitaxel; possible result of cisplatin decreasing paclitaxel clearance | 1. Monitor for paclitaxel side effects (e.g., neutropenia) |
| procarbazine (Matulane) | Activity of monoamine oxidase, enzyme responsible for degradation of sympathomimetic agents, may be inhibited; accumulation of these agents has potential to cause hypertensive crisis | 1. Concomitant administration with products such as decongestants or diet aids that contain sympathomimetic agents should be avoided 2. Avoid concomitant administration with aged foods, such as wine, beer, and cheese, that contain tyramine, an amino acid with sympathomimetic activity |

BUN = blood urea nitrogen.
*Source:* King, R. (1995). Drug interactions with cancer chemotherapy. *Cancer Practice* 3(1): 58–59. Reprinted with permission.

acid, bumetanide, furosemide), and possibly acyclovir, trimethoprim/sulfamethoxazole (Septra, Bactrim), and erythromycin. In addition, streptozocin (Zanosar) and MTX are two antineoplastic agents that can be nephrotoxic. Streptozocin is not likely to be administered with cisplatin. Methotrexate, however, may be used with cisplatin in several regimens used to treat bladder cancer.

The severity of these additive toxicities is extremely patient specific and may not be avoidable in certain instances. Typical measures used to prevent cisplatin-induced renal impairment include vigorous prehydration, concurrent hydration, and posthydration with a loop diuretic such as furosemide or an osmotic diuretic such as mannitol. Monitoring of serum levels of vancomycin and aminoglycosides, often given concurrently during neutropenia following chemotherapy, will aid in dosage adjustments if necessary, thus decreasing the incidence of toxic drug levels. Discontinuation of the causative agent(s) is common, given that an appropriate alternative is available.

In addition to nephrotoxicity and ototoxicity, electrolyte wasting, especially of potassium and magnesium, is another toxicity of several of these agents that can be additive. For example, concurrent therapy with amphotericin B, cyclosporine, and a loop diuretic is very common in the allogeneic BMT recipient. Chronic electrolyte replacement becomes standard care in these patients.

*L-asparaginase (Elspar).* Asparaginase therapy is frequently associated with impairment of pancreatic function that may be a result of decreased insulin synthesis or necrosis and inflammation of pancreatic cells. Hyperglycemia is usually temporary and should resolve once the effects of asparaginase have diminished, usually within several weeks. In patients receiving both asparaginase and prednisone, likely to occur in patients with ALL, the potential for increased hyperglycemic effects needs to be considered because of the decreased glucose tolerance associated with corticosteroids. Sliding-scale insulin therapy may need to be temporarily initiated for glucose control.

*Trastuzumab (Herceptin).* Herceptin is a monoclonal antibody directed against human epidermal growth factor receptor 2 (HER2). Metastatic breast cancer patients whose tumors overexpress HER2 are indicated to receive Herceptin as a single agent if they have received one or more prior chemotherapy regimens. The product information for Herceptin contains a black box warning emphasizing the possibility of developing ventricular dysfunction and congestive heart failure with Herceptin use. In clinical trials, patients who received Herceptin in combination with an anthracycline and cyclophosphamide experienced a higher incidence and severity of cardiac dysfunction (Herceptin Product Information 1999). Although Herceptin is not indicated for use in this manner, prior use of anthracyclines and cyclophosphamide, especially in the elderly or those with preexisting cardiac dysfunction, can put patients at higher risk of developing or worsening cardiac dysfunction. Prior radiation therapy to the chest should also be considered a risk factor. Clearly, any patient initiated on Herceptin needs to have a baseline cardiac assessment and continued follow-up during therapy.

## Administration Sequence-Dependent Interactions

Chemotherapy regimens commonly include three or four agents. Often these are administered in a fashion that is most convenient with regard to availability of intravenous (IV) line access. IV push medications may be given first, followed by those that require a continuous infusion, especially if over 24 hours

Alternatively, IV push medications may be administered while another agent is infusing. Sequence of administration usually is not an issue, but there are several instances in which a specific sequence of administration of two chemotherapy agents may be more beneficial to the patient with respect to optimal antineoplastic effects and decreased severity of adverse effects.

*L-asparaginase and Methotrexate.* Since MTX requires actively dividing cells for its effects, the administration of asparaginase immediately prior to or with MTX may decrease or prevent the antineoplastic effects of MTX (McEvoy 1994). The inhibition of protein synthesis in tumor cells by asparaginase is thought to prevent the entry of these cells into the S phase, which is the phase during which MTX has its maximum activity. In contrast, when asparaginase is given to leukemia patients 9–10 days prior to or shortly after MTX, the antitumor effects appear to be enhanced (McEvoy 1994). Gastrointestinal (GI) and hematologic toxicity also may be reduced in these patients (McEvoy 1994).

Therapy that involves both of these agents is limited to only one setting, since asparaginase is used exclusively in ALL. Thus, in patients scheduled to receive asparaginase and MTX in close proximity, an attempt should be made to administer MTX prior to asparaginase to decrease the potential for an interaction.

*Paclitaxel (Taxol) and Cisplatin.* When cisplatin administration is followed by paclitaxel, more severe myelosuppression has been demonstrated (Rowinsky et al. 1991). The mechanism for this interaction is not clearly defined. However, one postulation is that cisplatin induces a decrease in paclitaxel clearance, resulting in an increased exposure to paclitaxel and its well-documented neutropenia. Paclitaxel-associated neutropenia is typically brief in duration. A more severe

myelosuppression increases the period during which a patient is at risk for infection. Consequently, the sequence of paclitaxel followed by cisplatin was selected for ongoing and planned studies and should be considered the most optimal sequence until more information is obtained.

## Therapeutic Interactions

Therapeutic interactions are those that are prescribed intentionally for specific reasons. The three classic interactions of this type are the use of mesna for protection against hemorrhagic cystitis induced by either ifosfamide or cyclophosphamide, leucovorin rescue following methotrexate infusions, and potentiation of 5-fluorouracil's antineoplastic activity by leucovorin.

*Ifosfamide/Cyclophosphamide and Mesna.* The alkylating agents ifosfamide and cyclophosphamide share a common toxic metabolite, acrolein, that does not possess antitumor activity but is associated with bladder damage, specifically hemorrhagic cystitis. As a result of acrolein's irritant properties, patients can develop this complication, manifestations of which range from microscopic hematuria to frank hemorrhage. The risk of hemorrhagic cystitis with cyclophosphamide has increased with the advent of high-dose infusions as part of BMT preparative chemotherapy regimens. Mesna is a compound that protects the bladder epithelium by complexing with acrolein in the bladder to form an inactive product that can be readily eliminated. Other measures used to lessen the incidence or potential severity of hemorrhagic cystitis include vigorous hydration with or without urinary alkalinization to ensure frequent voiding and/or high-volume bladder irrigations.

*Methotrexate and Leucovorin.* The mechanism by which MTX interferes with DNA, RNA, and protein synthesis is via inhibition of the enzyme dihydrofolate reductase. This enzyme is responsible for the production of the tetrahydrofolate cofactors required for major cellular biosynthetic reactions. When MTX is administered in high doses for malignancies such as ALL and osteosarcoma, excessive toxicity can be expected to affect bone marrow and GI mucosa, both sites of rapid cell turnover. In an attempt to circumvent these toxicities, manifested as leukopenia, thrombocytopenia, anemia, and mucositis (stomatitis), leucovorin calcium is given as "rescue" therapy. Leucovorin, the active form of folic acid, is metabolized to tetrahydrofolate, the synthesis of which MTX prevents. Therefore, leucovorin competes with MTX for transport into human cells and is able to bypass the enzymatic block caused by MTX and allow DNA synthesis to resume. Leucovorin is typically initiated immediately following infusions of high-dose MTX and continued until serum levels of the agent have returned to a safe level, as discussed earlier.

*5-Fluorouracil (5-FU) and Leucovorin.* In the palliative treatment of advanced colorectal carcinoma, leucovorin has been used in combination with 5-FU to potentiate its antineoplastic activity. Improved response to 5-FU and prolonged survival are the goals of this therapeutic, or intentional, drug interaction. Elevated intracellular concentrations of reduced folates, such as leucovorin, appear to stabilize the complex formed between 5-FU and the enzyme it inhibits, thymidylate synthetase. The inhibition of thymidylate synthesis is one of the postulated mechanisms by which 5-FU interferes with DNA synthesis. Stabilization of the 5-FU-thymidylate synthetase complex is believed to enhance 5-FU's inhibition of the enzyme, thus increasing its efficacy. Increased efficacy of 5-FU would be expected to result in a potentiation of its adverse effects as well. GI toxicity in the form of diar-

rhea, nausea, stomatitis, and vomiting is most likely to be more pronounced. The myelosuppression commonly associated with 5-FU may also be enhanced. Patients must be monitored for symptoms of severe toxicity to determine those that are dose limiting and avoid any potential fatalities.

*Amphotericin B and potassium-sparing diuretics.* Amphotericin B often is used as empiric or specific therapy for highly suspected or documented systemic fungal infections. These infections can range from *Candida* to *Aspergillus*, mucor and other severe infections. Doses can range from 0.5 mg/kg/day up to 1.5 mg/kg/day, depending on severity of infection. One of amphotericin B's major toxicities is nephrotoxicity, manifested by increases in serum creatinine and a renal tubular acidosis (RTA). Hypomagnesemia and hypokalemia often are severe. Adequate magnesium replacement is clearly necessary when trying to maintain normal potassium levels. Increasing the potassium content in a patient's maintenance fluid or total nutrient admixture (TNA) commonly is needed to minimize the number of time-consuming potassium challenges that are given. Some patients may not require TNA, or their maintenance fluid requirements are minimal or constantly changing. Combined with the fact that oral potassium intake can be very difficult in a patient with mucositis, potassium replacement becomes a challenge. Initiation of a potassium-sparing diuretic, such as amiloride, triameterene, or spironolactone, can be extremely helpful. The renal damage induced by amphotericin B often is reversible but can take time, sometimes months or even longer. Patients may be discharged on oral potassium supplements along with a potassium-sparing diuretic.

In an allogeneic BMT patient who is also taking CSA or FK506, caution must be exercised. These immunosuppressants predispose a patient to hyperkalemia; in addition, some patients who have difficulty maintaining adequate hydration at home become dehydrated, further increasing the risk of developing hyperkalemia. With the advent of less nephrotoxic, lipid-based (amphotericin B lipid complex, Abelcet) and liposomal (Ambisome) preparations of amphotericin B, hypokalemia sometimes can be minimized. If a patient has received conventional amphotericin B prior to one of the special preparations, the RTA may have already been caused; using a lipid or liposomal amphotericin B product may or may not offer the advantage of a decreased incidence of hypokalemia.

## MISCELLANEOUS

*Procarbazine.* Procarbazine has been shown to possess the ability to inhibit monoamine oxidase (MAO) activity. MAO is an enzyme responsible for the degradation of neurotransmitters as well as other sympathomimetic agents such as ephedrine or pseudoephedrine, epinephrine, and phenylpropanolamine. Products containing these ingredients, such as decongestants and diet aids, should be avoided in patients receiving procarbazine. Accumulation of sympathomimetic agents has the potential to cause hypertensive crisis. Tyramine, an amino acid contained in certain foods, also has sympathomimetic activity that can be enhanced by the concurrent ingestion of procarbazine. The majority of these foods are those that are aged, such as wine, beer, and cheese, which should be avoided in patients receiving procarbazine.

In addition, procarbazine has been reported to have some disulfiram-like activity (McEvoy 1994). Disulfiram (Antabuse) is an alcohol deterrent used in the management of alcohol dependence. Thus, the simultaneous ingestion of alcohol, including that found in many medicinal preparations such as cough and cold products, should be avoided to prevent severe GI toxicity.

Finally, procarbazine crosses the blood-brain barrier and distributes into the cerebrospinal fluid. Thus, it has the potential to cause central nervous system (CNS) effects such as sedation. The administration of other CNS depressants with procarbazine needs to be avoided to prevent additive CNS toxicity. These agents include narcotic analgesics, antihistamines, phenothiazines, and barbiturates, among others.

*Alternative therapy.* Cancer patients increasingly are using more alternative therapies to combat their malignancies as well as other health problems. These patients should be questioned routinely about their use of nontraditional products, which may include high-dose vitamins, antioxidants, and other herbal preparations. Garlic, gingko, ginseng, St. John's wort, milk thistle, echinacea, and coenzyme $Q_{10}$ are some commonly used alternative therapies. Chinese herbs probably comprise another category. When a patient is scheduled to receive chemotherapy, the above information may be very useful in helping to ascertain whether there may be an interaction between prescribed and nonprescribed therapies. Traditional health care professionals may even want to communicate with their patients' herbalists and nutritionists in deciding on the best approach to providing optimal therapy. Although more information is being made available on alternative therapies, there remains a paucity of data regarding potential interactions.

Oncology patients often receive anticoagulant therapy with warfarin or a low molecular weight heparin to treat deep vein thrombosis, pulmonary embolus, or maintain catheter patency. In addition, these patients may be hypercoagulable or profoundly thrombocytopenic. Clearly, these are scenarios in which a drug interaction with an alternative therapy, such as garlic or ginseng, may prove to be detrimental. One of garlic's proven mechanisms of action is its ability to inhibit platelet function (Klepser and Klepser

1999); if used concomitantly with an anticoagulant, garlic may increase bleeding potential. One report described a probable interaction between warfarin and a ginseng product (Ginsana) (Janetzky and Morreale 1997). Although no mechanism was postulated, the concurrent use of these two agents resulted in a decrease in the international normalized ratios.

St. John's wort is thought to work by inhibiting MAO. Thus, it may be subject to the same drug and food interactions found with prescription MAO inhibitors and that described above with procarbazine. In the cancer patient who may be receiving a serotonin-reuptake inhibitor, such as fluoxetine, sertraline, or paroxetine, for depression, the simultaneous use of St. John's wort may be problematic if serotonin syndrome develops secondary to increased serotonin-mediated neurotransmission.

Since echinacea is believed to be an immune system stimulant, cancer patients may use it to help fight their disease. When allogeneic BMT is used to cure a hematologic malignancy such as chronic myelogenous leukemia, immunosuppressive agents are used to prevent or treat GVHD. It is probable that an antagonistic interaction would occur between echinacea and these immunosuppressants. Caution should definitely be exercised if concurrent use of these agents were to be considered.

## CONCLUSION

Drug interactions with cancer chemotherapy often can be very difficult to assess, given the polypharmacy that exists in cancer patients and the frequent inability to distinguish which drug is responsible for a certain toxicity. Discussed in this chapter are some of the classic interactions that have been described, as well as newer interactions that will be more clearly elucidated over time. Reported drug interactions may not present exactly as described in the literature in all patients. Available literature should be used as a guide in identifying potential drug interactions, the management of which will vary in each individual. Finally, numerous other potential interactions with cancer chemotherapy have been cited in the literature (see Table 6.3), but the clinical significance of these has not been established.

**Table 6.3   Drug Interactions with Cytoxic Chemotherapeutic Agents**

The material on the following pages should serve as a reference for interactions with cytotoxic chemotherapeutic agents, both between two cytotoxic agents and between a cytotoxic agent and another type of drug. Only those interactions that have been documented to occur in humans are included. To gain the most possible benefit from this material, please keep the following in mind:

- The chart is only a quick index to the written material discussing the interactions; it is not intended to be (and should not be) used without reading the accompanying discussions.
- The codes on the chart (A, B, C) indicate the likelihood that some action will need to be

taken by the pharmacist; they are not necessarily indications of the clinical importance of the interaction. You need to read the discussions following the chart to get a sense of the clinical importance.

- A blank on the chart simply means that there is no information about an interaction between the two drugs; it is not a guarantee that the two drugs will not be shown to interact in the future.

For more information and references, consult the standard textbooks of drug interactions and/or chemotherapeutic agents.[1-3]

*(continued)*

[1]Hansten P.D., and Horn, J.R. (1994). *Drug Interactions & Updates*. Vancouver, Wash.: Applied Therapeutics.
[2]Tatro, D.S. (1993). *Drug Interaction Facts*. St. Louis, Mo.: Facts and Comparisons.
[3]Dorr R.T., and Von Hoff, D.D. (1994). *Cancer Chemotherapy Handbook*. 2nd ed. Norwalk, Conn.: Appleton and Lange.

**Table 6.3** Drug Interactions with Cytoxic Chemotherapeutic Agents (continued)

| | Altretamine | Asparaginase | Bleomycin | Carboplastin | Carmustine | Cisplatin | Cyclophosphamide | Cytarabine | Dacarbazine | Doxorubicin | Etoposide | Fludarabine | Fluorouracil | Ifosfamide | Lomustine | Melphalan | Mercaptopurine | Methotrexate | Mitomycin | Mitotane | Procarbazine | Streptozocin | Teniposide | Thiotepa | Vinblastine | Vincristine |
|---|---|---|---|---|---|---|---|---|---|---|---|---|---|---|---|---|---|---|---|---|---|---|---|---|---|---|
| Allopurinol | | | | C[8] | | | C[18] | | | | | | | | | | A[41] | | | | | | | | | |
| Aminoglycoside antibiotics | | | | | | B[13] | | | | | | | | | | | | | | | | | | | | |
| Amiodarone | | | | | | | | | | | | | | | | | | B[45] | | | | | | | | |
| Azathioprine | | | | | | | B[19] | | | | | | | | | | | | | | | | | | | |
| Bleomycin | | | | | | B[4] | | | | | | | | | | | | | | | | | B[5] | | | |
| Carmustine | | | | | | | C[20] | | | | B[11] | | | | | | | | | | | | | | | |
| Chloramphenicol | | | | | | | | | | | | | | | | | | B[46] | | | | | | | | |
| Cholestyramine | | | | | | | | | | | | | | | B[5] | | | | | | | | | | | |
| Cimetidine | | | | | A[10] | | | | | | | | C[33] | | B[38] | C[39] | | | | | | | | | | |
| Cisplatin | | | B[4] | | | | | | | | | | | | | | | A[47] | | | | | | | | |
| Co-trimoxazole | | | | | | | | | | | | | | | | | | C[48] | | | | | | | | |
| Cyclosporine | | | | | | | | | | B[28] | C[32] | | | | | B[40] | | | | | | | | | | |
| Cytarabine | | | | | | C[14] | | | | | | C[25] | | | | | | | | | | | | | | |
| Diazoxide | | | | | | | | | | | | | | | | | | | | | | | | | | |
| Digoxin | | | | | | | B[21] | | | | | | | | | | | | | | | | | | | |
| Doxorubicin | | | | | | | | | | | | | | | | | | | | | | B[31] | | | | B[66] |
| Ethanol | | | | | | | | | | | | | | | | | | | | | A[57] | | | | | |
| Etoposide | | | | | B[11] | | | | | | | | | | | | | B[49] | | | | | | | | |
| Fludarabine | | | | | | | | C[25] | | | | | | | | | | | | | | | | | | |
| Interferon-α | | | | | | | | | | | | | | | | | | | | | | | | | B[64] | |
| Interleukin-2 | | | | | | | | | C[26] | | | | | | | | | | | | | | | | | |
| Leucovorin | | | | | | | | | | | | | A[34] | | | | | | | | | | | | | |
| Levodopa | | | | | | | | | B[27] | | | | | | | | | | | | | | | | | |
| Lithium | | | | | | C[15] | | | | | | | | | | | | | | | | | | | | |
| Lomustine | | | | | | | | | | | | | | | | | | | | | | | B[5] | | | |
| MAO inhibitors | B[1] | | | | | | | | | | | | | | | | | | | | | | | | | |
| Methotrexate | | | | | | C[16] | | | | | | | | | | | C[42] | | | | | | | | | |
| Metoclopramide | | | | | | | | | | | | | | | | | | | | | | | | | | |
| Metronidazole | | | | | | | | | | | | | B[35] | | | | | | | | | | | | | |
| Mitomycin | | | | | | | | | | | | | | | | | | | | | | | | | A[54] | |
| Nifedipine | | | | | | | | | | | | | | | | | | | | | | | | | | C[67] |
| NSAIDs | | | | | | | | | | | | | | | | | | A[50] | | | | | | | | |
| Oral nonabsorbable antibiotics | | | | | | | | | | | | | | | | | | B[51] | | | | | | | | |
| Oxygen | | | A[6] | | | | | | | | | | | | | | | | | | | | | | | |

(continued)

**Table 6.3  Drug Interactions with Cytoxic Chemotherapeutic Agents (continued)**

| | Altretamine | Asparaginase | Bleomycin | Carboplastin | Carmustine | Cisplatin | Cyclophosphamide | Cytarabine | Dacarbazine | Doxorubicin | Etoposide | Fludarabine | Fluorouracil | Ifosfamide | Lomustine | Melphalan | Mercaptopurine | Methotrexate | Mitomycin | Mitotane | Procarbazine | Streptozocin | Teniposide | Thiotepa | Vinblastine | Vincristine |
|---|---|---|---|---|---|---|---|---|---|---|---|---|---|---|---|---|---|---|---|---|---|---|---|---|---|---|
| Phenobarbital | | | | | | | C[22] | | | C[29] | | | | B[37] | | | | | | | | | C[61] | | | |
| Phenytoin | | | B[7] | B[9] | B[12] | A[17] | | | | B[30] | | | | | | | B[43] | B[52] | | | B[58] | B[60] | C[62] | | B[65] | |
| Probenecid | | | | | | | | | | | | | | | | | | A[53] | | | | | | | | |
| Spironolactone | | | | | | | | | | | | | | | | | | | | B[55] | | | | | | |
| Streptozocin | | | | | | | | | | B[31] | | | | | | | | | | | | | | A[63] | | |
| Succinylcholine | | | | | | | A[23] | | | | | | | | | | | | | | | | | A[63] | | |
| Sympathomimetic agents | | | | | | | | | | | | | | | | | | | | | B[59] | | | | | |
| Teniposide | B[2] | | B[5] | | | | | | | | | | | | B[5] | | | | | | | | | | | |
| Tricyclic antidepressants | | | | | | | | | | | | | | | | | | | | | | | | | | |
| Vaccines | A[68] | A[68] | A[68] | A[68] | A[68] | A[68] | A[68] | A[68] | A[68] | A[68] | A[68] | A[68] | A[68] | A[68] | A[68] | A[68] | A[68] | A[68] | A[68] | | A[68] | A[68] | A[68] | A[68] | A[68] | A[68] |
| Vinblastine | | B[3] | | | | | | | | | | | | | | | | | A[54] | | | | | | | |
| Vincristine | | B[3] | | | | | | | | | | | | | | | | | | | | | | | | |
| Warfarin | | | | | | | C[24] | | | | | | C[36] | | | | B[44] | | | B[56] | | | | | | |

A = Frequent significant interaction. Action usually needed. B = Moderately frequent significant interaction. Action needed in some cases. C = Infrequent or clinically insignificant interaction. Action usually not needed. (Blank) = No interaction information available to date.

**Table 6.3**   Drug Interactions with Cytoxic Chemotherapeutic Agents *(continued)*

**Discussions**

1. **Altretamine-Monoamine Oxidase (MAO) Inhibitors:** Administration of altretamine (Hexalen, US Bioscience) to patients receiving MAO inhibitors has been associated with symptomatic orthostatic hypotension.

2. **Altretamine-Tricyclic antidepressants:** Administration of altretamine (Hexalen, US Bioscience) to patients receiving tricyclic antidepressants has been associated with symptomatic orthostatic hypotension.

3. **Asparaginase-Vincristine:** Administration of asparaginase (Elspar, Merck) simultaneously or immediately before vincristine may lead to cumulative neuropathy and erythropoietic disorders. Asparaginase should be administered after vincristine.

4. **Bleomycin-Cisplatin:** The major route of elimination of bleomycin (Blenoxane, Bristol-Myers Squibb) is via the kidney. Patients who have received multiple courses of cisplatin (Platinol, Bristol-Myers Squibb) may develop renal dysfunction, which inhibits the elimination of bleomycin. This is especially likely with cumulative cisplatin doses of > 300 mg/m$^2$, even if the serum creatinine concentration is normal. Excessive toxicity, including pulmonary toxicity, may result.

5. **Bleomycin-Lomustine-Teniposide:** Administration of bleomycin to patients being treated with the combination of lomustine (CeeNU, Bristol-Myers Squibb) and teniposide (Vumon, Bristol-Myers Squibb) has been associated with an increased degree of bone marrow suppression.

6. **Bleomycin-Oxygen:** Bleomycin may cause acute inflammation and chronic fibrosis of the lungs. Acute pulmonary inflammation may be brought on by the administration of oxygen. When patients who have received bleomycin undergo surgery, it is recommended that the inspired oxygen concentration be as low as possible, preferably below 25%.

7. **Bleomycin-Phenytoin:** Bleomycin may decrease phenytoin levels, possibly through decreased oral absorption. All reported cases have involved coadministration of other antineoplastic agents. Patients receiving phenytoin should have serum concentrations

measured following administration of bleomycin.

8. **Carboplatin-Aminoglycosides:** The combination of carboplatin (Paraplatin, Bristol-Myers Squibb) and aminoglycoside antibiotics causes more hearing loss than would be expected with either agent alone. Alternatives to aminoglycosides should be considered in patients receiving carboplatin.

9. **Carboplatin-Phenytoin:** Phenytoin levels may be decreased for several days following a dose of carboplatin. This is based on a single case, which occurred in a patient on other drugs that may affect phenytoin metabolism. Patients receiving phenytoin should have serum concentrations measured following administration of carboplatin.

10. **Carmustine-Cimetidine:** The combination of carmustine (BiCNU, Bristol-Myers Squibb) and cimetidine (Tagamet, SmithKline Beecham) may increase the degree of bone marrow suppression beyond that which normally occurs with carmustine. Cimetidine should be avoided in patients receiving carmustine.

11. **Carmustine-Etoposide:** Coadministration of the maximum-tolerated doses of carmustine and etoposide (Vepesid, Bristol-Myers Squibb) in patients undergoing bone marrow transplantation has been associated with frequent hepatotoxicity.

12. **Carmustine-Phenytoin:** Phenytoin levels may be decreased by carmustine. All reported cases have involved coadministration of other antineoplastic agents. Patients receiving phenytoin should have serum concentrations measured following administration of carmustine.

13. **Cisplatin-Aminoglycosides:** Administration of gentamicin to patients undergoing cisplatin therapy may increase the incidence of nephrotoxicity; however, clinical evidence of this interaction in humans is lacking. Until more is known about this possible interaction, aminoglycosides should be avoided in patients being treated with cisplatin.

14. **Cisplatin-Diazoxide:** The combination of cisplatin and diazoxide (Proglycem, Baker

*(continued)*

**Table 6.3   Drug Interactions with Cytoxic Chemotherapeutic Agents** *(continued)*

## Discussions

Norton) may result in an increased degree of nephrotoxicity. Caution should be used when treating high blood pressure with diazoxide in patients receiving cisplatin.

15. **Cisplatin-Lithium:** Plasma lithium levels may be decreased in patients receiving cisplatin, usually to an insignificant degree. This may be related to more changes in fluid status of patients receiving cisplatin due to the extensive hydration required.

16. **Cisplatin-Metoclopramide:** Metoclopramide may alter responsiveness to cisplatin. In a single study in patients with head and neck cancer being treated with fluorouracil and cisplatin, radiation and surgery showed decreased response in patients in whom nausea was treated with metoclopramide compared to droperidol. The overall incidence and true significance of this interaction is unknown.

17. **Cisplatin-Phenytoin:** Cisplatin frequently causes a decrease in plasma phenytoin concentrations. Patients should have phenytoin concentrations monitored and phenytoin doses adjusted for one to two weeks after a dose of cisplatin. The mechanism may involve a combination of decreased absorption, altered plasma protein binding, and hepatic enzyme induction.

18. **Cyclophosphamide-Allopurinol:** Allopurinol may increase the concentration of active cyclophosphamide metabolites, however, there is conflicting evidence as to whether this results in increased bone marrow suppression. Until more is known about this interaction, allopurinol should be used with caution in patients receiving cyclophosphamide.

19. **Cyclophosphamide-Azathioprine:** Cyclophosphamide may cause hepatotoxicity when it follows azathioprine (Imuran, Burroughs Wellcome) therapy. One series reported four patients receiving this combination who developed biopsy-proven hepatic necrosis. The incidence of this interaction is unknown. If cyclophosphamide must be administered to a patient who has been treated with azathioprine, liver function should be monitored.

20. **Cyclophosphamide-Chloramphenicol:** Chloramphenicol may decrease the activity of the hepatic enzymes responsible for converting cyclophosphamide, which is inactive, into its active metabolites. However, this does not appear to result in any clinically significant change in cyclophosphamide activity or toxicity.

21. **Cyclophosphamide-Digoxin:** Cyclophosphamide may decrease the absorption of digoxin tablets by 20–45% but appears to have no effect on the absorption of digoxin capsules. This interaction was reported in patients receiving digoxin when cyclophosphamide was coadministered with other cytotoxic agents.

22. **Cyclophosphamide-Phenobarbital:** Phenobarbital increases the activity of the enzymes responsible for metabolizing cyclophosphamide, which is inactive, into its active metabolites; however, the metabolites are also cleared more rapidly. This does not appear to result in any clinically significant change in cyclophosphamide activity or toxicity.

23. **Cyclophosphamide-Succinylcholine:** Cyclophosphamide inhibits the enzyme pseudocholinesterase, which is responsible for metabolizing succinylcholine. Patients receiving cyclophosphamide may have a prolonged response to succinylcholine, which could result in prolonged apnea.

24. **Cyclophosphamide-Warfarin:** Cyclophosphamide may affect warfarin anticoagulation; however, reports are conflicting as to whether the degree of anticoagulation is increased or decreased. Patients receiving warfarin should have prothrombin times measured when beginning or discontinuing cyclophosphamide, and warfarin dosages adjusted accordingly.

25. **Cytarabine-Fludarabine:** Cytarabine increases the levels of fludarabine (Fludara, Berlex) in plasma. Both agents must be phosphorylated to be active, and there may be competition between the two agents for the enzymes responsible for phosphorylation. It is not known whether this results in any change in the activity or toxicity of either agent.

26. **Dacarbazine–Interleukin-2:** Interleukin-2 may decrease the levels of dacarbazine

*(continued)*

**Table 6.3**  Drug Interactions with Cytoxic Chemotherapeutic Agents *(continued)*

## Discussions

(DTIC-Dome, Miles) when administered prior to a dacarbazine dose. There does not appear to be any effect on the level of the metabolite of dacarbazine responsible for its antineoplastic activity. It is not known whether this changes the activity or toxicity of dacarbazine.

27. **Dacarbazine-Levodopa:** In a single reported case, dacarbazine impaired the response to levodopa without affecting plasma dopamine levels.

28. **Doxorubicin-Cyclosporine:** Administration of doxorubicin to patients receiving cyclosporine (Sandimmune, Sandoz) may induce coma and/or seizures. This is based on a single case report and does not necessarily preclude coadministration of the agents; however, caution should be used whenever patients are administered both agents.

29. **Doxorubicin-Phenobarbital:** Barbiturates increase the elimination of doxorubicin. It is not known whether this results in any clinically significant change in doxorubicin activity or toxicity.

30. **Doxorubicin-Phenytoin:** Phenytoin levels may be decreased by doxorubicin. All reported cases have involved coadministration of other antineoplastic agents. Patients receiving phenytoin should have serum concentrations measured following administration of doxorubicin.

31. **Doxorubicin-Streptozocin:** Streptozocin (Zanosar, Upjohn) may inhibit the hepatic metabolism and elimination of doxorubicin. This may result in increased mucositis and myelosuppression in patients receiving both agents.

32. **Etoposide-Cyclosporine:** High-dose cyclosporine (5–10 times conventional doses) causes increased bone marrow suppression when given with etoposide. This is due to decreased clearance of etoposide. Reduction of etoposide dosage by 50% is recommended if high-dose cyclosporine is used concurrently with etoposide.

33. **Fluorouracil-Cimetidine:** Cimetidine increases the plasma concentration and area under the plasma concentration time curve of fluorouracil, which increases the exposure to

fluorouracil. It is not known whether this changes the activity or toxicity of fluorouracil.

34. **Fluorouracil-Leucovorin:** Leucovorin increases the activity of fluorouracil biochemically. The combination is used therapeutically to enhance the activity of fluorouracil, however, when the two are used in combination, gastrointestinal toxicity, including mucositis and diarrhea, is increased over that seen when fluorouracil is used alone.

35. **Fluorouracil-Metronidazole:** Coadministration of fluorouracil and metronidazole may cause enhanced granulocytopenia. This effect is due to decreased clearance of fluorouracil. There is no corresponding increase in fluorouracil efficacy.

36. **Fluorouracil-Warfarin:** Continuous infusion fluorouracil may cause increased prothrombin time in patients stabilized on warfarin. There has been a single reported case of this interaction. Patients receiving warfarin therapy in whom continuous infusion fluorouracil is instituted should undergo frequent prothrombin time measurement.

37. **Ifosfamide-Phenobarbital:** Administration of ifosfamide (Ifex, Bristol-Myers Squibb) to patients receiving phenobarbital may be associated with neurotoxicity, including coma. There has been a single reported case of this interaction. The true incidence of this interaction is unknown.

38. **Lomustine-Cimetidine:** The combination of lomustine and cimetidine may increase the degree and duration of bone marrow suppression beyond that which normally occurs with lomustine.

39. **Melphalan-Cimetidine:** Cimetidine may decrease the absorption or increase the elimination of melphalan (Alkeran, Burroughs Wellcome). It is not known whether this affects the activity or toxicity of melphalan.

40. **Melphalan-Cyclosporine:** The combination of high-dose melphalan and cyclosporine in bone marrow transplant patients has been associated with an increased incidence of nephrotoxicity.

41. **Mercaptopurine-Allopurinol:** Allopurinol significantly decreases the hepatic first-pass metabolism of mercaptopurine (Purinethol, Burroughs Wellcome), causing a marked increase in mercaptopurine levels and increased

*(continued)*

**Table 6.3      Drug Interactions with Cytoxic Chemotherapeutic Agents** *(continued)*

### Discussions

myelosuppression. Allopurinol should be avoided in patients receiving mercaptopurine. If this is not possible, the mercaptopurine dose should be decreased to 25% of the original dose.

42. **Mercaptopurine-Methotrexate:** Oral methotrexate increases the area under the plasma concentration-time curve and increases the peak concentration of mercaptopurine. With conventional oral methotrexate doses this increase is generally not clinically significant.

43. **Mercaptopurine-Phenytoin:** Phenytoin levels may be decreased by mercaptopurine. All reported cases have involved coadministration of other antineoplastic agents. Patients receiving phenytoin should have serum concentrations measured when beginning or discontinuing mercaptopurine therapy.

44. **Mercaptopurine-Warfarin:** Mercaptopurine decreases the prothrombin time in patients receiving warfarin therapy, requiring an increased dose of warfarin to maintain therapeutic anticoagulation. Patients receiving warfarin anticoagulation should have prothrombin times monitored frequently when beginning or discontinuing mercaptopurine therapy.

45. **Methotrexate-Amiodarone:** Coadministration of methotrexate and amiodarone (Cordarone, Wyeth-Ayerst) has been associated with skin necrosis in a single case report.

46. **Methotrexate-Cholestyramine:** Oral cholestyramine (Questran, Bristol) decreases the plasma concentration of high-dose methotrexate by increasing the nonrenal excretion of methotrexate. This may be due to binding of methotrexate by cholestyramine in the gastrointestinal tract and elimination in the feces.

47. **Methotrexate-Co-trimoxazole:** The combination of methotrexate and co-trimoxazole is associated with greatly increased pancytopenia. This may be due to additive inhibition of the enzyme dihydrofolate reductase, decreased plasma protein binding of methotrexate, and decreased tubular secretion of methotrexate. Co-trimoxazole should not be administered to patients receiving methotrexate.

48. **Methotrexate-Cyclosporine:** Coadministration of methotrexate and cyclosporine decreases the elimination of both drugs. It is not known whether this results in any change in the activity or toxicity of either agent.

49. **Methotrexate-Ethanol:** The incidence of methotrexate-induced hepatotoxicity is increased in patients who consume alcohol. It is appropriate for patients receiving methotrexate to limit alcohol intake.

50. **Methotrexate-Nonsteroidal Anti-Inflammatory Drugs (NSAIDs):** Severe myelosuppression and mucositis due to decreased renal elimination of methotrexate has been associated with the following NSAIDs: aspirin, azapropazone, diclofenac (Voltaren, Ciba-Geigy), ibuprofen, indomethacin, ketoprofen (Orudis, Wyeth-Ayerst), naproxen (Naprosyn, Syntex), phenylbutazone, and salicylates. These drugs should not be given within 10 days of methotrexate. Other NSAIDs might produce a similar effect, and should be avoided in patients receiving methotrexate.

51. **Methotrexate–Oral Nonabsorbable Antibiotics:** Oral absorption of methotrexate is decreased by 30–50% in patients receiving oral antibiotic mixtures including neomycin, nystatin, and vancomycin.

52. **Methotrexate-Phenytoin:** Methotrexate may decrease phenytoin levels. All reported cases have involved coadministration of other antineoplastic agents.

53. **Methotrexate-Probenecid:** Probenecid may increase the myelosuppression and mucositis caused by methotrexate by decreasing the renal elimination of methotrexate. Probenecid should not be administered to patients receiving methotrexate.

54. **Mitomycin-Vinblastine:** The combination of mitomycin (Mutamycin, Bristol-Myers Squibb) and vinblastine has been associated with abrupt pulmonary toxicity. Coadministration of these agents should be avoided. In instances in which the combination is felt to be necessary, both drugs should be discontinued at the first sign of pulmonary compromise.

*(continued)*

**Table 6.3**     Drug Interactions with Cytoxic Chemotherapeutic Agents *(continued)*

**Discussions**

55. **Mitotane-Spironolactone:** Mitotane (Lysodren, Bristol-Myers Squibb) activity may be completely inhibited by the administration of spironolactone (Aldactone, Searle). Spironolactone should not be administered to patients receiving mitotane.

56. **Mitotane-Warfarin:** Mitotane may decrease the prothrombin time in patients receiving warfarin, requiring increased warfarin dosage to maintain a therapeutic degree of anticoagulation. Patients receiving warfarin anticoagulation should have prothrombin times closely monitored when starting or stopping mitotane.

57. **Procarbazine-Ethanol:** Ingestion of ethanol by patients receiving procarbazine (Matulane, Hoffman-La Roche) may result in a disulfiram-like reaction: flushing, headache, nausea, and hypotension. Patients receiving procarbazine should be advised to avoid alcohol.

58. **Procarbazine-Phenytoin:** Phenytoin levels may be decreased by procarbazine. All reported cases have involved coadministration of other antineoplastic agents. Patients receiving phenytoin should have serum concentrations measured when beginning or discontinuing procarbazine therapy.

59. **Procarbazine-Sympathomimetic Agents:** Procarbazine is a weak inhibitor of MAO. There is little evidence to support typical MAO drug interactions with procarbazine; however, sympathomimetic agents should be used with caution in patients receiving procarbazine to reduce the risk of extreme hypertension.

60. **Streptozocin-Phenytoin:** Pretreatment with phenytoin may inhibit the activity of streptozocin on pancreatic beta cells. Phenytoin should be avoided in patients receiving streptozocin.

61. **Teniposide-Phenobarbital:** Phenobarbital may increase the hepatic metabolism and elimination of teniposide. It is not known whether this affects the activity or toxicity of teniposide.

62. **Teniposide-Phenytoin:** Phenytoin may increase the hepatic metabolism and elimination of teniposide. It is not known whether this affects the activity or toxicity of teniposide.

63. **Thiotepa-Succinylcholine:** Thiotepa inhibits the enzyme pseudocholinesterase, which is responsible for metabolizing succinylcholine. Patients receiving thiotepa may have a prolonged response to succinylcholine. This could result in prolonged apnea.

64. **Vinblastine-Interferon** α: Patients receiving both vinblastine and interferon alpha may be at increased risk of developing peripheral neuropathy.

65. **Vinblastine-Phenytoin:** Phenytoin levels may be decreased by vinblastine. All reported cases have involved coadministration of other antineoplastic agents. Patients receiving phenytoin should have serum concentrations measured following administration of vinblastine.

66. **Vincristine-Digoxin:** Vincristine may decrease the absorption of digoxin tablets by 20–45% but appears to have no effect on the absorption of digoxin capsules. This interaction was reported in patients receiving digoxin when vincristine was coadministered with other cytotoxic agents.

67. **Vincristine-Nifedipine:** Nifedipine may decrease vincristine elimination. It is not known whether this affects the activity or toxicity of vincristine.

68. **Vaccines:** Administration of live vaccines to immunosuppressed patients, including those undergoing cytotoxic chemotherapy, may be hazardous. Patients receiving cytotoxic chemotherapy should not receive: BCG, measles vaccine, mumps vaccine, rubella vaccine, or yellow fever vaccine. Immunization with other vaccines may result in decreased levels of protective antibodies. However, current recommendations are that patients undergoing cancer chemotherapy may receive other vaccines.

## BIBLIOGRAPHY

Balis, F.M. (1986). Pharmacokinetic drug interactions of commonly used anticancer drugs. *Clinical Pharmacokinetics* 11(3): 223–235.

Balmer, C., and Valley, A.W. (1994). Basic principles of cancer treatment and cancer chemotherapy. In J.T. DiPiro, R.L. Talbert, P.E. Hayes, et al. (eds.): *Pharmacotherapy: A Pathophysiologic Approach.* 2nd ed. Norwalk, Conn.: Appleton and Lange

Bosanquet, A.G., and Gilby, E.D. (1984). Comparison of the fed and fasting states on the absorption of melphalan in multiple myeloma. *Cancer Chemotherapy and Pharmacology* 12(3): 183–186.

Brown, M.C. (1997). Multisite mucous membrane bleeding due to a possible interaction between warfarin and 5-Fluorouracil. *Pharmacotherapy* 17(3): 631–633.

Dorr, R.T., and von Hoff, D.D. (1994). *Cancer Chemotherapy Handbook.* 2nd ed. Norwalk, Conn.: Appleton and Lange.

Finley, R.S. (1992). Drug interactions in the oncology patient. *Seminars in Oncology Nursing* 8(2): 95–101.

Gunnarsson, P.O., Davidsson, T., Andersson, S.B., et al. (1990). Impairment of estramustine phosphate absorption by concurrent intake of milk and food. *European Journal of Clinical Pharmacology* 38(2): 189–193.

Hansten, P.D., and Horn, J.R. (1994). *Drug Interactions & Updates.* Vancouver, Wash.: Applied Therapeutics.

Herceptin (Trastuzumab). (1999). Product Information. San Francisco: Genentech, Inc.

Ignoffo, R.J. (1989). Drug interactions with antineoplastic agents. *Highlights on Antineoplastic Drugs* 7(1): 2–7.

Inman, W., and Kubota, K. (1992). Tachycardia during cisapride treatment. *BMJ* 305(6860): 1019.

Janetzky, K., and Morreale, A.P. (1997). Probable interaction between warfarin and ginseng. *Am J Health-Syst Pharm* 54(6): 692–693.

Klepser, T.B., and Klepser, M.E. (1999). Unsafe and potentially safe herbal therapies. *Am J Health-Syst Pharm* 56: 125–138.

King, R. (1995). Drug interactions with cancer chemotherapy. *Cancer Practice* 3(1): 58–59.

Kolesar, J.M., Johnson, C.L., Freeberg, B.L., Berlin, J.D., and Schiller, J.H. (1999). Warfarin-5-Fu interaction—A consecutive case series. *Pharmacotherapy* 19(12): 1445–1449.

Lien, E.A., Anker, G., Lonning, P.E., Solheim, E., and Ueland, P.M. (1990). Decreased serum concentrations of tamoxifen and its metabolites induced by aminoglutethimide. *Cancer Research* 50(18): 5851–5857.

Lonning, P.E., Kvinnsland, S., and Bakke, O.M. (1984). Effect of aminoglutethimide on antipyrine, theophylline, and digitoxin disposition in breast cancer. *Clinical Pharmacology Therapy* 36(6): 796–802.

Lonning, P.E., Kvinnsland, S., and Jahren, G. (1984). Aminoglutethimide and warfarin: A new important drug interaction. *Cancer Chemotherapy and Pharmacology* 12(1): 10–12.

McEvoy, G.K. (ed.). (1994). *AHFS Drug Information 94.* Bethesda, Md.: American Society of Health-System Pharmacists.

Michalets, E.L. (1998). Update: Clinically significant cytochrome P-450 drug interactions. *Pharmacotherapy* 18(1): 84–112.

Reece, P.A., Kotasek, D., Morris, R.G., et al. (1986). The effect of food on oral melphalan absorption. *Cancer Chemotherapy and Pharmacology* 16(2): 194–197.

Rowinsky, E.K., Gilbert, M.R., McGuire, W.P., Noe, D.A., Grochow, L.B., Forastiere, A.A., Ettinger, D.S., Lubejko, B.G., Clark, B., and Sartorious, S.E. (1991). Sequences of taxol and cisplatin: A phase I and pharmacologic study. *Journal of Clinical Oncology* 9(9): 1692–1703.

Stevens, D.A. (1999). Itraconazole in cyclodextrin solution. *Pharmacotherapy* 19(5): 603–611.

Synercid I.V. (quinupristin and dalfopristin). Product Information Collegeville, Penn.: Rhone-Poulenc Rorer Pharmaceuticals, Inc.

Tatro, D.S. (1990). *Drug Interaction Facts.* St. Louis, Mo.: Facts and Comparisons.

Tatro, D.S. (1991). *Drug Interaction Facts.* St. Louis, Mo.: Facts and Comparisons.

Tatro, D.S. (1993). *Drug Interaction Facts.* St. Louis, Mo.: Facts and Comparisons.

Xeloda, Capecitabine Product Information. (1991). Nutley, N.J.: Roche Laboratories, Inc.

# Part III

# *Clinical Application*

# Chapter 7

# Pediatric Aspects of Cancer Chemotherapy

**Vanessa C. Howard, RN, MSN, FNP**
**Martha May, RN, MSN, FNP**

## INTRODUCTION

Statistics reveal that each year in the United States more than 12,000 children and adolescents under the age of 20 are found to have cancer. Overall, cancer ranks fourth as a cause of death for persons in this age group, behind injuries, homicides, and suicides; however, it is the leading cause of disease-related death. During the last four decades, great strides have been made in the treatment of pediatric cancers and in the supportive care of patients with these diseases. In fact, it is estimated that, as the new millennium unfolds, one in 900 young adults will be a survivor of childhood cancer, a statistic unimaginable in the early 1900s when children died of more common childhood illnesses, such as pneumonia, influenza, and diarrhea. Today, the cure rates for most childhood cancers are greater than 70 percent (Ries, Percy, and Bunin 1999, DeLaat, and Lampkin 1992; Landis, Murray, Bolden, and Wingo 1999; Foley and Fergusson 1993).

Pediatric oncology nurses must be aware of the advances in the treatment of cancer that have been made through improved complexity of care and research. This chapter will provide the nurse with an overview of the history of pediatric oncology and pediatric oncology nurs-ing, with a discussion of diseases and research in pediatric oncology. Applicable standards of care for the child with cancer will be included.

## HISTORICAL ASPECTS

In the 1940s, Dr. Sidney Farber discovered the importance of folic acid antagonists in the treatment of pediatric acute leukemia. He found that certain folic acid compounds enhance the leukemic process within the patient's bone marrow and that certain folic acid antagonists induce a hypocellular process. When aminopterin, an antimetabolite, became available, Dr. Farber gave the drug to 16 children with acute lymphoblastic leukemia (ALL), 10 of whom experienced disease remission. In 1949, a similar compound amethopterin, methotrexate, was first used to induce remission in a child with leukemia; this compound continues to be used in therapeutic regimens today. In the 1950s, Dr. Farber introduced additional drugs classified as anti-tumor antibiotics. The successful use of one such drug, actinomycin D, to treat children with Wilms' tumor led to the development of additional antitumor antibiotics. Today, these drugs continue to be important in the treatment of many pediatric cancers (Pratt, Ruddon, Ensminger, and Maybaum 1994; Balis, Holcenberg, and Poplack 1997).

Drug development continued throughout the 1950s and 1960s; however, it became evident that single-drug therapies for childhood cancer were only moderately successful. Combination therapies were introduced and these regimens proved more valuable, particularly in the treatment of ALL in the 1960s (Rivera, Pinkel, Simon, Hancock, and Crist 1993).

With the development of anticancer drugs came the development of national cooperative study groups. The first such group, an outgrowth of a multidisciplinary approach to childhood cancer treatment initiated by Dr. Sidney Farber in the 1950s, was called the National Wilms' Tumor Study Group (NWTSG). This group was devoted to treatment for children with Wilms' tumors. The beginnings of the Children's Cancer Group (CCG) and the Pediatric Oncology Group (POG) were also formed in the 1950s. These groups are still in existence today and have now merged to form the Children's Oncology Group (COG). These collaborative groups were formed to enroll pediatric cancer patients in clinical research studies at various cancer centers across the country so that more could be learned about the treatment of pediatric cancer and the responses to specific therapies. Clinical trials involving combination chemotherapy, adjunct therapies, and collaboration among investigators were pioneered by pediatric oncology researchers and subsequently influenced the care of the adult with cancer. Nurses are an important part of these cooperative groups; they serve as a liaison between those who provide care to pediatric cancer patients and the patients and families (Foley and Fergusson 1993; Ungerlieder and Ellenberg 1997; Jenkins and Hubbard 1991; Bru 1998; Craig 1998).

The 1960s saw the rapid development of many chemotherapeutic agents. Combination therapy including multiple systemic chemotherapeutic agents and multimodal therapy, including craniospinal irradiation and intrathecal methotrexate for the treatment of ALL, was introduced in this era. The use of four drugs, vincristine, doxorubicin, prednisone, and methotrexate, all with different mechanisms of action, was initiated to induce remission in patients with ALL and is still in use today (Rivera et al. 1993; Craig 1998).

In the 1970s, drug development slowed. However, important discoveries were made about cancer cell biology in the fields of molecular biology, genetic engineering, and immunology, which led to the current practice of determining immunophenotyping and cytogenetics of the cancer cell. The use of adjuvant chemotherapy to destroy residual tumor cells after surgery or radiotherapy emerged during this era and it was noted that systemic chemotherapy could improve survival estimates. In addition, the NCI designed a screening program to assess the antitumor activity of compounds thought to be beneficial in cancer treatment (Craig 1998).

In the 1980s, such growth factors as granulocyte colony stimulating factor (GCSF), erythropoietin (EPO), and granulocyte macrophage colony stimulating factor (GMCSF) were developed and incorporated into pediatric clinical trials. In addition, several new chemotherapeutic agents were introduced, including Taxol, paclitaxel, and Topotecan, a topoisomerase inhibitor. Cancer cell biology continues to be at the forefront of cancer research.

The last decade of the twentieth century yielded many exciting discoveries in pediatric oncology. The fields of molecular biology, biochemistry, and immunology brought insights into the probable causes and pathogenesis of childhood cancer. Additionally, specific genetic abnormalities identified in some pediatric cancers have had important prognostic and therapeutic implications.

Today, the role of gene therapy in pediatric oncology is being explored. Efforts in gene therapy are directed at providing tailored therapy based on biologic findings of the cancer cell in order to minimize toxicity in individual patients (Balis, Holcenberg, and Poplack 1997; Craig 1998; Yarbro 1996; Pui 1998; Hasenauer 1998).

## HISTORY OF PEDIATRIC ONCOLOGY NURSING

Initially, the role of the pediatric oncology nurse was to comfort the child and to provide support to the family in the child's final days. Children were less likely to survive the treatment of their cancers because supportive care, such as antibiotic therapy and blood products, was not sufficiently developed. The role of the nurse expanded as the cure rates for childhood cancers increased. Children were living longer and the nurse needed a specialized body of knowledge as well as a solid foundation in pediatric nursing (Bru 1998).

With these developments, nurses began providing family-centered care and expanding their role within the setting of the cancer center. This change created specialized roles for the oncology nurse; these roles include nurse practitioner, clinical nurse specialist, data manager, research nurse, and chemotherapy nurse.

The professional organization for this specialized area of nursing is the Association of Pediatric Oncology Nursing (APON). It stemmed from a meeting held at the conference of the Association for the Care of Children's Health (ACCH) in 1973. A small group of pediatric oncology pioneers joined together that year and planned a special-interest session to be held at the 1974 ACCH meeting. They realized their need to join forces with other pediatric oncology nurses across the country so they could share experiences and promote education regarding the care of the child with cancer.

Today, APON has more than 1,900 members from the United States, Canada, and around the world. A quarterly publication, the *Journal of Pediatric Oncology Nursing (JOPON)*, and educational information for nurses and families are available. In 1982, the Association of Pediatric Oncology Nursing also was responsible for the publication of the book *Nursing Care of the Child with Cancer*, the first text devoted entirely to pediatric oncology nursing. A second edition of this book was published in 1993.

Also in 1993, APON in conjunction with Certification Corporation of Pediatric Oncology Nursing (CCPON) offered the first pediatric oncology certification examination. More than 500 nurses sat for this examination. Following this event, nurses have become compelled to show their expertise within the specialty by achieving certification. Today, certification is possible through the Oncology Nursing Certification Corporation (ONCC). Nurses who pass the examination demonstrate a level of competence in the area of pediatric oncology nursing and earn the credential of Certified Pediatric Oncology Nurse (CPON), which indicates competence in the area of pediatric oncology nursing.

The Association of Pediatric Oncology Nursing recognizes the importance of working with other professional nursing organizations and in doing so the organization has established national standards of care. This organization also supports nursing research and provides educational opportunities to improve nursing practice (Bru 1998; Walker 1998).

In 1987, in collaboration with the American Nurses Association (ANA), APON developed and published the Scope of Practice and Outcome Standards of Practice for Pediatric

Oncology Nursing (see Table 7.1). Nurses taking care of pediatric oncology patients are to use APON's standards in conjunction with the ANA's Standards of Maternal Child Health Nursing. This requirement reinforces the commitment of pediatric oncology nurses to child and family health (Bru 1998; Hockenberry-Eaton and Kline 1997).

Planning care for the child receiving chemotherapy entails the involvement not only of the child but the family unit as well. Two extensive care plans (Table 7.2 and Table 7.3) illustrate the complicated care required by the child and family. Children with cancer are not just small adults who require a reduced dose of chemotherapy for their care. Children are complex individuals with physical, psychological, social, informational, and developmental needs. Nurses and nursing become the cornerstone for the care of the pediatric cancer patient.

## OVERVIEW OF PRIMARY TYPES OF DISEASES

Pediatric cancers are very different from adult cancers with regard to physiology, sites of occurrence, and response to therapy. Most childhood cancers arise from the mesodermal germ layer, which in embryonic development becomes connective tissue, bone, cartilage, muscle, blood, blood vessels, sex organs, kidneys, and lymphatic and lymphoid organs. Sarcomas, leukemia, and lymphomas are found to arise from embryonal tissue, whereas central nervous system tumors are found in the neuroectodermal tissue. In contrast, the most common adult cancers, carcinomas, are epithelial in origin and are rare in children (Mooney 1993).

General statistics show that the risk of childhood cancers, such as ALL, lymphomas, and medulloblastoma, is higher among males. Within the United States, white children are at a higher risk of cancer than black children. The incidence of childhood cancers throughout the world varies markedly by race and geographic location. The highest rates are seen in Israel and Nigeria and the lowest in India and Japan. The reasons for these differences in incidence are not fully understood but may be related to numerous influences, including racial, genetic, and environmental factors (Mooney 1993).

Acute lymphoblastic leukemia (ALL), which affects approximately 2,400 children per year, is the most common childhood cancer. Table 7.4 shows the incidence and relative proportion of specific diagnostic categories by 5-year age groups. For children younger than 15 years of age, ALL represented 78% of leukemia cases, whereas the AML subgroup (Ib) represented 16% of cases. The relative frequency of AML increased in the second decade of life as that of ALL decreased. Although AML represented only 13–14% of leukemia cases in the first 10 years of life, it accounted for 36% of leukemia cases among 15–19-year-olds. The incidence and relative contribution of the chronic myeloid leukemia also increased with age, representing about 9% of cases among 15–19 year olds (SEER Data, 1999).

The treatment of ALL is a true success story of pediatric oncology; some of the most remarkable cure rates have been achieved with this disease. Although the different types of childhood leukemia may cause similar symptoms, the treatment and response rates vary (Ries, Percy, and Bunin 1999; Rasco 1998; Cohen 1998).

Central nervous system (CNS) tumors are the second most frequently occurring malignancy and the most common solid tumor in the pediatric population. Of the CNS malignancies, the most common are astrocytoma (52%), primitive neuroectodermal tumors (21%), gliomas (15%), and ependymomas (9%). Figure 7.1 shows further expansion of these data.

**Table 7.1** Outcome Standards of Pediatric Oncology Practice

## I. Information Regarding Disease and Therapy

*Standard*

The child and family possess accurate current information about the disease, options for treatment, consequences or side effects of treatment, potential oncologic emergencies, alternative care settings, and resources in order to be fully informed partners in the health care team. Information should be specific to the developmental level of the child and family.

*Rationale*

1. Securing adequate information is a prerequisite to decision-making concerning therapy, especially if investigational therapy is considered.
2. Assessment of a child's developmental stage is essential when informing a child about treatment, particularly when obtaining assent from the child for investigative therapy.
3. The child and family are informed and prepared before an actual event in order to participate in selecting an option specific to their needs.

*Nursing Process Criteria*

The nurse:

1. Facilitates an environment in which the child and family can receive and discuss information regarding the disease.
2. Is available to the child and family to clarify and expand on information received.
3. Responds as a patient advocate in all informational matters.
4. Uses appropriate teaching and learning strategies with the child and family.
5. Explains therapy schedules.
6. Serves as a resource to the child and family regarding community resources and services that can assist the family to meet the demands of treatment.
7. Uses appropriate resources when ethical dilemmas, such as DNR, option of no treatment, or use of unproven methods of treatment, are identified and addressed.

8. Presents information to the child and family about possible dysfunctional late consequences of the original cancer, complications of the cancer, or the treatment of cancer. Information is to be provided at appropriate times throughout the course of illness.
9. Evaluates nursing interventions on the basis of patient outcome criteria.
10. Revises the patient and family teaching plan as indicated from ongoing evaluation.

*Patient Outcome Criteria*

The child and family:

1. Describe the disease, therapy, and possible complications at a level consistent with their developmental, intellectual, and emotional states.
2. Participate at desired level in decision-making, care, and plans for activities of daily living.
3. Identify community, personal, and institutional resources and/or services.
4. Describe therapy schedule during treatment.
5. Identify the option of home care for terminal care in the event of final and certain therapy failure.
6. Acknowledge the right of the child to assent when consent from parents for investigational therapy is indicated.

## II. Growth and Development

*Standard*

The child and family possess adequate information regarding the psychological and physiological effects of the diagnosis and treatment of cancer on the normal growth and developmental level of the child and family.

*Rationale*

1. The majority of children diagnosed with cancer achieve long-term survival.
2. The diagnosis of cancer in a child creates a stressful, disruptive situation for the family.

*(continued)*

**Table 7.1** Outcome Standards of Pediatric Oncology Practice *(continued)*

This may be evidenced by chronic disruption in normal family routine and lack of age-appropriate activities for the child.

3. Therapy and its side effects can cause significant psychological stress for the child and/or family member(s) in society, school, and community.

4. Disruption of normal activities, e.g., school and association with peers, may take place due to acute episodic events during therapy.

5. Death of the child produces alterations in the family's ongoing growth and development.

*Nursing Process Criteria*

The nurse:

1. Assesses the child's growth and development throughout treatment and during follow-up.

2. Assesses the degree to which the diagnosis of cancer in a child has disrupted individual and family functioning.

3. Helps the family and child establish a routine that is appropriate to the developmental level of the child.

4. Provides information to the family regarding the child's growth and development needs.

5. Consults and collaborates with other professionals, such as psychologists, psychiatrists, and social workers, to provide normal growth and development information to the family and child.

6. Uses principles of normal growth and development when preparing the child and family for invasive procedures.

7. Incorporates knowledge of normal growth and development and family dynamics into the nursing care plan.

8. Uses principles of growth and development in all stages of treatment in order to alleviate long-term effects that diagnosis and treatment of cancer can have on growth and development.

9. Identifies resources and provides

information to families whose child has died.

10. Evaluates nursing interventions on the basis of patient outcome criteria.

11. Revises the care plan as indicated by evaluation data.

*Patient Outcome Criteria*

The child and family:

1. Participate in decision-making and care on an ongoing basis in ways appropriate to their developmental levels.

2. Modify the family routine as necessary to accommodate acute and chronic aspects of therapy.

3. Provide age-appropriate activities for the child.

4. Demonstrate use of appropriate resources to cope with maintaining normal growth and development for the child.

5. Demonstrate modifications in the child's activities of daily living to take into consideration the effects of cancer on normal growth and development.

6. Identify the effects of the diagnosis and treatment of cancer on the well-being of the sibling(s).

7. Use the nurse as a resource during and after the terminal phase to integrate the experience into the growth and development of the family.

### III. Physical Care

*Standard*

The child's physical care is provided by the nurse in collaboration with the child and family. The nurse is responsible for assessing and determining the child's and family's participation in the physical care of the child. The nurse selects interventions that facilitate an appropriate level of self-care.

*Rationale*

1. Physical care is provided by the nurse with recognition of the interrelatedness of the physical, psychological, and spiritual needs of the child. The family is the constellation within which these needs interact.

*(continued)*

**Table 7.1    Outcome Standards of Pediatric Oncology Practice (continued)**

2. During acute episodic events the child may be hospitalized. Depending upon the child's age, rooming-in and parental participation in physical care may be appropriate and necessary.

3. During the chronic phase of cancer therapy the child is encouraged to pursue normal activities whenever possible; this sometimes requires a large degree of parental participation in physical care in the home.

4. In the event of terminal illness, home care for the dying child may be an appropriate option. Family participation in physical care can be most intensive at that time.

*Nursing Process Criteria*

The nurse:

1. Recognizes chronic and acute physical care needs of the child with cancer.

2. Assesses the child and family developmentally, psychosocially, and cognitively when teaching self-care and/or parental participation in physical care.

3. Uses knowledge of common childhood illnesses and their management.

4. Uses knowledge of well-child health maintenance issues as they pertain to the child with cancer.

5. Provides physical nursing care of the child in the inpatient or outpatient setting as determined by the child's physical state and the role of the nurse, i.e., expanded role practitioner, staff nurse.

6. Monitors the physical condition of the child based on knowledge of common side effects of childhood cancer and its therapies in order to provide early assessment and intervention.

7. Develops a patient care plan in collaboration with all members of the health care team, which is evaluated at regular intervals and revised when alteration in physical status occurs.

8. Serves as a resource to child and family and health care professionals regarding management of the effects of cancer, the therapies, and the side effects of each.

9. Evaluates nursing interventions on the basis of patient outcome criteria.

10. Revises the care plan as indicated by evaluation data.

*Patient Outcome Criteria*

The child and family:

1. Use the nurse as a resource for information regarding physical care needs of the child related to the disease and treatment protocol.

2. Identify physical care needs of the child related to the effects of the disease and treatment protocol.

3. Identify measures necessary to prevent and care for specific side effects of the disease and treatment including skin breakdown, mucosal trauma, infections, bleeding, nutritional deficiencies, anemia, fever, nausea, and vomiting.

4. Demonstrate ability to care for special devices, e.g., central venous catheters, prostheses.

5. Demonstrate ability to manage common childhood illnesses and major health care issues of the child's age group.

## IV. Psychosocial Care

*Standard*

The child and family maintain psychological, social, and spiritual integrity while living with a diagnosis of cancer.

*Rationale*

1. Discomfort and stress may be experienced due to psychological, social, spiritual, or developmental disruptions at the time of diagnosis, during therapy, during long-term survival, or at the time of death.

*(continued)*

**Table 7.1** Outcome Standards of Pediatric Oncology Practice *(continued)*

2. The psychosocial health of the child is closely related to the psychosocial health of the family as a whole.

3. Healthy long-term adaptation is dependent upon maintenance of psychosocial equilibrium for the child and family early in diagnosis and throughout treatment.

*Nursing Process Criteria*

The nurse:

1. Assesses each family member's perceptions of how the diagnosis and treatment of cancer impact upon their psychological, social, and spiritual well-being.

2. Identifies cultural and belief systems that influence the child's and family's psychological, social, or spiritual functioning.

3. Assesses role relationships and interaction patterns of the family members.

4. Assesses stressors and coping strategies of family members.

5. Assesses adequacy of family support systems and mobilizes sources of support when needed.

6. Diagnoses alterations, disturbances, or deficits in psychological, social, or spiritual responses related to the diagnosis and treatment of cancer.

7. Consults and collaborates with other professionals, such as physician, clinical nurse specialist, psychologist, psychiatrist, social worker, and clergy as appropriate.

8. Develops a patient care plan in collaboration with all members of the health care team that is evaluated at regular intervals and supports growth and adaptation.

9. Provides opportunities for the child and family during diagnosis and treatment to verbalize thoughts and feelings in a nonjudgmental atmosphere.

10. Provides psychosocial support for the child and family throughout the illness experience.

11. Provides information for the child and family with regard to medical, spiritual, and community resources that could either decrease stressors or increase adaptive coping strategies.

12. Participates in child and family support groups.

13. Monitors child and family psychological, social, and spiritual needs on an ongoing basis throughout the illness experience.

14. Evaluates nursing interventions on the basis of patient outcome criteria.

15. Revises the care plan as indicated by evaluation data.

*Patient Outcome Criteria*

The child and family:

1. Identify psychological, social, and spiritual concerns about living with cancer.

2. Use appropriate psychological, social, and spiritual resources for support.

3. Participate in decision-making concerning psychosocial care and health.

4. Continue to grow and develop toward their full psychological, social, and spiritual potential.

**V. Prevention and Early Detection of Secondary Cancers and Malignancies in Adulthood**

*Standard*

The child and family possess appropriate knowledge with regard to prevention and early detection of secondary cancer and adult malignancies.

*Rationale*

1. In relationship to the general population, a child who survives childhood cancer is at a much greater risk for the development of a second malignancy.

2. The incidence of secondary cancers—those related to treatment for primary cancer—may increase as childhood cancer survival rates increase.

3. The earlier individuals are aware of environmental, personal, and therapy-related

*(continued)*

**Table 7.1    Outcome Standards of Pediatric Oncology Practice** *(continued)*

carcinogenic risk factors, the greater the possibility of early detection and treatment.

*Nursing Process Criteria*

The nurse:

1. Is knowledgeable of carcinogenic risk factors related to lifestyle, environment, genetics, and cancer therapy.
2. Identifies actual and potential factors that place individuals at risk for secondary cancers.
3. Monitors changes in environment and behaviors that may alter risk potential for primary malignancies in adulthood.
4. Teaches the child and family those warning signs of cancer.
5. Teaches the child and family the lifestyle behaviors known to decrease the risk of cancer.
6. Evaluates nursing interventions on the basis of patient outcome criteria.
7. Revises the care plan as indicated by evaluation data.

*Patient Outcome Criteria*

The child and family:

1. Recognize factors that place an individual at risk and may lead to cancer, such as smoking, immunosuppressive agents, and environmental hazards.
2. Seek preventive health care.
3. Identify resources and appropriate plan for assistance in the event of an alteration in health status.
4. Identify warning signals of cancer.
5. Identify behavior known to decrease the risk of cancer, such as a high-fiber diet, no smoking, and limited exposure to the sun.
6. Maintain routine follow-up activities after completion of therapy.

**VI. Long-Term Survival**

*Standard*

The child and family demonstrate optimal adaptation to long-term survival. This is demonstrated by integration into the family's usual health care practice of current information about possible later psychological and/or physical consequences from a diagnosis and treatment of cancer in childhood. The child and family also participate in long-term follow-up activities.

*Rationale*

1. Physical late consequences may be related to the cancer itself, complications of the disease, or its treatment.
2. Some and/or many late consequences of diagnosis and treatment of cancer can be alleviated or avoided with specific preventive intervention that is begun at the time of diagnosis.
3. Later consequences can be physical in nature, related to alterations in body structure or function.
4. Late consequences can be emotional in nature, related to disruption in normal patterns of growth and development during and after therapy or fears related to long-term consequences of therapy.
5. Late consequences may be related to discrimination after therapy as evidenced by difficulty securing employment, obtaining insurance, etc.
6. Learning disabilities and changes in cognitive ability can be related to late consequences of therapy.

*Nursing Process Criteria*

The nurse:

1. Uses anticipatory guidance and support to assist the patient and family to identify late consequences of therapy.
2. Identifies a plan with the child and family to provide follow-up health status evaluations at regular intervals and especially when alterations in health status occur.
3. Applies knowledge of risk factors to provide early assessment and intervention for the child at risk.

*(continued)*

**Table 7.1** Outcome Standards of Pediatric Oncology Practice *(continued)*

4. Assesses normal growth and development as well as psychosocial and cognitive function in the long-term survivor or ascertains that appropriate assessment is performed by other team members.

5. Diagnoses alterations in the child's responses to his or her own physical, psychosocial, and/or cognitive development.

6. Institutes a collaborative plan of care with the child, family, and health care team to maximize health care status and level of functioning in the long-term survivor.

7. Functions as a resource to the child and family and other health professionals who are concerned with late consequences of therapy for childhood cancer.

8. Acts as a child advocate and supports others who are active in maintaining a social atmosphere free of discrimination for long-term survivors of childhood cancer.

9. Is an advocate for the child in the school system for development of special resources as needed due to cognitive late effects.

10. Monitors legislative changes and incorporates into the practice the use of legislative changes that affect long-term survivors of childhood cancer.

11. Evaluates nursing interventions on the basis of patient outcome criteria.

12. Revises the care plan as indicated by evaluation data.

*Patient Outcome Criteria*

The child and family:

1. Identify possible late consequences of childhood cancer or therapy.

2. Use appropriate resources for maintenance of normal patterns of growth and development within the child's capacities.

3. State measures to manage possible or actual dysfunction in the future, e.g., sperm banking, hormonal replacement therapy, and special schooling.

4. Participate in long-term follow-up activities with the oncology health care team.

**VII. Professional Development**

*Standard*

The nurse assumes responsibility for improving pediatric oncology nursing practice through evaluation of practice and an ongoing involvement in continuing education, professional development, and research.

*Rationale*

1. The patient and family benefit from the nurse's commitment to improvement of pediatric oncology nursing practice obtained through increased clinical, professional, political, and legislative knowledge.

2. Optimal performance standards of pediatric oncology nursing practice depend on continual and regular evaluation of the quality of nursing care provided.

*Nursing Process Criteria*

The nurse:

1. Examines and evaluates models of practice.

2. Applies new knowledge to practice to improve patient care.

3. Uses research methodology to address identified clinical nursing problems.

4. Consults with and is a consultant to other nursing professionals in order to enhance standards of pediatric oncology nursing practice.

5. Maintains current knowledge of legislative and political issues affecting the nursing profession and pediatric oncology.

*Outcome Criteria*

The nurse:

1. Participates regularly in continuing education programs in pediatric oncology nursing.

2. Demonstrates familiarity with legislative issues related to pediatric oncology.

3. Shares new knowledge with colleagues in nursing through consultation, presentations, and/or publications.

4. Participates in research.

5. Applies research findings to nursing practice.

6. Serves as an active member in one or more professional organizations.

*Source:* O'Neill, J.B., et al. (2000). *Scope and Standards of Pediatric Oncology Nursing Practice.* Washington, D.C.: American Nurses Publishing.

**Table 7.2** Standardized Nursing Care Plan for Physical Care of the Child

| Nursing Diagnosis | Defining Characteristics | Expected Outcomes | Nursing Interventions |
|---|---|---|---|
| I. *Potential for injury related to bone marrow depression* | I. A. Leukopenia<br>B. Thrombocytopenia | I. A. Pt remains without s/s of infection or hemorrhage<br>B. Infection or bleeding is minimized by early detection and treatment | I. A. Avoid invasive procedures, such as urinary catheterization or bone marrow aspiration/biopsy if possible<br>B. Use careful hand washing in any contact with pt<br>C. Monitor absolute neutrophil count and platelet count<br>D. Assess for potential sites of infection (i.e., mouth, rectum, IV site, exit site for venous access devices)<br>E. Teach parents ways to prevent infection and injury<br>F. Teach parents to identify s/s of infection or bleeding and to notify appropriate health care provider<br>G. Have parents modify home environment to prevent injury from falls and other accidents<br>H. Have parents control exposure to potential infections, especially childhood communicable diseases<br>I. Teach pt to carry out mouth care using soft toothbrush or sponge appliance as prescribed by health care provider; have pt avoid flossing<br>J. Avoid rectal temperatures and suppositories<br>K. Teach pt to avoid contact sports, bicycle riding, diving, gymnastics, and skating<br>L. Advocate for use of car seat and seat belt |
| II. *Activity intolerance related to fatigue or anemia* | II. A. Pt reports being tired<br>B. Pt has dyspnea after playing or activity<br>C. Pt exhibits decreased energy levels<br>D. Anemia | II. A. Pt learns limits of activity tolerance and rest when tired<br>B. Anemia is minimized by early detection and treatment | II. A. Educate parents about potential for activity intolerance due to disease and treatment<br>B. Educate parents about need to modify activities until recovery from treatment side effects has been achieved<br>C. Monitor hemoglobin and hematocrit |

*(continued)*

**Table 7.2** Standardized Nursing Care Plan for Physical Care of the Child (continued)

| Nursing Diagnosis | Defining Characteristics | Expected Outcomes | Nursing Interventions |
|---|---|---|---|
| III. *Impairment of skin integrity* | III. A. Local infiltration or failure to aspirate blood flow through IV line<br>B. Hyperpigmentation<br>C. Erythema<br>D. Burning<br>E. Inflammation<br>F. Pain<br>G. Tissue sloughing<br>H. Loss of mobility | III. A. No tissue injury occurs<br>B. Tissue injury is minimized | III. A. Be knowledgeable about vesicant drugs and institutional policy and procedure for administration and management of extravasation<br>B. Use careful technique in administering vesicants<br>C. Use central line if administering continuous infusions of vesicants<br>D. Administer drugs through free-flowing IV and constantly monitor site<br>E. Recognize signs of infiltration and respond immediately according to institutional policy and procedure<br>F. Treat extravasation according to recommended antidotes<br>G. Document occurrence of extravasation according to institutional policy |
| IV. *Alteration in oral mucous membrane* | IV. A. Pt complains of dry mouth or being thirsty<br>B. Oral pain<br>C. Coated tongue related to candidiasis<br>D. Oral lesions or ulcers<br>E. Decreased salivation or lack of salivation<br>F. Oral plaque<br>G. Erythema | IV. A. Oral mucous membrane remains intact<br>B. Mucositis is minimized by early detection and treatment<br>C. Parent and pt are able to describe care that prevents and/or minimizes mucositis | IV. A. Assess oral cavity for presence of erythema, ulceration, plaque<br>B. Pt practices good dental hygiene<br>C. If mucositis present, encourage pt to follow prescribed mouth care<br>D. Assess for presence of pain<br>E. Teach parent and pt about importance of good pain control<br>F. Teach parent dietary measures to control pain, such as nonacidic liquids, popsicles, soft foods |
| V. *Potential for alteration in comfort related to bone pain disease or treatment* | V. A. Bone pain<br>1. Can result from packed marrow in leukemia patients<br>2. Can result from tumor growth in osteosarcoma and Ewing's sarcoma<br>B. Myalgia and dysarthralgia resulting from growth factors<br>C. Neurotoxicity from drugs such as vincristine | V. A. Pain is minimized or controlled through effective assessment and treatment<br>B. Pt verbalizes pain relief<br>C. Pt is able to engage in age-appropriate activities | V. A. Use age-appropriate pain scales, such as the FACES scale, to assess pain and effectiveness of interventions<br>B. Acknowledge that whatever pain is reported is accepted as the most important criteria in assessing pain<br>C. Educate parents about the importance of pain assessment and control<br>D. Use nonpharmacologic methods to relieve pain, including distraction, music, imagery, humor, touch |

D. Symptoms can include:
1. Pt complains of pain even when involved in activities
2. Pt exhibits facial grimaces
3. Pt avoids usual activities
4. Pt limps or refuses to walk
5. Pt cries, moans, or has difficulty falling asleep
E. Blood pressure and pulse rate increase
F. Increased respiration
G. Pupil dilation
H. Irritability
I. Lethargy

| | | | |
|---|---|---|---|
| VI. *Potential for alteration in comfort related to pain from invasive procedures* | VI. A. Pt exhibits facial grimaces<br>B. Pt avoids usual activities<br>C. Pt cries or moans<br>D. Blood pressure and pulse rate increase<br>E. Increased respiration<br>F. Pupil dilation<br>G. Irritability<br>H. Pt exhibits anticipatory anxiety to pain, including crying, withdrawal, or insomnia the night before procedures<br>I. Pt exhibits combative behavior during procedures | VI. A. Pain is minimized or controlled through effective assessment and treatment<br>B. Pt verbalizes pain relief<br>C. Pt is able to cooperate with procedure | VI. A. Use age-appropriate pain scales, such as the FACES scale, to assess effectiveness of interventions<br>B. Acknowledge that whatever pain is reported is accepted as the most important criteria in assessing pain<br>C. Educate parents about the importance of pain assessment and control<br>D. Educate parents and pt about procedures using booklets, videos, medical play<br>E. Use nonpharmacologic methods to relieve pain, including imagery, humor, touch, hypnosis<br>F. Use behavioral strategies such as distraction, blowing bubbles, music, pop-up books, positive reinforcement systems |
| VII. *Altered nutrition related to*<br>A. Anorexia | VII. A. 1. Weight loss of more than 10% of prediagnosis weight<br>2. Failure to eat well-balanced diet<br>3. Reported changes in taste of food or food aversions | VII. A. 1. Maintain or improve overall nutritional status<br>2. Weight is maintained within normal levels for age and size<br>3. Complications of poor nutrition are minimized through early detection and treatment | VII. A. 1. Obtain pt and family diet history<br>2. Monitor weight and height using growth chart<br>3. Educate pt and family about increased importance of good nutrition to fight disease, heal body, and promote growth<br>4. Monitor food intake if problems are identified<br>5. Monitor CBC and blood chemistry studies |

*(continued)*

**Table 7.2** Standardized Nursing Care Plan for Physical Care of the Child (*continued*)

| Nursing Diagnosis | Defining Characteristics | Expected Outcomes | Nursing Interventions |
|---|---|---|---|
| | B. Nausea and vomiting | | B. 1. Assess for excessive anxiety, which could lead to conditioned nausea and vomiting<br>2. Premedicate with antiemetic and repeat as needed; assess therapeutic response to medication<br>3. Encourage small meals 6 times a day using cool, bland foods<br>4. Refer pt for hypnosis and imagery sessions, especially adolescents<br>5. Educate pt to observe and report amount of fluid loss and s/s of dehydration |
| | C. Weight loss | | C. 1. Use good pain management if from mucositis<br>2. Identify any food aversions and modify diet accordingly<br>3. Encourage parents to make meals and foods fun and different and to allow pt to help with meal preparation<br>4. Recommend using citrus juices to flavor foods<br>5. Recommend using a variety of flavors in foods<br>6. Assess for underlying psychological processes that may contribute to loss of appetite (e.g., loss of control)<br>7. Refer to dietitian<br>8. Encourage high-protein, high-calorie foods or diet supplements<br>9. Develop and implement positive reinforcements to encourage intake<br>10. Assess need for TPN or feeding tube |
| VIII. *Alteration in bowel elimination, constipation related to loss of appetite, poor dietary habits, and side effects of drugs* | VIII. A. Pt reports changes in bowel habits<br>B. Decreased bowel sounds<br>C. Abdominal distention<br>D. Decreased appetite<br>E. Abdominal pain<br>F. Hard stools | VIII. A. Pt maintains prediagnosis bowel pattern<br>B. Problems with constipation are minimized by early identification and treatment | VIII. A. Obtain bowel history and assess current bowel habits<br>B. Use stool softeners if pt is receiving pain medication or chemotherapy known to cause constipation<br>C. Educate family about importance of normal bowel habits and potential problems (e.g., impaction and bowel obstruction related to constipation) |

| | | | D. Educate parents in assessment of constipation |
| | | | E. Educate parents in dietary methods to prevent constipation |
| | | | F. Encourage increased intake of fluids and high-fiber foods |
| | | | G. Encourage pt to drink warm liquids, soups, etc. |
| | | | H. Encourage pt to drink apple juice |
| | | | I. Avoid use of suppositories and enemas due to potential for bleeding and infection if immunosuppressed; teach parents same |
| IX. *Alteration in bowel elimination, diarrhea related to side effects of chemotherapy and changed intestinal flora due to antibiotics* | IX. A. Pt reports changes in bowel habits <br> B. Increased bowel sounds <br> C. Abdominal pain and cramping <br> D. Loose, frequent stools <br> E. Urgency | IX. A. Pt maintains prediagnosis bowel pattern <br> B. Problems with diarrhea are minimized by early identification and treatment | IX. A. Obtain bowel history and assess current bowel habits |
| | | | B. Educate family about importance of normal bowel habits and potential problems (e.g., dehydration and weight loss related to diarrhea) |
| | | | C. Educate parents in assessment of diarrhea |
| | | | D. Educate parents in dietary methods to control and prevent worsening of diarrhea |
| | | | E. Encourage increased intake of fluids |
| | | | F. Encourage such foods as rice, bananas, yogurt, toast |
| | | | G. Teach parents to observe for skin breakdown in anal area and follow rectal care guidelines |
| | | | H. Use over-the-counter diaper rash products for red and irritated skin |
| | | | I. Teach parents to call MD if bleeding or skin tears are noted |
| | | | J. Teach parents to avoid antidiarrheal drugs unless prescribed |

*(continued)*

**Table 7.2**  Standardized Nursing Care Plan for Physical Care of the Child *(continued)*

| Nursing Diagnosis | Defining Characteristics | Expected Outcomes | Nursing Interventions |
|---|---|---|---|
| X. *Potential for fluid and electrolyte imbalance related to tumor lysis syndrome (TLS)* Tumor lysis occurs when cancer cells are quickly killed due to their high sensitivity to chemotherapy. The metabolic breakdown of the cells releases intracellular ions into the bloodstream, changing the fluid and electrolyte balance. | X. A. Commonly seen in Burkitt's lymphoma, T-cell lymphoma, and leukemia<br>B. Large tumor burden at initiation of chemotherapy treatment<br>C. Hyperkalemia<br>D. Hyperuricemia<br>E. Hyperphosphatemia<br>F. Hypocalcemia<br>G. Changes in level of consciousness and mental status<br>H. Changes in neurological status<br>I. Seizures<br>J. Weakness<br>K. Changes in pulse and cardiac rhythm<br>L. Changes in blood pressure | X. A. Urinary output is maintained at 1 ml/kg/hr or greater<br>B. Urine pH is equal to or greater than 7<br>C. Absence of uric acid crystals<br>D. Fluid and electrolyte imbalance will be minimized by early detection and treatment | X. A. Be knowledgeable about the assessment and management of TLS, especially use of IV fluids and allopurinol<br>B. Identify pts at risk for developing TLS<br>C. Notify MD immediately of any s/s in pts at risk for developing TLS<br>D. Maintain adequate hydration<br>E. Monitor electrolytes and urinary alkalinization levels<br>F. Maintain accurate I & O records<br>G. Monitor vital signs |
| XI. *Potential for fluid and electrolyte imbalance related to overwhelming sepsis* | XI. A. Changes in electrolytes<br>B. Changes in level of consciousness and mental status<br>C. Changes in neurological status<br>D. Seizures<br>E. Weakness<br>F. Change in body temperature<br>G. Changes in pulse and cardiac rhythm<br>H. Change in blood pressure | XI. A. Fluid and electrolyte imbalance will be minimized by early detection and treatment | XI. A. Be knowledgeable about the assessment and management of sepsis<br>B. Identify pts at risk for developing sepsis<br>C. Notify MD immediately of any s/s in pts at risk for developing sepsis<br>D. Maintain appropriate hydration<br>E. Monitor electrolytes<br>F. Maintain accurate I & O records<br>G. Monitor vital signs<br>H. Educate parents about s/s of sepsis and emergency nature of the problem |

| | Assessment | Outcome | Intervention |
|---|---|---|---|
| XII. ...related for fluid and electrolyte imbalance related to side effects of chemotherapy | XII. A. Signs and symptoms of dehydration<br>B. Weakness<br>C. Thirst<br>D. Diarrhea<br>E. Electrolyte imbalance<br>F. Excessive vomiting<br>G. Major change in weight loss or weight gain | XII. A. Fluid and electrolyte balance is maintained<br>B. Fluid and electrolyte imbalance is minimized by early detection and treatment | XII. A. Monitor for dehydration or edema<br>B. Monitor vital signs<br>C. Monitor electrolytes<br>D. Monitor I & O<br>E. Assess for signs of fluid overload and educate parents about the same if receiving IV fluids at home<br>F. Educate parents about potential for fluid and electrolyte imbalance and emergency nature of the problem, especially if on home IV fluids or experiencing nausea and vomiting |
| XIII. *Impaired mobility related to disease or treatment* | XIII. A. Impaired ability or complete inability to move purposefully<br>B. Presence of amputation<br>C. Presence of peripheral neuropathy<br>D. Pt complains of difficulty with ambulation and/or movement | XIII. A. Pt adapts to limitations in movement<br>B. Complications are minimized or prevented<br>C. Pt verbalizes willingness to participate in rehabilitation<br>D. Pt participates in age-appropriate activities with modifications related to loss of movement and/or function<br>E. If limb salvage, pt complies with treatment regimen and adapts to movement limitation | XIII. A. Determine pt's functional ability<br>B. Determine cause of neuropathy and educate pt and family<br>C. Assess degree of pain and treat<br>D. Assess for emotional responses to loss of limb and grief reactions<br>E. Refer pt to physical or occupational therapy and involve in exercise program<br>F. Encourage pt to wear prosthesis<br>G. Educate about limb loss or limb salvage<br>H. Refer pt to rehabilitation program<br>I. Support pt in dealing with changed body image, grief, and peer reactions<br>J. Link pt to other pts with amputations or limb salvage |

*Source:* Heiney, S.P., and Wells, L.M. (1996). Care of the pediatric oncology patient. In M. Barton-Burke, G. Wilkes, and K. Ingwersen, *Cancer Chemotherapy: A Nursing Process Approach.* 2nd ed. Sudbury, Mass.: Jones & Bartlett, 496–504. Reprinted with permission.

**Table 7.3** Standardized Nursing Care Plan for Psychosocial Care of the Family and the Child

### Family

| Nursing Diagnosis | Defining Characteristics | Expected Outcomes | Nursing Interventions |
|---|---|---|---|
| I. *Alteration in family process* | I. A. Family expresses concern over impact of pt's diagnosis on family functioning and ability to cope<br>B. Family demonstrates temporary dysfunction; increased mood lability in one or both parents<br>C. Parents have difficulty making decisions<br>D. Family has difficulty appropriately disciplining ill child | I. A. Family appropriately expresses emotions<br>B. Family establishes equilibrium and function better than before diagnosis<br>C. Family uses good problem-solving skills<br>D. Family members are able to support each other without any members being scapegoated or feeling excessive guilt<br>E. Family promotes growth and independence in sick child, siblings, and parents<br>F. Family maintains rules and sets limits with children<br>G. Family attains developmental tasks appropriate for family life<br>H. Family adapts to situation and is able to verbalize meaning the experience has for them | I. A. Assess family's strengths and weaknesses<br>B. Determine family's previous experience with crisis and method of coping<br>C. Assess family's support systems (extended family and community)<br>D. Assess boundaries of family members and presence of negative family dynamics, such as rigidity, decreased emotional expression<br>E. Promote positive resolution of crisis<br>F. Link with support systems |
| II. *Potential for growth through effective family coping* | II. A. Cancer is perceived as crisis for family<br>B. Family seeks to find meaning in cancer diagnosis<br>C. Mood lability<br>D. Temporary cognitive disturbances<br>E. Temporary impairment in usual daily functioning<br>F. Family uses positive behaviors to deal with feelings and change in family life | II. A. Family's level of functioning improves<br>B. Family expresses willingness to cope with diagnosis and its impact on family members<br>C. Family members identify their ability to cope, especially in previous stressful situations<br>D. Family members accept individual responsibilities to deal with changes brought about by diagnosis | II. A. Assess family's level of functioning and family dynamics<br>B. Assess for previous crisis situations, especially natural disasters and previous major losses, including deaths<br>C. Support parents and primary caregivers and priority focus of interventions<br>D. Promote family mental health; identify and highlight strengths<br>E. Model positive communication<br>F. Educate about s/s of crisis and time-limited nature<br>G. Discourage precipitate decision-making<br>H. Refer to support groups, educational programs, retreats |

| Nursing Diagnosis | Defining Characteristics | Expected Outcomes | Interventions |
|---|---|---|---|
| III. *Potential for anxiety and other negative emotions such as anger related to fear of death, the unknown, disease treatment* | III. A. Parents report feeling scared, overwhelmed, helpless, being in a dream, having nightmares<br>B. Parents exhibit mood lability<br>C. Restlessness<br>D. Insomnia<br>E. Sympathetic stimulation<br>F. Inability to concentrate or focus | III. A. Parents verbalize understanding about disease<br>B. Parents exhibit reduced anxiety<br>C. Parents verbalize feelings of anxiety<br>D. Anxiety is be minimized or controlled<br>E. Parents verbalize coping strategies<br>F. Parents effectively use educational and supportive resources, such as parent groups, booklets | I. Refer to educational resources<br>J. Actively listen for feelings and assist parents in identifying ways to channel feelings (e.g., journals, photo albums)<br>K. Connect families with others going through similar experience<br><br>III. A. Observe behavior and define level of anxiety<br>B. Establish rapport with family; use therapeutic communication techniques<br>C. Identify methods that parents have used in the past to deal with anxiety-producing situations<br>D. Discourage parents from precipitate decisions, such as moving closer to treatment center<br>E. Acknowledge feelings and educate about crisis reaction<br>F. Provide information about disease, procedures<br>G. Teach methods for dealing with anxiety, such as relaxation, imagery, hypnosis<br>H. Encourage physical activity and involvement in leisure and recreational activities<br>I. Encourage involvement of extended family and community groups for support<br>J. Refer parents to counseling if stress seems overwhelming |
| IV. *Knowledge deficit related to childhood cancer and care* | IV. A. Statement of concern over caring for child at home<br>B. Parents request information<br>C. Parents unable to verbalize care instructions | IV. A. Family participates actively in learning about disease and care<br>B. Parents verbalize understanding of disease and treatment and major components of care at home<br>C. Parents verbalize emergency situations and ways to deal with them | IV. A. Assess readiness to learn and learning needs<br>B. Identify other caregivers who may need to be taught care routines (baby-sitters, extended family)<br>C. Assess blocks to learning, including reading comprehension, language barriers<br>D. Assess family's motivation to learn<br>E. Establish learning priorities in conjunction with parents |

*(continued)*

**Table 7.3**   Standardized Nursing Care Plan for Psychosocial Care of the Family and the Child *(continued)*

### Family

| Nursing Diagnosis | Defining Characteristics | Expected Outcomes | Nursing Interventions |
|---|---|---|---|
| | | D. Parents correctly perform care routines, such as flushing of venous device access<br><br>E. Parents make sure that other care providers are identified to the health care team and receive appropriate education | F. Identify content of teaching sessions and separate into cognitive, affective, and psychomotor domains of learning<br><br>G. Develop objectives of teaching sessions using child's protocol, age, and stage of development<br><br>H. Identify teaching methods, including one-on-one sessions, booklets, videos ·<br><br>I. Involve parents in cancer education programs and support groups<br><br>J. Facilitate learning by providing written guidelines regarding emergency situations, anemia, thrombocytopenia, neutropenia<br><br>K. Begin teaching as soon as diagnosis is confirmed and treatment protocol has been established<br><br>L. Monitor parents' level of anxiety and provide appropriate support, time-outs, etc.<br><br>M. Provide feedback frequently<br><br>N. Assure parents of availability of backup and encourage calling about problems<br><br>O. Personalize teaching tools as much as possible; use highlighters, fill-in-the-blanks |

### Child

| Nursing Diagnosis | Defining Characteristics | Expected Outcomes | Nursing Interventions |
|---|---|---|---|
| V. *Potential for mental status changes due to prednisone or high anxiety* | V. A. Affect<br>　1. Irritability<br>　2. Exaggerated emotional responses<br>　3. Rapid mood swings<br>B. Behavior<br>　1. Altered communication patterns<br>　2. Changes in behavior patterns<br>　3. Restlessness<br>　4. Changes in sleep patterns | V. A. Early s/s of mental status changes are identified | V. A. Observe for behavioral responses<br><br>B. Listen to family concerns related to pt's mental status<br><br>C. Provide environment with minimal stimuli<br><br>D. Explain new events in simple terms<br><br>E. Provide visual and auditory diversion if pt is actively hallucinating |

C. Cognition
1. Poor concentration
2. Disordered thought sequencing
3. Disoriented to time, place, or person
4. Change in problem-solving ability
5. Bizarre thinking
6. Hallucinations
7. Delusions

| Nursing Diagnosis | Signs/Symptoms | Expected Outcomes | Interventions |
|---|---|---|---|
| VI. *Potential for somnolence syndrome* Somnolence syndrome is a condition that may occur 6–8 weeks after cranial radiation and is characterized by excessive sleepiness and other mental status and physical changes. | VI. A. Nausea and vomiting<br>B. Lethargy<br>C. Diarrhea<br>D. Low-grade fever<br>E. Weight loss<br>F. Fussiness<br>G. Changes in sleep patterns | VI. A. Pt returns to normal functioning<br>B. Parents verbalize understanding of syndrome | VI. A. Monitor for s/s of somnolence syndrome within 4–10 weeks after completion of XRT<br>B. Educate parents about syndrome<br>C. Help parents understand that time is the only treatment<br>D. Refer pt for rehabilitation if permanent brain damage is noted<br>E. Maintain nutritional status |
| VII. *Potential for sensory/perceptual alterations related to* Temporary cranial edema due to radiation CNS tumor site Specific side effects of drug | VII. A. Reported or measured changes in sensory acuity<br>B. Decreased motor coordination<br>C. Problems communicating<br>D. Changes in usual response to stimuli | VII. A. Sensory impairments are recognized or treated<br>B. Early s/s of neurological toxicity are identified<br>C. Late effects of CNS toxicity are identified | VII. A. Monitor for peripheral neurotoxicities of chemotherapy<br>B. Monitor for s/s of increased CNS pressure (e.g., seizures)<br>C. Assist pt and parents with learning effective ways of coping with deficits<br>D. Refer parents to appropriate agencies for dealing with perceptual deficits<br>E. Teach family safety measures that need to be instituted in the home<br>F. Educate family about potential for late effects, especially learning difficulties |

*(continued)*

**Table 7.3** Standardized Nursing Care Plan for Psychosocial Care of the Family and the Child (*continued*)

*Child*

| Nursing Diagnosis | Defining Characteristics | Expected Outcomes | Nursing Interventions |
|---|---|---|---|
| VIII. *Potential for alteration in self-concept related to* Alopecia Weight changes Acne Loss of body part Scars Loss of function | VIII. A. Fear of peer rejection<br>B. Focus on past strengths, appearance, or function<br>C. Negative feelings about body, especially adolescents<br>D. Feeling of helplessness, hopelessness, powerlessness<br>E. Preoccupation with change or loss, especially adolescents<br>F. Personalization of part or loss by name<br>G. Amputation or enucleation<br>H. Not looking at body part<br>I. Actual change in structure or function<br>J. Change in social involvement, especially adolescents<br>K. Change in degree of independence<br>L. Overcompensating for loss<br>M. Greatest risk for poor psychosocial adaptation for females who have lost a body part | VIII. A. Pt verbalizes acceptance of self in light of loss of body part or function<br>B. Pt verbalizes relief of anxiety regarding altered body image<br>C. Pt seeks knowledge and skills to cope with loss<br>D. Pt maintains or improves self-esteem<br>E. Side effects of chemotherapy are reduced or eliminated | VIII. A. Assess for potential changes in body image and self-concept<br>B. Assess pt's interaction with family and peer network and note problem areas<br>C. Assist pt in identifying major component of body image and impact of loss in that area<br>D. Incorporate ethnic and cultural aspects of body image into plan of care<br>E. Encourage pt to verbalize perceptions of changes, their meaning, and feelings, as well as impact on life; promote discussions about these<br>F. Assess for changes in mood and/or mood lability or s/s of depression; refer for counseling<br>G. Educate pt and family about body image changes, especially temporary ones related to hair loss, acne, weight changes<br>H. Assist pt to deal with changes; teach ways to cope with changes and refer to image-building programs<br>I. Encourage family to allow pt to be independent, especially adolescents |
| IX. *Knowledge deficit related to childhood cancer and care* | IX. A. Statement of concern about disease<br>B. Questions about disease and treatment<br>C. Inability to verbalize care instructions | IX. A. Pt participate actively in learning about disease and care<br>B. Pt verbalizes understanding of disease and treatment and major components of care at home<br>C. Pt identifies situations that are considered emergencies (e.g., temperature of 101°F) and ways to deal with them | IX. A. Assess pt's readiness to learn and learning needs<br>B. Assess blocks to learning, including reading comprehension, language barriers, anxiety<br>C. Assess pt's motivation to learn<br>D. Establish learning priorities in conjunction with pt<br>E. Identify content of teaching sessions and separate into cognitive, affective, and psychomotor domains of learning<br>F. Identify teaching methods, including one-on-one sessions, booklets, videos<br>G. Involve pt in cancer education programs |

| Nursing Diagnosis | Signs and Symptoms | Expected Outcomes | Interventions |
|---|---|---|---|
| | | | D. Pt appropriately participates in any care routines, such as mouth care |
| | | | and support groups |
| | | | H. Facilitate learning by providing age-appropriate tools such as coloring books, videos, games |
| | | | I. Begin teaching as soon as diagnosis is confirmed and treatment protocol has been established |
| | | | J. Monitor pt's level of anxiety and provide appropriate support, time-outs, etc. |
| | | | K. Provide feedback frequently |
| X. Potential for non-compliance with self-care, especially in adolescents, related to oral chemotherapy regimens and prophylactic antibiotics | X. A. Subtherapeutic levels of drug<br>B. Blood counts do not reflect expected changes<br>C. Failure to keep appointments<br>D. High anxiety | X. A. Pt and family participate in educational sessions about disease and treatment<br>B. Pt and family agree who has responsibility for administration home drug<br>C. Pt reports drug compliance<br>D. Pt evidences compliance based on drug calendar and/or drug levels<br>E. Pt and family report compliance with neutropenic and thrombocytopenic guidelines | X. A. Educate pt and family using written material about disease, treatment, potential for recurrence, and problems, as well as home care routine<br>B. Periodically recheck level of understanding<br>C. Determine potential cultural, familial, and personal factors that may contribute to noncompliance<br>D. Listen and respond to pt and family concerns about treatment<br>E. Assess level of anxiety and any underlying psychosocial processes that may be contributing to noncompliance<br>F. Work with pt and family regarding ways to improve compliance and develop written contract to improve compliance<br>G. Develop and implement positive reinforcement system to improve compliance, especially in young children<br>H. Refer to individual or family counseling if origins of compliance appear to be family or personality related<br>I. Refer for imagery or hypnosis if noncompliance is related to nausea or difficulty swallowing |
| XI. Potential for anxiety and other negative emotions such as anger | XI. A. Pt reports feeling scared<br>B. Pt reports nightmares<br>C. Pt tells stories with content that reflects worry or concern<br>D. Pt draws pictures that contain references to disease that reflect worry<br>E. Pt's imaginative play reflects worry or concern | XI. A. Pt verbalizes understanding about disease<br>B. Pt exhibits reduced anxiety<br>C. Pt verbalizes feelings of anxiety<br>D. Pt verbalizes age-appropriate coping strategies | XI. A. Observe behavior and define level of anxiety<br>B. Identify methods pt has used in the past to deal with anxiety-producing situations<br>C. Encourage pt to use projective techniques for expressing and working through anxiety (i.e., therapeutic play, art therapy, music therapy)<br>D. Acknowledge feelings |

*(continued)*

**Table 7.3** Standardized Nursing Care Plan for Psychosocial Care of the Family and the Child *(continued)*

### Child

| Nursing Diagnosis | Defining Characteristics | Expected Outcomes | Nursing Interventions |
|---|---|---|---|
| | F. Pt verbalizes fear<br>G. Pt reports vague somatic complaints, such as stomachache, headache<br>H. Hyperactivity<br>I. Restlessness<br>J. Insomnia, night wakening<br>K. Sympathetic stimulation | E. Pt uses educational and support resources effectively | E. Provide information about disease, procedures, etc., using puppets, play, videos<br>F. Teach methods for dealing with anxiety, such as relaxation, imagery, hypnosis<br>G. Encourage physical activity and normal developmental tasks<br>H. Encourage use of punching bag and other means for acting out negative emotions in noninjurious ways<br>I. Refer pt to play groups and oncology camps |
| XII. *Potential for alterations in behavior* | XII. A. Return to earlier developmental stage or activity, such as bed-wetting or use of pacifier, that lasts longer than several weeks<br>B. Notable personality changes<br>C. Decreased school performance<br>D. Behavioral acting out in social situations and school<br>E. Temper tantrums<br>F. Increased sibling arguments<br>G. Dysfunctional family dynamics<br>H. Inappropriate reactions to health care provider or evidence of knowledge about sexual activity beyond age level | XII. A. Pt maintains or improves behavior<br>B. Pt's school performance is maintained or improved<br>C. Pt demonstrates age-appropriate developmental behavior<br>D. Family maintains or improves discipline<br>E. Family uses positive parenting skills | XII. A. Educate family about importance of maintaining normal life, limits, discipline<br>B. Educate family about importance of promoting normal growth and development and school participation<br>C. Involve pt in school reentry program<br>D. Refer pt to counseling if inappropriate behaviors persist<br>E. Develop and implement positive reinforcement systems to improve behavior<br>F. Assess pt for physical and sexual abuse<br>G. Encourage independence in pt<br>H. Encourage pt and family participation in support groups<br>I. Refer family to parent education programs<br>J. Refer to family therapy |

## *Siblings*

| Nursing Diagnosis | Defining Characteristics | Expected Outcomes | Nursing Interventions |
| --- | --- | --- | --- |
| XIII. *Potential for anxiety and other negative emotions such as anger* | XIII. A. Sibling verbalizes variety of feelings about situation, especially resentment<br>B. Sibling reports feeling scared<br>C. Sibling reports nightmares<br>D. School-aged sibling develops behavioral problems, decreased school performance<br>E. Sibling reports vague somatic complaints, such as stomachache, headache<br>F. Hyperactivity<br>G. Restlessness<br>H. Insomnia<br>I. Sympathetic stimulation | XIII. A. Sibling verbalizes understanding about disease<br>B. Sibling exhibits reduced anxiety<br>C. Sibling verbalizes feelings of anxiety<br>D. Sibling verbalizes age-appropriate coping strategies<br>E. Sibling uses educational and support resources effectively | XIII. A. Observe behavior and define level of anxiety<br>B. Identify methods that sibling has used in the past to deal with anxiety-producing situations<br>C. Encourage sibling to use projective techniques for expressing and working through anxiety (i.e., therapeutic play, art therapy, music therapy)<br>D. Acknowledge feelings<br>E. Provide information about disease, procedures, etc., using puppets, play, videos<br>F. Teach methods for dealing with anxiety, such as relaxation, imagery, hypnosis<br>G. Encourage physical activity and fulfillment of normal developmental tasks<br>H. Encourage use of punching bag and other means for acting out negative emotions in noninjurious ways<br>I. Refer to siblings programs and cancer camps if available |
| XIV. *Knowledge deficit related to childhood cancer and care* | XIV. A. Statement of concern about disease<br>B. Questions about disease and treatment<br>C. Inability to verbalize care instructions<br>D. Sibling avoids asking about pt or disease; refuses to visit pt in hospital | XIV. A. Sibling participates actively in learning about disease<br>B. Sibling verbalizes understanding of disease and treatment<br>C. Sibling identifies situations that are considered emergencies (e.g., temperature of 101°F) and what to do if one occurs | XIV. A. Assess readiness to learn and learning needs<br>B. Assess blocks to learning, including reading comprehension, language barriers, anxiety<br>C. Assess motivation to learn<br>D. Establish learning priorities in conjunction with sibling<br>E. Identify content of teaching sessions and separate into cognitive, affective, and psychomotor domains of learning<br>F. Identify teaching methods, including one-on-one sessions, booklets, videos<br>G. Involve sibling in sibling teaching groups, cancer education programs, support groups<br>H. Facilitate learning by providing age-appropriate tools such as coloring books, videos, games |

*(continued)*

**Table 7.3** Standardized Nursing Care Plan for Psychosocial Care of the Family and the Child (*continued*)

### Siblings

| Nursing Diagnosis | Defining Characteristics | Expected Outcomes | Nursing Interventions |
|---|---|---|---|
| | | | I. Begin teaching as soon as diagnosis is confirmed and treatment protocol has been established |
| | | | J. Assure sibling that disease is not catching and that he or she did nothing to cause disease |
| | | | K. Monitor sibling's level of anxiety and provide appropriate support, time-outs, etc. |
| | | | L. Provide feedback frequently |

*Source:* Heiney, S.P., and Wells, L.M. (1996). Care of the pediatric oncology patient. In M. Barton-Burke, G. Wilkes, and K. Ingwersen. *Cancer Chemotherapy: A Nursing Process Approach.* 2nd ed. Sudbury, Mass.: Jones & Bartlett, 505–516. Reprinted with permission.

**Table 7.4** Age-Adjusted Incidence Rates Per Million for Specific Leukemia by Age Groups All Races, Both Sexes, SEER, 1990–95

| Age (in Years) at Diagnosis | < 5 | 5–9 | 10–14 | 15–19 | < 15* |
|---|---|---|---|---|---|
| Total leukemia | 72.4 (100%) | 38.0 (100%) | 25.9 (100%) | 26.0 (100%) | 43.8 (100%) |
| ALL | 58.1 (80%) | 30.6 (81%) | 17.4 (67%) | 13.0 (50%) | 34.0 (78%) |
| AML (Ib) | 10.3 (14%) | 5.0 (13%) | 6.2 (24%) | 9.3 (36%) | 7.0 (16%) |
| CML (Ic) | 1.1 (2%) | 0.7 (2%) | 1.1 (4%) | 2.2 (9%) | 1.0 (2%) |
| Other specified leukemias (Id) | 0.3 (–) | 0.3 (1%) | 0.1 (–) | 0.1 (–) | 0.2 (1%) |
| Unspecified leukemias (Ie) | 2.2 (3%) | 1.0 (3%) | 0.6 (2%) | 1.1 (4%) | 1.2 (3%) |

* Rates are adjusted to the 1970 US standard population. Numbers in parentheses represent the percentage of the total cases for the specific age group.

*Source:* Smith, M.A., Ries, L.A.G., Gurney, J.G., and Ross, J.A. (1999). Leukemia. In L.A.G. Ries, M.A. Smith, J.G. Gurney, M. Linet, T. Tamra, J.L. Young, and G.R. Buni (eds.): *Cancer Incidence and Survival among Children and Adolescents: United States SEER Program 1975–1995.* Bethesda, Md.: National Cancer Institute, SEER Program. NIH Publication 99-4649.

The incidence rates by location within the brain and other CNS sites as a function of age are shown in Figure 7.2. Unlike adults and older children who have higher rates in the cerebrum, young children have a relatively high occurrence of malignancies in the cerebellum and the brain stem. In fact, in children between the ages of 5 and 9, the brain stem malignancies were nearly as common as cerebral malignancies and cerebellum malignancies were far more common than cerebral malignancies. The pattern shifts among children between the ages of 10 and 19; the incidence of both brain stem and cerebellar cancers decreased, whereas cerebral cancers malignancies increased slightly. The "other" brain site group included the ventricles where ependymomas generally develop and malignancies with brain sites not otherwise specified. The "Other CNS" category found in the illustration includes malignancies of the meninges, cranial nerves, and spinal cord (SEER Data 1999).

Unfortunately, patients with these tumors continue to have an unfavorable prognosis. Even though not all brain tumors are malignant, a benign tumor that requires intensive therapy can have a devastating effect on the immature brain of the child (Rasco 1998; Ries, Percy, and Bunin 1999).

Lymphomas are the third most common malignancy in the pediatric population. Non-Hodgkin's lymphoma accounts for 60% of diagnosed pediatric lymphomas and includes small noncleaved cell (Burkitt's), lymphoblastic, and large cell types. Hodgkin's disease accounts for the remaining 40 percent. Lymphomas are seen in both the pediatric population and the adult population; however, the subtypes are treated very differently (Sandlund, Downing, and Crist 1996).

## Clinical Trials in Pediatric Oncology

A clinical trial is a research study designed to answer a specific medical question. The conduct of clinical trials requires the development of a protocol that contains background information and specific instructions about how to carry out all the elements of the clinical study.

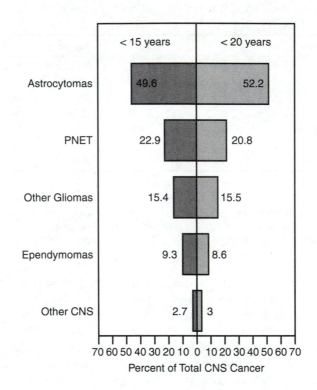

**Figure 7.1** **Percent Distribution of Malignant CNS Tumors by Age and Histologic Group, All Races, Both Sexes, SEER, 1975–95.**
*Source:* Gurney, J.G., Smith, M.A., and Bunin, G.R. (1999). CNS and miscellaneous intracranial and intraspinal neoplasms. In L.A.G. Ries, M.A. Smith, J.G. Gurney, M. Linet, T. Tamra, J.L. Young, and G.R. Bunin (eds.): *Cancer Incidence and Survival among Children and Adolescents: United States SEER Program 1975–1995.* Bethesda, Md.: National Cancer Institute, SEER Program. NIH Publication 99-4649.

If a clinical trial is well designed, it answers the research question and provides reliable data that are easy to interpret (Cheson 1991; Ungerleider and Ellenberg 1997).

Clinical trials can be divided into three phases. A phase I study determines the maximum tolerated dose (MTD) of a certain chemotherapeutic agent or combination of agents and determines the toxicity associated with treatment. A phase II study determines the effectiveness of the agent against particular types of diseases. A phase III study assesses the activity of the agent in comparison to that of the current or standard therapy (Craig 1998; Jenkins and Hubbard 1991; Ungerleider and Ellenberg 1997).

Before participants are enrolled in a clinical trial, they must give written informed consent. However, because children have limited autonomy, they require special consideration from those conducting pediatric trials. Children are considered vulnerable subjects.

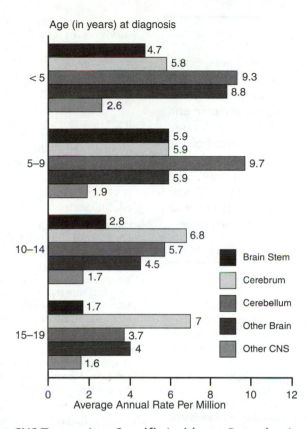

Age (in years) at diagnosis

**Figure 7.2**   Malignant CNS Tumor Age-Specific Incidence Rates by Anatomic Site and Age All Races, Both Sexes, SEER, 1975–95.

*Source:* Gurney, J.G., Smith, M.A., and Bunin, G.R. (1999). CNS and miscellaneous intracranial and intraspinal neoplasms. In L.A.G. Ries, M.A. Smith, J.G. Gurney, M. Linet, T. Tamra, J.L. Young, and G.R. Bunin (eds.): *Cancer Incidence and Survival among Children and Adolescents: United States SEER Program 1975–1995.* Bethesda, Md.: National Cancer Institute, SEER Program. NIH Publication 99-4649.

Because the child cannot legally give consent for research or treatment, parents must give their "permission" for a child to participate in a study. Pediatric patients between the ages of 7 and 14 years should be allowed to indicate their willingness (assent) or unwillingness (dissent) to participate in the study. Children should be given an age-appropriate explanation of the study, including any risks and benefits. For the very young child (preschool or younger), the parent's permission is generally the only consent required. It is advisable to have children sign an age-appropriate consent document, in addition to the standard detailed consent form that is signed by the parent or guardian. Today, more than 80% of pediatric oncology patients are enrolled in clinical trials. If a clinical trial is well designed, it answers the research question and provides reliable data that are easy to interpret (Cheson 1991; Dunn and Chadwick 1999).

## CONCLUSION

This chapter presents just one small perspective of the oncology nursing subspecialty, pediatric oncology. The authors have attempted to give a brief overview of this area of cancer care and the chemotherapy-related issues. For a more in-depth and comprehensive discussion of the care of the pediatric oncology patient, the reader is directed to Foley, Fochtman, and Mooney (1993) *Nursing Care of the Child with Cancer* and Hockenberry-Eaton (1998) *Essentials of Pediatric Oncology Nursing: A Core Curriculum.*

## BIBLIOGRAPHY

Balis, F.M., Holcenberg, J.S., and Poplack, D.G. (1997). General principles of chemotherapy. In P.A. Pizzo and D.G. Poplack (eds.): *Principles and Practice of Pediatric Oncology.* 3rd ed. Philadelphia: Lippincott-Raven, 215–272.

Bru, G.D. (1998). History and philosophy of pediatric oncology nursing. In M. Hockenberry-Eaton (ed.): *Essentials of Pediatric Oncology Nursing: A Core Curriculum.* Glenview, Ill.: Association of Pediatric Oncology Nursing, 2–5.

Cheson, B.D. (1991). Cancer clinical trials. Clinical trials programs. *Seminars in Oncology Nursing* 7(4): 235–242.

Cohen, D.G. (1998). Leukemia in children and adolescents. In G. Foley, D. Fochtman, and K. Mooney (eds.): *Nursing Care and the Child with Cancer.* 2nd ed. Philadelphia: W.B. Saunders, 208–225.

Craig, C.E. (1998). Clinical trials. In M. Hockenberry-Eaton (ed.): *Essentials of Pediatric Oncology Nursing: A Core Curriculum.* Glenview, Ill.: Association of Pediatric Oncology Nursing, 77–78.

———. (1998). History of chemotherapy. In M. Hockenberry-Eaton (ed.): *Essentials of Pediatric Oncology Nursing: A Core Curriculum.* Glenview, Ill.: of Pediatric Oncology Nursing, 75–76.

DeLaat, C., and Lampkin, B.C. (1992). Long-term survivors of childhood cancer: Evaluation and identification of sequelae of treatment. *CA—Cancer Journal for Clinicians* 42(5): 263–282.

Dunn, C.M., and Chadwick, G. (1999). Ethics and federal regulations. In *Protecting Study Volunteers in Research.* Boston: CenterWatch, Inc., 15–32.

Foley, G., and Fergusson, J. (1993). History, issues and trends. In G. Foley, D. Fochtman, and K. Mooney (eds.): *Nursing Care of the Child with Cancer.* 2nd ed. Philadelphia: W.B. Saunders, 1–24.

Foley, G., Fochtman, D. and Mooney, K. (eds.): (1993). *Nursing Care of the Child with Cancer.* 2nd ed. Philadelphia: W.B. Saunders.

Gurney, J.G., Smith, M.A., and Bunin, G.R. (1999). CNS and miscellaneous intracranial and intraspinal neoplasms. In L.A.G. Ries, M.A. Smith, J.G. Gurney, M. Linet, T. Tamra, J.L. Young, and G.R. Bunin (eds.): *Cancer Incidence and Survival among Children and Adolescents: United States SEER Program 1975–1995.* Bethesda, Md.: National Cancer Institute, SEER Program. NIH Publication 99-4649.

Hasenauer, B.F. (1998). Gene therapy. In M. Hockenberry-Eaton (ed.): *Essentials of Pediatric Oncology Nursing: A Core Curriculum.* Glenview, Ill.: Association of Pediatric Oncology Nursing, 112–15.

Heiney, S.P., and Wells, L.M. (1996). Care of the pediatric oncology patient. In M. Barton-Burke, G. Wilkes, and K. Ingwersen. *Cancer Chemotherapy. A Nursing Approach.* 2nd ed. Sudbury, Mass.: Jones & Bartlett, 496–504.

Hockenberry-Eaton, M. (1998). *Essentials of Pediatric Oncology Nursing: A Core Curriculum.* Glenview, Ill.: Association of Pediatric Oncology Nursing.

Hockenberry-Eaton, M., and Kline, N.E. (1997). Nursing support of the child with cancer. In P.A. Pizzo and D.G. Poplack (eds.): *Principles and Practice of Pediatric Oncology.* 3rd ed. Philadelphia: Lippincott-Raven, 1209–1239.

Jenkins, J., and Hubbard, S. (1991). History of clinical trials. *Seminars in Oncology Nursing* 7(4): 228–234.

Landis, S.H., Murray T., Bolden S., and Wingo, P.A. (1999). Cancer statistics, 1999. *CA—Cancer Journal for Clinicians* 49(1): 8–31.

Mooney, K.H. (1993). Biologic basis of childhood cancer. In G. Foley, D. Fochtman, and K. Mooney (eds.): *Nursing Care and the Child with Cancer.* 2nd ed. Philadelphia: W.B. Saunders, 25–55.

O'Neill, J.B., Cleveland, M.J., Forte, K., Harvey, J., Hooke, C., Kelly, K.P., Mosher, R., and Siever, J.D. (2000). *Scope and Standards of Pediatric Oncology Nursing Practice.* Washington, D.C.: American Nurses Publishing.

Pratt, W.B., Ruddon, R.W., Ensminger, W.D., and Maybaum, J. (1994). Some milestones in the development of cancer chemotherapy. In *The Anticancer Drugs.* 2nd ed. New York: University Press, 18–25.

Pui, C.H. (1998). Recent advances in the biology and the treatment of childhood acute lymphoblastic leukemia. *Current Opinions in Hematology* 5(4): 292–301.

Rasco, C. (1998). Overview of childhood cancer. In M. Hockenberry-Eaton (ed.): *Essentials of Pediatric Oncology Nursing: A Core Curriculum.* Glenview, Ill.: Association of Pediatric Oncology Nursing, 11–12.

Ries, L.A.G., Percy, C., and Bunin, G.R. (1999). Cancer incidence and survival among children and adolescents: United States SEER program 1975–1995. Bethesda, Md.: National Institutes of Health, http://www-seer.ims.nci.nih.gov/Publications/PedMono/

Rivera, G.K., Pinkel, D., Simone, J.V., Hancock, M.L., and Crist, W.M. (1993). Treatment of acute lymphoblastic leukemia. Thirty years' experience at St. Jude Children's Research Hospital. *New England Journal of Medicine* 329(18): 1289–1295.

Sandlund, J.T., Downing, J.R., and Crist, W.M. (1996). Non-Hodgkin's lymphoma in childhood. *New England Journal of Medicine* 334: 1238–48.

Smith, M.A., Ries, L.A.G., Gurney, J.G., and Ross, J.A. (1999). Leukemia. In L.A.G. Ries, M.A. Smith, J.G. Gurney, M. Linet, T. Tamra, J.L. Young, and G.R. Bunin (eds.): *Cancer Incidence and Survival among Children and Adolescents: United States SEER Program 1975–1995.* Bethesda, Md.: National Cancer Institute, SEER Program. NIH Publication 99–4649.

Ungerleider, R.S., and Ellenberg, S.S. (1997). Cancer clinical trials: Design, conduct, analysis, and reporting. In P.A. Pizzo and D.G. Poplack (eds.): *Principles and Practice of Pediatric Oncology.* 3rd ed. Philadelphia: Lippincott-Raven, 385–406.

Walker, C. (1998). Association of pediatric oncology nurses. In M. Hockenberry-Eaton (ed.): *Essentials of Pediatric Oncology Nursing: A Core Curriculum.* Glenview, Ill.: Association of Pediatric Oncology Nursing, 5–7.

Yarbro, J.W. (1996). The scientific basis of chemotherapy. In M.C. Perry (ed.): *The Chemotherapy Source Book.* Baltimore: Williams and Wilkins, 3–18.

# Chapter 8

# Chemotherapy in the Elderly
## Considerations for Clinical Practice

### Constance Engelking, RN, MS, OCN

## INTRODUCTION

Caring for older adults with cancer is analogous to being on the crest of a wave. That analogy is especially relevant because it reflects two stunning surges germane to gero-oncology: the surge in our geriatric population and the surge in cancer incidence among the elderly. The population of those 65 years of age and older is undergoing dramatic, even explosive expansion. Currently accounting for 12.5% of the U.S. population (i.e., 31.1 million), the 65+ year age group is projected to grow to about 16% of our population by the year 2010. As longevity continues to increase in the next century, the elderly are expected to account for one in five Americans by 2033 (double our current number) and will encompass fully one-quarter of the total population by 2050 (Trimble et al. 1994; U.S. Census Bureau 1990). Of particular note is the observation that 5-year survival has become considerably more important for 65-year-olds, who are expected to live an additional 20 years (Lichtman 1995), and even for 85-year-olds, who currently have a 5.5-year (men) to 7-year (women) life expectancy (Cohen 1995).

The surge in our geriatric population and increasing longevity hold special significance in light of the fact that cancer incidence increases logarithmically after age 40, thus making age the single most important risk factor for the development of malignant disease. Currently, more than half of all cancers are diagnosed in those over the age of 65. Comparatively, according to the National Cancer Institute Surveillance, Epidemiology, and End Results (SEER) program, the occurrence of cancer in those over 65 years of age is 10 times greater than in their younger counterparts. Mortality rates also are significantly higher in older adults with cancer, documented to account for more than two-thirds of all deaths attributable to neoplastic diseases in 1994 (American Cancer Society 1995; Boyle et al. 1992; Giovanazzi-Bannon, Rademaker, Lai, and Benson 1994; Miller, Ries, Hankey et al. 1993).

Because these intersecting trends will result in a sizable population of geriatric cancer patients in need of treatment, the elderly are an especially appropriate target group for cancer control activities and for cancer clinical trials focused on defining optimal therapy for this age group (Yancik and Ries 1994). In fact, the elderly have been identified as "one of the most important groups for future cancer treatment trials" (Trimble et al. 1994). Moreover, the Oncology Nursing Society position paper on cancer and aging mandates, among other things, attention to building a knowledge base about the interrelationship between cancer and aging, incorporating gerontologic aspects into cancer nursing assessment, and implementing interventions to ameliorate age-specific sequelae of cancer treatment (Table 8.1). Yet the elderly continue to face an array of barriers to optimal cancer treatment and care (Boyle et al. 1992; Giovanazzi-Bannon et al. 1994; McKenna 1994).

The intent of this chapter is to provide an overview of philosophic and physiologic treatment barriers encountered by older adults with cancer and to highlight considerations for the modification of assessment, planning, and implementation of nursing care for elderly patients undergoing chemotherapy alone or in combination with other modalities for the treatment of cancer.

## BARRIERS TO TREATMENT

### Effects of Ageism

The issue of age bias has a particularly dramatic negative impact on both the recommendation and the administration of antineoplastic drug therapy, as well as on the post therapy care received by older adults with cancer. *Ageism* is a term applied to the stigmatizing effects of societal prejudice toward the aging process and older individuals. This prejudice causes people to make stereotypic assumptions about, discriminate against, ignore, isolate, and otherwise disassociate from those considered to be elderly. Ageist views have traditionally hindered the older adult's access to aggressive but optimal cancer therapies, thus interfering with the achievement of positive treatment outcomes and, perhaps, contributing to higher cancer mortality rates among the elderly.

**Table 8.1**    Oncology Nursing Society Position Statements on Cancer and Aging

1. It is imperative for oncology nurses to recognize personal biases toward aging and the elderly that may interfere with the delivery of quality nursing care.
2. It is imperative that oncology nurses advocate cancer prevention and early detection activities for older adults.
3. It is imperative that oncology nurses acknowledge the dynamic and complex interrelationships between cancer and aging that affect cancer nursing care.
4. It is imperative that oncology nurses intervene to prevent or minimize the unique age-specific sequelae of cancer and its management.
5. It is imperative that oncology nurses integrate comprehensive gerontologic assessment into the nursing care of older adults.
6. It is imperative that oncology nurses assess the availability and capability of the support networks of elderly patients and their significant others.
7. It is imperative that oncology nurses increase communication with colleagues to enhance problem-solving in a variety of settings and at different points along the cancer continuum.
8. It is imperative that oncology nurses consider age-related factors that affect learning and performance of self-care activities related to the cancer experience.
9. It is imperative that oncology nurses maximize their advocacy role in ethical decision-making relative to quality of life of elderly people with cancer.
10. It is imperative that oncology nurses recognize the effects of health care policy on the nursing care of older adults who have or who are at risk of cancer.

*Source:* Boyle, D.M., et al. (1992). Oncology Nursing Society position paper on cancer and aging: The mandate for oncology nursing. *Oncology Nursing Forum* 19(6): 913–933.

The practice of using chronologic rather than biologic age as a component of the eligibility criteria for treatment is a direct outgrowth of ageism and the associated perspective that equates chronologic age with poor prognosis, frailty, cognitive impairment, and limited life expectancy. This view regards the elderly as a homogeneous group; it rules out consideration of an individual's actual physiologic status, demonstrated stamina, and other unique personal characteristics when formulating treatment recommendations; and it contributes heavily to the widely held opinion that the elderly, by virtue of age alone, are unable to withstand the physiologic rigors of aggressive anticancer therapy (Berkman, Rohan, and Sampson 1994; Boyle et al. 1992; McKenna 1994).

### State-of-the-Art

Evidence that age bias exists and that it dictates practice is clear (Koeller 1993; McKenna 1994). Although studies targeting the elderly are gradually being introduced, older adults have been significantly underrepresented in cancer treatment trials. A review of 8,000 elderly patients accrued to National Cancer Institute–sponsored trials for cancers with the highest mortality rates in 1992 was compared with 1990 SEER incidence data to determine representation of those over the age of 65 years. Of all patients accrued, only 39% of men and 29.5 of women accrued to the trials were older adults (Trimble et al. 1994). Indicators of underrepresentation also are evident in studies targeting specific tumor types. For example, an evaluation of 11,450 women who underwent chemotherapy for breast cancer by the Early Breast Cancer Trialists' Collaborative Group (1992) determined that only 274 of those women were older than 70 years. Similarly, a review of accrual to two breast cancer studies of the Cancer and Leukemia Group B revealed that fewer than 40% of subjects were women 70 years of age or older despite the high incidence of breast cancer in that age group (Wood et al. 1994). These results confirm earlier findings of the Southwest Oncology Group (Goodwin, Hunt, and Humble 1988) that those over 70 years of age are rarely accrued to cancer treatment trials that the group sponsors. Trimble and colleagues (1994) propose six possible explanations for low accrual of older patients to cancer clinical trials (Table 8.2). Each of the reasons cited is based on an ageist perspective on the part of either providers or consumers of cancer care.

Despite limited study of chemotherapy toxicity and efficacy in the elderly, investigational drug protocols have traditionally imposed the arbitrary age limit of 65 or 70 years as an eligibility standard. Other exclusion criteria that put clinical trials out of reach for most older adults are those related to having a history of previous malignancy or other chronic illnesses (including Alzheimer's and depression), presentation with late-stage cancer, and inadequacy of func-

**Table 8.2    Possible Reasons for Ineligibility and Subsequent Underrepresentation of Older Adults in Cancer Treatment Trials**

Increased risk for history of prior malignancy

Presence of one or more comorbid illnesses

Present with advanced-stage disease

Decreased likelihood of seeking out or considering enrollment in clinical trials

Perceptions of clinicians, family members, and patients that the benefit of and ability to tolerate aggressive anticancer regimens are low

Lack of Medicare reimbursement for cancer treatment and supportive care deemed to be "experimental"

*Source*: Trimble, E.L., et al. (1994). Representation of older patients in cancer treatment trials. *Cancer* 74 (7 Suppl): 2208–2214. Reprinted with permission.

tional status and organ function, all of which are common in the elderly. Although the exclusion of older adults from receiving aggressive experimental drug regimens was discontinued in the mid-1980s, when age eligibility was loosened on paper, age bias subsequently expanded to conventional regimens, and exclusionary practices still exist today. In one recent university-based study, more than half the physicians surveyed reported using age as the sole exclusionary criterion for anticancer treatment (Benson et al. 1991).

Several other studies comparing cancer treatment among older and younger patients revealed that those over 65 years of age were less likely to be considered for or to receive postsurgical chemotherapy or radiotherapy (Mor, Masterson-Allen, Goldberg et al. 1985; Silliman, Guadagnoli, Weitberg et al. 1989). Less rigorous pursuit of adjuvant therapies also has been documented. Markman and colleagues (1993) found that older patients with ovarian cancer were less frequently referred to a major cancer center for either adjuvant or salvage therapy. Similarly, the number of older women entered into ovarian cancer treatment trials sponsored by the Gynecologic Oncology Group constituted only 18% of the total accrual despite the fact that 48% of ovarian cancer occurs in women over the age of 65 years (Young et al. 1993).

Undertreatment (i.e., receiving lower than optimal drug dosages), resulting in poorer survival, has been documented among the elderly as well (Bonadonna and Valagussa 1981; Samet, Hunt, Key, Humble, and Goodwin 1986). In the treatment of non-Hodgkin's lymphoma, for example, a 25% dosage reduction for those over the age of 65 has been a general rule of thumb even in the absence of comorbid illness (Byrne and Carney 1993). Although reduced dosing of chemotherapeutic agents will comprise tumor response and survival in the elderly, it will not necessarily produce significant reductions in the incidence and severity of toxicity (Knopf, Fulmer, and Mion 1993).

The unfortunate result of age bias is that those who are 65 years of age or older are often denied both the opportunity to participate in clinical trials that could ultimately define optimal treatment for cancer patients in this age group, as well as the opportunity to receive therapies that might ensure enhanced survival and, possibly, cure. At the same time, clinicians responsible for recommending cancer treatment for the elderly are faced with the serious clinical dilemma of how to choose suitable therapy for this group in the absence of scientific data. Byrne and Carney (1993) relate the dilemma primarily to (1) the lack of pharmacokinetic data regarding chemotherapy in older adults, (2) the biases inherent in the retrospective study design, and (3) low accrual in the relatively few geriatric cancer treatment trials that have been conducted. Kennedy and Balducci (1995) cite the paucity of research that includes people older than 70 years of age as a "major obstacle in determining appropriate treatment for older cancer patients" (p. 35). The current state-of-the-art for geriatric cancer treatment is well summarized in the key points made by Fentiman and colleagues (1990):

- Despite the magnitude of the problem, cancer in the elderly is poorly treated and the behavior of cancer in older patients is not well understood.

- Because of historical exclusion of the elderly from entry into randomized cancer clinical trials, data to formulate appropriate treatment selection are nonexistent.

- In current practice, the elderly, disfranchised from entry into clinical trials, receive untested treatment, inadequate treatment, or even none at all, "at the whim of their clinician."

## State-of-the-Knowledge

Contrary to the ageist beliefs and attitudes that limit the use of chemotherapy in older adults with cancer, there is a growing body of data to support the appropriateness of antineoplastic drug therapy in the elderly, provided existing physiologic deficits have been taken into consideration and planned for. According to Cohen (1995), although a great deal of research documenting the efficacy of chemotherapy in the elderly is still necessary, current data suggest that in the absence of comorbid illness, older individuals treated with mild to moderately aggressive drug regimens are likely to experience responses and toxicities similar to those expected in comparable younger patients. It is only with regimens that are highly aggressive (i.e., in complexity, dose intensity, and potential toxicity) or in the presence of poor performance status that the ability of older adults to tolerate antieoplastic drug therapy declines.

Specific data exist to support the concept that age alone does not place patients at higher risk for poor outcome. An early review of trials conducted by the Eastern Cooperative Oncology Group revealed that with the exception of myelosuppression, patients 70 years of age or older generally experienced chemotherapy-induced toxicity that was similar to patients in younger age groups (Begg and Carbone 1983). A more recent comparative analysis of treatment tolerance by patients entered into a variety of phase II cancer clinical trails (including some relatively aggressive regimens) in a major cancer center, revealed no significant differences between older and younger patients for seven of nine identified treatment-related variables, including performance status, number of dose reductions, treatment interruptions, days of treatment delay, incidence of grade 3–4 toxicity, best disease response, and reasons for discontinuation of treatment (Giovanazzi-Bannon et al. 1994). Comparing women over 70 years of age without comorbid illness and their younger counterparts undergoing therapy for breast cancer, Christman and colleagues (1992) documented similar outcomes for both groups in age-related response rates, time to disease progression, median survival, and profile of major toxicities (i.e., hematologic and emetic). Although none of these research groups generalizes its findings to all elderly patients with cancer, these data help to make the case for inclusion of older patients in the candidate pool for clinical drug trials and more than minimally aggressive antineoplastic therapies.

Data also are available to support the use of more aggressive chemotherapy in selected older patients as a way of increasing survival without sacrificing quality of life. Comparing survival among elderly patients with acute myelogenous leukemia (AML) managed with either a supportive care approach (i.e., low-dose chemotherapy, blood transfusions, and antibiotics) or standard to high-dose chemotherapy (i.e., cytarabine in combination with mitoxantrone or idarubicin), median survival was 11 weeks with supportive interventions versus 6–12 months with more aggressive drug therapy (Champlin, Gajewski, and Golde 1989; Lowenberg et al. 1989). In an attempt to ameliorate hematopoietic toxicity and subsequently permit the administration of full drug dosages on schedule while simultaneously decreasing drug-related morbidity and mortality among the elderly, a few studies have examined the use of cytokines (G-CSF, GM-CSF) in patients over 65 years of age. Findings indicate that the introduction of a growth factor early on may be beneficial for elderly patients with lymphoma and AML and with limited marrow reserves who are receiving dose-intensive regimens, and even with less myelosuppressive regimens if initiated in later drug cycles (Vose 1995).

Seeking additional strategies to preserve quality of life, another trial evaluating the efficacy of low-dose (36 mg/m$^2$) versus high-dose (80 mg/m$^2$) mitoxantrone as an element of the induction regimen for "good risk" elderly patients (e.g., favorable cytogenetic patterns, good performance status, negative history for antecedent hematologic disorders) is currently in progress. Preliminary results indicate that survival is enhanced in the group receiving high-dose mitoxantrone, the toxicity profile is similar in patients younger and older than 60 years of age, and, most important, the overall number of hospital days during survival is significantly reduced (i.e., 30 versus 60 days of 300-day survival) (Feldman 1995). Given that the elderly are a heterogeneous group, additional research of this type is required to define the therapies that not only optimize survival but also ensure quality of life for discrete subpopulations of elderly patients undergoing treatment with cancer chemotherapy.

## Other Treatment Hurdles

In addition to ageism, a variety of other treatment hurdles associated with aging exists for older adults diagnosed with cancer. These hurdles arise from various phenomena related to aging that include not only the physiologic realities of the aging process, the occurrence of comorbid illness, and the potential for drug interactions associated with "polypharmacy syndrome," but also the practical issues of education about, consent for, and compliance with anticancer treatment. Oncology nurses involved in the administration of chemotherapy to the elderly must be aware of how these realities and issues are related to patient needs so that they can plan and deliver care that is sensitive to the idiosyncrasies of old age.

## Normal Aging Changes

Normal aging constitutes a universal and progressive deterioration of physiologic processes. Defined broadly, it is a generalized loss of cellular and extracellular function manifested by observable structural changes in various cells, tissues, and organ systems (Dieckman 1988) and a subsequent decline in overall organ function. Blesch (1988) characterizes the process of aging in relation to alterations in bodily structure and composition and in physiologic function that result in diminished capacity to respond to or recover from stress. Many authors describe the changes of aging from the viewpoint of diminished protective mechanisms. Both perspectives have relevance to the older adult's overall ability to respond to and tolerate the effects of antineoplastic agents. The normative decline in baseline physiologic function of the cardiac, pulmonary, and renal systems is illustrated in Figure 8.1. Hepatic mass, circulation, and oxidative metabolism, as well as hematologic reserves and CNS function, also are known to deteriorate with age (Blesch 1988; Byrne and Carney 1993; Cohen 1995).

The most important changes of aging associated with the older adult's ability to respond to and tolerate chemotherapy, however, are those that affect pharmacokinetic and pharmacodynamic processes. These processes are depicted graphically in Figure 8.2. *Pharmacokinetic* effects relate to the processing of drugs, from their entry into the body through excretion, and include effects on absorption, distribution, metabolism, and elimination. Changes in these processes can influence or determine the bioavailability of drugs administered. Although these effects are not well described for the elderly, the normal changes of aging have the potential to alter these processes in various ways. Gastrointestinal absorptive

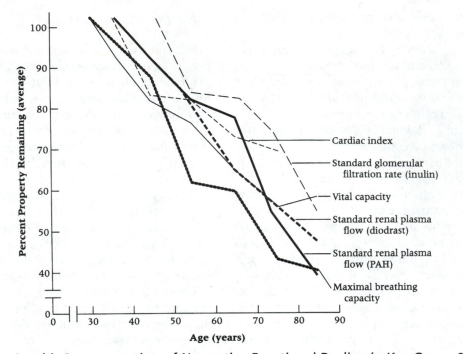

**Figure 8.1** Graphic Representation of Normative Functional Decline in Key Organ Systems Typical of the Aging Process

*Source*: Rowe, J.W., and Bradley, E.C. (1983). The elderly cancer patient: Pathophysiological considerations. In R. Yancik (ed.): *Perspectives on Prevention and Treatment of Cancer in the Elderly*. New York, Raven. Reprinted with permission.

capacity (important with oral agents) may be reduced, volume distribution to target tissues may be impaired, and metabolism and excretion may be delayed (Balducci, Parker, Sexton and Tantranard 1989; Byrne and Carney 1993; Soefje and Koeller 1993). The specific physiologic changes of aging most commonly associated with antineoplastic drug response and tolerability are outlined in Table 8.3.

In contrast, *pharmacodynamic* effects are associated with a drug's specific interactions with its target organs and tissues. For antineoplastic agents to have their maximal tumor effect, certain biochemical mechanisms must be intact, including those related to (1) drug transport across cell membranes, (2) capacity for intracellular drug accumulation, and

(3) drug biotransformation or activation once inside the cell. It is speculated that aging may impair the integrity of these mechanisms in various ways, hence inhibiting the activity of chemotherapeutic agents in the elderly. The ability of drugs to cross the cell membrane may be counteracted by age-dependent alterations in membrane receptors. Overall intracellular drug concentration may be inhibited by reduced transport across cell membranes or by expulsion from the cell as a result of certain mechanisms that may be more active in older adults. One such mechanism mediated by the multidrug resistance gene (MDR1) is the existence of a type of cellular efflux pump that extrudes selected antineoplastics (e.g., vinca alkaloids, doxorubicin) out of the cell on con-

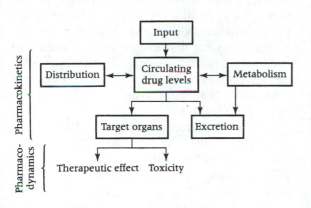

**Figure 8.2** Relationship of Pharmaco-kinetic and Pharmacodynamic Processes

*Source*: Balducci, et al. (1989). Pharmacology of antineo-plastic agents in the elderly patient. *Seminars in Oncology* 16(1): 77. Reprinted with permission.

tact and results in tumor resistance. In addition, age-associated abnormalities in protein synthesis may alter enzyme activity necessary for intracellular activation of drugs. Lower enzyme concentrations may potentiate drug activity, while higher concentrations exert an opposite effect (Balducci et al. 1989; Soefje and Koeller 1993). At this point, however, the possibilities are only theoretical and speculative. Considerable research is necessary to elucidate the specific impact of aging on pharmaco-dynamic processes and their interaction with the antineoplastic agents in the setting of geri-atric cancer drug therapy.

## Comorbid Illness and "Polypharmacy Syndrome"

Besides cancer, the majority of older adults are dealing with at least two other concurrent chronic illnesses for which multiple medica-tions are prescribed. Yancik and Ries (1994) state, "Cancer is [often] diagnosed in bodies already rife with comorbid conditions. There-fore, there are competing diseases for treat-ment" (p. 2002). The most common comorbid illnesses include cardiac problems such as con-gestive heart failure, stroke, and hyperten-sion, pulmonary diseases, diabetes, and arthritis. In addition, acute confusional states, depression, and Alzheimer's disease are preva-lent among the elderly (Boyle et al. 1992; Sarna and Weinrich 1994; Stone and Chenitz 1991). The coexistence of any of these condi-tions with cancer can significantly increase the patient's risk for adverse drug effects, thereby limiting specific chemotherapeutic agents or drug dosages that can safely be administered to treat the malignancy. Comorbid illness also makes monitoring for adverse antineoplastic drug effects a challenge, since drug-related symptoms often overlap with the manifesta-tions of various clinical conditions.

Moreover, because the elderly experience multiple coexisting chronic illnesses, they are typically heavy drug users, accounting for 30% of all prescription drug usage; although 60% of those residing in the community consume over-the-counter medications, they represent little more than 12% of the total population (Ali 1992). Up to 90% of the elderly take at least one medication, and the majority take more than two. The most common pharmaco-logic agents used by older adults are anti-hypertensives and other cardiovascular agents, analgesics, antiarthritic preparations, sedatives, tranquilizers, laxatives, and antacids (Roberts and Turner 1988).

This "polypharmacy syndrome" can be prob-lematic in the elderly patient receiving anti-cancer drug therapy for several reasons. First, the number of medication errors attributable to either care providers or patients themselves is directly proportionate to the total number of drugs prescribed. Instructions about drug scheduling, self-administration techniques, and/or in-home monitoring parameters from clinicians who do not coordinate with one another may be unclear or conflicting; the patient's own interpretation of instructions may be faulty because of visual or hearing impairments or other barriers to information processing; or the responsibility for creating an accurate drug administration schedule to accommodate multiple agents in a 24-hour period may simply be beyond patient/family capability. For instance, coordinating the oral steroid component of a cytotoxic regimen for lymphoma with ranitidine and antacids along with antiemetic agents may be a particularly tall order for an older person who has visual disturbances, sleep/rest alterations, or impaired memory and is also taking an anti-inflammatory agent for arthritis.

The incidence of adverse drug interactions stemming from pharmacokinetic or pharmacodynamic alterations, potentiation, synergism, or incompatibility also will rise as the total number of drugs being taken increases. For example, antimetabolites known to impair gastric mucosa may indirectly inhibit absorption of oral agents such as digoxin, which are typically prescribed for and critical to the management of nonmalignant comorbid illnesses in elderly patients. An array of other pharmacologic agents, including salicylates, meperidine, warfarin, probenecid, and certain antibiotics, may displace antineoplastic drugs from protein-binding sites, producing increased levels of circulating free drug that can result in enhanced toxicity (Balducci et al. 1989). Other examples include propananol, which may potentiate the cardiotoxic effects of doxorubicin; phenytoin and tolbutamide, which are both documented to enhance

methotrexate toxicity; combining hypotensives, barbiturates, or antihistamines with procarbazine, which can enhance central nervous system depression; and concomitant prednisone and L-asparaginase, which may augment hyperglycemic reactions (Dorr and Von Hoff 1994). For further discussion of this topic, see Chapter 6.

Finally, the accurate determination of the causative factor(s) for an older patient's often vaguely described symptomatology becomes difficult when symptoms can be either disease or drug induced, and the etiology is further confounded by a pharmacologic profile characterized by multiple agents prescribed to treat various medical conditions or manage specific symptoms. The vicious cycle continues, as there is a marked tendency among clinicians to ascribe new symptoms to new disease states, exacerbation of existing conditions, or aging itself rather than to the effects of medications being taken by the patient. Ultimately, additional drugs that further complicate the patient's clinical situation are often prescribed (Stone and Chenitz 1991).

Clearly, in this setting, comprehensive assessment to identify all currently prescribed or over-the-counter medications being taken and to establish baseline function and a preexisting symptom profile at the outset of therapy is critical to accurate evaluation of drug reactions and responses throughout the course of chemotherapy. Oncology nurses who recognize and respond to this critical need can use the data from focused patient assessment to collaborate with the physician and pharmacist in planning a customized anticancer drug regimen designed to minimize existing risk for toxicity while at the same time maximizing potential for disease response.

**Table 8.3** Aging Changes with Potential Impact on Antineoplastic Drug Processing by Older Adults*

| Aging Changes | Possible Effects | Specific Agents |
|---|---|---|
| *Absorption*<br>↓ acid production→ ↑ pH<br>↓ motility→slowed gastic emptying<br>↓ microvilli→absorptive surface<br>↓ splanchnic blood flow | ↓ GI tract absorption† | 6-mercaptopurine<br>hexamethylmelamine<br>melphalan |
| ↓ active transport mechanism | ↓ drug movement across cell membrane | methotrexate<br>leucovorin<br>procarbazine |
| *Distribution*<br>Altered body composition<br>↓ lean body mass<br>↑ adipose tissue<br>↓ intracellular water | ↓ vD of hydrophilic drugs→ ↑ serum concentration<br>↑ vD of lipophilic drugs→ ↑ tissue accumulation | liposomal preparations<br>(e.g., doxorubicin) |
| Altered plasma protein levels<br>↓ serum albumin | ↓ bioavailability of protein-bound drugs→ ↑ free fraction of drug and ↑ therapeutic or toxic effects | cisplatin<br>doxorubicin<br>etoposide<br>methotrexate<br>melphalan<br>nitrosoureas<br>paclitaxel<br>vinca alkaloids |
| *Metabolism/excretion*<br>Altered hepatic function<br>↓ hepatic mass<br>↓ hepatic circulation<br>↓ hepatic enzyme activity | ↓ biotransformation of drug to active form<br>↓ formation of active metabolites<br>↓ inactivation of drug<br>↓ drug clearance | 5-fluorouracil<br>amsacrine<br>anthracyclines<br>cyclophosphamide<br>dacarbazine<br>lomustine<br>vinca alkaloids |
| Altered renal function<br>↓ renal mass<br>↓ renal circulation<br>↓ glomerular filtration rate<br>↓ tubular reabsorption | ↓ drug clearance | bleomycin<br>cis-/carboplatin<br>methotrexate<br>streptozocin |

vD = volume distribution

*Because there is little supporting scientific data, the information presented is theoretical.

†No significant change in absorption of oral agents via the aging gastrointestinal tract is thought to occur, with the exception of the identified agents.

*Source*: Derived from Balducci et al. (1989). Pharmacology of antineoplastic agents in the elderly patient. *Seminars in Oncology* 16(1): 76–84; Blesch, K.S. (1988). The normal physiological changes of aging and their impact on the response to cancer treatment. *Seminars in Oncology Nursing* 4: 178–188; Byrne, A., and Carney, D.N. (1993). Cancer in the elderly. *Current Problems in Cancer* 17(3): 145–220 (May/June); Soefje, S.A., and Koeller, J. (1994). Pharmacology and toxicology of cancer chemotherapy in the elderly. *Highlights on Antineoplastic Drugs* 11: 68–75; Egorin, M.J. (1993). Cancer pharmacology in the elderly. *Seminars in Oncology* 20(1): 43–49.

## Education, Consent, and Compliance Issues

Older adults face a variety of challenges to information processing, treatment decision-making, and self-management of their pre-scribed cancer care regimen. Boyle and colleagues (1992) postulate four factors that interfere with the elderly care patient's ability to receive and process the relatively complex information typically provided when anti-cancer treatment is proposed:

- high rate of functional illiteracy among the over-65 age group
- presence of age-related neurosensory compromise
- misconceptions about or fear of cancers common in older adults
- lack of appropriate educational approaches and materials

About one-third of all people over the age of 65 have formal education to the eighth grade or less. In addition, the elderly often have diminished sensory perceptual and motor function (e.g., acuity of vision, hearing, touch, fine motor coordination) necessary for the reception and processing of information, "can-cerphobia," and negative past experiences with cancer, which can influence hopefulness and motivation to acquire information or skills. There is also an absence of a geriatric focus in available teaching materials (e.g., high reading levels, print and graphic limitations, factual congestion). These factors all combine to make the task of applying what has been taught to daily life overwhelming. Often the net result is limited understanding of proposed therapeutic options and their implications, which may sub-sequently hamper the clinician's ability to obtain truly informed consent. Further compli-cating the process of informed consent is the general acceptance of surrogate treatment decision-making by adult children or other family members, even when the older person is perfectly capable of choosing among the options independently. Consider your own observations or participation in clinician/patient/family interactions involving the pres-entation of treatment options to older patients. How often is the interaction automatically directed to family members rather than to the patient or the information delivered at a level that gives the patient no alternative but to turn to family members for clarification? These are common scenarios that promote dependency among the elderly and foster surrogate decision-making. The oncology nurse can advocate for older adults faced with decisions about pursuing therapy in two ways: (1) by engaging in interventions to ensure that a bal-ance is reached between older patients' right to self-determination and their desire for a desig-nated surrogate to make those decisions for them, and (2) by raising awareness among health care team and family members as to ageist perspectives that may interfere with the presentation of all options for treatment and care to the patient.

In addition to consent issues, the teaching/learning barriers cited can contribute to the geriatric patient's inability to comply with required post treatment monitoring and symp-tom management without some level of super-vision or assistance. Studies examining compliance among community-residing eld-erly have revealed that 26–59% of patients are not compliant with their prescribed regimens (Spagnoli et al. 1989). In light of the changing profile of social support as individuals age (i.e., decrease in size and capacity of support net-work) and decreasing reimbursement for pro-fessional health care, the need for support to manage health care needs posed by anticancer therapy presents special challenges for the elderly. Comprehensive assessment that includes not only availability and capability of the patient's support network but also motivation of its members to provide assistance is a prerequisite to the mobilization of available support or the expansion of deficient networks. To avoid posttreatment problems, this evaluation should occur prior to the initiation of therapy in order to anticipate needs unique to aging, and it should be communicated to the physician or other involved team members with the intent of constructing a workable plan for the patient.

## AGE-RELATED DRUG TOXICITIES

Functional competence of major body organs and systems is necessary for patients to meet the physical challenges imposed by antineoplastic drugs. Although normal aging alters baseline organ function, in the absence of illness older adults generally retain sufficient reserves for the routine activities of daily living. Collectively, however, changes in organ function reduce the older person's ability to withstand stressors that draw on that reserve (Cohen 1995). This is particularly true when the stress is of protracted duration (e.g., as with cancer and its treatment) or is intense in nature (e.g., sepsis).

Depending on the degree of age-related physiologic compromise exhibited and the particular chemotherapy regimen, the older adult may potentially be at risk for an array of drug-induced toxicities. Reduced cardiac index at baseline, for example, increases the risk for cardiotoxic effects associated with the anthracyclines, especially when combined with chest irradiation. An undetected cardiac electrical conduction defect could predispose the older patient to bradyrhythmia, generally docu-

mented as a rare occurrence with paclitaxel. A decrease in vital lung capacity could increase the patient's risk for pulmonary compromise with agents such as bleomycin in doses exceeding 450 IU or high-dose methotrexate. Diminished glomerular filtration rate and renal blood flow heighten the risk of nephrotoxicity with platinol and its analogues, particularly after multiple doses or in conjunction with other agents also known to be nephrotoxic. Slowed bladder emptying ability could predispose to alkylator-induced hemorrhagic cystitis. Reduced hepatic circulation delays clearance of agents metabolized by the liver (e.g., antimetabolites), thereby prolonging exposure to the drug and subsequently increasing both the probability and the severity of toxicities such as mucositis. Brain atrophy could result in increased dementia with platinol, cerebellar dysfunction with cytarabine, or heightened peripheral neuropathies with the vinca alkaloids. Diminished protective mechanisms, including hematopoietic reserves, skin and mucous membrane integrity, and central nervous system competency, also may contribute to enhanced risk for antineoplastic drug toxicity. Knowledge of the potential age-related risks for adverse antineoplastic drug effects prepares the clinician to build in allowances for altered organ function and to target monitoring activities more specifically to high-risk systems. Antineoplastic agents associated with high risk for toxicity in elderly patients are listed in Table 8.4 and are described in greater detail elsewhere (Balducci et al. 1989; Blesch 1988; Byrne and Carney 1993; Soefje and Koeller 1993; Walsh, Begg, and Carbone 1989).

Although the changes of aging have been described in general for older adults, the elderly are known to be a highly heterogeneous group and should therefore be evaluated as individuals. Wide variation in the rate and character of aging among those considered to

**Table 8.4** Antineoplastic Agents Associated with Increased Risk for Toxicity in the Elderly

|  | High-Risk Agents | Potential Toxicities |
|---|---|---|
| *Hematologic* | etoposide<br>dactinomycin<br>doxo/daunorubicin<br>lomustine<br>methotrexate<br>semustine<br>vinblastine | Protracted marrow suppression |
| *Cardiac* | cyclophosphamide (HD)<br>doxo/daunorubicin<br>fluorouracil<br>mitoxantrone | Cardiomyopathy<br>Angina 2° coronary spasm<br>Congestive heart failure |
| *Pulmonary* | bleomycin | Pulmonary fibrosis |
| *Neurologic (CNS)* | cytarabine (HD)<br>fluorouracil<br>methotrexate<br>nitrosoureas | Cerebellar dysfunction; ataxia<br>Delerium; dementia<br>Cortical atrophy |
| *(PNS)* | cisplatin<br>vincristine<br>paclitaxel | Ototoxicity<br>Peripheral neuropathy<br>Paralytic ileus<br>Bradyrhythmia |
| *Renal* | carboplatin (HD)<br>cisplatin<br>methotrexate<br>mitomycin-C<br>nitrosoureas | Nephrotoxicity in varying degrees |
| *Hepatic*\* | carmustine<br>cyclophosphamide<br>dacarbazine<br>epirubicin<br>fluorouracil<br>ifosfamide<br>lomustine<br>methotrexate<br>vinca alkaloids | Delayed clearance with subsequent enhanced toxicity in other organ systems |

*Theorized but not supported with scientific data.
HD = high dose; CNS = central nervous system; PNS = peripheral nervous system
*Sources*: Soefje, S.A., and Koeller, J. (1994). Pharmacology and toxicology of cancer chemotherapy in the elderly. *Highlights on Antineoplastic Drugs* 11: 68–75; Walsh, S.J., Begg, C.B., and Carbone, P. (1989). Cancer chemotherapy in the elderly. *Seminars in Oncology* 16(1): 66–75; Byrne, A., and Carney, D.N. (1993). Cancer in the elderly. *Current Problems in Cancer* 17(3): 145–220 (May/June); Cohen, H.J. (1995). Geriatric principles of treatment applied to medical oncology: An overview. *Seminars in Oncology* 22(1 Suppl1): 1–2.

be elderly has been documented. Rather than age, it is the degree of compromise in organ function that dictates both the incidence and severity of drug toxicity. For that reason, blanket guidelines for dosage modifications based solely on age should be avoided (Koeller 1993). Guidelines established to accommodate for diminished renal function (Table 8.5), for example, emphasize the level of kidney function rather than age in recommendations for drug dose modification (Soefje and Koeller 1993). The absence of criteria for the objective measurement of organ function, physiologic deficits and needs, and functional status unique to geriatric patients undergoing cancer treatment has been noted. To fill that gap, the development of guidelines for targeted monitoring of response and toxicity (with special emphasis on hematologic toxicity) associated with chemotherapy in the older cancer patient has been recommended (Knopf, Fulmer, and Mion 1993).

## NURSING CONSIDERATIONS

The trends associated with cancer and aging are clear. The American public is aging at a rapid pace; cancer incidence among the elderly is rising dramatically; and scientific data are demonstrating that, in the absence of comorbid disease, a select group of older Americans with cancer can tolerate moderate to aggressive multiagent antineoplastic treatment regimens. As these trends continue to mature and new strategies for ameliorating drug-induced toxicity are introduced, oncology nurses will find themselves administering chemotherapeutic drugs to a growing population of elderly patients with cancer. Several considerations will help to guide clinical nursing practice in relation to that population of patients.

- *Ageist attitudes are invalid and serve only to undermine the appropriateness and quality of care delivered to the elderly.* In reality, the elderly are a highly heterogeneous group comprising individuals with diverse abilities to tolerate chemotherapy physically, to receive and process information, and to follow through on the prescribed health care regimen. Conducting a comprehensive nursing assessment that addresses each of these capabilities prior to administering chemotherapy is critical to minimizing toxicity and maximizing tumor responsiveness. Assessment strategies targeting elderly patients receiving chemotherapy should build on the elements of gerontologic assessment frameworks already in existence.

- *Alterations in pharmacokinetic and pharmacodynamic processes associated with aging play a major role in the response of older patients to antineoplastic drug therapy.* Although few studies focusing on the effects of antineoplastic agents have been conducted, changes in pharmacokinetic and pharmacodynamic processes due either to the phenomenon of normal aging or to other factors such as comorbid illnesses and polypharmacy syndrome can theoretically influence drug delivery to the site of tumor as well as the degree of toxicity experienced by the older patient. According to Cohen (1994), the elderly patient's potential for tumor response and associated toxicity constitute a broad spectrum that depends primarily on the aggressiveness of the regimen and host constitution. Developing an understanding of the impact of aging on pharmacokinetic and pharmacodynamic processes is critical to the ability of the nurse to anticipate and plan for potential toxicities in older

**Table 8.5** Parameters for Modification of Antineoplastic Drug Dosages to Accommodate for Compromised Renal or Hepatic Function Typical Among Elderly Patients

| Drug | Route of Elimination | Creatinine Clearance (ml/min) | Dose Reduction (%) | Major Toxicities |
|---|---|---|---|---|
| bleomycin | Renal | < 10 | 50 | Lung fibrosis<br>Mucositis |
| carmustine | Hepatic<br>Renal | < 10 | 25 | Renal<br>BM suppression<br>Lung fibrosis |
| carboplatin | Renal | 41–59<br>16–40<br>< 16 | 40<br>50<br>Avoid | Renal<br>Peripheral neuropathy<br>BM suppression |
| cisplatin* | Renal | 10–50<br>< 10 | 25<br>50 | Renal<br>Peripheral neuropathy |
| cyclophosphamide | Hepatic<br>Renal | < 10 | 50 | Hemorrhagic cystitis<br>BM suppression |
| cytarabine | Hepatic | — | None | BM suppression<br>Cerebellar toxicity<br>Increase in liver enzymes |
| daunorubicin | Hepatic | < 10 | 25 | Cardiac<br>Severe mucositis<br>BM suppression |
| doxorubicin | Hepatic | 10–50 | 25 | Cardiac<br>Severe mucositis<br>BM suppression |
| etoposide* | Hepatic<br>Renal | 10–50<br>< 10 | 25<br>50 | |
| fluorouracil | Hepatic<br>Renal | — | None | Mucositis<br>Diarrhea<br>BM suppression |
| hydroxyurea | Renal | 10–50<br>< 10 | 50<br>10 | BM suppression |
| methotrexate | Renal<br>Hepatic (minor) | 10–50<br>< 10 | 50<br>Avoid | Renal<br>Mucostitis<br>BM suppression |
| mitomycin | Hepatic | < 10 | 25 | |
| vinca alkaloids | Hepatic | — | None | Peripheral neuropathy (paralytic ileus)<br>SIADH<br>BM suppression |

*Dosage reductions in renal impairment are not clearly defined.

BM = bone marrow; SIADH = Syndrome of Inappropriate Antidiuretic Hormone.

*Source*: Soefje, S.A, and Koeller, J. (1994). Pharmacology and toxicology of cancer chemotherapy in the elderly. *Highlights on Antineoplastic Drugs* 11: 68–75. Reprinted with permission.

patients. Further, that knowledge will provide a sound base from which to individualize the content of patient/family education for the elderly.

- *With the exception of hematopoietic toxicity, chemotherapy-induced toxicity profiles observed in certain subsets of older adults appear to be similar to those demonstrated by younger patients.* Currently, there are few scientific data upon which to base drug treatment recommendations for older adults with cancer. The new thrust among investigators to design drug trials specifically targeting older patients with cancer and raising age eligibility for accrual to more general trials, however, is now producing data that are beginning to change the common practice of underdosing or excluding older patients from anticancer treatment options available to younger patients. Emerging data suggest that select subpopulations of older cancer patients (e.g., those without comorbid disease) can tolerate significantly more aggressive chemotherapy regimens than was previously believed, provided that there is a plan in place to meet the challenge of diminished hematopoietic reserves common among the elderly. Oncology nurses can make a valuable contribution to this fledgling database by developing, conducting, or participating in clinical nursing research or companion studies (to medical research) designed to describe chemotherapy-associated symptomatology specific to the elderly and subsequently to examine the impact of those responses on quality of life for the older patient.

- *Patient/family education, the process of informed consent, and compliance with the therapeutic regimen pose unique problems for many older patients.* These functions rely on information intake and processing capabilities, which often are impaired to varying degrees among older patients for a variety of reasons, including limited education, neurosensory compromise, faulty perceptions about cancer, dependency on adult children, and inadequate availability of targeted educational materials. Oncology nurses must remain cognizant of the education, consent, and compliance issues unique to the elderly and customize their approaches when managing these aspects of care for older patients undergoing cancer chemotherapy.

## BIBLIOGRAPHY

Ali, N.S. (1992). Promoting safe use of multiple medications by elderly persons. *Geriatric Nursing* 13 (3): 157–159.

American Cancer Society. (1995). *Facts & Figures.* Atlanta: American Cancer Society.

Balducci, L., Parker, M., Sexton, W., and Tantranond, P. (1989). Pharmacology of antineoplastic agents in the elderly patient. *Seminars in Oncology* 16(1): 76–84.

Begg, C.B., and Carbone, P.P. (1983). Clinical trials and drug toxicity in the elderly. *Cancer* 52(11): 1986–1992.

Benson III, A.B., Pregler, J.P., Bean, J.A., Rademaker, A.W., Eshler, B., and Anderson, K. (1991). Oncologists' reluctance to accrue patients onto clinical trials: An Illinois Cancer Center study. *Journal of Clinical Oncology* 9(11): 2067–2075.

Berkman, B., Rohan, B., and Sampson, S. (1994). Myths and biases related to cancer in the elderly. *Cancer* 74(suppl): 2004–2008 (October).

Blesch, K.S. (1988). The normal physiological changes of aging and their impact on the response to cancer treatment. *Seminars in Oncology Nursing* 4: 178–188.

Bonadonna, G., and Valagussa, P. (1981). Dose-response effect of adjuvant chemotherapy in breast cancer. *New England Journal of Medicine* 304: 10–15.

Boyle, D.M., Engelking, C., Blesch, K., Dodge, J., Sarna, L., and Weinrich, S. (1992). Oncology Nursing Society position paper on cancer an aging: The mandate for oncology nursing. *Oncology Nursing Forum* 19(6): 913–933.

Byrne, A., and Carney, D.N. (1993). Cancer in the elderly. *Current Problems in Cancer* 17(3): 145–220 (May/June).

Champlin, R.E., Gajewski, J.L., and Golde, D.W. (1989). Treatment of acute myelogenous leukemia in the elderly. *Seminars in Oncology* 16(1): 51–56.

Christman, K., Muss, H.B., Case, L.D., et al. (1992). Chemotherapy of metastic breast cancer in the elderly: The Piedmont Oncology Association experience [comment]. *Journal of the American Medical Association* 268: 57–62.

Cohen, H.J. (1995). Geriatric principles of treatment applied to medical oncology: An overview. *Seminars in Oncology* 22(1 Suppl1): 1–2.

———. (1994). Biology of aging as related to cancer. Cancer 74(7 Suppl): 2092–2100 (October).

Dieckman, J.M. (1989). Cancer in the elderly: Systems overview. *Seminars in Oncology Nursing* 4: 169–177.

Dorr, R.T., and Von Hoff, D.D. (1994). *Cancer Chemotherapy Handbook.* Norwalk, Conn.: Appleton and Lange.

Early Breast Cancer Trialists' Collaborative Group (1992). Systemic treatment of early breast cancer by hormonal, cytotoxic or immune therapy: 133 randomised trials involving 31,000 recurrences and 24,000 deaths among 75,000 women. *Lancet* 339: 1–15, 71–85.

Egorin, M.J. (1993). Cancer pharmacology in the elderly. *Seminars in Oncology* 20(1): 43–49.

Feldman, E.J. (1995). Acute myelogenous leukemia in the older patient. *Seminars in Oncology* 22(1 Suppl1): 21–24.

Fentiman, I.S., Tirelli, U., Monfardini, S., Schneider, M., Festen, J., Cognetti, F., and Aapro, M.S. (1990). Cancer in the elderly: Why so badly treated? *Lancet* 335(8696): 1020–1022.

Giovanazzi-Bannon, S., Rademaker, A., Lai, G., and Benson III, A.B. (1994). Treatment tolerance of elderly cancer patients entered onto phase II clinical trials: An Illinois Cancer Center study. *Journal of Clinical Oncology* 12(11): 2247–2452.

Given, C.W., Given, B.A., and Stommel, M. (1994). The impact of age, treatment, and symptoms on the physical and mental health of cancer patients: A longitudinal perspective. *Cancer* 74(7 Suppl): 2128–2138 (October).

Goodwin, J.S., Hunt, W.C., Humble, C.G., Key, C.R., and Samet, J.M. (1988). Cancer treatment protocols: Who gets chosen? *Archives of Internal Medicine* 148(10): 2258–2260.

Kennedy, B.J., and Balducci, L. (1995). Closing remarks. *Seminars in Oncology* 22(Suppl): 35.

Knopf, T., Fulmer, T.T., and Mion, L.C. (1993). Geriatric perspective for oncology nursing practice. *Current Issues in Cancer Nursing Practice* 3: 1–14.

Koeller, J. (1993). Are you ever too old to receive chemotherapy? *Highlights on Antineoplastic Drugs* 11: 57.

Lichtman, S.M. (1995). Lymphoma in the older patient. *Seminars in Oncology* 22(1 Suppl1): 25–28.

Lowenberg, B., Zittoun, R., Kerkhofs, H., Jehn, U., Abels, J., Debusscher, L., Cauchie, C., Peetermans, M., Solbu, G., and Suciu, S. (1989). On the value of intensive remission-induction chemotherapy in elderly patients of 65+ years with acute myeloid leukemia: A randomised phase III study of the European Organization for Research and Treatment of Cancer Leukemia Group. *Journal of Clinical Oncology* 7(9): 1268–1274.

Markman, M., Lewis, J.L. Saio, P., Hakes, T., Jones, W., Rubin, S., Reichman, B., Barakat, R., Curtin, J., and Almadrones, L. (1993). Epithelial ovarian cancer in the elderly: The Memorial Sloan-Kettering Cancer Center experience. *Cancer* 71(2 Suppl): 634–637.

McKenna, R.J. (1994). Clinical aspects of cancer in the elderly: Treatment decisions, treatment choices, and follow-up. *Cancer* 74(7 Suppl): 2107–2117 (October).

Miller, B.A., Ries, L.A.G., Hankey, B.F., et al. (eds.). (1993). Surveillance, epidemiology and end results program. National Institutes of Health, Bethesda, Md. NIH Report 94-3074.

Mor, V., Masterson-Allen, S., Goldberg, R.J., et al. (1985). Relationship between age at diagnosis and treatments received by cancer patients. *Journal of the American Geriatric Society* 33: 585–589.

Mortenson, L.E. (1994). Health care policies affecting the treatment of patients with cancer and cancer research. *Cancer* 74(7 Suppl): 2204–2207 (October).

Roberts, J., and Turner, N. (1988). Pharmacodynamic basis for altered drug action in the elderly. *Clinics in Geriatric Medicine* 4(1): 127–149.

Rowe, J.W., and Bradley, E.C. (1983). The elderly cancer patient: Pathophysiological considerations. In R. Yancik (ed.): *Perspectives on Prevention and Treatment of Cancer in the Elderly.* New York: Raven.

Samet, J., Hunt, W.C., Key, C., Humble, C.G. and Goodwin, J.S. (1986). Choice of cancer therapy varies with age of patient. *Journal of the American Medical Association* 255(24): 3385–3390.

Silliman, R.A., Guadagnoli, E., Weitberg, A.B., et al. (1989). Age as a predictor of diagnostic and initial treatment intensity in newly diagnosed breast cancer patients. *Journal of Gerontology* 4: 46–50.

Soefje, S.A., and Koeller, J. (1994). Pharmacology and toxicology of cancer chemotherapy in the elderly. *Highlights on Antineoplastic Drugs* 11: 68–75.

Spagnoli, A., Ostino, G., Borga, A.D., et al. (1989). Drug compliance and unreported drugs in the elderly. *Journal of American Geriatric Society* 37: 619–624.

Stone, J.T., and Chenitz, W.C. (1991). An overview of gerontological nursing. In W. Chenitz, J.T. Stone, and S.A. Salisbury (eds.): *Clinical Gerontological Nursing: A Guide to Advanced Practice.* Philadelphia: W.B. Saunders.

Trimble, E.L., Carter, C.L., Cain, D., Freidlin, B., Ungerleider, R.S., and Friedman, M.A. (1994). Representation of older patients in cancer treatment trials. *Cancer* 74(7 Suppl): 2208–2214.

United States Bureau of the Census (prepared by Spencer, G.). (1990). Projections of the population of the United States by age, sex and race: 1988–2080. Washington, D.C.: United States Bureau of the Census, Current Population Reports, Series P-25, No. 1018.

Vose, J. (1995). Cytokine use in the older patient. *Seminars in Oncology* 22(1 Suppl1): 6–8 (February).

Walsh, S.J., Begg, C.B., and Carbone, P. (1989). Cancer chemotherapy in the elderly. *Seminars in Oncology* 16(1): 66–75.

Weinrich, S., and Sarna, L. (1994). Delirium in the older person with cancer. *Cancer* 74(7 Suppl): 2079–2091.

Wood, W.C., Budman, D.R., Korzun, A.H., et al. (1994). Dose and dose intensity of adjuvant chemotherapy for stage II, node-positive breast carcinoma. *New England Journal of Medicine* 330: 1258–1259.

Yancik, R., and Ries, L.A. (1994). Cancer in older persons: Magnitude of the problem—How do we apply what we know? *Cancer* 74(7 Suppl): 1995–2003 (October).

Young, R.C., Brady, M.F. Walton, L.A., Homestey, H.D., Averette, H.E., and Long, H.J. (1993). Localized ovarian cancer in the elderly: The gynecologic oncology group experience. *Cancer* 71(2 Suppl): 524–529.

# Chapter 9

# Chemotherapy Administration: General Principles for Nursing Practice

**Martha Langhorne MSN, RN, FNP, AOCN**
**and Margaret Barton-Burke PhD (c), RN, AOCN**

## INTRODUCTION

Chemotherapy administration has changed markedly. In the past, physicians administered the drugs, nurses cared for the patient's side effects, and the pharmacist was involved in a variety of ways. Currently, this multidisciplinary team still works together to administer chemotherapeutic drugs but the roles have changed markedly. The practice of chemotherapy administration varies according to institutional policies and procedures, state professional practice acts, i.e., pharmacy and nurse practice acts, and national organizations. For example, the formal, national organization for oncology nurses, the Oncology Nursing Society (ONS), regularly publishes and revises guidelines and recommendations for chemotherapy administration. Also, the ONS (1999) recommends that specialized preparation of the professional registered nurses can ensure a safe level of care for the individual receiving chemotherapy.

To prepare nurses to administer chemotherapy, the educational programs should include both didactic theory and supervised clinical experience. The didactic component should include a review of cancer pathophysiology, focusing on the pharmacology of antineoplastic agents, principles of safe handling and drug administration, and management of potential treatment side effects and complications related to drug administration. The clinical aspects must provide skills in intravenous therapy (e.g., venipuncture and site selection; administration techniques and guidelines; management of various venous access devices, such as silastic catheters, implantable ports) and, as appropriate, the more complex drug delivery techniques of intraperitoneal, intracavitary, and intrathecal therapies; arterial lines; and internal and external infusion pumps. Although the nurse should be able to recall the side effects listed for a particular drug, it is more important that she or he anticipate and prevent side effects that the patient is actually at risk of developing. Pain, nausea, and vomiting can interfere with successful treatment and therefore should be minimized or precluded (Barton-Burke, Wilkes, and Ingwersen 1996).

Current events within the field of oncology have underscored the importance of all members of the multidisciplinary team in the safe administration of cancer chemotherapy and although this chapter focuses on nurses and chemotherapy administration, some emphasis should be given to the team. In the mid-1990s, national attention was given to the tragic consequences of cancer chemotherapy overdoses at one of the leading comprehensive cancer centers in the United States. This episode emphasized the reality of the risk of drug errors and heightened the awareness of the public, media, patients, and health care professionals. (Fischer, Alfano, Knobf, Donovan, and Beaulieu 1996).

Guidelines are recommended to establish safe and effective use of chemotherapy in patients treated for cancer. The incidence of chemotherapy-related errors should be zero, but it is human to make mistakes. With guidelines such as those proposed, it is hoped that the error rate will approach zero. Clinical practice guidelines should be reviewed and updated as needed, and at least yearly, by a multidisciplinary team (Fischer et al. 1996). Table 9.1 provides a list of multidisciplinary practice guidelines that should be considered before, during, and after chemotherapy administration for all members of the multidisciplinary team.

Various guidelines from different organizations proposed by different groups, such as the Oncology Nursing Society (ONS), offer suggestions for chemotherapy administration. This chapter is an attempt to synthesize material from several sources in an effort to present scientifically based information that provides a basis for safe nursing practice and comprehensive nursing care.

## CHEMOTHERAPY ADMINISTRATION

Chemotherapy may be the therapy of choice for certain cancers, may only control or palliate the cancer, or at times may have no therapeutic effect at all (Berman 1999). More than one-half of all patients diagnosed with cancer receive chemotherapy treatment, with the volume of treatment activity set to increase as cytotoxic agents become more powerful and numerous (Sitzia and Wood 1998). In most cases, chemotherapy is administered through a systemic route (e.g., oral or intravenous) out of concern that a cancer has spread from the primary tumor through the lymphatic or vascular system to distant sites in the body (Berman 1999).

The role of the oncology nurse in relation to chemotherapy administration is one of enormous responsibility, as mentioned previously. In addition to considerable knowledge about the drugs to be administered, oncology nurses require substantial technical skills in and knowledge of drug administration. The management of chemotherapy administration includes such technical information as prescription (as mentioned in Table 9.1), assessment—including patient information, specific steps to take prior to administration, and venous access, the actual administration of the drug, and postchemotherapy evaluation—including observation and management of side effects (Bertolone 1997).

Assessment of the patient about to receive the chemotherapy involves gathering unique data about the individual, about the chemotherapeutic agent, and about the knowledge and skill that the nurse has in order that the drug or drugs may be given safely. In Table 9.2, a nursing assessment is proposed for both pre- and postchemotherapy.

Table 9.3 provides in-depth guidelines for nursing assessment, expanding the information provided in Table 9.2. These guidelines provide a step-by-step assessment that can be used by the nurse before the actual administration, whereas Table 9.4 is a detailed checklist that could be used for technical assessment prior to actual chemotherapy administration. In addition to a thorough medical history, it must be ascertained

## Table 9.1   Multidisciplinary Practice Guidelines

I. Baseline professional training
   A. There are three primary disciplines involved in the chemotherapy process. Each professional should have a baseline knowledge of cancer chemotherapy before practicing.
      1. Physicians authorized to write chemotherapy orders for neoplastic disease states should be board-certified and/or board-eligible hematologists or medical, pediatric, radiation (for specified drugs on protocol), or gynecologic oncologists and the oncology fellows who have been deemed capable by the section chief. An attending physician thus qualified should routinely check and countersign chemotherapy orders written by an oncology fellow during the first two months on the clinical service.
      2. In acute-care hospitals, which are not solely cancer centers, many nononcology specialties use antineoplastic drugs for treatment of nonmalignant conditions in dermatology (e.g., methotrexate for psoriasis) or rheumatology (cyclophosphamide for patients with lupus nephritis). The recommendations for these non-oncology specialties that use cytotoxic chemotherapy include having the department or section register with the pharmacy department the usual agents, dose ranges, and indicated diseases, with provision of published reference sources and/or institutional review board–approved protocols for these treatments.
      3. Registered nurses who will handle and administer chemotherapy need to be cancer chemotherapy–certified. Certification includes:
         - attending a chemotherapy certification course
         - successful completion of a written examination
         - demonstrated competency in administering chemotherapy
         - attendance at a yearly update session to remain certified
      4. Pharmacists involved in chemotherapy practice must complete the departmental staff development chemotherapy lecture series. Completion includes:
         - successful completion of a written examination
         - demonstrated competency in safe and accurate chemotherapy compounding and handling
         - attendance at a yearly update session to remain certified

II. Standard practice
   A. Oncologists or oncology fellows should be solely responsible for writing chemotherapy orders and/or entering them into a computer or specially authorized chemotherapy order form. To maintain a system of checks, it is imperative that the physicians complete the first step of order-writing—which includes dose calculations and modifications. This also encompasses a practice of limiting verbal chemotherapy orders to dose reduction in modification of an existing order.
   B. The chemotherapy order should be composed in a standard format. Computer order sets should be created and/or order sheets preprinted with standard and commonly used regimens. Drugs should always be ordered by the generic or US Assigned Name, consistent with usage in the hospital formulary, and the three federally recognized compendia. Although the trade name or an abbreviation or jargon name may be placed in parentheses if it will add to the clarity of the order, it is not an acceptable substitute for the generic name even though a cooperative group protocol uses it. When free-form chemotherapy orders are written for unusual or nonstandard drug regimens, a reference to the source(s) that provided the basis for the order must be cited and, when possible, a copy of the relevant source placed in the

*(continued)*

**Table 9.1**    Multidisciplinary Practice Guidelines *(continued)*

chart and an explanation given in writing as to why this particular therapy was chosen. Initial creation of preprinted orders or order sets should be the responsibility of one discipline and verified independently by the other two. This would include a formal sign-off when the check is complete.

C. Journal articles, abstracts, outside institutional protocols, and any other potential treatment references that represent the source of the orders or clarify them should be made known to all involved professionals by placement of a direct copy in the patient's chart before treatment. Copies of outside institutional protocols should also be made available to the pharmacist. This direct copy should contain at least the following information: generic drug name, dose, dosage schedule, side effects or toxicity, rationale for the regimen, necessary dose reductions, and administration guidelines.

D. All orders should be written using the following format: generic drug name, dose to be given (in milligrams), dosage used (milligrams per meter squared or per kilogram), frequency, days of administration, and infusion guidelines. Ordinarily, the total dose for the course should not be listed on the order sheet or the computer order screen, lest it be misinterpreted as a single dose to be administered. (For continuous infusion pump delivery, the total dose to be infused over the set period must be included, but there should be a notation of how much is to be delivered each day.) All pertinent information must be supplied to ensure a safe and accurate order capable of verification.

E. Standard chemotherapy reference texts and handbooks and standard drug references should be readily available to physicians, nurses, and pharmacists on all patient-care areas and the central and decentralized pharmacy.

F. An increasing number of patients are being treated on protocols. Any protocol that

accrues patients must be approved by the institutional review board. When a new protocol is instituted, multidisciplinary education must take place before patient enrollment. This is especially important when protocols involve investigational agents, high-dose therapy, and unusual or new combination therapies. This education must ensure adequate communication between the principle investigator, clinic nurses, research nurses, inpatient nurses, and all oncology pharmacists. Copies of all new protocols and amendments must be placed in designated patient-care areas, clinics, and central and decentralized pharmacies. Preprinted or computer order sets should be configured and in place before patient enrollment to avoid order variability and ambiguity. New protocols or unusual therapies should not begin off-hours or on weekends unless it is an acute emergency situation. They should be initiated on weekdays when appropriate specialists and clinicians are available.

G. Order verification and/or double-checking enhances safe chemotherapy practice, and there should not be any exceptions to this. The nurse and pharmacist are each independently responsible for the following:
- check entire order set against an acceptable reference (protocol, journal article, chemotherapy text or handbook, abstract, computer hard copy of order set, etc.)
- verify that current body surface area, height, and weight are correct
- verify the final dose of each drug
- check the rate of administration, amount, and type of solution
- check the antiemetic regimen, prehydration and posthydration, for omissions or additions of ancillary medication therapy
- compare current orders with previous therapy—consider any radical changes
- check that an X-ray has been read to confirm central venous access for new

*(continued)*

**Table 9.1** Multidisciplinary Practice Guidelines *(continued)*

line placements for continuous vesicant infusions

- if dose modification has been made, confirm parameters with reference or research protocol and then consult with prescriber to verify rationale if nonstandard modification was made

- determine if appropriate laboratory values are within normal parameters, based on known organ-specific toxicity of each drug, in addition to hematologic parameters; abnormal values should be called to the attention of the prescriber and treatment modifications made after adequate discussion

The nursing verification should be completed by two nurses, one of whom is a certified chemotherapy nurse. Each should sign each chemotherapy order. Nurses must also verify availability of progenitor cells with attending oncologist or oncology fellows in situations that involve bone marrow transplant or stem cell transplant. Research nurses are also responsible for checking laboratory parameters dictated by the research protocol. In addition to the above expectations for pharmacy, pharmacists must ensure that the prescribed solution and administration parameters will enable adequate drug delivery, and ensure compatibility of chemotherapy with intravenous solutions and/or additives. Once orders are double-checked, they should be prepared and labeled following pharmacy compounding policies and safe handling procedures.

H. Chemotherapy administration may begin once the final product, which has been checked by a pharmacist, arrives in the designated patient care area. Two nurses, one of whom must be chemotherapy-certified, must check the final product against the original order before administration. In the clinic setting, one certified nurse and pharmacist should check the final product before administration. The check should take place at the patient's bedside so that the two professionals can ensure that the correct drug is being given to the appropriate patient by checking the identification band in the same fashion that a blood transfusion is checked. The attending oncologist and/or oncology fellow may also administer chemotherapy when necessary after following comparable procedures.

I. Chemotherapy administration should occur on dedicated oncology inpatient units and ambulatory oncology sites that are staffed by certified chemotherapy nurses. On occasion, patients are on other units or must be transferred, such as a patient on continuous infusion to an intensive care unit. That nursing staff should then be educated by a certified chemotherapy nurse. All oncology settings should have a standard oncology text, chemotherapy handbook, copies of approved protocols, and a standard drug reference.

J. The attending physician who writes the chemotherapy order should be required to include the cumulative dose of anthracycline, bleomycin, and mitomycin previously received by the patient. It should be noted that the system instituted to require notation of previously received cumulative doses should not require current dose and previous dose to be noted on the same screen or together as part of the order, to avoid confusion and potential error.

*Source:* Fischer, D.S., Alfano, S., Knobf, M.T., Donovan, C., and Beaulieu, N. (1996). Improving the cancer chemotherapy use process. *Journal of Chemical Oncology* 14(12), 3148–3155. Reprinted with permission.

**Table 9.2** Nursing Assessment for Chemotherapy

I. Prechemotherapy assessment

   A. Physical evaluation
      1. Pertinent past history
         a. Diagnosis and disease presentation
         b. Concomitant health conditions and allergies
      2. System review
         a. Pertinent laboratory data (hematopoietic function)
         b. Neurologic function
         c. Oral cavity and integumentary status
         d. Cardiovascular function
         e. Respiratory function
         f. Urologic function
         g. Gastrointestinal function
         h. Sexual function
         i. Dermatologic status
      3. Presence of prior cancer therapy toxicities
         a. Surgery
         b. Radiation therapy
         c. Chemotherapy

   B. Psychosocial evaluation
      1. Knowledge of cancer and chemotherapy
         a. Dispel myths
         b. Address feelings of anxiety and fear
      2. Prior (personal) experience with chemotherapy
      3. Support system and significant others
      4. Informed consent (see Chapter 1)

   C. Patient and family education

II. Postchemotherapy assessment

   A. Review assessment as above for changes
      1. Tumor response
      2. Status improvements
      3. Abnormal findings

   B. Management of side effects (see Chapter 4)

   C. Patient/family education

*Source:* Berg, D. (1996). Principles of chemotherapy administration. In M. Barton-Burke, G. Wilkes, and K. Ingwersen, *Cancer Chemotherapy: A Nursing Process Approach.* 2nd ed. Sudbury, Mass.: Jones & Bartlett.

**Table 9.3**  Prechemotherapy Nursing Assessment Guidelines

| Potential Problems/ Nursing Diagnoses | Physical Status: Assessment Parameters/ Signs and Symptoms | Drug- and Dose-Limiting Factors |
|---|---|---|
| *Hematopoietic system* | | |
| A. Impaired tissue perfusion related to chemotherapy-induced anemia | • Hgb g (norms 12–14; 14–16)<br>• Hct% (norms 32–36; 36–40)<br>• Vital signs (BP, pulse, respiration)<br>• Pallor (face, palms, conjunctiva)<br>• Fatigue or weakness<br>• Vertigo | • Hgb < 8 g<br>• Hct < 20%<br>• Blood transfusions not initiated |
| B. Impaired immuno-competence and potential for infection related to chemotherapy-induced leukopenia | • WBC (norm 4500–9000/mm$^3$)<br>• Pyrexia/rigor, erythema, swelling, pain any site<br>• Abnormal discharges, draining wounds, skin/mucous membrane lesions<br>• Productive cough, SOB, rectal pain, urinary frequency | • WBC < 3,000/mm$^3$<br>• Fever > 101°F<br>– Hold all myelosuppressive agents (exceptions may include leukemia, lymphoma, and/or situations in which there is neoplastic marrow infiltration) |
| C. Potential for injury (bleeding) related to chemotherapy-induced thrombocytopenia | • Platelet count (150,000–400,000/mm$^3$)<br>• Spontaneous gingival bleeding or epistaxis<br>• Presence of petechiae or easy bruisability<br>• Hematuria, melena, hematemesis, hemoptysis<br>• Hypermenorrhea<br>• S/s of intracranial bleeding (irritability, sensory loss, unequal pupils, headache, ataxis) | • Platelet count < 100,000/mm$^3$<br>– Hold all myelosuppressive agents (exceptions may include leukemia, lymphoma, and/or situations in which there is neoplastic marrow infiltration) |
| *Integumentary system* | | |
| Alteration in mucous membrane of mouth, nasopharynx, esophagus, rectum, anus, or ostomy stoma related to chemotherapy-induced tissue changes | Mucositis Scale<br>  0 = pink, moist, intact mucosa; absence of pain or burning<br>+ 1 = generalized erythema with or without pain or burning<br>+ 2 = isolated small ulcerations and/or white patches<br>+ 3 = confluent ulcerations with white patches on 25% mucosa<br>+ 4 = hemorrhagic ulcerations | • + 2 mucositis<br>– Hold antimetabolites (esp. methotrexate, 5-FU)<br>– Hold antitumor antibiotics (esp. doxorubicin, dactinomycin) |
| *Gastrointestinal system* | | |
| Discomfort, nutritional deficiency, and/or fluid and electrolyte disturbances related to chemotherapy-induced: | | |
| A. Anorexia | • Lab values: albumin and total protein<br>• Normal weight/present weight and % of body weight loss<br>• Normal diet pattern/changes in diet pattern | |

*(continued)*

**Table 9.3**  Prechemotherapy Nursing Assessment Guidelines *(continued)*

| Potential Problems/ Nursing Diagnoses | Physical Status: Assessment Parameters/ Signs and Symptoms | Drug- and Dose-Limiting Factors |
|---|---|---|
| A. Anorexia (continued) | • Alterations in taste sensation<br>• Early satiety | |
| B. Nausea and vomiting | • Lab values: electrolytes<br>• Pattern of nausea/vomiting (incidence, duration, severity)<br>• Antiemetic plan<br>  Drug(s), dosage(s), schedule, efficacy<br>• Other (dietary adjustments, relaxation techniques, environmental manipulation) | • Intractable nausea/ vomiting × 24 hrs if IV hydration not initiated |
| C. Bowel disturbances<br>  1. Diarrhea | • Normal pattern of bowel elimination<br>• Consistency (loose, watery/bloody stools)<br>• Frequency and duration (#/day and # of days)<br>• Antidiarrheal drug(s), dosage(s), efficacy | • Diarrheal stools × 3 per 24 hrs<br>– Hold antimetabolites (esp. methotrexate, 5-FU) |
|   2. Constipation | • Normal pattern of bowel elimination<br>• Consistency (hard, dry, small stools)<br>• Frequency (hours or days beyond normal pattern)<br>• Stool softener(s), laxative(s), efficacy | • No BM × 48 hrs past normal bowel patterns<br>– Hold vinca alkaloids (vinblastine, vincristine) |
| D. Hepatotoxicity | • Lab values: LDH, SGOT, alk phos, bilirubin<br>• Pain/tenderness over liver, feeling of fullness<br>• Increase in nausea/vomiting or anorexia<br>• Changes in mental status<br>• Jaundice<br>• High-risk factors<br>  –Hepatic metastasis<br>  –Viral hepatitis<br>  –Abdominal XRT<br>  –Concurrent hepatotoxic drugs<br>  –Graft vs. host disease<br>  –Blood transfusions | • Evidence of chemical hepatitis<br>– Hold hepatotoxic agents (esp. methotrexate, 6-MP) until differential dx established |
| *Respiratory system* | | |
| Impaired gas exchange or ineffective breathing pattern related to chemotherapy-induced pulmonary fibrosis | • Lab values: PFTs, CXR<br>• Respiration (rate, rhythm, depth)<br>• Chest pain<br>• Nonproductive cough<br>• Progressive dyspnea<br>• Wheezing/stridor<br>• High-risk factors<br>  –Total cumulative dose of bleomycin<br>  –Preexisting lung disease<br>  –Prior/concomitant XRT<br>  –Age > 60 yrs<br>  –Concomitant use of other pulmonary toxic drugs<br>  –Smoking hx | • Acute unexplained onset respiratory symptoms<br>– Hold all antineoplastic agents until differential dx established |

*(continued)*

**Table 9.3** Prechemotherapy Nursing Assessment Guidelines *(continued)*

| Potential Problems/ Nursing Diagnoses | Physical Status: Assessment Parameters/ Signs and Symptoms | Drug- and Dose-Limiting Factors |
|---|---|---|
| *Cardiovascular system* | | |
| Decreased cardiac output related to chemotherapy-induced:<br>A. Cardiac arrhythmias<br>B. Cardiomyopathy | • Lab values: cardiac enzymes, electrolytes, EKG, ECHO, MUGA<br>• Vital signs<br>• Presence of arrhythmia (irregular radial/apical)<br>• S/s of CHF (dyspnea, ankle edema, nonproductive cough, rales, cyanosis)<br>• Hold anthracyclines<br>• High-risk factors<br>  –Total cumulative dose anthracyclines<br>  –Preexisting cardiac disease<br>  –Prior/concurrent mediastinal XRT<br>  –Bolus administration higher drug doses | • Acute s/s of CHF and/or cardiac arrhythmia<br><br>– Hold all antineoplastic agents until differential dx established<br>• Total dose doxorubicin or daunorubicin > 550 mg/m$^2$ |
| *Genitourinary system* | | |
| A. Alteration in fluid volume (excess) related to chemotherapy-induced:<br>1. Glomerular or renal tubule damage<br>2. Hyperuricemic nephropathy<br>B. Alteration in comfort related to chemotherapy-induced hemorrhagic cystitis | • Lab values: BUN, creatinine clearance, serum creatinine, uric acid, electrolytes, urinalysis<br>• Color, odor, clarity of urine<br>• 24-hr fluid I&O (estimate/actual)<br>• Hematuria; proteinuria<br>• Development of oliguria or anuria<br>• High-risk factors<br>  –Preexisting renal disease<br>  –Concurrent treatment with nephrotoxic drugs (esp. aminoglycoside antibiotics) | • Hematuria<br>– Hold cyclophosphamide Serum creatinine > 2.0 and/or creatinine clearance < 70 ml/min<br>– Hold Cis-platinum, streptozocin Anuria × 24 hrs<br>– Hold all antineoplastic agents |
| *Nervous system* | | |
| A. Impaired sensory/ motor function related to chemotherapy-induced:<br>1. Peripheral neuropathy<br>2. Cranial nerve neuropathy | • Paresthesias (numbness, tingling in feet, fingertips)<br>• Trigeminal nerve toxicity (severe jaw pain)<br>• Diminished or absent deep tendon reflexes (ankle and knee jerks)<br>• Motor weakness, slapping gait, ataxia<br>• Visual and auditory disturbances | • Presence of any neurologic s/s<br>– Hold vinca alkaloids, Cis-platinum, hexamethylmelamine, procarbazine until differential dx established |
| B. Impaired bowel and bladder elimination related to chemotherapy-induced autonomic nerve dysfunction | • Urinary retention<br>• Constipation, abdominal cramping and distention<br>• High-risk factors<br>  –Changes in diet or mobility<br>  –Frequent use of narcotic analgesics<br>  –Obstructive disease process | • Presence of any neurologic s/s<br>– Hold vinca alkaloids until differential dx established |

*Source:* Adapted from Engelking, C. (1988). Prechemotherapy nursing assessment in outpatient settings. *Outpatient Chemotherapy* 3(1): 9–11. Reprinted with permission from World Health Communications, Inc.

whether the patient has received prior chemotherapy or had recent surgery, and what the disease course has been thus far. A review of systems, including allergies, changes in the overall physical condition, including physical performance status (see Table 9.5), height and weight (see Appendices 6 and 7), and laboratory values should be evaluated also. These assessments should be followed by a calculation of the body surface area (m$^2$), as shown in Figure 9.1.

The assessment process should include the patient, the partner, and the family members or caregiver when possible. Documentation in the medical record is fundamental and should include all information covered during the prechemotherapy assessment, as well as the patient's understanding of disease, treatments,

**Table 9.4  Chemotherapy Checklist**

1. Verify informed consent: may be written or oral depending on institution policy, but it is required before chemotherapy administration.
2. Know the drug pharmacology: mechanism of action; usual dosage; route of administration; acute and long-term side effects; and route of excretion.
3. Review laboratory data keeping in mind acceptable parameters. Report abnormalities to the physician.
4. Complete prechemotherapy assessment of patient, medical history, and prior chemotherapy.
5. Check physician order for name of drug(s): dosage; route; rate; and timing of drug(s) administration. (Question anything that seems out of the ordinary.)
6. Recalculate dosage: check height and weight; calculate body surface area (BSA).
7. Verify physician orders and dosage calculations with another nurse.
8. Premedication: administer most premedications at least 20–30 minutes before chemotherapy starts. In some cases, may want to start the patient on antiemetic therapy the night before or the morning of therapy.
9. Patient education: teach and review with the patient and family details of the chemotherapy schedule, expected side effects, and self-care preventive management suggestions to minimize untoward side effects. Provide written explanations the patient can refer to later because this information may be overwhelming. Refer questions to physician as necessary.
10. Provide patient with telephone numbers for physician, clinic, as appropriate.
11. Reconstitute drug(s) according to manufacturer suggestions, OSHA guidelines, and institution procedures. May be the responsibility of the nursing or the pharmacy department depending on the institution's policy.
12. Gather appropriate equipment: D$_5$W or normal saline (NS) are commonly used to infuse chemotherapy, but not exclusively. Use the correct solution and volume. Protect from direct sunlight if applicable.
13. Administer chemotherapy agents according to written policies and procedures using proficient intravenous therapy skills and techniques.
    a. Administer all medications using the five rights:
       (1) Right Patient
       (2) Right Drug
       (3) Right Dose
       (4) Right Route
       (5) Right Time

*(continued)*

**Table 9.4** Chemotherapy Checklist *(continued)*

    b. If no information is available, assume the drug you are giving is a vesicant and administer it with caution, according to institutional policy and procedure.

    c. Avoid drug infiltration: if unsure whether the IV is infiltrated, discontinue it, and restart another IV rather than risk extravasation. WHEN IN DOUBT, PULL IT OUT.

    d. Do not mix drugs together when administering combination therapy. Use syringe or intravenous of NS to flush before first drug, in between drugs, and upon completion of all drugs.

    e. It is not optimal to administer vesicant drugs through an indwelling peripheral IV (one that has been in place 4–6 hours or more). It is important to preserve veins, but it is more important to prevent potential extravasation.

    f. Nonvesicant chemotherapy drugs may be administered through an existing IV, once the site has been fully assessed for patency and lack of infiltration.

    g. If unable to start an IV after two attempts, consult a colleague for assistance.

14. Do not allow anyone to interrupt you during the preparation or administration of chemotherapy.

15. Do not foster a patient's dependency on one nurse.

16. Always have emergency drugs and an extravasation kit readily available should an adverse reaction occur.

17. Always listen to the patient: the patient's knowledge and preference should be utilized as frequently as possible. As the patient becomes more knowledgeable regarding IV techniques, his or her personal experience with successful IV sites, methods, and sensations can be a great aid to the nurse. There are times when the patient's preference may not be the best choice, but his or her participation should always be encouraged.

18. Dispose of intravenous supplies according to OSHA guidelines, and institution policy and procedure. (See Chapter 11.)

19. Document drug administration according to institution policy and procedures. Use time savers in documentation, e.g., instead of writing step-by-step how a vesicant was given, write "(Name of drug) administered according to institution policy and procedure for vesicants."

20. Observe for adverse reactions.

21. Use the opportunity to teach and counsel the patient and the family while administering the chemotherapy.

*Sources:* Oncology Nursing Society. (1988). *Cancer Chemotherapy Guidelines: Module II. Recommendations for Nursing Practice in the Acute Care Setting.* Pittsburgh: Oncology Nursing Society Press; Morra, M.E. (ed). (1981). *Cancer Chemotherapy Treatment and Care.* Boston: G.K. Hall Medical; Miller, S.A. (1980). Nursing actions in cancer chemotherapy administration. *Oncology Nursing Forum* 7(4): 8–16.

and particular aspects of care in which the individual and the family members will participate. The family and patient should be given resource materials that can assist them during the treatment of their disease with chemotherapy. If the patient's first language is not English or if other cultural or religious barriers exist that hinder the ability to comprehend the "process involved in receiving chemotherapy therapy treatment," an interpreter, a clergy member, or a community member should be involved from the beginning to keep the patient completely informed about the disease and the treatment.

Family members play a significant role throughout the entire process but particularly if chemotherapy is administered in the home. Although the technical aspects of this service usually are provided by a proprietary home care company, nurses employed by these companies should be held to the same standard

**Table 9.5** Karnofsky Performance Status Scale

| Condition | Percentage | Comments |
|---|---|---|
| Able to carry on normal activity and to work; no special care is needed | 100 | Normal; no complaints; no evidence of disease |
| | 90 | Able to carry on normal activity; minor signs or symptoms of disease |
| | 80 | Normal activity with effort; some signs or symptoms of disease |
| Unable to work; able to live at home; able to care for most personal needs; a varying degree of assistance is needed | 70 | Cares for self; unable to carry on normal activity or to do active work |
| | 60 | Requires occasional assistance but is able to care for most needs |
| | 50 | Requires considerable assistance and frequent medical care |
| Unable to care for self; requires equivalent of institutional or hospital care; disease may be progressing rapidly | 40 | Disabled; requires special care and assistance |
| | 30 | Severely disabled; hospitalization is indicated, although death is not imminent |
| | 20 | Hospitalization is necessary; very sick; active supportive treatment necessary |
| | 10 | Moribund; fatal processes progressing rapidly |
| | 0 | Dead |

*Sources:* Karnofsky and Burchenal (1949). In S.L. Groenwald (1990). *Cancer Nursing Principle and Practice.* Boston: Jones & Bartlett.

mentioned earlier in this chapter. That is, they should be trained specifically in oncology, certified in chemotherapy administration, and work in collaboration with the patient's multidisciplinary team.

Many patients prefer being treated at home because of increased privacy, convenience, and less individual anxiety (McPhail 1999). The nurse working in oncology home care must possess highly developed assessment and communication skills because this person may be the only health care provider observing the patient's reaction to chemotherapy.

Patient selection is an important factor in determining the success of chemotherapy outside the hospital. The health care team must be confident that all potential complications and side effects can be managed safely before a patient is selected for outpatient therapy. If the team is not confident of the patient's ability to tolerate chemotherapy, it may be better for the patient to receive one course of therapy in the hospital or to receive one course of therapy as an inpatient so the team can assess drug tolerance. The nurse's assessment of the patient and his or her environment must be continuous so that the health care team has a basis for clinical judgments relating to continued therapy in an ambulatory setting (Berg 1996).

At present, various chemotherapeutic agents are being successfully administered in ambulatory and home settings. As providers become more sophisticated in side effect management and can rely on more innovative equipment, the number of drugs will

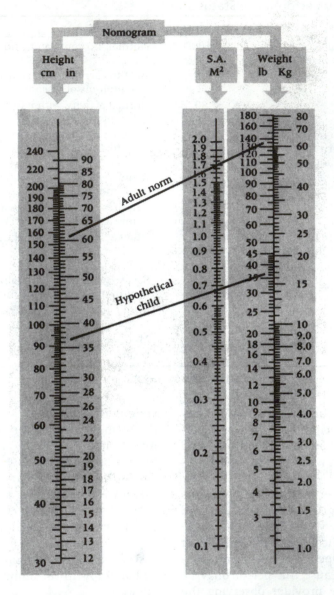

## Figure 9.1   Body Surface Area Determination

The patient's body surface area (m²) is calculated from his or her height and weight. In the figure, body surface area is the point of intersection on the middle scale when a straight line joins the height and weight scales. For example, if a patient's weight is 109 kg and height is 161 cm, the patient's BSA is 2.1.

*Source:* Behrman, R.E., and Vaughn, V.C. (eds.) (1983). *Nelson Textbook of Pediatrics.* 12th ed. Philadelphia: W.B. Saunders. Reprinted with permission.

increase. Ambulatory and home care nurses also administer blood products, antibiotics, nutritional support products, and pain medications, but they cannot do so successfully in an outpatient or home setting without the support of family caregivers. The patient and family must be capable of assuming care measures to minimize side effects and must be taught reactions and how to report them. The assistance of other community-based support services also may be required (Berg 1996).

## SPECIFIC REACTIONS TO CHEMOTHERAPY: EXTRAVASATION, HYPERSENSITIVITY, AND ANAPHYLAXIS EXTRAVASATION

Several local reactions, venospasm, irritation, and flare reaction, can occur when infusing cancer chemotherapeutic agents. Table 9.6 highlights the various differences between these local skin reactions and Table 9.7 specifies current knowledge about vesicants,

**Table 9.6**   Nursing Assessment of Extravasation Versus Other Reactions

| Assessment Parameter | Extravasation Immediate Manifestations | Delayed Manifestations | Irritation of the Vein | Flare Reaction |
|---|---|---|---|---|
| Pain | Severe pain or burning that lasts minutes or hours and eventually subsides; usually occurs while the drug is being given and around the needle site | Hours–48 | Aching and tightness along the vein | No pain |
| Redness | Blotchy redness around the needle site; not always present at time of extravasation | Later occurrence | The full length of the vein may be reddened or darkened. | Immediate blotches or streaks along the vein, which usually subside within 30 minutes with or without treatment |
| Ulceration | Develops insidiously; usually occurs 48–96 hours later | Later occurrence | Not usually | Not usually |
| Swelling | Severe swelling; usually occurs immediately | Hours–48 | Not likely | Not likely; wheals may appear along vein line |
| Blood return | Inability to obtain blood return | Good blood return during drug administration | Usually | Usually |
| Other | Change in the quality of infusion | Local tingling and sensory deficits | | Urticaria |

*Source:* Oncology Nursing Society. (1999). *Cancer Chemotherapy Guidelines and Recommendations for Practice.* 2nd ed. Pittsburgh: Oncology Nursing Society Press. Reprinted with permission.

**Table 9.7** Vesicants and Irritants

| | | Vesicants | | |
|---|---|---|---|---|
| **Chemotherapeutic Agents** | **Antidote** | **Antidote Preparation** | **Local Care** | **Comments** |
| **Alkylating agents**<br>mechlorethamine hydrochloride (nitrogen mustard) | Isotonic sodium (Na) thiosulfate | Prepare 1/6 molar solution:<br>a. If 10% Na thiosulfate solution, mix 4 ml with 6 ml sterile water for injection<br>b. If 25% Na thiosulfate solution, mix 1.6 ml with 8.4 ml sterile water | 1. Immediately inject Na thiosulfate through IV cannula, 2 ml for every mg extravasated<br>2. Remove needle<br>3. Inject antidote into subcutaneous (SC) tissue | 1. Na thiosulfate neutralizes nitrogen mustard, which then is excreted via the kidneys<br>2. Time is essential in treating extravasation<br>3. Heat and cold not proven effective (Dorr 1990, 1994)<br>4. Although clinically accepted, reports of the benefits are scant (Ignoffo and Friedman 1980) |
| cisplatin (Platinol[a]) | Same as above | Same as above | 1. Use 2 ml of the 10% Na thiosulfate for each 100 mg of cisplatin<br>2. Remove needle<br>3. Inject SC | 1. Vesicant potential seen with a concentration of more than 20 cc of 0.5 mg/ml extravasates. If less than this, drug is an irritant; no treatment recommended (Dorr 1994) |
| **Antitumor antibiotics**<br>doxorubicin (Adriamycin[b]) | None | | 1. Apply cold pad with circulating ice water, ice pack, or cryogel pack for 15–20 minutes at least four times per day for the first 24–48 hours (Harwood and Govin 1994) | 1. Extravasations of less than 1–2 cc often will heal spontaneously; if greater than 3 cc, ulceration often results (Goodman and Riley 1997)<br>2. Protect from sunlight and heat<br>3. Studies suggest benefit of 99% dimethyl sulfoxide (DMSO) 1–2 ml applied to site every six hours (Olver et al. 1988; St. Germain, Houlihan, and D'Amato 1994). Other studies show delayed healing with DMSO (Harwood and Bachur 1987). |

| Drug | Antidote | Local care | Special considerations |
|---|---|---|---|
| daunorubicin (Cerubidine[c]) | None | | 1. Little information known. 2. In mouse experiments, some benefit from topical DMSO (Olver et al. 1988) |
| mitomycin-C (Mitomycin) | None | | 1. Protect from sunlight 2. Delayed skin reactions have occurred in areas far from original IV site 3. Some research studies show benefit with use of 99% DMSO 1–2 ml applied to site every six hrs for 14 days. More studies needed (Alberts and Dorr 1991) |
| dactinomycin (Actinomycin-D) | None | 1. Apply ice to increase comfort at the site. 2. Elevate for 48 hrs then resume normal activity. (Goodman and Riley 1997) | 1. Heat may enhance tissue damage |
| mitoxantrone | Unknown | | 1. Antidote or local care measures unknown (Dorr 1990) 2. Ulceration rare unless concentrated dose infiltrates |
| epirubicin Idarubicin (Idamycin[d]) esorubicin | None | | 1. Antidote and local care measures unknown 2. Cold, DMSO, and corticosteroids ineffective in experiments with mice (Soble, Dorr, Plezia, and Breckenridge 1987). Esorubicin-phlebitis common (Dorr 1990). |

*(continued)*

**Table 9.7** Vesicants and Irritants *(continued)*

Vesicants

| Chemotherapeutic Agents | Antidote | Antidote Preparation | Local Care | Comments |
|---|---|---|---|---|
| **Vinca alkaloids/ microtubular inhibiting agents** | | | | |
| vincristine (Oncovin[e]) | hyaluronidase* | Mix 150 units hyaluronidase with 1–3 ml saline | 1. Apply warm pack for 15–20 mins at least 4 times per day for the first 24–48 hrs and elevate (Larson 1985; Rudolph and Larson 1987) | 1. Administer hyaluronidase and apply heat for 15–20 mins at least 4 times per day for the first 24–48 hrs <br> 2. These two methods of treatment are very effective for rapid absorption of drug (Bellone 1981; Laurie, Wilson, Kernahan, Bauer, and Vistnes 1984; Dorr 1994; Goodman and Riley, 1997) |
| vinblastine (Velban[e]) | Same as above | Same as above | Same as above | Same as above |
| vindesine | Same as above | Same as above | Same as above | Same as above |
| vinorelbine (Navelbine[f]) | Same as above | Same as above | Same as above | 1. Same treatment as vincristine/vinblastine (Dorr and Bool 1995) <br> 2. Moderate vesicant <br> 3. Manufacturer recommends administering drug over 6–10 mins into side port of freeflowing IV closest to the IV bag, followed by flush of 75–125 ml of IV solution to reduce incidence of phlebitis and severe back pain |

**Taxanes**

| Chemotherapeutic Agents | Antidote | Antidote Preparation | Local Care | Comments |
|---|---|---|---|---|
| Paclitaxel (Taxol)[a] | Hyaluronidase* Ice | | 1. Apply ice pack for 15–20 mins at least 4 times per day for the first 24 hrs | 1. Recent documentation of vesicant potential (Harrington and Figueroa 1997; Ajani, Dodd, Daugherty, Warkentin, and Ilson 1994) 2. Paclitaxel has rare vesicant potential (probably due to dilution in 500 cc diluent) (Dorr, Snead, and Liddil 1996) 3. Ice and hyaluronidase have been effective in decreasing local tissue damage in a mouse model (Dorr, Snead, and Liddil 1996) |

**Irritants**

| Chemotherapeutic Agents | Antidote | Antidote Preparation | Local Care | Comments |
|---|---|---|---|---|
| **Alkylating agents** | | | | |
| dacarbazine (DTIC) | | | | 1. May cause phlebitis 2. Protect from sunlight (Dorr, Alberts, Einspahr, Mason-Liddil, and Soble 1987) |
| ifosfamide carboplatin | | | | 1. May cause phlebitis 2. Antidote or local care measures unknown |
| **Nitrosoureas** | | | | |
| carmustine (BCNU) | | | | 1. May cause phlebitis 2. Antidote and local care measures unknown |

*(continued)*

**Table 9.7**  Vesicants and Irritants *(continued)*

|  | Irritants | | | |
| --- | --- | --- | --- | --- |
| **Chemotherapeutic Agents** | **Antidote** | **Antidote Preparation** | **Local Care** | **Comments** |
| **Antitumor antibiotics** | | | | |
| doxorubicin liposome | | | | 1. May produce redness and tissue edema 2. Low ulceration potential 3. If ulceration begins or pain, redness, or swelling persist, treat like doxorubicin |
| bleomycin | | | | 1. May cause irritation to tissue 2. Little information known |
| menogaril | | | | 1. May cause phlebitis, venous edema, and induration 2. Increased incidence if concentrations greater than 1 mg/ml infiltrates or administration occurs in more than 2 hours (Dorr 1994) |
| **Vinca alkaloids** | | | | |
| etoposide (VP-16) | hyaluronidase* | | 1. Apply warm pack | 1. Treatment necessary only if large amount of a concentrated solution extravasates. In this case, treat like vincristine or vinblastine (Dorr 1994) 2. May cause phlebitis, urticaria, and redness |
| teniposide (VM-26) | | | | Same as above |

[a] Bristol-Myers Squibb Oncology, Princeton, NJ; [b] Pharmacia & Upjohn Co., Kalamazoo, MI; [c] Chiron Therapeutics, Emeryville, CA; [d] Adria Laboratories, Dublin, OH; [e] Eli Lilly and Co., Indianapolis, IN; [f] Glaxo Wellcome Oncology/HIV, Research Triangle Park, NC

\* Hyaluronidase is no longer manufactured.

*Note:* Based on information from Bertelli, G. et al. (1995). Topical dimethylsulfoxide for the prevention of soft tissue injury after extravasation of vesicant cytotoxic drugs: A prospective clinical study. *Journal of Clinical Oncology* 13(11): 2851–2855; Lebredo, L., Barrie, R., and Woltering, E.A. (1992). DMSO protection against adriamycin-induced tissue necrosis. *Journal of Surgery Research* 53(1): 26–65; Rospond, E.M., and Engel, L.M. (1993). Dimethyl sulfoxide for treating anthracycline extravasation. *Clinical Pharmatherapeutics* 12(8): 560–561.

*Source:* Oncology Nursing Society. (1999). *Cancer Chemotherapy Guidelines and Recommendations for Practice.* 2nd ed. Pittsburgh: Oncology Nursing Society Press. Reprinted with permission.

irritants, and their antidotes and treatment. Occasionally, venospasm occurs at the beginning of an intravenous injection and the patient experiences pain, which subsides within a few minutes. However, this type of reaction makes it difficult to distinguish a venous spasm from an extravasation because both have similar symptoms. Extravasation, the more serious reaction, is discussed in detail in this section.

Certain chemotherapeutic agents irritate the injection site or the lining of the vein. An irritant is an agent that can cause aching, tightness, and phlebitis at the injection site or along the vein with or without an inflammatory reaction. Finally, a flare reaction is a local, benign, allergic reaction that usually is accompanied by red blotches or streaking along the vein but there is no pain. It too can be confused with an extravasation; however, in a flare reaction, symptoms subside within 30 minutes with or without treatment (Camp-Sorell 1998; Ellenberger 1999).

The most serious reaction is an extravasation of a chemotherapeutic vesicant. Vesicants are medications that cause blisters, severe tissue injury, or necrosis when they extravasate into surrounding tissues. Vesicant extravasation is the leakage of a drug that causes pain, necrosis, or sloughing of tissue into the subcutaneous space. The extent of injury that occurs when a vesicant infiltrates depends on many factors: the agent used, the concentration, the dosage, the pH, the osmolarity, and the molecular weight (McCaffrey-Boyle and Engelking 1995). Delayed extravasation refers to an infiltration of a cancer chemotherapeutic agent with symptoms occurring in a delayed pattern, after 48 hours of drug administration.

Extravasation results from certain chemotherapeutic agents that infiltrate into surrounding tissue and potentiate a serious clinical situation. Cancer patients at high risk for extravasation have fragile veins, lymphedema, repeated venapuncture procedures, and are given specific types and kinds of chemotherapeutic agents (refer to Table 9.7) (Camp-Sorrel 1998; Chrystal 1997). Risk factors are compounded if blood vessels are thrombosed (consequently limiting the number of accessible veins), if complications from the disease are present (i.e., superior vena cava syndrome), or if decreased sensation or parasthesias are present (Camp-Sorrel 1998; How and Brown 1998). Medical conditions, such as Raynaud's disease and diabetes with accompanying neuropathy, can be additional compounding factors (Camp-Sorrel 1998; How and Brown 1998). Administration of previous chemotherapy increases the risk of extravasation due to many of the factors mentioned previously. Also, a patient who received previous radiotherapy at the vein site may experience a severe local reaction in the event of an extravasation (McCaffrey-Boyle and Engleking 1995). The presence of any preexisting conditions that might influence site selection or make a patient prone to an extravasation should be documented in the patient's chart (Ellenberger 1999).

In addition to pain, a vesicant infiltration can result in hyperpigmentation, induration, burning, inflammation, sloughing, necrosis, and ulceration. Severe infiltrations may result in damage to underlying structures such as muscles, tendons, and nerves. Severe tissue destruction will interfere ultimately with the affected extremity's function, and if severe enough, may lead to the loss of a limb. In the case of an extravasation from a vascular access device, one could possibly lose a breast (Oncology Nursing Society). Table 9.8 presents a standardized care plan for the patient experiencing an extravasation.

Extravasation has long been a concern to those administering chemotherapy agents. Usually, unique institutional policies and procedures are to be followed when administering such agents. Prevention (Table 9.9) is the key when administering a chemotherapeutic agent with a high likelihood of extravasation. With an extravasation, it may not always be obvious that a problem exists initially. Both

**Table 9.8** Standardized Nursing Care Plan for Patient Experiencing Extravasation (Based on 1999 ONS Cancer Chemotherapy Guidelines)

| Nursing Diagnosis | Defining Characteristics | Expected Outcomes | Nursing Interventions |
|---|---|---|---|
| I. Potential alteration in skin integrity related to extravasation | I. Vesicant drugs may cause erythema, burning, tissue necrosis, tissue sloughing | I. Extravasation, if it occurs, will be detected early with early intervention | I. Careful technique is used during venipuncture (see Chapter 10). A. Select venipuncture site away from underlying tendons and blood vessels. B. Secure IV so that catheter/needle site is visible at all times. C. Administer vesicant through freely flowing IV, constantly monitoring IV site and pt response. Nurse should be thoroughly familiar with institutional policy and procedure for administration of a vesicant agent. D. If vesicant drug is administered as a continuous infusion, drug must be given through a patent central line. |
| II. Potential pain at site of extravasation | II. Vesicant drugs include A. Commercial agents 1. dactinomycin 2. daunorubicin 3. doxorubicin 4. mitomycin C 5. mechlorethamine 6. vinblastine 7. vincristine 8. vinorelbine 9. idarubicin 10. vindesine 11. epirubicin 12. esorubicin 13. cisplatin 14. mitoxantrone 15. paclitaxel | II. Skin and underlying tissue damage will be minimized | II. If extravasation is suspected: A. Stop drug administration. B. Aspirate any residual drug and blood from IV tubing, IV catheter/needle, and IV site if possible. C. Instill antidote if one exists through needle if able to remove remaining drug in previous step. If standing orders are not available, notify MD and obtain order. D. Remove needle. E. Inject antidote into area of apparent infiltration if antidote is recommended, using 25-gauge needle into subcutaneous tissue. F. Apply topical cream if recommended. G. Cover lightly with occlusive sterile dressing. H. Apply warm or cold applications as prescribed. I. Elevate arm. |

J. Assess site regularly for pain, progression of erythema, induration, and for evidence of necrosis:

1. If outpatient, arrange to assess site or teach pt to and to notify provider if condition worsens. Arrange next visit for assessment of site depending on drug, amount infiltrated, extent of potential injury, and pt variables.

2. Discuss with MD the need for plastic-surgical consult if erythema, induration, pain, tissue breakdown occurs.

K. When in doubt about whether drug is infiltrating, treat as an infiltration.

L. Document precise, concise information in patient's chart.

1. Date, time
2. Insertion site, needle size and type
3. Drug administration technique, drug sequence, and approximate amount of drug extravasated
4. Appearance of site, patient's subjective response
5. Nursing interventions performed to manage extravasation, and notification of MD
6. Photo documentation if possible
7. Follow-up plan
8. Nurse's signature
9. Institutional policy and procedure for documentation should be adhered to

B. Investigational agents

1. amsacrine
2. maytansine
3. bisantrene
4. pyrazofurin
5. adozelesin
6. anti-B4-blocked ricin

III. *Potential loss of function of extremity related to extravasation*

IV. *Potential infection related to skin breakdown*

*Source:* Berg, D. (1996). Principles of chemotherapy administration. In M. Barton-Burke, G. Wilkes, and K. Ingwersen, *Cancer Chemotherapy: A Nursing Process Approach.* 2nd ed. Sudbury, Mass.: Jones & Bartlett.

patients and nurses have reported that often the first indication of an extravasation is a vague feeling or complaint that "something feels different this time," or that there is a burning sensation, tenderness, or pain when receiving the chemotherapy treatment (How and Brown 1998; McCaffrey-Boyle and Engelking 1995). The patient may experience a mild redness, blotchy skin, swelling, or temperature change. The nurse administering the drug may have a feeling that something is different during this intravenous injection, there may be increased resistance to the intravenous flow and no blood flashback (McCaffrey-Boyle and Engelking 1995). If the extravasation is missed, then discoloration, induration, dry desquamation, and blistering can occur, all of which can be accompanied by discomfort or pain. If no action is taken, the extravasation can develop into an ulcerative necrotic lesion that may require surgical intervention to heal (McCaffrey-Boyle and Engelking 1995).

Should an extravasation occur or even be suspected, the management (see Table 9.10) and documentation of the incident per institutional policy is imperative. Figure 9.2 is one example of a chemotherapy drug extravasation record. In the case of a suspected extravasation,

the chemotherapeutic agent must be discontinued immediately, the institution's extravasation protocol must be initiated, and the physician must be notified at once. The patient and family must be well informed that extravasation is a possible outcome of vesicant administration and should be instructed to report immediately any sensation of warmth, burning, tingling, pain at the injection site, pain along the vein, pain in the area of their port, or pain across the chest wall.

The variability in symptoms and indolent nature of tissue destruction requires that nurses thoroughly educate patients and family members regarding extravasation. Follow-up care after a suspected or actual vesicant extravasation is crucial. The nurse should develop a consistent, continuous format for documentation of nursing assessments, evaluations, and interventions.

Finally, upon discharge, written instructions should be given to patients regarding what observable changes should be reported and how to notify their health care provider 24 hours a day. Institutions also should provide patient information sheets on extravasation site care and follow-up, if necessary.

As mentioned earlier, the severity of an extravasation is usually proportional to the

**Table 9.9  Prevention of Extravasation**

Use experienced personnel.

Use patient education.

Use single venipuncture—new site.

Avoid areas of compromised circulation (phlebitis, lymphedema, mastectomy side, lower extremities, hematomas).

Avoid areas with underlying tendons and nerves.

Ensure adequate drug dilution—sidearm injection through freely flowing IV.

Maintain careful observation—visualize entire limb continuously throughout procedure.

Consider the use of venous access devices in cases of difficult peripheral access.

*Source:* Adapted from Montrose, P.A. (1987). Extravasation management. *Seminars in Oncology Nursing* 3: 128–132. Reprinted with permission of W.B. Saunders.

**Table 9.10    Management of Extravasation**

1. Assess site for signs and symptoms of extravasation (see Table 9.6)
2. Manage extravasation of drugs with known intravenous antidotes (see Table 9.7) or with subcutaneous antidote.
   a. Stop the chemotherapy administration.
   b. Leave the needle in place.
   c. Aspirate any residual drug and blood in the intravenous tubing, needle, and infiltration site.
   d. Instill the intravenous antidote (see Table 9.7).

**NB:** If unable to aspirate the residual drug from the intravenous tubing, **DO NOT** instill the antidote through the needle. Proceed directly to the next step.

   e. Remove the needle.
   f. Inject the subcutaneous antidote in a clockwise fashion into the infiltrated area, using a 25-gauge needle.
   g. Avoid applying pressure to the suspected infiltration site.
   h. Apply topical ointment as needed, if ordered.
   i. Cover lightly with an occlusive sterile dressing.
   j. Apply warm or cold compresses as indicated (see Table 9.7).
   k. Elevate the arm.
   l. Observe the site regularly for reaction.
   m. Document the following information in the patient's medical record:
      (1) Date
      (2) Time
      (3) Needle size and type
      (4) Insertion site
      (5) Drug sequence
      (6) Drug administration technique
      (7) Approximate amount of drug extravasated
      (8) Nursing management of extravasation
      (9) Patient complaints and statement
      (10) Appearance of the site
      (11) Physician notification
      (12) Follow-up measures
   n. Document the incident on a report form according to institution policy and procedures (see Figure 9.2).

*Source:* Oncology Nursing Society. (1992b). *Cancer Chemotherapy Guidelines: Recommendations for the Management of Vesicant Extravasation, Hypersensitivity, and Anaphylaxis.* Pittsburgh: Oncology Nursing Society Press. Oncology Nursing Society Press. (1992a). *Cancer Chemotherapy Guidelines: Module V. Recommendations for the Management of Extravasation and Anaphylaxis.* Pittsburgh: Oncology Nursing Society Press.

quantity of the drug extravasated, as well as cellular toxicity, high osmolarity, pH, and the ability of the agent to cause tissue ischemia and to bind directly with DNA (How and Brown 1998). It is well known that the DNA-binding properties of anthracylines will continue to cause tissue damage until the drug is completely removed (McCaffrey-Boyle and Engelking 1995). The actual drug uptake into the soft tissue can influence the severity and the progression of an ulcer. Anthracyclines produce immediate damage characterized by a

Date _____

Time _____

Patient _____

Drug _____ Dilution mg/ml _____

Method of Administration: Piggy Back _____

Side-arm _____

VAD: Port _____ Tunnel _____ PICC _____

Type of needle/size _____

Other: _____

Amount infiltrated _____ Amount aspirated _____

Size of infiltration (note size in cm) _____

**Location of extravasation**

*Hand:* dorsal surface                              *Arm:* ventral surface

hand _____ rt _____ lt _____              forearm _____ rt _____ lt _____

forearm _____ rt _____ lt _____           wrist _____ rt _____ lt _____

wrist _____ rt _____ lt _____             ac fossa _____ rt _____ lt _____

VAD: Describe _____

other _____ Photograph yes _____ no _____

**Process Documentation**

Patient symptoms _____

Assessment of site _____

Suspected extravasation _____ Definite extravasation _____

Physician notified: _____ Date _____ Time _____

Interventions _____ Antidote _____ Cold/warm application _____

Follow-up (document with serial photographs): _____

**Patient Instructions**

1. Continue with warm/cold compresses for the first 24–48 hours, then as needed.
2. Avoid pressure to the original IV site.
3. Rest and elevate the site for the first 48 hours, then you can resume your normal activities.
4. Call if you experience any of the following.
   - Pain, burning, redness, swelling at the original IV site
   - Skin breakdown or areas of blackness anywhere on skin
   - Difficulty moving hand, wrist, elbow or shoulder
5. Names and numbers to call 24 hours a day

   MD _____

   RN _____

   Other _____

6. Return appointments with _____

   Date/time: _____

Keep main copy in clinical record and duplicate to patient.

*Note.* From "Delivery of Cancer Chemotherapy," by M. Goodman, in S.B. Baird, R. McCorkle, and M. Grant (Eds.), *Cancer Nursing: A Comprehensive Textbook* (p. 304), 1991, Philadelphia: W.B. Saunders. Copyright 1991 by W.B. Saunders. Adapted with permission.

**Figure 9.2   Chemotherapy Drug Extravasation Record**

*Source:* Oncology Nursing Society. (1999). *Cancer Chemotherapy Guidelines and Recommendations for Practice.* 2nd ed. Pittsburgh: Oncology Nursing Society Press. Reprinted with permission.

prolonged binding effect causing a necrotic process that destroys cells over time. Anthracyclines can remain active even after being released from the dying or necrotic cells and can damage adjacent cells, causing progression of the necrosis (How and Brown 1998). Some agents, such as vincristine or vinblastine, cause rapid tissue damage with the clinical characteristics of a burn (How and Brown 1998). Adequate flushing with a neutral solution at the termination of a vesicant infusion may decrease the potential for a residual drug to be distributed in subcutaneous tissue or at the needle insertion site, where it can result in tissue damage (Ingle 1995).

Extravasation kits and accompanying policies and procedures must be available in whatever setting chemotherapy is administered. These kits must be checked on a regular basis for outdated supplies, and supplies must be replaced immediately after use. Standards of care, policies, and procedures must be updated as new drugs are released or at least annually. In most settings, there is a close working relationship between the oncology staff and the quality assurance department to ensure and safeguard patient safety, efficacy, and follow-up study with the issue of chemotherapy extravasation.

## HYPERSENSITIVITY REACTIONS AND ANAPHYLAXIS

Cancer chemotherapy drugs are foreign substances able to induce hypersensitivity reactions (HSRs). Hypersensitivity reactions range from mild cutaneous symptoms to severe respiratory distress and cardiovascular collapse. The incidence of acute hypersensitivity is reduced greatly when the agent is administered orally. Conversely, these events are more frequent and severe when the causal agent is injected (Liberman 1995a; Liberman 1995b;

Labovich 1999). Factors that influence the development of HSR include gender, age, genetic makeup, nutritional status, individual stress level, and immune system along with hormonal and environmental influences (Labovich 1999). Patients with cancer often have poor protein caloric intake, are immunosuppressed, and may be receiving ionizing radiation or chemotherapy. All these factors have the potential to interfere with the functional ability of the immune system and possibly put patients at greater risk for HSR (Ewan 1998).

Hypersensitivity reactions are those reactions of the immune system that occur in response to a foreign substance. Hypersensitivity reactions are rated as Types I–IV by the Gell and Coombs Classification System (see Table 9.11) (Oncology Nursing Society 1999; Labovich 1999).

HSRs are believed to be antigen-antibody Type I hypersensitivity reactions mediated by IgE and are defined as local reactions. Hypersensitivity reactions can occur with all chemotherapy agents except the nitrosoureas and have occurred in 5–15% of patients receiving chemotherapy. Hypersensitivity reactions to paclitaxel were observed in early Phase 1 clinical trials. Eight percent of these reactions were classified as major reactions, and minor hypersensitivity reactions have not been associated with subsequent development of a major reaction. With premedication, the incidence of major hypersensitivity reactions has decreased to 1–3% (Ciesielski-Carlucci 1997). A HSR differs from a normal immune response because of the exaggerated or inappropriate immune response. The exact mechanism of what transpires when a particular drug is infused and an HSR occurs is unclear. Table 9.12 provides a list of chemotherapeutic agents with a high incidence of hypersensitivity reactions.

Skin testing for immediate HSR is an established diagnostic tool in the study of allergies

**Table 9.11** Types of Hypersensitivity Reactions (Gell and Coombs Classification)

| Type | Major Signs and Symptoms | Example of Reaction | Mechanism of Action |
|------|--------------------------|---------------------|---------------------|
| I | Anaphylactic symptoms: urticaria, angioedema, rash, bronchospasm, abdominal cramping, respiratory collapse and cardiovascular collapse | Anaphylaxis to chemotherapy, bee stings, food allergies | IgE-mediated HSR; antigen-IgE antibody interaction on basophil and mast cell surfaces causing degranulation |
| II | Hemolytic anemia, cardiovascular collapse, and possibly death | Massive hemolysis from transfusion of incompatible blood | Cell surface antigens interacting with IgG or IgM antibodies with destruction (lysis) of target cell |
| III | Deposition of immune complexes in tissues resulting in various forms of tissue injury and manifestations | Systemic lupus, rheumatoid arthritis, horse serum sickness; may produce a maculopapular eruption or vasculitic lesions | Antigen-antibody interaction, forming immune complexes; anaphylactoid reaction from complement activation via classical pathway, may mimic type I reaction |
| IV | Stomatitis, pneumonitis, contact dermatitis, granuloma formation, and homograft rejection | Tuberculosis, poison ivy, contact sensitivity from mechlorethamine topical application for mycosis fungoides | Sensitized T lymphocytes react with antigen and release lymphokines |

*Source:* Labovich, T.M. (1999). Acute hypersensitivity reactions to chemotherapy. *Seminars in Oncology Nursing* 11(3): 225. Reprinted with permission.

and remains the most sensitive tool in the evaluation of Type I, IgE mediated HSR. In oncology, performing a scratch test, intradermal skin test, or administering a test dose prior to the initial dose of a drug with incidence of hypersensitivity reactions are accepted methods of determining an individual's reactivity, i.e., bleomycin (Oncology Nursing Society 1999; Labovich 1999). Guidelines for patient care during skin testing are: (1) to observe the patient for a local or systemic reaction (which can occur up to one hour or more after the test is performed); (2) if no sign of a hypersensitivity reaction appears proceed with the initial dosing; and (3) when administering an IV bolus drug with an incidence of hypersensitivity, infuse slowly and continue to observe the patient for shortness or breath, flushing, or a change in vital signs, and have an emergency cart in close proximity (Oncology Nursing Society 1999).

## ANAPHYLAXIS AND ANAPHYLACTOID REACTIONS

Anaphylaxis and anaphylactoid reactions with cancer chemotherapy occur through a variety of mechanisms ranging from mild cutaneous reactions to fatal shock. Anaphylaxis is a generalized, immediate hypersensitivity reaction and involves the activation of many different inflammation pathways, most commonly mast cells and basophil degranulation. This mediator release causes increased vascular permeability, vasodilation, smooth muscle contraction, stimulation of sensory and autonomic nerves, and

**Table 9.12**  Summary of Chemotherapy Agents With a High Incidence of Hypersensitivity Reactions

| Drug | Factors Increasing Risk of HSRs | Comments |
|---|---|---|
| L-asparaginase | Administered as a single agent<br>After fourth dose | HSR most likely IgE-mediated<br>*Erwinia* asparaginase can be substituted if reaction occurs |
| | Hiatus of > 1 month between doses<br>Weekly administration versus daily or 3×/week<br>Prior exposure to L-asparaginase, months or even years previously<br>Intravenous route of administration<br>High doses | Pegasparaginase under investigation as a substitute |
| paclitaxel | Faster infusion rate<br>Higher dosage | Premedication with dexamethasone, diphenhydramine, HCI, and cimetadine, famotadine, or ranitadine ± ephedrine to prevent reaction |
| etoposide<br>teniposide | | Can occur with the first dose or subsequent doses<br>HSR can occur shortly after or several hours after infusion<br>No published reports of HSR to oral etoposide |
| cisplatin | Six or more doses<br>Intravesicular route of administration* | HSRs are less common now compared with their initial use; may be attributed to fewer courses and current trends of antiemetic use with diphenhydramine and dexamethasone<br>Cross-reactivity exists between carboplatin and cisplatin |
| procarbazine | | Pulmonary toxicity has been reported in anecdotal form |
| melphalan and chlorambucil | At least 2 prior doses of melphalan | Chlorambucil has a few type I reactions with urticaria and angioedema but no hypotension |
| anthracycline antibiotics | Intravesical administration of doxorubicin | Flare reactions usually do not progress to acute HSR†<br>Sudden cardiac arrest during infusion, although rare, is considered a direct cardiac toxicity versus an acute HSR |
| cyclophosphamide and ifosfamide | | Can occur with both oral and intravenous administration<br>Mesna also has been reported to cause type I HSRs |

\* Intravesicular administration typically has a higher number of courses of treatment; premedication for nausea and vomiting is not needed as with intravenous administration.
†Acute HSR involves serum sickness, bronchospasm, parental medication administration, and/or anaphylaxis.
*Source:* Labovich, T.M. (1999). Acute hypersensitivity reactions to chemotherapy. *Seminars in Oncology Nursing* 11(3): 224. Reprinted with permission.

myocardial depression. Anaphylaxis is IgE mediated and occurs in three phases: sensitization, activation, and effector (Liberman 1995a; Labovich 1999; Ewan 1998).

An anaphylactoid reaction is an event similar to anaphylaxis and has an identical presentation to a Type I anaphylactic reaction; however, it is not mediated by IgE. Anaphylactoid reactions that involve chemotherapy are thought to result for the following two ways: direct stimulation of the mast cell surface (which results in the degranulation of mast cells and a release of vasoactive substances), and uncontrolled activation of the complement cascade system (Liberman 1995a; Labovich 1999).

Four crucial factors that influence the development of anaphylaxis are the route of entry, the amount of antigen introduced, the rate of absorption, and the individual's degree of hypersensitivity to that agent. Anaphylactic reactions to chemotherapy, although not completely understood, currently are ranked as immediate immunoglobulin E (IgE)-mediated HSR (TypeI) in the Gell and Coombs classification system (Labovich 1999).

Risk factors for anaphylaxis in patients receiving chemotherapy include receiving a drug known to cause hypersensitivity reactions, a history of allergies (particularly a drug allergy), previous exposure to the agent, failure to administer prophylactic premedications, and previous exposure to metals. A thorough allergy history is important, and a detailed history of allergic medication encounters is essential. Prior history of HSR, even to structurally unrelated pharmacologic agents, increases the patient's risk of subsequent HSR and anaphylaxis. Additional risk factors include: (1) a history of atopy or allergies to normally harmless substances; (2) prior exposure to the medication; and (3) administration of chemotherapeutic agents with a known history of HSR (Liberman 1995a; Labovich 1999).

When anaphylaxis occurs, four organ systems are involved: cutaneous, gastrointestinal, respiratory, and cardiovascular (Labovich 1999). A working definition for anaphylaxis involves one or both of two severe features: respiratory difficulty (due to laryngeal edema or asthma) and hypotension (which can present as fainting, collapse, or loss of consciousness). The most common causes of death from anaphylaxis are cardiovascular collapse and asphyxiation manifested by angioedema of the airway, bronchospasm, and shock (Liberman 1995a). The major factors in this reaction include the initation of mast cells, the shift of fluid from intravascular space to extravascular space, vasodilation followed by compensatory vasoconstriction, and myocardial depression. The increased vascular permeability can produce a rapid profound loss of intravascular volume of up to 50% in 10 minutes (Labovich 1999). This cardiovascular collapse and shock also can occur without any cutaneous or respiratory symptoms. The absence of cutaneous symptoms (uticaria, angioedema, and flush) places the diagnosis of anaphylaxis in question (Labovich 1999; Liberman 1995a).

Symptoms usually begin within 5–30 minutes after the chemotherapy (antigen) begins infusing (Oncology Nursing Society 1999; Labovich 1999). There may be a direct relationship between onset and the severity of symptoms, i.e., the more rapid the onset the more severe the episode (Liberman 1995a). Patients usually exhibit urticaria, angioedema, upper airway edema, dyspnea, wheezing, flushing, dizziness, syncope, and hypotension. Less common symptoms of anaphylaxis include nausea, vomiting, diarrhea, cramping, abdominal pain, rhinitis, headache, substernal pain, and seizure (Labovich 1999). The likelihood of a fatal event is dependent on several factors: (1) the amount of drug (antigen) absorbed; (2) the time lapsed between the onset of the reaction and the initiation of appropriate treatment; and (3) the degree of hypersensitivity to the offending drug (Labovich 1999). One of the most important steps in managing anaphylaxis is rapid recognition, with immediate care being the critical factor in the event (Oncology Nursing Society 1999; Labovich 1999; Liberman 1995a). Tables 9.13 and 9.14 outline the management and nursing care for the patient who experiences either hypersensitivity or anaphylactic reactions.

Premedication protocols for patients were developed initially for the prevention of reactions to radiocontrast materials. These protocols have reduced the incidence of chemotherapy anaphylaxis (Labovich 1999). For chemotherapy agent hypersensitivity prophylaxis the protocol usually consists of a triad of dexamethasone, H-2 antagonist (cimetidine, famotidine, or ranitidine), and diphenhydramine. Institutional policies and procedures regarding hypersensitivity reactions should include prewritten doctor's orders as to how to proceed with care for a hypersensitivity reaction. These policies should be reviewed frequently, updated regularly, and made readily available to all members of the multidisciplinary team. An emergency drug box, fully stocked, with written instructions for anaphylaxis management should be at hand, readily refilled, and checked on a regular basis for outdated medications.

If possible, patients with a history of anaphylaxis should avoid taking B-adrenergic blocking agents, angiotensin converting enzyme (ACE) inhibitors, monoamine oxidase (MAO) inhibitors, or certain tricyclic antidepressants, such as amitriptyline (Oncology Nursing Society 1999; Labovich 1999; Liberman 1995a). The B-adrenergic blocking agents can increase the severity of an allergic attack and can inhibit the therapeutic effect of epinephrine. While MAO inhibitors and certain tricyclic antidepressants make the use of epinephrine hazardous because they interfere with its degradation and ACE inhibitors prevent the release of angiotensin II, an endogenous compensatory mechanism (Labovich 1999; Liberman 1995a).

Finally, teach the patient to recognize the signs and the symptoms of hypersensitivity and anaphylactic reactions that may occur with chemotherapeutic drug administration and to report those signs, symptoms, or any change immediately (Oncology Nursing Society 1999; Labovich 1999). It is also important to note that some reactions are protracted or biphasic, with symptoms being delayed for several hours or possibly recurring hours after the initial reaction. Due to this possibility, hospitalization is recommended for at least 24 hours after an acute HSR even with the cessation of all symptoms (Liberman 1995a; Liberman 1995b; Labovich 1999). Death has been known to occur at any time during protracted anaphylaxis (Liberman 1995a).

## CONCLUSION

From this chapter, it can be determined that the administration of cancer chemotherapeutic agents is more than just "pushing poisons." It is both an art and a science that requires didactic knowledge and technical skills. The process of chemotherapy administration involves the entire team, including the patient and the family, and covers the gamut of informed consent through prescription writing, dose calculation, assessment, and evaluation of the patient for side effect management. It is medication administration at its very finest. It involves every aspect of the nursing process and working with every member of the multidisciplinary team. It is a very humbling experience for every nurse who ventures to care for the cancer patient requiring this type of treatment.

## Table 9.13 Management of Hypersensitivity and Anaphylactic Reactions

1. Review the pt's allergy history.
2. Consider prophylactic medications with hydrocortisone or an antihistamine in atopic/allergic individuals (this requires a physician's order).
3. Pt and family education: Assess the pt's readiness to learn. Inform pt of the potential of an allergic reaction and report any unusual symptoms such as:
   a. Uneasiness or agitation
   b. Abdominal cramping
   c. Itching
   d. Chest tightness
   e. Lightheadedness or dizziness
   f. Chills
4. Ensure emergency equipment and medications are readily available.
5. Obtain baseline vital signs and note pt's mental status.
6. As appropriate, perform a scratch test, intradermal skin test, or test dose before administering the full dosage (this requires a physician's order). If there is no reaction, the remaining dose can be administered. If an allergic response is suspected, discontinue the test dose (unless it has been completed), maintain the intravenous line, and notify the physician.
7. For a localized allergic response:
   a. Evaluate symptoms; observe for urticaria, wheals, localized erythema.
   b. Administer diphenhydramine or hydrocortisone as per physician's order.
   c. Monitor vital signs every 15 minutes for 1 hour.
   d. Continue subsequent dosing or desensitization program according to a physician's order.
   e. If a "flare" reaction appears along the vein with doxorubicin (Adriamycin) or daunorubicin (see Table 10.11), flush the line with saline.
      (1) Ensure that extravasation has not occurred.
      (2) Administer hydrocortisone 25–50 mg intravenously with a physician's order followed by a normal saline flush. This may be adequate to resolve the "flare" reaction.
      (3) After the "flare" reaction has resolved, continue slow infusion of the drug.
      (4) Monitor for repeated "flare" episodes. It is preferable to change the intravenous site if possible.
8. For a generalized allergic response, anaphylaxis may be suspected if the following signs or symptoms

occur (usually within the first 15 minutes of the start of the infusion or injection):
   a. Subjective signs and symptoms
      (1) Generalized itching
      (2) Chest tightness
      (3) Difficulty speaking
      (4) Agitation
      (5) Uneasiness
      (6) Dizziness
      (7) Nausea
      (8) Crampy abdominal pain
      (9) Anxiety
      (10) Sense of impending doom
      (11) Desire to urinate or defecate
      (12) Chills
   b. Objective signs
      (1) Flushed appearance (edema of face, hands, or feet)
      (2) Localized or generalized urticaria
      (3) Respiratory distress with or without wheezing
      (4) Hypotension
      (5) Cyanosis
9. For a generalized allergic response:
   a. Stop the infusion immediately and notify the physician.
   b. Maintain the intravenous line with appropriate solution to expand the vascular space, e.g., normal saline.
   c. If not contraindicated, ensure maximum rate of infusion if the pt is hypotensive.
   d. Position the pt to promote perfusion of the vital organs; the supine position is preferred.
   e. Monitor vital signs every 2 minutes until stable, then every 5 minutes for 30 minutes, then every 15 minutes as ordered.
   f. Reassure the pt and the family.
   g. Maintain the airway and anticipate the need for cardiopulmonary resuscitation.
   h. All medications must be administered with a physician's order.
10. Document the incident in the medical record according to institution policy and procedures.
11. Physician-guided desensitization may be necessary for subsequent dosing.

*Source:* Berg, D. (1996). Principles of chemotherapy administration. In M. Barton-Burke, G. Wilkes, and K. Ingwersen, *Cancer Chemotherapy: A Nursing Process Approach*. Sudbury, Mass.: Jones & Bartlett. Reprinted with permission.

**Table 9.14** Standardized Nursing Care Plan for Patient Experiencing Hypersensitivity or Anaphylaxis

| Nursing Diagnosis | Defining Characteristics | Expected Outcomes | Nursing Interventions |
|---|---|---|---|
| I. *Potential for injury related to hypersensitivity or anaphylaxis* | I. A. Allergic or hypersensitivity reactions to chemotherapy vary from simple allergic reactions to life-threatening ones<br>B. The reactions are the result of a foreign substance being introduced into the body, with resultant antibody formation<br>C. The reactions may worsen with subsequent exposure to the foreign substance (chemotherapeutic agent) | I. A. Allergic reactions (hypersensitivity and anaphylaxis), if they occur, will be detected early<br>B. Airway will remain patent<br>C. BP will remain within 20 mmHg of baseline<br>D. Future allergic responses will be prevented | I. A. Review standing orders for management of allergic reactions (hypersensitivity and anaphylaxis) per institutional policy and procedure<br>B. Identify location of anaphylaxis kit; the kit should contain:<br>  1. epinephrine 1:1000<br>  2. hydrocortisone sodium succinate (SoluCortef)<br>  3. diphenhydramine HCl (Benadryl)<br>  4. aminophylline<br>  5. similar emergency drugs<br>C. Prior to drug administration, obtain baseline vital signs and record mental status<br>D. Observe for following s/s, usually occurring within the first 15 mins of infusion<br>  1. *Subjective*<br>    a. nausea<br>    b. generalized itching<br>    c. crampy abdominal pain<br>    d. chest tightness<br>    e. anxiety<br>    f. agitation<br>    g. sense of impending doom<br>    h. wheeziness/shortness of breath<br>    i. desire to urinate/defecate<br>    j. dizziness<br>    k. chills<br>  2. *Objective*<br>    a. flushed appearance (angioedema of the face, neck, eyelids, hands, feet)<br>    b. localized or generalized urticaria<br>    c. respiratory distress and wheezing<br>    d. hypotension<br>    e. cyanosis |

*(continued)*

**Table 9.14** Standardized Nursing Care Plan for Patient Experiencing Hypersensitivity or Anaphylaxis *(continued)*

| Nursing Diagnosis | Defining Characteristics | Expected Outcomes | Nursing Interventions |
|---|---|---|---|
| | | | E. ONS recommendations for generalized allergic response<br>1. Stop infusion and notify MD<br>2. Obtain orders for infusion of NS to maintain vascular volume and titrate infusion rate to maintain adequate BP (i.e., within 20 mmHg of baseline systolic BP)<br>3. Place pt in supine position to promote perfusion of visceral organs<br>4. Monitor vital signs q 2 mins until stable, then q 5 mins for 30 mins, then q 15 mins<br>5. Provide emotional reassurance to pt and family<br>6. Maintain patent airway and have equipment ready for CPR if needed<br>7. Medications per MD order and institutional policy and procedure<br>F. Document incident<br>G. Discuss with MD desensitization versus drug discontinuance for further dose |

*Source:* Berg, D. (1996). Principles of chemotherapy administration. In M. Barton-Burke, G. Wilkes, and K. Ingwersen, *Cancer Chemotherapy: A Nursing Process Approach.* Sudbury, Mass.: Jones & Bartlett.

# BIBLIOGRAPHY

Ajani, J.A., Dodd, L.G. Daugherty, K., Warkentin, D., and Ilson, D.H. (1994). Taxol-induced soft-tissue injury secondary to extravasation: Characterization by histopathology and clinical course. *Journal of the National Cancer Institute* 86(1): 51–53.

Alberts, D.S., and Dorr, R.T. (1991a). Case report: Topical DMSO for mitomycin-C induced skin ulceration. *Oncology Nursing Forum* 18(4): 693–695.

Alberts, D.S., and Dorr, R.T. (1991b). Symptomatic cardiotoxicity with high-dose 5-fluorouracil infusion: A prospective study. *Oncology* 50: 441–444.

Barton-Burke, M., Wilkes, G., and Ingwersen, K. (1996). *Cancer Chemotherapy: A Nursing Process Approach.* 2nd ed. Sudbury, Mass.: Jones & Bartlett.

Behrman, R.E., and Vaughn, V.C. (eds.) (1983). *Nelson Textbook of Pediatrics.* 12th ed. Philadelphia: W.B. Saunders.

Bellone, J.D. (1981). Treatment of vincristine extravasation. [Letter to the editor]. *Journal of the American Medical Association* 245: 343.

Berg, D. (1996). Principles of chemotherapy administration. In M. Barton-Burke, G. Wilkes, and K. Ingwersen, *Cancer Chemotherapy: A Nursing Process Approach.* 2nd ed. Sudbury, Mass.: Jones & Bartlett.

Berman, A. (1999). Supporting the home care client receiving chemotherapy. *Home Care Provider* 4(2): 81–85.

Bertelli, G., Gozzo, A., Forno, G.B., Vidili, M.G., Silvestro, S., Venturini, M., DelMastro, L., Garrone, O., Rosso, R., and Dini, D. (1995). Topical dimethylsulfoxide for the prevention of soft tissue injury after extravasation of vesicant cytotoxic drugs: A prospective clinical study. *Journal of Clinical Oncology* 13(11): 2851–2855.

Bertolone, K. (1997). Pediatric oncology: Past, present and new modalities of treatment. *Journal of Intravenous Nursing* 20(3): 136–140.

Camp-Sorrell, D. (1998). Developing extravasation protocols and monitoring outcomes. *Journal of Intravenous Nursing* 21(4): 232–239.

Chrystal, C. (1997). Administering continuous vesicant chemotherapy in the ambulatory setting. *Journal of Intravenous Nursing* 20(2): 78–88.

Ciesielski-Carlucci, C. (1997). Case report of anaphylaxis from cisplatin/paclitaxel and a review of their hypersensitivity reaction profiles. *American Journal of Clinical Oncology* 20(4): 373–375.

Davis, M.E., DeSantis, D., and Klemm, K. (1995). A flow sheet for follow-up after chemotherapy extravasation. *Oncology Nursing Forum* 22(6): 979–983.

Dorr, R.T. (1994). Pharmocologic management of vesicant chemotherapy extravasations. In R.T. Dorr and D.D. von Hoff (eds.): *Cancer Chemotherapy Handbook.* 2nd ed. Norwalk, Conn.: Appleton and Lange.

Dorr, R.T. (1990). Antidotes to vesicant chemotherapy extravasation. *Blood Review* 4(1): 41–60.

Dorr, R.T., Alberts, D.S., Einsphar, J., Mason-Liddil, N., and Soble, M. (1987). Experimental dacarbazine antitumor activity and skin toxicity in relation to light exposure and pharmacologic antidotes. *Cancer Treatment Reports* 71: 267–272.

Dorr, R.T., and Bool, K.L. (1995). Antidote studies of vinorelbine-induced skin ulceration in the mouse. *Cancer Chemotherapy Pharmacology* 36(4): 290–292.

Dorr, R.T., Snead, K., and Liddil, J.D. (1996). Skin ulceration potential of paclitaxel in a mouse skin model in vivo. *Cancer* 78: 152–156.

Dorr, R.T., and Von Hoff, D.D. (1994). *Cancer Chemotherapy Handbook.* Norwalk, Conn.: Appleton and Lange.

Ellenberger, A. (1999). Starting an IV line. *Nursing 99* (March): 56–59.

Engelking, C. (1988). Prechemotherapy nursing assessment in outpatient settings. *Outpatient Chemotherapy* 3(1): 9–11.

Ewan, P. (1998). Anaphylaxis. *British Medical Journal* 316(7142): 1442–1445.

Fisher, D.S., Alfano, S., Knobf, M.T., Donovan, C., and Beaulieu, N. (1996). Improving the cancer chemotherapy use process. *Journal of Chemical Oncology* 14(12): 3148–3155.

Goodman, M., and Riley, M.B. (1997). Chemotherapy: Principles of administration. In S.L. Groenwald, M.H. Frogge, M. Goodman, and C.H. Yarbro (eds.): *Cancer Nursing: Principles and Practice*. 4th ed. Sudbury, Mass.: Jones & Bartlett, 317–384.

Groenwald, S.L. (1987). *Cancer Nursing: Principles and Practice*. Boston: Jones & Bartlett.

Harrington, J., and Figueroa, J. (1997). Severe necrosis due to paclitaxel extravasation. *Pharmacotherapy* 17(1): 163–165.

Harwood, K.L., Vito, B., Brady, P., Much, J., Krzysko-Depew, A., Wagler, K., and Strauman, J. (1989). Management of doxorubicin extravasation. *Oncology Nursing Forum* 16(1): 10–11.

Harwood, K., and Bachur, N. (1987). Evaluation of dimethyl sulfoxide and local cooling as antidotes for doxorubicin extravasation in a pig model. *Oncology Nursing Forum* 14(1): 39–44.

Harwood, K., and Govin, R. (1994). Short term vs. long term local cooling after doxorubicin (Dox) extravasation: An Eastern Cooperative Oncology Group (ECOG) study [Abstract]. *Program/Proceedings of the American Society of Clinical Oncology* 13: 447.

How, C., and Brown, J. (1998). Extravasation of cytotoxic chemotherapy from peripheral veins. *European Journal of Oncology Nursing* 2(1): 51–58.

Ignoffo, R., and Friedman, M.A. (1980). Therapy of local toxicities caused by extravasation of cancer chemotherapeutic drugs. *Cancer Treatment Review* 7(1): 17–27.

Ingle, R. (1995). Rare complications of vascular access devices. *Seminars in Oncology Nursing* 11(3): 184–193.

Karnofsky, D.A., and Burchenal, J.H. (1949). The clinical evaluation of therapeutic agents used in cancer. In C.M. MacLeod (ed.): *Evaluation of Chemotherapeutic Agents*. New York: Columbia University Press, 196.

Labovich, T.M. (1999). Acute hypersensitivity reactions to chemotherapy. *Seminars in Oncology Nursing* 11(3): 222–231.

Laurie, S.W., Wilson, K.L., Kernahan, D.A., Bauer, B.S., and Vistnes, L.M. (1984). Intravenous extravasation injuries: The effectiveness of hyaluronidase in their treatment. *Annals of Plastic Surgery* 13(3): 191–194.

Lebredo, L., Barrie, R., and Woltering, E.A. (1992). DMSO protection against adriamycin-induced tissue necrosis. *Journal of Surgery Research* 53(1): 26–65.

Liberman, P. (1995a). Distinguishing anaphylaxis from other serious disorders. *Journal of Respiratory Diseases* 16(4): 411–420.

———. (1995b). Anaphylaxis: Guidelines for prevention and management. *Journal of Respiratory Diseases* 16(5): 456–462.

McCaffrey-Boyle, D., and Engelking, C. (1995). Vesicant extravasation: Myths and realities. *Oncology Nursing Forum* 22(1): 57–66.

McPhail, G. (1999). Chemotherapy in palliative cancer: Changing perspectives. *International Journal of Palliative Nursing* 5(2): 81–85.

Miller, S.A. (1980). Nursing actions in cancer chemotherapy administration. *Oncology Nursing Forum* 7(4): 8–16.

Montrose, P.A. (1987). Extravasation management. *Seminars in Oncology Nursing* 3(2): 128–132.

Morra, M.E. (ed.) (1981). *Cancer Chemotherapy Treatment and Care*. Boston: G.K. Hall Medical.

Olver, I.N., Aisner, J., Hament, A., Buchanan, L., Bishop, J.F., and Kaplan, R.S. (1988). A prospective study of topical dimethyl sulfoxide for treating anthracycline extravasation. *Journal of Clinical Oncology* 6(11): 1732–1735.

Oncology Nursing Society. (1999). *Cancer Chemotherapy Guidelines and Recommendations for Practice*. 2nd ed. Pittsburgh: Oncology Nursing Society Press.

———. (1992a). *Cancer Chemotherapy Guidelines: Module V. Recommendations for the Management of Extravasation and Anaphylaxis*. Pittsburgh: Oncology Nursing Society Press.

———. (1992b). *Cancer Chemotherapy Guidelines: Recommendations for the Management of Vesicant Extravasation, Hypersensitivity, and Anaphylaxis*. Pittsburgh: Oncology Nursing Society Press.

———. (1988). *Cancer Chemotherapy Guidelines: Module II. Recommendations for Nursing Practice in the Acute Care Setting*. Pittsburgh: Oncology Nursing Society Press.

Rospond, E.M., and Engel, L.M. (1993). Dimethyl sulfoxide for treating anthracycline extravasation. *Clinical Pharmatherapeutics* 12(8): 560–561.

Sitzia, J., and Wood, N. (1998). Patient satisfaction with cancer chemotherapy nursing: A review of the literature. *International Journal of Nursing Studies* 35 (1–2): 1–12.

Soble, M.J., Dorr, R.T., Plezia, P., and Breckenridge, S. (1987). Dose-dependent skin ulcers in mice treated with DNA binding antitumor antibiotics. *Cancer Chemotherapy & Pharmacology* 20(1): 86–98.

St.Germain, B., Houlihan, N., and D'Amato, S. (1994). Dimethyl sulfoxide therapy in the treatment of vesicant extravasation: Two case presentations. *Journal of Intravenous Nursing* 17(5): 261–266.

# Chapter 10

# Chemotherapy Administration: General Principles for Vascular Access

**Gail Esan Sansivero, MS, ANP, AOCN and**
**Margaret Barton-Burke, PhD (c), RN, AOCN**

## INTRODUCTION

The goal of chemotherapy administration is to optimize drug availability and thus maximize neoplastic cell death. Many routes of drug administration are used in an attempt to deliver drugs to areas of disease (sites known or suspected), to improve the antitumor effects, and to decrease toxicity. In general, chemotherapeutic drugs are administered either systemically or regionally. Table 10.1 identifies the various routes of administration, as well as the advantages, disadvantages, complications, and nursing implications. The current routes of administration are:

| Regional Routes | Systemic Routes |
|---|---|
| Intrathecal (IT) | Subcutaneous (SQ) |
| Intra-arterial (IA) | Intramuscular (IM) |
| Intracavitary (IC) | Oral (PO) |
| | Intravenous (IV) |

The three regional routes of administration allow for high drug concentrations in the disease area while minimizing systemic concentrations and thus side effects: intrathecal, intra-arterial, and intracavitary.

Administering chemotherapy *intrathecally* allows the drug to reach the central nervous system and thus to prevent or treat local dis-ease. The majority of chemotherapeutic agents do not cross the blood-brain barrier, so they must be delivered directly into the cerebrospinal fluid. This is accomplished by either a lumbar puncture or the use of an indwelling subcutaneous cerebrospinal fluid reservoir, such as the Ommaya reservoir (Heyer-Schulte del Caribe, Anasco, Puerto Rico). The benefits and risks to the patient must be determined before either method of administration is chosen and include: (1) having a lumbar puncture performed for each treatment (weighing the pain and the potential complications the procedure involves) and (2) the potential complications of surgically inserting an Ommaya reservoir but using a consistent port for each treatment.

*Intra-arterial* infusions treat an isolated organ or inoperable tumor. The chemotherapeutic agent is administered through a catheter inserted into an artery, usually in the liver, head, neck, or brain. The celiac artery is used to treat the liver, the external carotid artery for the head and neck area, and the internal carotid artery for brain tumors (Johnston and Pratt 1981). Catheters are inserted into the artery surgically using general anesthesia or angiographic catheterization and a local anesthetic. They then are connected to either an implanted or a

**Table 10.1  Routes of Administration of Antineoplastic Agents**

| Route | Advantages | Disadvantages | Potential Complications | Nursing Implications |
|---|---|---|---|---|
| Oral | Ease of administration | Inconsistency of absorption | Drug-specific complications | Evaluate compliance with medication schedule. Teach patient handling techniques. |
| Subcutaneous Intramuscular | Ease of administration Decreased side effects | Inconsistency of absorption Requires adequate muscle mass and tissue for absorption | Infection Bleeding | Evaluate platelet count (> 50,000). Use smallest gauge needle possible. Prepare injection site with an antiseptic solution. Assess injection site for signs and symptoms of infection or bleeding. |
| IV | Consistent absorption Required for vesicants | Sclerosing of veins over time | Infection Phlebitis Extravasation | Check for blood return before and after administration of drugs. |
| *Intra-arterial | Increased doses to tumor with decreased systemic toxic effects | Requires surgical procedure or special radiography equipment for catheter/port placement; patient lies flat for 3–7 days during drug infusion | Bleeding Embolism Pain | Monitor for signs and symptoms of bleeding. Monitor partial thromboplastin time, prothrombin time. Monitor catheter site. Intense patient education needed for pump and catheter care. |
| Internal (implanted) pump | | Cost-effective only with long-term therapy (i.e., 3–6 months) | Pump occlusion malfunction As above | Specialized nursing education needed regarding arterial pumps. |
| *Intrathecal Intraventricular | More consistent drug levels in cerebro-spinal fluid | Requires lumbar puncture or surgical placement of reservoir or implanted pump for drug delivery | Increased ICP Headaches Confusion Lethargy Nausea and vomiting Seizures Infection | Observe site for signs of infection. Monitor functioning of reservoir or pump. Assess patient for headache or signs of increased intracranial pressure. |

INTRODUCTION **647**

| Route | Rationale | Considerations | Complications | Nursing interventions |
|---|---|---|---|---|
| *Intraperitoneal | Direct exposure of intra-abdominal metastases to drug | Requires placement of Tenckhoff catheter or intraperitoneal port | Abdominal pain Abdominal distention Bleeding Ileus Intestinal perforation Infection | Warm chemotherapy solution to body temperature. Check patency of catheter or port. Instill solution according to protocol-infuse, dwell, and drain or continuous infusion. |
| Intrapleural | Sclerosing of pleural lining to prevent recurrence of effusions | Requires insertion of a thoracotomy tube Usually not in nurse practice act to administer | Pain Infection | Monitor for complete drainage from pleural cavity before instillation of drug. Following instillation, clamp tubing and reposition patient every 10–15 mins × 2 hours or according to protocol. Attach tubing to suction × 18 hrs. Assess patient for pain or anxiety. Provide analgesia and emotional support. |
| Intravesicular | Direct exposure of bladder surfaces to drug | Requires insertion of Foley catheter | Urinary tract infections Cystitis Bladder contracture Urinary urgency | Maintain sterile technique when inserting Foley catheter. Instill solution, clamp catheter for one hour, and unclamp to drain or according to protocol. |

* Specialized nursing education is required for certain administration methods. Refer to individual state nurse practice acts and agency policies and procedures, or see Camp-Sorrell (1996).

*Note:* From Bender, C. (1998). Nursing implications of antineoplastic therapy. In J.K. Itano and K.N. Taoka (eds.): *Core Curriculum for Oncology Nursing.* 3rd ed. Philadelphia: W.B. Saunders, 641–656. Adapted with permission.

*Source:* Oncology Nursing Society. (1999). *Cancer Chemotherapy Guidelines and Recommendations for Practice.* 2nd ed. Pittsburgh: Oncology Nursing Press. Reprinted with permission.

portable pump. The chemotherapeutic agents then are pumped directly to the affected area.

*Intracavitary* administration is a broad term used to describe the administration of chemotherapy directly into a body cavity. Commonly this is done to treat malignant effusions or microscopic localized disease in the bladder, peritoneum, or pleura. Chemotherapy is infused via a catheter placed directly into one of these areas. The drug remains in the area for a specific amount of time and then may or may not be drained out via the same catheter. Either an external catheter, such as the Tenckhoff catheter (Cobe Laboratory, Lakewood, CO), or a subcutaneous intravenous port, such as the Port-A-Cath (SIMS Deltec, Inc., St. Paul, MN) is used in intraperitoneal chemotherapy. Foley catheters are used for bladder instillations, and a chest tube is used to treat the pleura.

The less frequently used modes of drug administration are subcutaneous and intramuscular. Many of the antineoplastic agents are irritating or damaging to body tissue and thus are inappropriate for either the subcutaneous or intramuscular route. Some agents that can be given by the subcutaneous route are cytosine arabinoside (ARA-C), interleukin-2, granulocyte colony-stimulating factor (G-CSF), and the interferons. Bleomycin and methotrexate can be given intramuscularly. L-asparaginase may be given by either the subcutaneous or the intramuscular route.

The last two routes of chemotherapy administration are the most common: oral and intravenous. The oral route includes tablets, pills, and liquids. Several factors must be considered before choosing the oral route: patency and functioning of the GI tract; presence of nausea, vomiting, or dysphagia; the patient's state of consciousness; the patient's willingness to comply with the schedule; and the availability of the medication in oral form. Table 10.2 offers special tips for giving oral chemotherapy to children.

The intravenous (IV) route of administration is the most common method used to deliver chemotherapy. It allows easy absorption of the drug, thus providing predictable blood levels. IV drugs may be administered through a peripheral access (a vein in the patient's arm or hand) or through a central venous access device, such as a silicone silastic catheter or an implanted infusion port.

There are four methods of IV administration: push (IVP), piggy back (IVB), sidearm, and infusion (continuous or intermittent). IV push refers to administering the medication directly into the IV cannula, through either an angiocatheter or a butterfly needle. Piggy back denotes a main line of IV fluid connected to the IV cannula. The solution to be piggy backed is connected into the main IV line, usually in the port closest to the patient. The sidearm method of administration is the route of choice for chemotherapy with vesicant properties. Again, a main line of freely flowing IV fluid is connected directly into the cannula. The nurse administers the medication slowly into the port closest to the patient while continually assessing the peripheral IV site for redness, swelling, pain, rash, and extravasation. This method and the piggy back method allow for further dilution of the chemotherapeutic agent with the main fluid. The two solutions must be compatible (see Appendix 2). The infusion method delivers chemotherapy as the main line infusion over several minutes (bolus infusions), several hours (intermittent infusions), or 24 hours a day (continuous infusions) for 1 or more days.

## VASCULAR ACCESS

Accurate administration of antineoplastic agents through a suitable vascular access is a basic clinical practice issue in oncology care. Morbidity from infiltration, extravasation, and

**Table 10.2**   Special Tips for Giving Oral Chemotherapy to Children

| Approach | Problem |
|---|---|
| Administering oral medications to a child who cannot swallow | Ability to swallow pills is more dependent on the child's past experiences than age. Do not use a medication that has an unpleasant taste (e.g., prednisone) to teach the child how to swallow a tablet. |
| Tablets | Tablets may be chewed. Crush tablet into fine powder, dissolve in warm water. Mix solution with juice or food acceptable to the child (e.g., ice cream, applesauce). |
| Capsules | Open capsule (e.g., CCNU, PCB, HU) and sprinkle contents into food. Not all capsules should be opened; consult with pharmacist. |
| Administering liquid chemotherapy to an infant/ very young child | Place liquid in empty nipple, place nipple in infant's mouth, and allow child to suck. Draw medication up into syringe, place along inside of cheek, and administer slowly. Raise child's head slightly during administration to avoid aspiration. |
| Administering medications with an unpleasant taste (e.g., prednisone) | Discourage chewing of tablets. Mix crushed tablet in juice or food with a strong taste (e.g., peanut butter, maple syrup, fruit-flavored syrup). Mix crushed tablet with a small amount of juice or food. Child must take all to receive total dose. Do not mix with essential food items (e.g., milk, cereal, orange juice). Avoidance may develop through conditioned association. Crush pills and place in gelatin capsule. |
| Administering partial doses (e.g., 6-MP) | Break scored tablets only. Pharmacy will crush tablets and dispense in unit dose packages. Dissolve crushed tablet in premeasured amount of water; calculate portion that will give correct dose. |
| Administering oral medications to promote drug absorption | Notify physician if child vomits after oral administration of medication; drug may need to be repeated. (With prednisone, another form [liquid, pill, IV] or oral dexamethasone may be substituted). Control vomiting of oral medications with antiemetics. With single daily doses, administer all tablets at one time to achieve maximum blood level. Some medications should be given between meals on an empty stomach; consult with pharmacist. |
| Administering oral medications that are irritating to gastrointestinal mucosa (e.g., prednisone) | Give medications with milk or food. Antacids may promote comfort. |

*Source:* Meeske, K., and Ruccione, K. (1987). Cancer chemotherapy in children: Nursing issues and approaches. *Seminars in Oncology Nursing* 3(2): 118–127. Reprinted with permission.

intravascular sclerosis related to these agents may include tissue destruction; pain; erythema; loss of sensory and motor function; and destruction of vascular access sites for the remainder of the patient's life. Safe drug administration can also make the difference in a positive or negative treatment experience for patients and their families. Anxiety over obtaining vascular access, and maintaining venous patency are frequent concerns expressed by patients, particularly those who have experienced multiple therapies. An active nursing role in the selection, placement, use, and problem solving with vascular access and the use of devices is an important component of oncology nursing practice.

## CHALLENGES OF ACCESS IN ONCOLOGY PATIENTS

Patients with a cancer diagnosis often have several factors that contribute to the difficulty in obtaining or maintaining vascular access. Although these factors do not contraindicate vascular access placement, they may make conventional placement challenging.

### Site Selection

Vein selection is critical to the success of all intravenous therapy, including peripheral cannula. A suitable vein should be palpable, resilient, and soft. Figure 10.1 illustrates the various veins that may be selected for peripheral intravenous (IV) infusion and that may be used with a vascular access devices. The practitioner should select the target vessel being cognizant not only of the patient's immediate access needs, but also with thoughts to preserve future access sites. Tables 10.3 and 10.4 highlight the assessment factors to be considered when selecting a vein for a peripheral IV and establishing a new site.

Combining the placement of a peripheral device with sampling from this device is one way to reduce punctures and the inevitable damage to the patient's vasculature. The basilic vein is the largest vein in the upper extremities, providing the most hemodilution of peripheral access sites. It may be difficult to cannulate above the antecubital fossa, as it is located on the inner aspect of the arm. The cephalic vein in the forearm is generally long and more stable. However, at about half the size of the basilic, there is significantly less hemodilution. The cephalic vein above the antecubital fossa, although still small, is often palpable in young adults and is an ideal location for cannulation with a peripheral cannula. It makes a fairly sharp turn into the subclavian vein, however, and so is a more challenging selection for catheter advancement into central circulation.

The brachial vein, located on the inner aspect of the upper arm, is often paired and located in close proximity to the brachial artery and brachial nerve. For this reason, puncture of the brachial vein generally should be attempted only with image guidance.

Small veins of the hand and digits should be avoided because they are fragile and more likely to rupture. There is also little subcutaneous tissue surrounding these veins, so that placement can be more uncomfortable. All devices should be secured thoroughly to prevent accidental removal or partial removal from the selected vessel.

The internal jugular is the vein of choice for the placement of a tunneled, cuffed catheter, a short nontunneled catheter, or an implanted chest port. It is accessible just above the supraclavicular space, and provides short distance access to the brachiocephalic (also known as the inominate) vein and superior vena cava (SVC). The internal jugular vein is

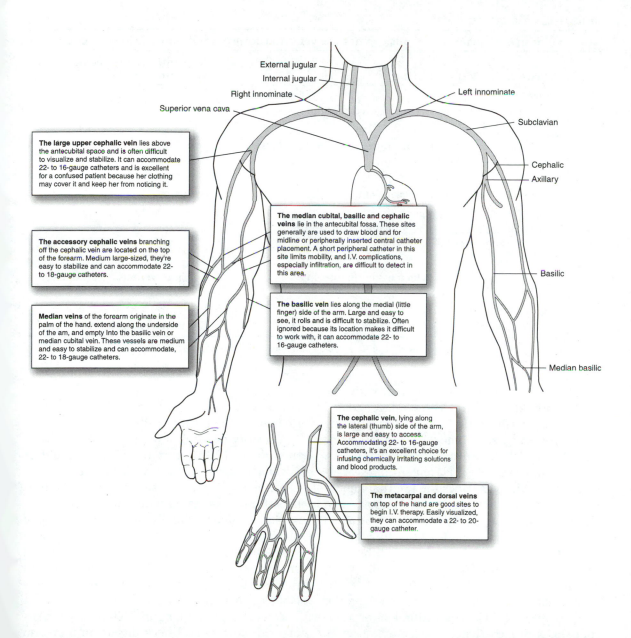

External jugular

Internal jugular

Right innominate

Superior vena cava

Left innominate

Subclavian

Cephalic

Axillary

Basilic

Median basilic

**The large upper cephalic vein** lies above the antecubital space and is often difficult to visualize and stabilize. It can accommodate 22- to 16-gauge catheters and is excellent for a confused patient because her clothing may cover it and keep her from noticing it.

**The accessory cephalic veins** branching off the cephalic vein are located on the top of the forearm. Medium large-sized, they're easy to stabilize and can accommodate 22- to 18-gauge catheters.

**Median veins** of the forearm originate in the palm of the hand. extend along the underside of the am, and empty Into the basilic vein or median cubital vein. These vessels are medium and easy to stabilize and can accommodate, 22- to 18-gauge catheters.

**The median cubital, basilic and cephalic veins** lie in the antecubital fossa. These sites generally are used to draw blood and for midline or peripherally inserted central catheter placement. A short peripheral catheter in this site limits mobility, and I.V. complications, especially infiltration, are difficult to detect in this area.

**The basilic vein** lies along the medial (little finger) side of the arm. Large and easy to see, it rolls and is difficult to stabilize. Often ignored because its location makes it difficult to work with, it can accommodate 22- to 16-gauge catheters.

**The cephalic vein**, lying along the lateral (thumb) side of the arm, is large and easy to access. Accommodating 22- to 16-gauge catheters, it's an excellent choice for infusing chemically irritating solutions and blood products.

**The metacarpal and dorsal veins** on top of the hand are good sites to begin I.V. therapy. Easily visualized, they can accommodate a 22- to 20-gauge catheter.

**Figure 10.1** Vein selection is critical to all intravenous therapy, including chemotherapy administration.

**Table 10.3**  Selecting a Vein

**Assess veins in both arms and hands. Do not use veins in compromised limbs or lower extremities.**

| Criteria for Vein Selection | Appropriate Choice of Venipuncture Site |
|---|---|
| IDEAL VEIN/BEST LOCATION | |
| Large, soft, resilient veins in forearm/hand | Forearm |
| IDEAL VEIN/UNDESIRABLE LOCATION | |
| Large, soft, resilient veins in hand/antecubital fossa; small, thin veins in forearm | Hand |
| SATISFACTORY VEIN/BEST LOCATION | |
| Small, thin veins in forearm/hand | Forearm |
| SATISFACTORY VEIN/UNDESIRABLE LOCATION | |
| Small, thin veins in hand; veins in forearm not palpable or visible | Hand |
| UNSATISFACTORY VEIN/UNDESIRABLE LOCATION | |
| Small, fragile veins, which easily rupture, in hand/forearm | Consider venous access device |
| UNSATISFACTORY VEIN/UNDESIRABLE LOCATION | |
| Veins in forearm/hand not palpable or visible | Consider venous access device |

*Source:* Hughes, C.B. (1986). Giving cancer drugs IV—some guidelines. *American Journal of Nursing* (January): 34–38. Reprinted with permission.

approached most successfully and with the least morbidity by employing image guided techniques, such as ultrasound, for targeting (Denys, Vretsky, and Ruddy 1993; Silberzweig and Mitty 1998; Gordon, Saliken, Johns, Owen, and Gray 1998). Placement of a vascular access device (VAD) via the internal jugular vein is associated with less thrombosis and stenosis than placement via the subclavian veins (Cimochowski, et al. 1990). In addition, the risk of pneumothorax and hemothorax is reduced substantially (MacDonald, Watt, McNally, Edwards, and Moss 2000).

Alternative sites of access are the inferior vena cava (IVC) via a translumbar or transhepatic approach (Patel 1998; Bennett, et al. 1997; Kazanjian and Kaufman 1994). These sites usually are reserved for patients with stenosis and thrombosis of the SVC not amenable to correction with angioplasty, stent placement, or thrombolysis. Exit sites for an IVC approach typically lie over the lower anterior ribs or the posterior ribs.

A history of surgical intervention at or near the intended VAD entry or exit site should be evaluated. In particular, vein harvesting may deplete an extremity of suitable sites. The ipsilateral limb associated with a lymph node dissection should optimally be avoided for VAD placement, as this limb is believed to be more susceptible to edema and infection. There is currently no data available regarding the use of the ipsilateral limb in a patient who has undergone sentinal node biopsy.

The internal jugular approach on the ipsilateral side to a radical neck dissection may also be difficult, because there may be limited tissue in the supraclavicular area, making a catheter tract prominent. Concurrent radiation to this site may also impede wound healing.

**Table 10.4    Establishing a New Intravenous Line**

I. Examine the patient's veins and elicit the patient's desire in selecting a peripheral access site.

A. Proceed distally (from the hand) to proximally (toward the forearm).

B. Avoid limbs with compromised circulation, impaired lymphatic drainage (e.g., the side of a prior mastectomy with lymph node dissection), phlebitis, invading neoplasms, hematomas, inflamed or sclerosing areas, the lower extremities and feet (due to an increased risk of phlebitis), and sites distal to a recent venipuncture.

C. When administering vesicant drugs, avoid using existing peripheral lines and sites of joint flexion for establishing new lines (e.g., antecubital fossa, wrist).

D. Alternate arms whenever possible.

E. Use heat or ask the patient to pump a fist to distend veins.

II. Select appropriate equipment depending upon the venous access route and the method of administration to be used.

III. Exercise safety during venipuncture, drug handling, and administration according to the established policies and procedures of the institution (i.e., wash hands, wear protective clothing, gloves).

IV. Perform venipuncture according to institutional policies and procedures.

*Source:* Berg, D. (1996). Drug delivery systems. In M. Barton-Burke, G. Wilkes, and K. Ingwersen: *Cancer Chemotherapy: A Nursing Process Approach*. 2nd ed. Sudbury, Mass.: Jones & Bartlett. Reprinted with permission.

Siting a tunneled VAD or implanted port on the contralateral side in a woman with breast cancer may be most appropriate so that the device does not impede breast exam.

Although not contraindications to placement, severe thrombocytopenia and leukopenia are predictors of procedural risk. A platelet count of less than 50,000 is associated with an increased risk of intra- and post-procedural bleeding. Transfusion with platelets may be necessary before and after device placement, particularly for tunneled and implanted devices. Concurrent anticoagulation and administration of anti-platelet agents should be stopped temporarily for device placement as well. Patients with fibrinogen deficiency or liver dysfunction may require administration of fresh frozen plasma and or Vitamin K before VAD placement.

Leukopenia is the primary predictor of device-related infection. Optimal timing of VAD placement, then, is prior to the initial chemotherapy treatment or just before a planned cycle.

Physical examination should include the evaluation for presence of prominent collateral vessels on the chest wall and the arms. If present, they are a clue to possible subclavian or superior vena cava stenosis or thrombosis. A history of previous central VAD placement increases the risk that a patient will have stenosis, particularly if the VADs were placed via a subclavian approach.

Consideration should be given to current or proposed radiation ports. Wound healing within a concurrent radiation port may be problematic, particularly for port placement. In patients with head and neck, lung, or metastatic pulmonary disease, potential radiation sites in the chest and neck area should be anticipated. In these cases, placement of a VAD via the arm may be prudent.

Many patients with cancer are hypercoagulable. There is extensive disagreement about the utility of prophylactic, low-dose anticoagulation in preventing VAD-related thrombosis and fibrin sheath formation.

## Intravenous Therapy Techniques

The choice of an angiocatheter or a butterfly needle must be based on the individual patient, the goal of the therapy, the length of time the needle is required to be in place, the risk of vein perforation with the steel cannula of a butterfly needle, and the type of therapy to be given. The size of the needle to be used is a result of the same factors as choosing the type of needle. Usually a 21-gauge needle is acceptable for most IV therapies. Large-bore 18- or 19-gauge needles usually are required for blood transfusions and viscous fluids. Small-bore 23- or 25-gauge needles are used for patients with small, fragile veins and for IV fluids of short duration.

Controversy exists within the oncology nursing community as to whether large-gauge needles are better than small-gauge needles for chemotherapy administration. Many believe that large-gauge needles provide more rapid access to the general circulation and decrease the potential of vein irritation. Small-gauge needles are believed to be less likely to cause vein perforation and scar tissue, while providing an increase in blood circulation and thus better drug dilution during administration.

After the vein has been selected and venipuncture has been performed, the next consideration becomes the preservation of the vein's integrity. Chemotherapy treatments may go on for many months. Therefore, it is important to guard the existing veins so as to prolong their quality for later use. A few steps that can be taken to maintain venous integrity follow:

- Prevent infections with the use of institutionally approved skin preparation and dressing procedures.

- Flush the IV line with normal saline before and after each medication in a combination and after the last medication. This prevents drug mixing, precipitates, and vein damage.
- Securely tape all junctures and tubing to avoid local trauma.
- Protect IV lines and needle placement with arm boards or other devices.
- To preserve the number of available quality veins:
  —Use veins sparingly.
  —Obtain all available laboratory work by finger stick or drawing blood at the time the IV is started (i.e., one single venipuncture).
  —Use veins sequentially, starting distally near the hand and proceeding proximally toward the elbow with each venipuncture.

## Dealing with the "Veinless" Patient

One of the most common dilemmas facing oncology nurses is trying to administer chemotherapy to the "veinless" patient, as described by Lokich (1978). With the variety of central venous access devices, including catheters and subcutaneous ports, this issue does not have to be a problem. However, there is always the patient who declines to have another surgical procedure until it is absolutely necessary, even if the benefits dramatically outweigh the risks. Patients, and in some cases their physicians, decline the procedure due to a variety of factors, including site of disease, anatomy, personal preference, or lack of conviction that a venous access device is required. The following list of suggestions may prove beneficial to ease the venipuncture experience for both the patient and the nurse.

- Help the patient assume a comfortable position.
- To allay patient anxiety about the procedure, provide emotional support and explanations of the actions to be taken.
- Teach the patient relaxation techniques as needed to ease the stress related to the procedure.
- Instruct the patient to exercise his or her hands with a rubber ball daily between treatments. This aids in vein development.
- Assess both arms before selecting the best vein. Visualize the standard venous patterns (see Figure 10.1). Assess the veins by palpation.
- To dilate the veins, apply moist heat to the patient's arms for 5–10 minutes. Remove the soaks and work efficiently while the veins are dilated.
- Local vein manipulation may also aid dilation:
  a. Appropriate use of a tourniquet or blood pressure cuff to encourage pooling of venous blood
  b. "Milking" the veins from proximal to distal (elbow to hand)
  c. Gently striking the surface of the vein
- Select an angiocatheter or butterfly carefully. Veins may be small, and an appropriate-size needle will decrease trauma.
- Perform the actual techniques and preparation for venipuncture according to the institution's policies and procedures.

- Request the assistance of a colleague after two unsuccessful attempts at venipuncture.

---

## ADDITIONAL ISSUES IN CHEMOTHERAPY ADMINISTRATION

The Oncology Nursing Society (ONS) has developed guidelines for chemotherapy administration, recognizing that there continue to be issues that are not easily resolved (e.g., the issue of the antecubital fossa being a reasonable vein to use in chemotherapy administration) (see Table 10.5). The authors are aware of these controversies, and our goal in this section is to acknowledge and present the issues, allowing readers to decide the best method of handling these concerns. Unfortunately, a review of the literature does not provide helpful answers.

### Dose Calculations and Modifications

Dosages of chemotherapeutic agents vary widely. *The standard dosage will vary from the current clinical trial dosage.* It is very important to know the *usual* dosage of each chemotherapy agent and to question any dose that seems incorrect. The physician must assess the following areas before prescribing the patient's chemotherapy dosage:

1. age
2. nutritional status
3. any prior chemotherapy or radiation therapy
4. current blood counts, both hematologic and chemistry profiles

**Table 10.5**  Controversial Issues and Arguments Pro and Con for Vesicant Chemotherapy Administration Practices

| Controversial Practices | Pro | Con |
|---|---|---|
| Vesicant first | Vascular integrity decreases over time. Initially, practitioner's assessment skills more accurate. Patient may become more sedated from antiemetics and less able to report burning, pain at infusion site (Otto 1997). | Vesicant is irritating, compromising integrity of vein. Nonvesicants are less irritating to veins. Venous spasm may occur early during injection, altering assessment of patency (Otto 1997). |
| Side-arm administration | Free-flowing IV lines allow for maximal dilution of drugs that could be potentially irritating and provide assessment of vein patency. | Integrity of vein can be assessed more easily and the early signs of extravasation can be noted more easily. |
| Direct push administration | Integrity of vein can be assessed more easily, and the early signs of extravasation can be noted more easily than with a piggy back infusion. | |
| Use of antecubital fossa | Larger veins permit more rapid infusion/administration of drug. Larger veins permit potentially irritating chemotherapeutic agents to reach the general circulation sooner with less irritation to small veins. | Arm mobility is restricted with a needle in place. The risk of extravasation is increased due to patient mobility (e.g., coughing, vomiting). Infiltration could require extensive reconstruction efforts with limited arm use during the healing process, resulting in increased morbidity and decreased function. Because of the subcutaneous tissues, early infiltration is more difficult to assess. |
| Large-gauge needles (e.g., #19 and #21 scalp vein needles) | Potentially irritating chemotherapeutic agents can reach the general circulation sooner, with reduced irritation to the peripheral veins. Drug administration time is decreased, which reduces the patient's exposure to a potentially stressful environment. | |
| Small-gauge needles (e.g., #23 and #25 scalp vein needles) | Smaller gauge needles are less likely to puncture the wall of a small vein. Scar tissue may be formed with needle insertion; small-gauge needles cause less scar tissue formation. The patient may experience less pain during the insertion of a smaller needle. Increased blood flow around a smaller-bore needle increases dilution of the chemotherapeutic agent. Mechanical phlebitis may be minimized with a smaller-bore needle. | |

*Source:* Oncology Nursing Society. (1999). *Cancer Chemotherapy Guidelines and Recommendations for Practice.* 2nd ed. Pittsburgh: Oncology Nursing Press. Reprinted with permission.

5. bone marrow reserve
6. renal and hepatic function
7. performance status (see Chapter 9, Table 9.5)
8. expected drug tolerance

Individual dosages take into consideration the above factors and are based on the patient's body surface area ($m^2$), which is calculated from his or her height and weight. See Chapter 9, Figure 9.1 for further explanation.

Dose modifications may be made in a case of renal or hepatic impairment or persistent bone marrow depression. The physician must weigh many issues when considering a dose modification:

- Goal of therapy: cure, control, or palliation. In the setting of cure, the patient may be asked to tolerate mild to moderate short-term toxicity to achieve a long-term disease-free state.

- Issues related to routes of metabolism, excretion, and potential interference by drug interactions.

- Desired antitumor effects: still achievable with a dose modification versus delaying therapy for a short period of time so that maximal doses can be maintained. A rest period is required for normal body cells to recover from the effects of chemotherapy, but the cancer cells that are still living also are able to replicate during this period.

- Reasons for relapse: sanctuary sites (e.g., CNS, testes) and the multiple factors of drug resistance (e.g., MDR, P-glycoprotein expression).

- The overall benefits and risks.

Unfortunately, this is not always an easy responsibility for the physician. Most chemotherapeutic agents do not have established guidelines for dose modifications. Instead, the patient's treatment protocol may be the only source of guidelines for when to decrease the dose of chemotherapy. There is a fine line between prescribing too little medication and prescribing too much with intolerable side effects.

## Drug Interactions

Numerous medications are being used today in the oncology setting. Various agents are being used to treat the disease; support the patient through their nadir; control pain, nausea, vomiting, and infections; and correct electrolyte imbalances. Because the median age for developing most cancers is in the sixth decade (Peters 1987), many patients also are taking other prescription and over-the-counter medications for concomitant medical problems. With so many different drugs potentially being used in the same person, it would be reasonable to expect a drug interaction. This interaction could be of benefit, worsen the toxicities, or decrease the chemotherapeutic drug's effectiveness. Some interactions are noticeable (e.g., drug precipitations in IV tubing), but reactions inside the body may not be "seen" at all. An interaction may be noted because of the resultant change, but the reaction itself is not obvious. It is important, but unrealistic, for both the nurse and the physician to know potential drug interactions with each medication administered and to be aware of every additional medication prescribed by a non-oncology physician or self-administered by the patient.

Rules of thumb related to drug interactions include the following (see Chapter 6 for further details):

- Chemotherapeutic agents should not be mixed with any IV additive (e.g., heparin, potassium).

- Only plain solutions (e.g., 5% dextrose in water, sodium chloride) should be used as main-line infusions for the sidearm and piggy back methods of administration.
- When a combination of drugs is being administered, normal saline should be used to flush the IV line before, between, and after the medications.
- When there is any doubt as to whether the medications are compatible, it is safest to assume that they are not unless there is information to show otherwise.
- A pharmacist experienced with chemotherapy agents is a good source of information.

## VASCULAR ACCESS DEVICES

Every patient should be assessed at or near diagnosis for a vascular access device. A proactive approach to vascular access assessment and planning can serve to prevent complications and to ease the treatment process.

The patient's typical activity level; occupational history; body habitus; self-care skills; handedness; ability to read and understand instructions; and personal preferences should be considered in VAD selection. A very active individual, for example, may prefer an implanted device in order to maintain the ability to swim, play tennis, or golf. Conversely, a patient who is very "needle phobic" may prefer a device that requires no needle access, such as a tunneled catheter or PICC.

A brief review of VAD options with risks and benefits may help the patient and family choose the best device for their particular situation. These VAD options include but are not limited to peripherally cannulas; midlines; peripherally inserted central catheters; non-

tunneled and noncuffed as as well as tunneled and cuffed catheters; and implantable ports. This section reviews the advantages, disadvantages, and uses of these devices (see Table 10.6). Table 10.7 highlights the assessment parameters for a patient's VAD.

### Peripheral Cannulas

Although a peripheral cannula may be what comes to mind when most people think of intravenous therapy. These devices are used widely in all health care settings, and are suitable for a variety of therapies. They are intended for short-term therapy of less than 72 hours. Extended dwell short catheters are now being studied. Health care practitioners from many settings are familiar with their insertion and maintenance. Placed in the peripheral veins of the upper extremities, cannulas come in a variety of sizes and lengths, and are now available in single and dual lumen.

### Midlines

Also known as "longlines" and "halfways," midlines are catheters inserted peripherally with the tip terminating in the proximal portion of the extremity (INS 1997). Midlines typically possess the same characteristics as their longer cousins, peripherally inserted central catheters (PICCs). They are made of silicone or polyurethane, are soft and flexible, and inserted in a vein of the upper extremity. Available in single and dual lumen, midlines are appropriate choices for intermediate term therapy of 2–4 weeks. A midline would be a good choice for the patient with limited peripheral access who requires administration of IV fluids or isotonic medications. Because the midline tip is in peripheral circulation, sampling capability is suboptimal and hemodilution of infusates minimal. Therefore, mid-

**Table 10.6** Advantages, Disadvantages, and Uses of Various VADs

|  | Advantages | Disadvantages |
|---|---|---|
| **Peripheral Cannulas** | Equipment readily available<br>Most professionals skilled at placement<br>Inexpensive<br>Good for isotonic, rapid infusions | Require frequent replacement<br>Painful to insert<br>Sites limited to palpable/visible veins<br>Not suitable for all infusates |
| **Midlines** | Bedside placement<br>Reliable<br>Cost effective<br>No X-ray confirmation required<br>Preserves access sites<br>Good complication profile<br>Minimal discomfort<br>Decreased patient anxiety | Requires training to place<br>Sites limited to palpable/visible veins<br>Can be mistaken for a PICC<br>Low hemodilution |
| **PICCs** | Cost effective<br>Bedside placement in many situations<br>Comfortable for patients<br>Reliable<br>Good complication profile<br>Suitable for most therapies | Requires training to place<br>X-ray confirmation of tip placement<br>Frequent maintenance required<br>Some activity restrictions |
| **Nontunneled, Noncuffed Catheters** | Quick placement<br>Cost effective<br>Suitable for most therapies<br>Useful for hemodynamic monitoring | May require MD to place<br>X-ray confirmation of tip placement<br>Polyurethane products may be stiff<br>Little protection against accidental removal<br>Some activity restrictions |
| **Tunneled, Cuffed Catheters** | Reliable for sampling, infusion<br>Long-term use appropriate<br>Available in multiple configurations<br>May be repaired | More invasive placement procedure<br>Requires regular maintenance<br>Some activity restrictions<br>Requires physician placement |
| **Implanted Ports** | Reliable for sampling, infusion<br>Long-term use appropriate<br>Minimal maintenance<br>Minimal body image distortion<br>Few activity restrictions | Most invasive placement procedure<br>Highest initial cost<br>Requires puncture to access<br>Requires physician placement |

lines are not appropriate for irritant or vesicant therapy.

## Peripherally Inserted Central Catheters (PICCs)

A PICC is a catheter inserted in a peripheral vein with the tip residing in the thoracic vena cava (INS 1997). PICCs most often are used for therapy required for less than 6 months, though patient acceptance is often so good that patients prefer to keep them, if needed, for longer periods. Made of silicone or polyurethane, and 50–60 cm in length, PICCs are placed via an upper extremity vein and are threaded to central circlution. A standard single view chest X-ray confirms tip position. Available in several configurations of French

**Table 10.7** Assessment of the Patient with a Vascular Access Device

Routine assessment of the oncology patient should include assessment of the patient's vascular access device and infusion system. The following parameters should be considered:

Site and Tract
    Skin condition
    Presence and character of drainage
    Skin color, temperature and sensation
    Integrity of Huber needles
    Dressing integrity
    Presence of edema, collateral vessels
    Device

Integrity (check for leaks, holes)
    Presence of clamps
    Tubing, cap, extension set security
    External length
    Presence of blood return prior to initiating infusion

Securing Devices
    Security of sutures
    Security of skin securing devices

Pumps
    Verify infusate, dose, volume
    Verify rate
    Assess for precipitation
    Confirm alarm and pressure settings

Assessment can be facilitated by the use of a VAD flow sheet (See Figure 10.6), which tracks catheter performance.

size and lumens (single, dual, and triple), PICCs provide a vascular access option that can be established quickly. Because they are small and easily inserted, PICCs can be placed in the sickest patients with less risk than tunneled catheter placement, so are sometimes used as a "bridge" VAD until the patient is more stable.

## Nontunneled, Noncuffed VADs

Although often thought of as critical care VADs, nontunneled, noncuffed VADs, such as Hohn catheters, can provide a safe alternative to other devices in patients who need intermediate-term therapy (weeks to a few months). Placed via the internal jugular or subclavian approach, the device tip is situated in the SVC. Because they are nontunneled and noncuffed, these single or dual lumen VADs may be removed quickly and easily.

## Tunneled, Cuffed VADs

Tunneled, cuffed VADs (e.g. Hickmans, Broviacs) are the typical catheters used for patients who require multiple infusions and frequent samplings. Silastic or polyurethane, single, dual, or triple lumen, these VADs are placed via the internal jugular, subclavian, or IVC routes. Optimal tip location is at the atriocaval junction.

Tunneling the VAD from the entry site in the vein to a more remote exit site accomplishes two objectives. First, the tunnel helps secure the VAD in position. Second, it is thought that the separation of the catheter's exit site from the vein entry site provides some protection from infection.

The dacron cuff is infiltrated with subcutaneous tissue over 6–8 weeks, forming a type of "lock" that helps secure the device against accidental removal. The cuff also is theorized to reduce infection risk by making it difficult for bacteria to travel from the exit site, through the cuff, and into circulation.

## Implanted Ports

Implanted ports are totally implanted devices that provide long-term access and are ideal for patients requiring intermittent therapy. Placed via a peripheral vein in the upper extremities, the internal jugular, subclavian, or IVC, the port's catheter is targeted to the atriocaval junction. Ports also can be placed for intra-arterial chemotherapy administration. Ports are available in single and dual lumen, with valved or end hole catheters. Because these devices are completely subcutaneous, maintenance requirements between chemotherapy cycles is minimal or nonexistent. The patient is able to maintain an active lifestyle, including such activities as swimming, golf, and tennis.

## VASCULAR ACCESS DEVICE–RELATED COMPLICATIONS

Vascular access device complications are associated not only with the VAD itself, but also the patient's immune status; maintenance and therapy regimen; and risk factors, such as thrombocytopenia. Each should be treated as an urgent problem requiring thorough investigation and prompt treatment.

### Withdrawal Occlusion

Withdrawal occlusion occurs when the VAD is functional for infusion but the practitioner is unable to obtain a blood return, a common problem with many potential causes that may require substantial investigation (Stephens, Haire, and Kotulak 1995). Although often presumed to be related to intraluminal thrombus, a drug precipitate may be the source. Drug precipitate occurs when two or more incompatible infusates come in contact, resulting in crystallization within the VAD. The patient's infusion plan should be assessed for incompatibilities and drug sequencing and VAD maintenance should be explored. For example, phenytoin is incompatible with heparin. If the occlusion occurred shortly after phenytoin administration in a heparinized catheter, steps can be taken to attempt to restore patency.

If occlusion occurred after sampling, or if a drug precipitate is not suspected, intraluminal thrombus may be the cause. Instillation of 1–2 mg tissue plasminogen activator (TPA, Alteplase) for 1 hour has been noted to be clin-ically effective in restoring patency in many VADs. Repeat instillation may be administered if the first dose is ineffective.

If administration of thrombolytic and other agents is ineffective, the patient should be referred for a dye study. A contrast medium injected through each lumen is examined fluoroscopically for evidence of filling defects consistent with pericatheter thrombus or retrograde flow typical of fibrin sheath formation. Depending on the extent of the fibrin sheath, retrograde infusate flow can extend to the catheter's exit site, resulting in extravasation (Mayo and Pearson 1995). Each can be treated with higher dose thrombolytic infusion, catheter exchange, or catheter stripping (Brady, Spence, Levitin, Mickdich, and Dolmatch 1999; Haskal et al. 1996).

### Thrombosis

Thrombosis, or clotting near the VAD tip or tract, may occur because of traumatic insertion, catheter irritation against the vein wall, inappropriate sizing between the catheter and vein, or infusion of irritating solutions in a small vein. Puel et al. (1993) evaluated the risk of VAD-related thrombosis in 379 adult patients with VADs receiving chemotherapy. They found that a shortened catheter tip position, inominate vein, or the upper third of the superior vena cava (SVC) was associated with a higher risk of thrombosis development, whereas catheter tips in the distal SVC or atrio-caval junction were less likely to develop thrombus. People with many cancers are also thought to be hypercoagulable with a higher risk for VAD-related thrombosis than patients with nonmalignant illnesses.

Catheter-related thromboses may be asymptomatic and discovered only when the target site is selected for VAD placement again. If symptomatic, the patient typically complains of swelling, tenderness, and erythema near the VAD. There may be obvious engorged collateral vessels if the target vessel is largely occluded. In SVC occlusion, the patient may complain of suffusion, a feeling of fullness in the head which is worse upon awakening. The force of gravity during the day promotes venous drainage into the chest from collateral pathways.

VAD-related thrombosis may be diagnosed with ultrasound or dye study. Ultrasound typically is used to examine the vein surrounding the catheter, especially in the extremities. It is less useful for examining deeper structures, such as the SVC. Contrast injection demonstrating typical peri-catheter thrombus is seen in Figure 10.2. If the vein surrounding the

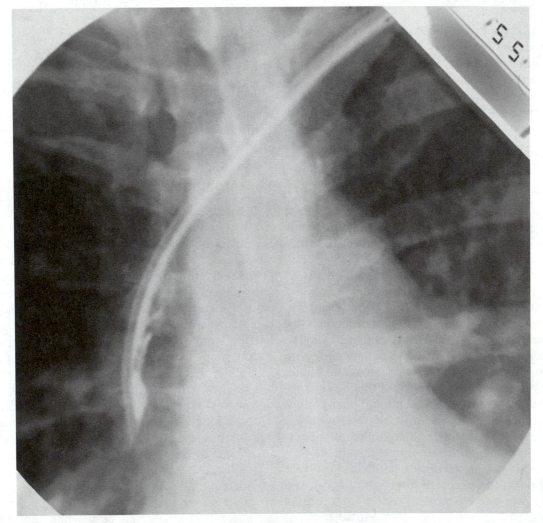

**Figure 10.2** Injection of contrast revealing fibrin sheath surrounding VAD tip with retrograde flow of contrast material.
*Source:* G. Sansivero. Used with permission.

entire length of the VAD is to be examined, a peripheral cannula must be placed distal to the origin of the VAD to opacify the entire tract.

The goals of treating VAD-related thrombosis should be to minimize the risk of pulmonary embolism, reduce the risk for infection (thrombus is a nidus for infection); maintain the vein and VAD patency; and to minimize patient discomfort. Thrombolysis may be accomplished by infusion of TPA at doses of 1–2 mg per lumen per hour for 2–4 hours. Another option is to administer a thrombolytic agent via a pulse spray catheter inserted into the thrombus. Chang, Horne, Mayo, and Doppman (1996) treated 12 patients with this approach, lysing 8 of the 12 patients and maintaining patency over 2 months in 4 of these. This approach was most likely to succeed in thrombi less than 2 weeks old.

Systemic anticoagulation first with heparin and then warfarin may be required with large or symptomatic thromboses. This can be particularly problematic because of the monitoring requirements of anticoagulant therapy. There is some evidence (Drakos et al. 1992) that low molecular weight heparin may be effective in treating catheter-related thrombosis. Drakos et al. (1992) treated 5 patients with catheter-related thrombus and profound thrombocytopenia undergoing bone marrow transplant. All patients recovered without hemorrhagic complications. Anticoagulation is contraindicated in patients with primary or metastatic brain malignancies, severe thrombocytopenia, or other bleeding disorders.

Thrombolysis may be paired with angioplasty and stent placement to achieve a widely open SVC (Perno, Putman, Cohen, and Bell 1999). Future VADs are then passed directly through the stent.

## Catheter Malposition and Embolus

According to the FDA's Central Venous Working Group, the correct tip placement for a central vascular access device is at the superior vena cava/atrial junction. Correct catheter tip position is critical for safe drug administration, optimal sampling performance, and contributes to a reduction in thrombosis, cardiac perforation, cardiac arrhythmias and extravasation. The catheter tip position is checked upon insertion and before the device is used.

Suboptimal tip position may occur on insertion or later in the life of the catheter when the catheter migrates or is dislodged. During insertion, catheter tips preferentially travel into collateral or neighboring vessels, such as the azygos or internal mammary veins, especially when there is stenosis or thrombosis of the brachiocephalic veins or SVC. These malpositions should be corrected before the VAD is cleared for use.

VAD placement via a medial approach into the subclavian veins may result in catheter pinch off (Krutchen et al. 1996). As the catheter passes through the costoclavicular space, it is compressed between the clavicle and first rib (Figure 10.3). If the angle is severe, the catheter may be fractured, with a fragment embolized (Nace and Ingle 1993). Avoidance of the subclavian approach, or lateral placement into the subclavian vein, can prevent most of these problems. If a catheter fractures, the embolized fragment must be retrieved using percutaneous angiographic techniques.

Delayed catheter malposition may occur because of increases in intrathoracic pressure during prolonged coughing or vomiting, where the catheter is pushed from the SVC into the internal jugular or brachiocephalic veins (Figure 10.4). Patients who do extensive upper arm exercises are also at risk. Some spontaneous

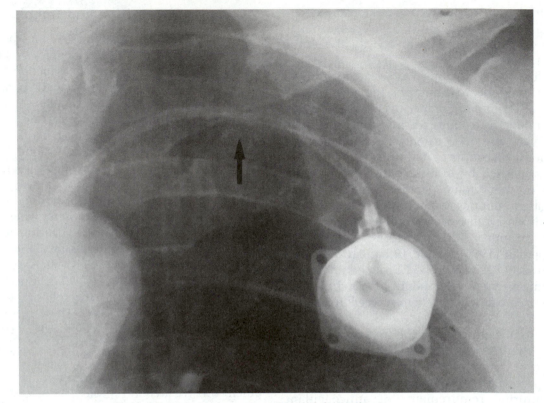

**Figure 10.3**  Pinch off catheter between clavicle and first rib.
*Source:* G. Sansivero. Used with permission.

catheter malpositions are never explained. In many cases, the malpositioned catheter can be snared and maneuvered into correct position (Figure 10.5).

Inaccurate tip positions can be detected on chest X-ray. Some patients will complain of a gurgling sound in their ear, or pain in the neck or ear, when a catheter is positioned in the internal jugular vein. Patients with an embolized fragment may complain of chest pain or a sense of irregular heartbeat. In some cases, evidence of malposition or embolization may be a change in catheter function, such as loss of blood return, signs of fluid leak along the catheter tract, or resistance to infusion.

## Needle Displacement

Needle displacement from the septum of implanted ports has occurred in both ambulatory and inpatient settings. The needle may become dislodged for a variety of reasons, such as failing to secure the needle by not taping the wing tips in place, slipage of the siliconized noncoring needles, failing to provide extension tubing of adequate length to allow for patient movement, and not selecting the correct size of needle to reach the port. The optimal positioning of a new port would be in the infraclavicular fossa, where it is over a firm surface and it is less mobile with movement. Port location should be marked before surgery. Ideally, in

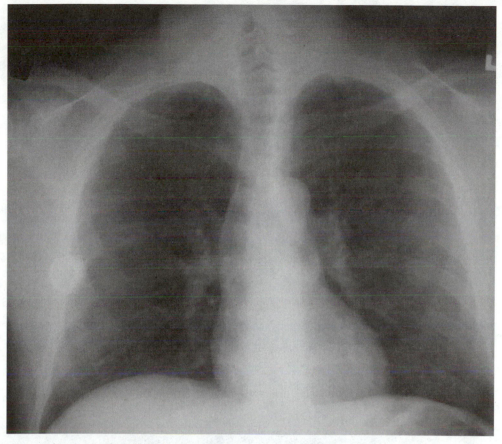

**Figure 10.4** Catheter malposition in right internal jugular vein.
*Source:* G. Sansivero. Used with permission.

women or obese people, the markings should be made while in an upright position to avoid implantation under breast or adipose tissue, which makes access difficult and increases the risk of extravasation (Mayo and Pearson 1995).

## Infection

Infection can be a life-threatening complication or a manageable exit site problem. Careful assessment of the etiology of infection and treatment options is essential. Those at highest risk for VAD-related infection include the very young, neutropenic patients, those with multiple lumen devices, and those whose VADs have been in place for extended periods of time. Figure 10.6 is one example of a VAD flowsheet. This tool can aid the nurse in assessing not only VAD-related infection but other complications also.

Erythema, drainage, and tenderness characterize exit site infections. Leukopenic and immunosuppressed patients may not exhibit the typical inflammatory response, however. Any drainage from the exit site should be

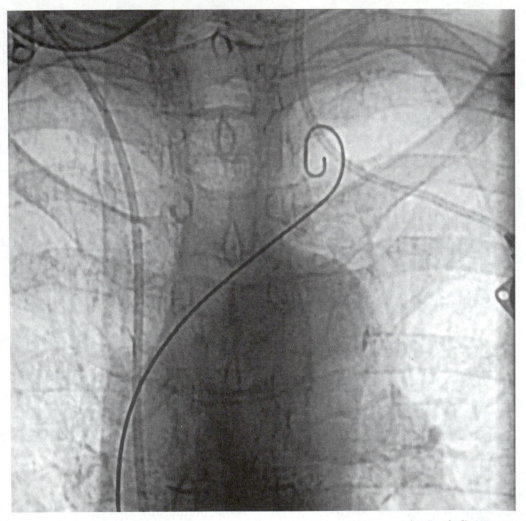

**Figure 10.5** Catheter malposition correction by securing catheter with tip deflecting wire.
*Source:* G. Sansivero. Used with permission.

cultured. The skin should be examined for signs of a possible allergic reaction to dressing materials. If suspected, the dressing technique could be altered. The tract, the tunnel, and the pocket of the VAD should be assessed for phlebitis and palpable cord, indicating a problem with vein wall inflammation and possible thrombus and fluctuance. Topical antimicrobial ointments or preparations may be used for exit site infections but they have not proven effective in preventing bacteremia. Tunnel and pocket infections are treated with systemic intravenous antibiotics although they typically are difficult to clear and often require VAD removal.

*Clinical Journal of Oncology Nursing*

Name _____ Type of Catheter _____ Insertion Date _____

| Questions | Date | Date | Date | Date | Date |
|---|---|---|---|---|---|
| Infection? | | | | | |
| Fevers/chills? If yes, did they occur after flushing? | | | | | |
| Any shortness of breath? | | | | | |
| Any swelling in face, head, neck, or eyes, especially after reclining? | | | | | |
| Any dizziness or vision changes? | | | | | |
| Any difficulty with function of catheter? | | | | | |
| Was urokinase or other drug used? | | | | | |
| **Physical Assessment** | | | | | |
| Obvious swelling of either arm? | | | | | |
| Edema of the face or neck? | | | | | |
| Distended external jugular veins? | | | | | |
| Visible collateral veins or the chest wall? | | | | | |
| Dressing dry and intact? | | | | | |
| Site red, edematous, or tender? | | | | | |
| Catheter intact? | | | | | |
| Catheter flushes easily with normal saline? | | | | | |
| Free-flowing blood return? | | | | | |
| Pain associated with a vigorous flush? | | | | | |

**Figure 10.6   Venous Access Device Flowsheet**

*Source:* Mayo, D.J., Pearson, D.C., and Horne, M.K. (1997). Superior vena cava thrombosis associated with a central venous device: A case report. *Clinical Journal of Oncology* 1(1): 9. Reprinted with permission.

There are several possible sources of VAD-related bacteremia, including contamination of the device on insertion, seeding of the catheter from an infection elsewhere in the body, contamination of the infusate or IV delivery system, or migration of bacteria from the exit site to the intravascular space. The three most common organisms cultured are *staphylococcus, streptococcus,* and *candida.* In patients with fever, tachycardia, hypotension, or unexplained malaise, infection should be considered.

If bacteremia is suspected, blood cultures should be drawn: one set drawn peripherally and one from the VAD. The initial sample from the VAD should be used; a discard specimen is unnecessary. Other sources of fever should be investigated. If the VAD is suspected to be the source, the catheter should be removed and its tip cultured. A temporary VAD should be placed to accommodate immediate vascular access needs. A permanent device should not be placed until the patient has been completely treated for the initial bacteremia.

## SUMMARY

Vascular access devices are one means to support quality of life and to enhance the safety of chemotherapy administration. Accurate placement, use, and maintenance can help minimize the risk of complications and optimize catheter performance.

Many unanswered questions remain and more research is needed in vascular access. Little data exists to support the optimal dressing and flushing regimen for VADs. Despite many types of silicone and polyurethane catheters, uncertainty still exists over what is the best catheter material and whether this material should be coated or impregnated with antimicrobial or anticoagulant solutions. New valved, positive pressure, and needleless systems are increasing in use, yet we are unsure of their impact on catheter patency and infection.

Patient education about device choices, maintenance, and troubleshooting should be a basic component of cancer care education. Consumers also should be invited to participate with manufacturers in the development of new vascular access devices and accessory products that are user-friendly.

Nurses have a unique opportunity as professionals involved in initial vascular access assessment and as end users to participate in the VAD design, development, and testing process. It is clearly within the scope of oncology nursing practice to examine novel strategies for VAD maintenance and complication management. Instruments for scoring risk for VAD complications should be developed. Vascular access research is in its infancy, and nursing is in a prime position to mature this clinical specialty.

## BIBLIOGRAPHY

Bakker, J., van Overhagen, H., Wielanga, J., de Marie, S., Nouwen, J., de Ridder, M.A.J., and Lameris, J.S. (1998). Infectious complications of radiologically inserted Hickman catheters in patients with hematologic disorders. *Cardiovascular and Interventional Radiology* 21(2): 116–121.

Bender, C. (1998). Nursing implications of antineoplastic therapy. In J.K. Itano and K.N. Taoka (eds.): *Core Curriculum for Oncology Nursing.* 3rd ed. Philadelphia: W.B. Saunders, 641–656.

Bennett, J.D., Papadouris, D., McGloughlin, R.F., Kribs, S., Kozak, R.I., Garvin, G., and Elliot, J. (1997). Percutaneous inferior vena caval approach for long-term central venous access. *Journal of Cardiovascular and Interventional Radiology* 8(5): 851–855.

Berg, D. (1996). Drug delivery systems. In M. Barton-Burke, G. Wilkes, and K. Ingwersen: *Cancer*

*Chemotherapy: A Nursing Process Approach.* 2nd ed. Sudbury, Mass.: Jones & Bartlett.

Brady, P.S., Spence, L.D., Levitin, A., Mickolich, C.T., and Dolmatch, B.L. (1999). Efficacy of percutaneous fibrin sheath stripping in restoring patency of tunneled hemodialysis catheters. *American Journal of Roentgenology* 173(4): 1023–1027.

Camp-Sorrell, D. (ed.) (1996). *Access Device Guidelines: Recommendations for Nursing Practice and Education.* Pittsburgh: Oncology Nursing Press.

Chang, R., Horne, M.K., Mayo, D.J., and Doppman, J.L. (1996). Pulse-spray treatment of subclavian and jugular venous thrombi with recombinant tissue plasminogen activator. *Journal of Cardiovascular and Interventional Radiology* 7(6): 845–851.

Cimochowski, G.E., Worley, E., Rutherford, W.E., Sartain, J., Blondin, J., and Harter, H. (1990). Superiority of the internal jugular over the subclavian access for temporary dialysis. *Nephron* 54(2): 154–161.

Denys, B.G., Uretsky, B.F., and Reddy, P.S. (1993). Ultrasound-assisted cannulation of the internal jugular vein. *Circulation* 87(5): 1557–1562.

Drakos, P.E., Nagler, A., Or, R., Gillis, S., Slavin, S. and Eldor, A. (1992). Low molecular weight heparin for Hickman catheter-induced thrombosis in thrombocytopenic patients undergoing bone marrow transplantation. *Cancer* 70(7): 1895–1898.

Eastridge, B.J., and Lefor, A.T. (1995). Complications of indwelling venous access devices in cancer patients. *Journal of Clinical Oncology* 13(1): 233–238.

Farber, A., Barbey, M.M., Grunert, J.H., and Gmelin, E. (1999). Access-related venous stenoses and occlusions: Treatment with percutaneous transluminal angioplasty and dacron-covered stents. *Cardiovascular and Interventional Radiology* 22(3): 214–218.

Gordon, A.C., Saliken, J.C., Johns, D., Owen, R., and Gray, R.R. (1998). U.S.-guided puncture of the internal jugular vein: Complications and anatomic considerations. *Journal of Vascular and Interventional Radiology* 9: 333–338.

Haskal, Z.J., Leen, V.H., Thomas-Hawkins, C., Shlansky-Goldberg, R.D., Baum, R.A., and

Soulen, M.C. (1996). Transvenous removal of fibrin sheaths from tunneled hemodialysis catheters. *Journal of Vascular and Interventional Radiology* 7(4): 513–517.

Hughes, C.B. (1986). Giving cancer drugs IV—Some guidelines. *American Journal of Nursing* (January): 34–38.

Ingle, R.J. (1995). Rare complications of vascular access devices. *Seminars in Oncology Nursing* 11: 184–193.

Johnston, S., and Pratt, Y.Z. (1981). Caring for the patient on intra-arterial chemotherapy . . . Are you ready? *Nursing 81* (November): 108–112.

Kaufman, J.A., Kazanjian, S.A., Rivitz, S.M., Geller, S.C., and Waltman, A.C. (1996). Long-term central venous catheterization in patients with limited access. *American Journal of Roentgenology* 167(5): 1327–1333.

Kazanjian, S.A., and Kaufman, J.A. (1994). Strategies for central venous catheter placement in patients with limited access. *Seminars in Interventional Radiology* 11(4): 377–387.

Krutchen, A.E., Bjarnason, H., Stackhouse, D.J., Nazarian, G.K., Magney, J.E., and Hunter, S.W. (1996). The mechanisms of positional dysfunction of subclavian venous catheters. *Radiology* 200(1): 159–163.

Lokich, J.J. (1978). *Primer of Cancer Management.* Boston: G. K. Hall.

MacDonald, S., Watt, A.J.B., McNally, D., Edwards, R.D., and Moss, J.G. (2000). Comparison of technical success and outcome of tunneled catheters inserted via the jugular and subclavian approaches. *Journal of Vascular and Interventional Radiology* 11(2): 225–231.

Mayo, D.J., and Pearson, D.C. (1995). Chemotherapy extravasation: A consequence of fibrin sheath formation around venous access devices. *Oncology Nursing Forum* 22(4): 675–680.

Mayo, D.J., Pearson, D.C., and Horne, M.K. (1997). Superior vena cava thrombosis associated with a central venous access device: A case report. *Clinical Journal of Oncology Nursing* 1(1): 5–10.

Meeske, K., and Ruccione, K. (1987). Cancer chemotherapy in children: Nursing issues and approaches. *Seminars in Oncology Nursing* 3(2): 118–127.

Nace, C.S., and Ingle, R.J. (1993). Central venous catheter "pinch off" and fracture: A review of two under-recognized complications. *Oncology Nursing Forum* 20(8): 1227–1235.

Oncology Nursing Society. (1999). *Cancer Chemotherapy Guidelines and Recommendations for Practice*. 2nd ed. Pittsburgh: Oncology Nursing Press.

———. (1996). *Cancer Chemotherapy Guidelines: Module II. Recommendations for Nursing Practice in the Acute Care Setting*. Pittsburgh: Oncology Nursing Press.

———. (1988). *Cancer Chemotherapy Guidelines and Recommendations for Practice*. Pittsburgh: Oncology Nursing Press.

Orr, M.E., and Ryder, M.A. (1993). Vascular access devices: Perspectives on designs, complications and management. *Nutrition in Clinical Practice* 8(4): 145–152.

Otto, S. (ed.) (1997). *Oncology Nursing*. St. Louis: Mosby.

Patel, N.H. (1998). Alternate approaches to central venous access. *Seminars in Interventional Radiology* 15(3): 325–333.

Perno, J., Putnam, S.G., Cohen, G.S., and Ball, D. (1999). Endovascular treatment of superior vena cava syndrome without removing a central venous catheter. *Journal of Interventional and Vascular Radiology* 10(7): 917–918.

Peters, P.S. (1987). Cancer incidence and trends. In C.R. Ziegfeld (ed.): *Core Curriculum for Oncology Nursing*. Philadelphia: W.B. Saunders, 35–38.

Puel, V., Caudry, M., Le Metayer, P.L., Baste, J.C., Midy, D., Marsault, C., Demeaux, H., and Maire, J.P. (1993). Superior vena cava thrombosis related to catheter malposition in cancer chemotherapy given through implanted ports. *Cancer* 72(7): 2249–2252.

Rumsey, K.A., and Richardson, D.K. (1995). Management of infection and occlusion associated with vascular access devices. *Seminars in Oncology Nursing* 11(3): 174–183.

Silberzweig, J.E., and Mitty, H.A. (1998). Central venous access: Low internal jugular vein approach using imaging guidance. *American Journal of Roentgenology* 170(6): 1617–1620.

Stephens, L.C., Haire, W.D., and Kotulak, G.D. (1995). Are clinical signs accurate indicators of the cause of central venous catheter occlusion? *Journal of Parenteral and Enteral Nutrition* 19(1): 75–79.

Teichgraber, U.K.M., Benter, T., Gebel, M., and Manns, M.P. (1997). A sonographically guided technique for central venous access. *American Journal of Roentgenology* 169(3): 731–733.

# Chapter 11

# Controlling Occupational Exposure to Hazardous Drugs: OSHA Guidelines*

Margaret Barton-Burke, PhD (c), RN, AOCN

## INTRODUCTION

I am going out on a limb! I have completely revised the previous chapter in this book on chemotherapy handling, and I am writing this introduction in the first person.

Why would an author completely revise a perfectly well-written, scientifically correct, and clinically sound chapter? Especially when she had worked so closely with the previous author to make the chapter fit so well within the frame work of this chemotherapy book. Well the answer to such a question is based on a scientific review of the literature on and about chemotherapy handling that I conducted while preparing to revise this chapter. In doing this literature review, I found out that there is not much new in the field, except for some new products for safe preparation, administration, and spills handling. Also, I have come to believe that, although we included the OSHA Guidelines as an appendix in the second edition, no one uses them unless a reader actually needs them as a primary source document.

So this is where I go out on my limb. I wanted to get those guidelines out of the appendices and into full view by anyone reading this book. Therefore, I have taken the lib-erty of editing, not changing, the OSHA guidelines to read as a chapter. Since these documents are within the public domain and for use by the public, editing them seemed perfectly logical. The OSHA guidelines are the foundation upon which the previous chapter is based. They are the basis for the current handling practices within institutions and the basis for organizational recommendations, for example, those of the Oncology Nursing Society. Finally, these guidelines cite all the research literature and clinical practice from an array of sources thus expanding the scope of the previous chapter.

So what is contained in the present chapter are the bare bones of the OSHA guidelines for handling chemotherapy, along with a few tables to supplement the text. I hope you find this chapter interesting and informative and I ask for feedback—from colleagues—regarding this revision and I am sure I will receive it!

## CATEGORIZATION OF DRUGS AS HAZARDOUS

A number of pharmaceuticals in the health care setting may pose occupational risk to

---

* Adapted and compiled from OSHA Guidelines. For complete OSHA Guidelines related to hazardous drugs, see http://www.osha-slc.gov/SLTC/hazardousdrugs/index.html

employees through acute and chronic workplace exposure. Past attention focused on drugs used to treat cancer. However, it is clear that many other agents also have toxicity profiles of concern. This recognition prompted the American Society of Hospital Pharmacists (ASHP) to define a class of agents as "hazardous drugs" (American Society of Hospital Pharmacists 1990). That report specified concerns about antineoplastic and nonantineoplastic hazardous drugs in use in most institutions throughout the country. Occupational Safety and Health Administration (OSHA) shares this concern. The ASHP Technical Assistance Bulletin (TAB) described four drug characteristics, each of which could be considered hazardous:

- genotoxicity
- carcinogenicity
- teratogenicity or fertility impairment
- serious organ or other toxic manifestation at low doses in experimental animals or treated patients

Table 11.1 lists some common drugs that are considered hazardous by the above criteria. There is no standardized reference for this information nor is there complete consensus on all agents listed. Professional judgment by personnel trained in pharmacology/toxicology is essential in designating drugs as hazardous. Some drugs, which have a long history of safe use in humans despite in vitro or animal evidence of toxicity, may be excluded by the institution's experts by considerations, such as those used to formulate GRAS (Generally Regarded as Safe) lists by the Federal Drug Administration (FDA) under the Food, Drug, and Cosmetics Act. In contrast, investigational drugs are new chemicals for which there is often little information

on potential toxicity. Structure or activity relationships with similar chemicals and in vitro data can be considered in determining potential toxic effects. Investigational drugs should be prudently handled as hazardous drugs (HDs) unless adequate information becomes available to exclude them.

## BACKGROUND: HAZARDOUS DRUGS AS OCCUPATIONAL RISKS

Preparation, administration, and disposal of HDs may expose pharmacists, nurses, physicians, and other health care workers to potentially significant workplace levels of these chemicals. The literature establishing these agents as occupational hazards deals primarily with cytotoxic drugs (CDs); however, documentation of adverse exposure effects from other HDs is rapidly accumulating (Chen, Vasquez-Padua, and Cheung 1990; International Agency for Research on Cancer 1982; International Agency for Research on Cancer 1990; Matthews and Boehme 1988). The degree of absorption that takes place during work and the significance of secondary early biological effects on each individual encounter are difficult to assess and may vary depending on the HD. As a result, it is difficult to set safe levels of exposure on the basis of current scientific information. However, there are several lines of evidence supporting the toxic potential of these drugs if handled improperly. Therefore, it is essential to minimize exposure to all HDs.

### Mechanism of Action

Most HDs either bind directly to genetic material in the cell nucleus or affect cellular protein synthesis. Cytotoxic drugs may not dis-

**Table 11.1    Some Common Drugs Considered Hazardous**

This table is not all inclusive, should not be construed as complete, and represents an assessment of some, but not all, marketed drugs at a fixed point in time. This table was developed through consultation with institutions that have assembled teams of pharmacists and other health care personnel to determine which drugs should be handled with caution. These teams reviewed product literature and drug information when considering each product.

Sources for this table are the Physician's Desk Reference, Section 10:00 in the American Hospital Formulary Service Drug Information, IARC publications (particularly Volume 50), the Johns Hopkins Hospital, and the National Institutes of Health, Clinical Center Nursing Department. No attempt to include investigational drugs was made, but they should be prudently handled as hazardous drugs until adequate information becomes available to exclude them. Any determination of the hazard status of a drug should be periodically reviewed and updated as new information becomes available. Importantly, new drugs should routinely undergo a hazard assessment.

| Chemical/Generic Name | Chemical/Generic Name | Chemical/Generic Name |
|---|---|---|
| altretamine | doxorubicin | melphalan |
| aminoglutethimide | estradiol | mercaptopurine |
| azathioprine | estramustine | methotrexate |
| L-asparaginase | ethinyl estradiol | mitomycin |
| bleomycin | etoposide | mitotane |
| busulfan | floxuridine | mitoxantrone |
| carboplatin | fluorouracil | nafarelin |
| carmustine | flutamide | pipobroman |
| chlorambucil | ganciclovir | plicamycin |
| chloramphenicol | hydroxyurea | procarbazine |
| chlorotrianisene | idarubicin | ribavirin |
| chlorozotocin | ifosfamide | streptozocin |
| cyclosporin | interferon-A | tamoxifen |
| cisplatin | isotretinoin | testolactone |
| cyclophosphamide | leuprolide | thioguanine |
| cytarabine | levamisole | thiotepa |
| dacarbazine | lomustine | uracil mustard |
| dactinomycin | mechlorethamine | vidarabine |
| daunorubicin | medroxyprogesterone | vinblastine |
| diethylstilbestrol | megestrol | vincristine |
| | | zidovudine |

*Source:* U.S. Department of Labor, Occupational Safety and Health Administration. (1996). *Controlling occupational exposure to hazardous drugs.* OSHA Instruction CPL2-2.20B. Washington, D.C.: Author.

tinguish between normal and cancerous cells. The growth and reproduction of the normal cells are often affected during treatment of cancerous cells.

Numerous studies document the carcinogenic, mutagenic, and teratogenic effects of HD exposure in animals. They are well summarized in the pertinent International Agency for

Research on Cancer (IARC) publications (1975 and 1990). Alkylating agents present the strongest evidence of carcinogenicity (e.g., cyclophosphamide, mechlorethamine hydrochloride [nitrogen mustard]). However, other classes, such as some antibiotics, have been implicated as well. Extensive evidence for mutagenic and reproductive effects can be found in all antineoplastic classes.

## Occupational Exposure—Human Effects

### Cytogenetic Effects

A number of studies have examined the relationship of exposure to CDs in the workplace to chromosomal aberrations. These studies have looked at a variety of markers for damage, including sister chromatid exchanges (SCE), structural aberrations (e.g., gaps, breaks, translocations), and micronuclei in peripheral blood lymphocytes. The results have been somewhat conflicting. Several authors found increases in one or more markers (Nikula, Kiviniitty, Leisti, and Taskinen 1984; Norppa et al. 1980; Pohlova, Cerna, and Rosner 1986; Waksvik, Klepp, and Brogger 1981). Increased mutation frequency has been reported as well (Chrysostomou, Morley, and Seshadri 1984). Other studies have failed to find a significant difference between workers and controls (Stiller, Obe, Bool, and Pribhilla 1983; Stucker et al. 1986). Some researchers have found higher individual elevations (Ferguson et al. 1988) or a relationship between number of drugs handled and SCEs (Benhamou, Pot-Deprun, Sancho-Garnier, and Chouroulinkov 1988). These disparate results are not unexpected. The difficulties in quantitating exposure have resulted in different exposure magnitudes between studies; workers in several negative studies appear to have a lower overall exposure (Stucker et al. 1986). In addition, differences in the use of Personal Protective Equipment (PPE) and work technique will alter absorption of CDs and resultant biologic effects.

Finally, techniques for SCE measurement may not be optimal. A recent study that looked at correlation of phosphoramide-induced SCE levels with duration of anticancer drug handling found a statistically significant correlation coefficient of 0.6. (McDiarmid, Kolodner, Humphrey, Putman, and Jacobson-Kram 1992).

Taken together, the evidence indicates an excess of markers of mutagenic exposure in unprotected workers.

### Reproductive Effects

Reproductive effects associated with occupational exposure to CDs have been well documented. Hemminki, Kyyronen, and Lindbohm (1985) found no difference in exposure between nurses who had spontaneous abortions and those who had normal pregnancies. However, the study group consisted of nurses who were employed in surgical or medical floors of a general hospital. When the relationship between CD exposure and congenital malformations was explored, the study group was expanded to include oncology nurses, among others, and an odds ratio of 4.7 was found for exposures of more than once per week. This observed odds ratio is statistically significant. Selevan, Lindbohm, Hormung, and Hemminki (1985) found a relationship between CD exposure and spontaneous abortion in a case-control study of Finnish nurses. This well-designed study reviewed the reproductive histories of 568 women (167 cases) and found a statistically significant odds ratio of 2.3. Similar results were obtained in another large case-control study of French nurses (Stucker et al. 1990), and a study of Baltimore area nurses found a significantly higher proportion of adverse pregnancy outcomes when exposure to antineoplastic agents occurred during the pregnancy (Rosner 1976). The nurses involved in these studies usually prepared and administered the drugs. Therefore, workplace exposure of these groups of professionals to such products has been associated with adverse reproductive outcomes in several investigations.

## Other Effects

Hepatocellular damage has been reported in nurses working in an oncology ward; the injury appeared to be related to intensity and duration of work exposure to CDs (Sotaniemi et al. 1983). Symptoms such as lightheadedness, dizziness, nausea, headache, and allergic reactions have also been described in employees after the preparation and administration of antineoplastic drugs in unventilated areas (Doll 1989; Rosner 1976). In occupational settings, these agents are known to be toxic to the skin and mucous membranes, including the cornea (McLendon and Bron 1978; Reich and Bachur 1975).

Many HDs are known human carcinogens, for which there is no safe level of exposure. The development of secondary malignancies is a well documented side-effect of chemotherapy treatment (Kyle 1984; Rosner 1976; Siever 1975; Weisburger et al. 1975). Leukemia has been observed most frequently. However, other secondary malignancies, such as bladder cancer and lymphoma, have been documented in patients treated for other, usually solid, primary malignancies (Kyle 1984; Wall and Clausen 1975).

Chromosomal aberrations can result from chemotherapy treatment as well. One study, on chlorambucil, reveals chromosomal damage in recipients to be cumulative and related to both dose and duration of therapy (Palmer, Dore, and Denman 1984).

Numerous case reports have linked chemotherapeutic treatment to adverse reproductive outcomes (Barber 1981; Schafer 1981; Sieber and Adamson 1975; Stephens, Golbus, Miller, Wilbur, and Epstein 1980). Testicular and ovarian dysfunction, including permanent sterility, have occurred in male and female patients who have received CDs either singly or in combination (Chapman 1984). In addition, some antineoplastic agents are known or suspected to be transmitted to infants through breast milk (Physicians Desk Reference 1991).

## Occupational Exposure—Airborne Levels

Concentrations of fluorouracil have been found during monitoring of drug preparation without a Biological Safety Cabinet (BSC) implying an opportunity for respiratory exposure (Neal, Wadden, and Chiou 1983). Elevated concentrations of cyclophosphamide were found by these authors as well. Cyclophosphamide has also been detected on the High Efficiency Particulate Air (HEPA) filters of flow hoods used in HD preparation demonstrating aerosolization of the drug and an exposure opportunity mitigated by effective engineering controls (Pyy, Sorsa, and Hakala 1988).

A recent study has reported wide samples of cyclophosphamide, on surfaces of work stations in an oncology pharmacy and outpatient treatment areas (sinks and countertops). Concentrations documented opportunity for dermal exposure (McDevitt, Lees, and McDiarmid 1992).

Administration of drugs via aerosolization can lead to measurable air concentrations in the breathing zone of workers providing treatment (Harrison, Bellows, and Rempel 1988).

## Occupational Exposure—Biological Evidence of Absorption

### Urinary Mutagenicity

Falck et al. (1979) were the first to note evidence of mutagenicity in the urine of nurses who handled cytotoxic drugs. The extent of this effect increased over the course of the work week. With improved handling practices, a decrease in mutagenic activity was seen (Falck, Sorsa, and Vainio 1981). Researchers have also studied pharmacy personnel who reconstitute antineoplastic drugs. These employees showed increasingly mutagenic urine over the period of exposure; when they stopped handling the drugs, activity fell within 2 days to the level of unexposed controls (Anderson et al. 1982; Nguyen, Theiss, and Matney 1982). They also found mutagenicity in workers using horizontal laminar flow BSCs that decreased to control levels with the use of vertical flow containment BSCs (Nguyen et al. 1982). Other studies have failed to find a relationship between exposure and urine mutagenicity (Everson et al. 1985). Sorsa et al. (1985) summarizes this information and discusses the factors, such as differences in urine collection timing and variations in the use of PPE, which could lead to disparate results. Differences may also be related to smoking status; smokers exposed to CDs exhibit greater urine mutagenicity than exposed nonsmokers or control smokers suggesting contamination of the work area by CDs and some contribution of smoking to their mutagenic profile (Bos, Leenars, Theuws, and Henderson 1982).

### Urinary Thioethers

Urinary thioethers are glutathione conjugated metabolites of alkylating agents which have been evaluated as an indirect means of measuring exposure. Workers who handle cytotoxic drugs have been reported to have increased levels compared to controls and also have increasing thioether levels over a five day work week (Jagun, Ryan, and Waldron 1982; Karakaya, Burgaz, and Bayhan 1989). Other studies of nurses who handle CDs and of treated patients have yielded variable results which could be due to confounding by smoking, PPE, and glutathione-S-transferase activity (Burgaz, Ozdamar, and Karakaya 1988).

### Urinary Metabolites

Venitt, Crofton-Sleigh, Hunt, Specchly, and Briggs (1984) assayed the urine of pharmacy and nursing personnel handling cisplatin and found platinum concentrations at or below the limit of detection for both workers and controls. Hirst, Tse, Mills, Levin, and White (1984) found cyclophosphamide in the urine of two nurses who handled the drug, documenting worker absorption. Hirst also documented skin absorption in human volunteers by using gas chromotography after topical application of the drug.

---

## WORK AREAS

### Pharmacy or Other Preparation Areas

In large oncology centers, HDs are usually prepared in the pharmacy. However, in small hospitals, outpatient treatment areas, and physicians' offices they have been prepared by physicians or nurses without appropriate engineering controls and protective apparel (Christensen, Lemasters, and Wakeman 1990; Crudi 1980). Many HDs must be reconstituted, transferred from one container to another, or manipulated before administration to patients. Even if care is taken, opportunity for absorption through inhalation or direct skin contact can occur (Hirst et al. 1984; Hoy and Stump 1984; Neal et al. 1983; Zimmerman, Larsen, Barkley, and Gallelli 1981). Examples of manipulations that can cause splattering, spraying, and aerosolization include:

- withdrawal of needles from drug vials
- drug transfer using syringes and needles or filter straws
- breaking open of ampules
- expulsion of air from a drug-filled syringe

Evaluation of these preparation techniques, using fluorescent dye solutions, has shown contamination of gloves and the sleeves and chest of gowns (Stellman 1987).

Horizontal airflow work benches provide an aseptic environment for the preparation of injectable drugs. However, these units provide a flow of filtered air originating at the back of the workspace and exiting toward the employee using the unit. Thus, they increase the likelihood of drug exposure to both the preparer and other personnel in the room. As a result, the use of horizontal BSCs is contraindicated in the preparation of HDs. Smoking, drinking, applying cosmetics, and eating while these drugs are prepared, stored, or used also increase the chance of exposure.

## Administration of Drugs to Patients

Administration of drugs to patients is generally performed by nurses or physicians. Drug injection into the IV line, clearing of air from the syringe or infusion line, and leakage at the tubing, syringe, or stopcock connection present opportunities for skin contact and aerosol generation. Clipping used needles and crushing used syringes can produce considerable aerosolization as well.

Such techniques where needles and syringes are contaminated with blood or other potentially infectious material are prohibited by the Occupational Exposure To Bloodborne Pathogens Standard (U.S. Department of Labor OSHA 1991). Prohibition of clipping or crushing of any needle or syringe is sound practice.

Excreta from patients who have received certain antineoplastic drugs may contain high concentrations of the drug or its hazardous metabolites. For example, patients receiving cyclophosphamide excrete large amounts of the drug and its mutagenic metabolites (Juma, Rogers, Trounce, and Bradbrook 1978; Siebert and Simon 1973). Patients treated with *cisplatin* have been shown to excrete potentially hazardous amounts of the drug (Venitt et al. 1984). Unprotected handling of urine or urine-soaked sheets by nursing or housekeeping personnel poses a source of exposure.

## Disposal of Drugs and Contaminated Materials

Contaminated materials used in the preparation and administration of HDs, such as gloves, gowns, syringes, and vials, present a hazard to support and housekeeping staff. The use of properly labeled, sealed, and covered disposal containers, handled by trained and protected personnel, should be routine, and is required under the Occupational Exposure To Bloodborne Pathogens Standard (U.S. Department of Labor, OSHA 1991) if such items are contaminated with blood or other potentially infectious materials. HDs and contaminated materials should be disposed of in accordance with federal, state, and local laws. Disposal of some of these drugs is regulated by the Environmental Protection Agency (EPA). Those drugs that are unused commercial chemical products and are considered by the EPA to be toxic wastes must be disposed of in accordance with 40CFR part 261.33 (EPA 1991). Spills can also represent a hazard; the employer should ensure that all employees are familiar with appropriate spill procedures.

## Drug Preparation Precautions

### Work Area

The ASHP recommends that HD preparation be performed in a restricted, preferably centralized area. Signs restricting the access of unauthorized personnel are to be prominently displayed. Eating, drinking, smoking, chewing gum, applying cosmetics, and storing food in the preparation area should be prohibited (National Study Commission on Cytotoxic Exposure 1983). The ASHP recommends that procedures for spills and emergencies, such as skin or eye contact, be available to workers, preferably posted in the area (ASHP 1990).

### Biological Safety Cabinets

Class II or III Biological Safety Cabinets BSC that meet the current National Sanitation Foundation Standard 49 (National Sanitation Foundation 1990; National Study Commission on Cytotoxic Exposure 1984) should minimize exposure to HDs during preparation. Although these cabinets are designed for biohazards, several studies have documented reduced urine mutagenicity in CD-exposed workers or reduced environmental levels after the institution of BSCs (Anderson et al. 1982; Kolmodin-Hedman, Hartvig, Sorsa, and Falck 1983; McDiarmid et al. 1988). If a BSC is unavailable, for example in a private practice office, accepted clinical practice is the sharing of a cabinet (e.g., several medical offices share a cabinet) or sending the patient to a center where HDs can be prepared in a BSC. Alternatively, preparation can be performed in a facility with a BSC and the drugs transported to the area of administration. Use of a dedicated BSC, where only HDs are prepared, is prudent clinical practice.

## Types of BSCs

Four main types of Class II BSCs are available. They all have downward airflow and HEPA filters. They are differentiated by the amount of air recirculated within the cabinet, whether this air is vented to the room or the outside, and whether contaminated ducts are under positive or negative pressure. These four types are:

- Type A cabinets recirculate approximately 70% of cabinet air through HEPA filters back into the cabinet; the rest is discharged through a HEPA filter into the preparation room. Contaminated ducts are under positive pressure.

- Type B1 cabinets have higher velocity air inflow, recirculate 30% of the cabinet air, and exhaust the rest to the outside through HEPA filters. They have negative pressure contaminated ducts and plenums.

- Type B2 systems are similar to Type B1 except that no air is recirculated.

- Type B3 cabinets are similar to Type A in that they recirculate approximately 70% of cabinet air. However, the other 30% is vented to the outside and the ducts are under negative pressure.

Class III cabinets are totally enclosed with gas-tight construction. The entire cabinet is under negative pressure, and operations are performed through attached gloves. All air is HEPA filtered.

Class II, type B or Class III BSCs are recommended since they vent to the outside (ASHP 1990). Those without air recirculation are the most protective. If the BSC has an outside exhaust, it should be vented away from air intake units.

The blower on the vertical airflow hood should be on at all times. If the BSC is turned off, it should be decontaminated and covered in plastic until airflow is resumed (ASHP 1990; National Study Commision On Cytotoxic Exposure 1984). Each BSC should be equipped with a continuous monitoring device to allow confirmation of adequate airflow and cabinet performance. The cabinet should be in an area with minimal air turbulence; this will reduce leakage to the environment (Avis and Levchuck 1984; NSF 1990).

Ventilation and biosafety cabinets installed should be maintained and evaluated for proper performance in accordance with the manufacturer's instructions.

## Decontamination

The cabinet should be cleaned according to the manufacturer's instructions. Some manufacturers have recommended weekly decontamination, as well as whenever spills occur, or when the cabinet requires moving, service, or certification.

## Personal Protective Equipment

**Gloves.** Research indicates that the thickness of the gloves used in handling HDs is more important than the type of material since all materials tested have been found to be permeable to some HDs (ASHP 1990; Connor et al. 1984; Laidlaw et al. 1984). The best results are seen with latex gloves. Therefore, latex gloves should be used for the preparation of HDs unless the drug-product manufacturer specifically stipulates that some other glove provides better protection (Connor et al. 1984; Laidlaw et al. 1984; National Study Commision On Cytotoxic Exposure 1984; Slevin, Ang, Johnston, and Turner 1984; Stoikes, Carlson, Farris,

and Walker 1987). Thicker, longer latex gloves that cover the gown cuff are recommended for use with HDs. Individuals with latex allergy should consider the use of vinyl or nitrile gloves or glove liners. Gloves with minimal or no powder are preferred since the powder may absorb contamination (ASHP, 1990; U.S. DHHS. National Institute for Occupational Safety and Health (NIOSH) 1988).

The above referenced sources have noted great variability in permeability within and between glove lots. Therefore, double gloving is recommended if it does not interfere with an individual's technique (ASHP 1990). Because all gloves are permeable to some extent and their permeability increases with time, they should be changed regularly (hourly) or immediately if they are torn, punctured, or contaminated with a spill. Hands should always be washed before gloves are put on and after they are removed. Employees need thorough training in proper methods for contaminated glove removal.

**Gowns.** A protective disposable gown made of lint-free, low permeability fabric with a closed front, long sleeves, and elastic or knit closed cuffs should be worn. The cuffs should be tucked under the gloves. If double gloves are worn, the outer glove should be over the gown cuff and the inner glove should be under the gown cuff. When the gown is removed, the inner glove should be removed last. Gowns and gloves in use in the HD preparation area should not be worn outside the HD preparation area (ASHP 1990).

As with gloves, there is *no ideal material*. Research has found nonporous Tyvek and Kaycel to be more permeable than Saranex-laminated Tyvek and polyethylene-coated Tyvek after 4 hours of exposure to the CDs tested (Laidlaw, Connor, and Theiss 1985). However, little airflow is allowed with the latter materials. As a result, manufacturers have produced gowns with Saranex or polyethylene reinforced sleeves and front in an effort to decrease permeability in the most exposure prone areas, but little data exists on decreasing exposure.

**Respiratory Protection.** A BSC is essential for the preparation of HDs. Where a BSC is not currently available, a NIOSH-approved respirator* appropriate for the hazard must be worn to afford protection until the BSC is installed. The use of respirators must comply with OSHA's Respiratory Protection Standard (U.S. Department of Labor, OSHA 1984), which outlines the aspects of a respirator program, including selection, fit testing, and worker training. Surgical masks are not *appropriate* since they *do not prevent* aerosol inhalation. Permanent respirator use, in lieu of BSCs, is imprudent practice and should not be a substitute for engineering controls.

**Eye and Face Protection.** Whenever splashes, sprays, or aerosols of HDs may be generated, which can result in eye, nose, or mouth contamination, chemical barrier face and eye protection must be provided and used in accordance with 29CFR 1910.133. Eyeglasses with temporary side shields are inadequate protection.

When a respirator is used to provide temporary protection as described above, and splashes, sprays, or aerosols are possible, employee protection should be:

- a respirator with a full face piece or
- a plastic face shield or splash goggles complying with ANSI standards

(American National Standards Institute 1968) when using a respirator of less than full face piece design

Eyewash facilities should also be made available.

**PPE Disposal and Decontamination.** All gowns, gloves, and disposable materials used in preparation should be disposed of according to the hospital's hazardous drug waste procedures and as described under this review's section on Waste Disposal. Goggles, face shields, and respirators may be cleaned with mild detergent and water for reuse.

### Work Equipment

National Institute of Health (NIH) has recommended the work with HDs be carried out in a BSC on a disposable, plastic-backed paper liner. The liner should be changed after preparation is completed for the day or after a shift, whichever comes first. Liners should also be changed after a spill (U.S. NIH 1992).

Syringes and IV sets with Luer-lock fittings should be used for HDs. Syringe size should be large enough so that they are not full when the entire drug dose is present.

A covered disposable container should be used to contain excess solution. A covered sharps container should be in the BSC.

The ASHP (1990) recommends that HD-labeled plastic bags be available for all contaminated materials (including gloves, gowns, and paper liners), so that contaminated material can be immediately placed in them and disposed of in accordance with ASHP recommendations.

---

* NIOSH recommendation at the time of this publication is for a respirator with a high-efficiency filter, preferably a powered air-purifying respirator.

## Work Practices

Correct work practices are essential to worker protection. *Aseptic technique* is assumed as a standard practice in drug preparation. The general principles of aseptic technique, therefore, will not be detailed here. It should be noted, however, that BSC benches differ from horizontal flow units in several ways that require special precautions. Manipulations should not be performed close to the work surface of a BSC. Unsterilized items, including liners and hands, should be kept downstream from the working area. Entry and exit of the cabinet should be perpendicular to the front. Rapid lateral hand movements should be avoided.

All PPE should be donned before work is started in the BSC. All items necessary for drug preparation should be placed within the BSC before work is begun. Extraneous items should be kept out of the work area.

**Labeling.** In addition to standard pharmacy labeling practices, all syringes and IV bags containing HDs should be labeled with a distinctive warning label such as:

| Special Handling/Disposal Precautions |
| --- |

**Needles.** The ASHP recommends that all syringes and needles used in the course of preparation be placed in "sharps" containers for disposal without being crushed, clipped or capped (ASHP 1990; U.S. NIH 1992).

**Priming.** Prudent practice dictates that drug administration sets be attached and primed within the BSC, prior to addition of the drug. This eliminates the need to prime the set in a less well controlled environment and ensures that any fluid that escapes during priming contains no drug. If priming must occur at the site of administration, the intravenous line should be primed with nondrug-containing fluid or a backflow closed system should be used (ASHP 1990).

**Handling Vials.** Extremes of positive and negative pressure in medication vials should be avoided, e.g., attempting to withdraw 10 cc of fluid from a 10 cc vial or placing 10 cc of a fluid into an air-filled 10 cc vial.

The use of large-bore needles, #18 or #20, avoids *high-pressure syringing* of solutions. However, some experienced personnel believe that large-bore needles are more likely to drip. Multi-use dispensing pins are recommended to avoid these problems.

Venting devices, such as filter needles or dispensing pins, permit outside air to replace the withdrawn liquid. Proper worker education is essential before using these devices (ASHP 1990). Although venting devices are recommended, another technique is to add diluent slowly to the vial by alternately injecting small amounts and allowing displaced air to escape into the syringe. When all diluent has been added, a small amount of additional air may be withdrawn to create a slight negative pressure in the vial. This should not be expelled into room air because it may contain drug residue. It should either be injected into a vacuum vial or remain in the syringe to be discarded.

If any negative pressure must be applied to withdraw a dosage from a stoppered vial and handling safety is compromised, an air-filled syringe should be used to equalize pressure in the stoppered vial.

The volume of the drug to be withdrawn can be replaced by injecting small amounts of air into the vial and withdrawing equal amounts of liquid until the required volume is withdrawn. The drug should be cleared from the needle and hub (neck) of the syringe before separating to reduce spraying on separation.

**Handling Ampules.** Prudent practice requires that ampules with dry materials should be *"gently tapped down"* before opening to move any material in the top of the ampule to the bottom quantity. A sterile gauze pad should be wrapped around the ampule neck before breaking the top (ASHP 1990). This can protect against cuts and catch airborne powder or aerosol. If diluent is to be added, it should be injected slowly down the inside wall of the ampule. The ampule should be tilted gently to ensure that all powder is wet before agitating it to dissolve the contents.

After the solution is withdrawn from the ampule with a syringe, the needle should be cleared of solution by holding it vertically with the point upwards; the syringe should be tapped to remove air bubbles. Any bubbles should be expelled into a closed container.

**Packaging HDs for Transport.** The outside of bags or bottles containing the prepared drug should be wiped with moist gauze. Entry ports should be wiped with moist alcohol pads and capped. Transport should occur in sealed plastic bags and transported in containers designed to avoid breakage.

HDs that are shipped and which are subject to EPA regulation as hazardous waste are also subject to Department of Transportation (DOT) regulations as specified in S49CFR part 172.101.

**Non-liquid HDs.** The handling of non-liquid forms of HDs requires special precautions as well. Tablets which may produce dust or potential exposure to the handler should be counted in a BSC. Capsules, i.e., gel caps or coated tablets, are unlikely to produce dust unless broken in handling.

These are counted in a BSC on equipment designated for HDs only, because even manual counting devices may be covered with dust from the drugs handled. Automated counting machines should not be used unless an enclosed process isolates the hazard from the employee(s).

Compounding should also occur in a BSC. A gown and gloves should be worn. If a BSC is unavailable, an appropriate NIOSH-approved respirator must be worn.

## Drug Administration

**Personal Protective Equipment.** The National Study Commission on Cytotoxic Exposure has recommended that personnel administering HDs wear gowns, latex gloves, and chemical splash goggles or equivalent safety glasses as described under the PPE section, preparation (National Study Commission On Cytotoxic Exposure 1983). NIOSH-approved respirators should be worn when administering aerosolized drugs.

**Administration Kit.** Protective and administration equipment may be packaged together and labeled as an HD administration kit. Such a kit could include:

- personal protective equipment
- gauze (4 x 4) for cleanup
- alcohol wipes
- disposable plastic-backed absorbent liner
- puncture-resistant container for needles and syringes
- a thick sealable plastic bag (with warning label)
- accessory warning labels

**Work Practices.** Safe work practices when handling HDs should include:

- Hands should be washed before donning and after removing gloves. Gowns or gloves that become contaminated should be changed immediately. Employees should be trained in proper methods to remove contaminated gloves and gowns. After use, gloves and gowns should be disposed of in accordance with ASHP recommendations.

- Infusion sets and pumps, which should have Luer-lock fittings, should be observed for leakage during use. A plastic-backed absorbent pad should be placed under the tubing during administration to catch any leakage. Sterile gauze should be placed around any push sites; IV tubing connection sites should be taped.

- Priming IV sets or expelling air from syringes should be carried out in a BSC. If done at the administration site, ASHP (1990) recommends that the line be primed with nondrug-containing solution or that a backflow closed system be used. IV containers with venting tubes should not be used.

- Syringes, IV bottles and bags, and pumps should be wiped clean of any drug contamination with sterile gauze. Needles and syringes should not be crushed or clipped. They should be placed in a puncture-resistant container, then into the HD disposal bag with all other HD-contaminated materials.

- Administration sets should be disposed of intact. Disposal of the waste bag should follow HD disposal requirements. Unused drugs should be returned to the pharmacy.

- Protective goggles should be cleaned with detergent and properly rinsed. All protective equipment should be disposed of upon leaving the patient care area.

- Nursing stations where these drugs will be administered should have spill and emergency skin and eye decontamination kits available and relevant Material Safety Data Sheets MSDSs for guidance. The Hazard Communication Standard (HCS) requires MSDSs to be readily available in the workplace to all employees working with hazardous chemicals.

- PPE should be used during the administration of oral HDs if splashing is possible.

Table 11.2 summarizes the OSHA guidelines into a simple-to-follow outline.

A large number of investigational HDs are under clinical study in health care facilities. Personnel not directly involved in the investigation should not administer these drugs unless they have received adequate instructions regarding safe handling procedures. Literature regarding potential toxic effects of investigational drugs should be evaluated prior to the drug's introduction into the workplace (McDiarmid, Gurley, and Arrington 1991).

The increased use of HDs in the home environment necessitates special precautions. Employees involved in home care delivery should follow the above work practices and employers should make administration and spill kits available. Home health care workers should have emergency protocols with them as well as phone numbers and addresses in the event emergency care becomes necessary. (ASHP, 1990) Waste disposal for drugs delivered for home use and other home contaminated material should also be considered by the employer and should follow applicable regulations.

**Table 11.2   Guidelines for Handling Cytotoxic Drugs**

## Preparation

- Wash hands thoroughly.
- Put on protective disposable gown made of lint-free, low-permeability material with long sleeves and elastic or knit-closed cuffs.
- Put on nonpowdered surgical latex gloves (powdered gloves may cause exposure to drug through the powder residue).
- Double-gloving has been recommended if it does not interfere with technique; gloves should be changed hourly or if they have a tear.
- *Surgical masks do not protect against the inhalation of aerosols.*
- A biological safety cabinet is essential. It should conform to OSHA guidelines. It should be inspected and cleaned according to guidelines.
- A respirator with a high-efficiency filter (powered air-purifying respirator) should be used if a BSC is unavailable.
- Plastic face shields and splash goggles should be used with the respirator if a BSC is unavailable.
- Disposable, plastic-backed absorbent pads should be used to protect the preparation area.
- A Leur-lock system for syringes, needles, tubing, and connectors should be used.
- Use aseptic technique when reconstituting cytotoxic drugs. Avoid overfilling containers; slowly add diluent. Use sterile gauze around the neck of glass ampules when opening.
- IV tubing should be primed with the solution before the cytotoxic drug is added.
- All syringes and containers should be wiped, cleaned, and labeled as cytotoxic drug.
- All needles and syringes should be discarded in a puncture-proof container labeled as harzardous waste.
- *Do not recap or clip needles.*
- Discard protective clothing and other contaminated equipment in appropriately labeled containers that conform to OSHA guidelines.
- Wash hands thoroughly after removing gloves.

## Administration

- Cytotoxic drugs should be labeled appropriately in clean, dry syringes or IV bags.

- Syringes should be kept in zip-closed plastic bags.
- For overt contamination of gloves or gowns, remove them immediately.
- For skin exposure, wash affected area with soap and water.
- For exposure to eyes, use water or an isotonic eyewash for at least 5 minutes. Obtain medical attention immediately.
- For small spills (less than 5 ml or 5 gm), personnel should wear gowns, double gloves, and facial protection. Care should be taken to remove any glass fragments and dispose of them in a properly labeled container. Spill pads should be used to absorb a liquid, and a dampened disposable gauze pad should be used to remove a powder. The area should then be rinsed with water and cleaned with a detergent. All the contaminated wastes should be disposed of properly.
- Wash hands thoroughly.
- Wear nonpowdered surgical latex gloves.
- Wear a disposable gown of low-permeable or nonpermeable fabric with a closed front and long sleeves with elastic or knit-closed cuffs.
- Use a disposable plastic-backed pad on the administration area to absorb any drips.
- Use Leur-lock IV tubing, syringes, and connector sites during administration.
- If tubing is not primed, it should be primed into a gauze pad inside a zip-closed plastic bag or piggybacked into a plain IV fluid and primed by retrograde flow ("back-primed").
- Tape all Leur-lock connections and Y-sites. Keep gauze available to wipe droplets of Y-sites and connectors.
- Watch infusion sets and pumps for signs of leakage.
- Do not expel air from syringes.
- Do not use venting tubing with IV bottles.
- Do not clip or recap needles.
- Discard needles and syringes into an appropriately labeled puncture-proof container.
- Wash hands thoroughly after removal of gloves.

*(continued*

**Table 11.2**   Guidelines for Handling Cytotoxic Drugs *(continued)*

**Disposing of body fluids**

- Surgical latex gloves and disposable gowns should be worn when handling body fluids (blood, urine, stool, emesis) up to 48 hours after the patient has received a cytotoxic agent.
- Provide urinals with a tight-fitting lid for male patients.
- Avoid back-splashing when disposing of urine and stool by placing a waterproof pad over the top of the bedpan or toilet.
- Use gloves when handling linens contaminated with cytotoxic drugs and body fluids for up to 48 hours after drug administration. Place contaminated linens in appropriately labeled double bags that are designated for separate laundering.

**Managing a cytotoxic drug spill**

- Know where the spill kit is located. Be knowledgeable about the proper procedure for managing a spill.

- For large spills, a respirator should be worn in case of aerosols or airborne powder. The spread should be limited by covering the spill with absorbent sheets or spill-control pillows. Damp towels or cloths can control a powder spill. Caution should be taken not to generate aerosols. Restrict access to the spill area. The area should be washed thoroughly with detergent and then wiped with clean water. All contaminated equipment and wastes should be disposed of properly.
- For spills in the BSC hood, follow the procedures for any spill. If the HEPA filter is contaminated, the BSC should be labeled "Contaminated: do not use." Changing and disposal of the filter must be done immediately by properly trained personnel.

---

**Aerosolized Drugs.** The administration of aerosolized HDs requires special engineering controls to prevent exposure to health care workers and others in the vicinity. Table 11.3 illustrates the modifications that can be made to OSHA guidelines in the home.

### Caring for Patients Receiving HDs

In accordance with the Occupational Exposure To Bloodborne Pathogens Standard, universal precautions must be observed to prevent contact with blood or other potentially infectious materials. Under circumstances in which differentiation between body fluid types is difficult or impossible, all body fluids should be considered potentially infectious materials and must be managed as dictated in the Occupational Exposure To Bloodborne Pathogens Standard (U.S. Department of Labor, OSHA 1991).

Personnel dealing with excreta, primarily urine, from patients who have received HDs in the last 48 hours should be provided with and wear latex or other appropriate gloves and disposable gowns, to be discarded after each use or whenever contaminated. Eye protection should be worn if splashing is possible. Such excreta contaminated with blood, or other potentially infectious materials as well, should be managed according to the Bloodborne Pathogen Standard. Hands should be washed after removal of gloves or after contact with the above substances.

Linen contaminated with HDs or excreta from patients who have received HDs in the past 48 hours is a potential source of exposure to employees. Linen soiled with blood or other potentially infectious materials as well as contaminated with excreta must also be managed

## Table 11.3    Safe Management of Chemotherapy in the Home

You are receiving chemotherapy to treat or control your cancer. In the past few years, people with cancer have been able to receive these drugs in the ambulatory oncology setting, the hospital, or at home. Chemotherapy can be administered by injection, intravenously, or orally. Its purpose is to kill or stop cancer cells from growing, but it also may damage normal cells. Special precautions must be taken to prevent chemotherapy from coming into accidental contact with you or others. This pamphlet teaches you and your family how to avoid exposure to chemotherapy and how to handle hazardous waste in your home.

### Chemotherapy Is Hazardous Waste

Chemotherapy medicine, equipment, or items that come into contact with the medicine (i.e., syringes, needles) at any time are considered contaminated with hazardous waste. Regardless of its administration method, chemotherapy remains in your body for many hours, sometimes days, after your treatment and is excreted in urine and stool. If you are vomiting, the vomitus may contain traces of chemotherapy.

### Hazardous Waste Disposal

Chemotherapy is considered hazardous waste. Materials contaminated with chemotherapy must be disposed of in specially marked containers. You will be given a hard plastic container labeled "Chemotherapy" or "Hazardous Waste." Equipment and gloves that have been in contact with chemotherapy should be placed into this container. If materials in contact with chemotherapy are too large to fit in the plastic container, place them in a special bag and seal it tightly with rubber bands. Sharp objects should only be placed in hard plastic containers. Ask your doctor or nurse which containers you should use. Containers or bags should be removed from your home when full. Either return waste containers to your physician's office or arrange for the company supplying your medicines and equipment to remove the waste.

### Body Wastes

You may use the toilet (septic tank or city sewage) as usual, just flush it twice after using for 48 hours after receiving chemotherapy. Wash your hands well with soap and water afterward, and wash your skin if urine or stool gets on it. Pregnant women should avoid direct contact with chemotherapy or contaminated wastes.

### Laundry

Items soiled with chemotherapy should be handled carefully to avoid getting the drug on your skin. Wear gloves to immediately place soiled sheets and clothing in the washer and wash as usual. If you do not have a washer, place soiled items in a plastic bag until they can be washed. Wash unsoiled clothes and linens in the usual manner. Also, dispose of plastic sheets as hazardous waste.

### Skin Care

Chemotherapy spilled on the skin may cause irritation. If this happens, thoroughly wash the area with soap and water, then dry. If redness persists more than one hour or if irritation occurs, call your doctor. Because chemotherapy is absorbed through the skin, gloves should be worn when working with the chemotherapy, equipment, or wastes.

### Eye Care

If any chemotherapy splashes into your eyes, flush them out with water for 10–15 minutes and notify your doctor.

### QUESTIONS AND ANSWERS

**Is it safe for family members to have contact with me during my chemotherapy?**

Yes. Being with your loved ones is an important part of life. Eating together, enjoying favorite activities, hugging, and kissing are all safe.

**Is it safe for my family to use the same toilet as I do?**

Yes. As long as any chemotherapy waste is cleaned from the toilet, sharing is safe.

**What should I do if I do not have control of my bladder or bowels?**

Use a disposable, plastic-backed pad, diaper, or sheet to absorb urine or stool. Change immediately when soiled and wash skin with soap and water. If you have an ostomy, your caregiver should wear gloves when emptying or changing appliances. Used ostomy supplies must be handled as hazardous waste.

**What if I use a bedpan, urinal, or commode?**

Your caregiver should wear gloves when emptying the wastes. Rinse the container with water after each use, and wash it with soap and water at least once a day.

*(continued)*

**Table 11.3   Safe Management of Chemotherapy in the Home** *(continued)*

**What if I vomit?**

Your caregiver should wear gloves when emptying the basin. Rinse it with water after each use. Wash the basin at least once a day with soap and water.

**Is if safe to be sexually active during my treatment?**

Most often, yes. Special precautions may need to be taken (ask your doctor or nurse). Chemotherapy is present in urine, stool, and vomitus, and it is probable that traces of chemotherapy are present in vaginal fluid and semen.

**Is it possible to become pregnant or father a child while receiving chemotherapy?**

Yes. A reliable method of birth control should be used while you are receiving chemotherapy.

**How should I store chemotherapy at home?**

Chemotherapy and equipment should be stored in a safe place, out of reach of children and pets. Do not store chemotherapy in the bathroom, as high humidity may damage the drugs. Check medicine labels to see if your chemotherapy should be kept in the refrigerator or away from light, and be sure all medicines are completely labeled.

**Is it safe to dispose of chemotherapy in the trash?**

No. Chemotherapy is hazardous waste that should be handled separately. If you are administering IV chemotherapy at home, you should have a special container in which to put all chemotherapy and equipment. This includes used syringes, needles, tubing, bags, cassettes, and vials. This container should be hard plastic and labeled "Hazardous Waste" or "Biohazard." Normally, you will not have extra oral chemotherapy medicine, but if you do, return it to your doctor or nurse for disposal. *Do not throw any hazardous wastes into the garbage!*

**Can I travel with my chemotherapy?**

Yes. Usually, traveling is no problem. However, because some chemotherapy requires special storage (e.g., refrigeration), you may need to make special arrangements. Check with your nurse, doctor, or medicine supplier for further instructions. Regardless of your means of travel (airplanes, cars, etc.), always seal your chemotherapy drugs in a plastic bag.

**What should I do if I spill some chemotherapy?**

In the event of a chemotherapy spill, clean the area wearing two pairs of gloves, a mask, gown, and goggles. Absorb the spill with a disposable sponge. Clean the area with soap and water. Dispose of materials in the chemotherapy hazardous waste container.

*Source:* From Sansivero, G., and Murray, S. (1989). Safe management of chemotherapy at home. *Oncology Nursing Forum* 16(5): 711–713. Copyright 1989 by the Oncology Nursing Press. Adapted with permission.

Oncology Nursing Society Clinical Practice Committee. (1997). *Cancer Chemotherapy Guidelines and Recommendations for Practice.* 2nd ed. Pittsburgh: Oncology Nursing Press.

according to the Occupational Exposure To Bloodborne Pathogens Standard (1991). Linen contaminated with HDs should be placed in specially marked laundry bags and then placed in a labeled impervious bag. The laundry bag and its contents should be prewashed, and then the linens added to other laundry for a second wash. Laundry personnel should wear latex gloves and gowns while handling prewashed material.

Glassware or other contaminated reusable items should be washed twice with detergent, by a trained employee wearing double latex gloves and a gown.

## Waste Disposal

Thick, leakproof plastic bags, colored differently from other hospital trash bags, should be used for routine accumulation and collection of used containers, discarded gloves, gowns, and any other disposable material. Labels should indicate that bags contain HD-related wastes.

Needles, syringes, and breakable items not contaminated with blood or other potentially infectious materials should be placed in a "sharps" container before they are stored in the waste bag. Such items that are contaminated with blood or other potentially infectious material must be placed in a "sharps" container. Similarly, needles should not be clipped or capped nor syringes crushed. If contaminated by blood or other potentially infectious material, such needles/syringes must not be clipped, capped, or crushed (except as on a rare instance where a medical procedure requires recapping). The waste bag should be kept inside a covered waste container clearly labeled "HD Waste Only." At least one such receptacle should be located in every area where the drugs are prepared or administered. Waste should not be moved from one area to another. The bag should be sealed when filled and the covered waste container taped.

Prudent practice dictates that every precaution be taken to prevent contamination of the exterior of the container. Personnel disposing of HD waste should wear gowns and protective gloves when handling waste containers with contaminated exteriors. Prudent practice further dictates that such a container with a contaminated exterior be placed in a second container in a manner which eliminates contamination of the second container.

Hazardous drug-related wastes should be handled separately from other hospital trash and disposed of in accordance with applicable EPA, state, and local regulations for hazardous waste (EPA 1991; Vaccari, Tonat, DeChristoforo, Gallelli, and Zimmerman 1984). This disposal can occur at either an incinerator or a licensed sanitary landfill for toxic wastes, as appropriate. Commercial waste disposal is performed by a licensed company. While awaiting removal, the waste should be held in a secure area in covered, labeled drums with plastic liners.

## Spills

Incidental spills and breakages should be cleaned up immediately by a properly protected person trained in the appropriate procedures. The area should be identified with a warning sign to limit access to the area. Incident Reports should be filed to document the spill and those exposed.

Contamination of protective equipment or clothing, or direct skin or eye contact, should be treated by

- Immediately removing the gloves or gown.
- Immediate cleansing of the affected skin with soap and water.
- Flooding an affected eye at an eyewash fountain or with water or isotonic eyewash designated for that purpose for at least 15 minutes, for eye exposure.
- Obtaining medical attention. Protocols for emergency procedures should be maintained at the designated sites for such medical care. Medical attention should also be sought for inhalation of HDs in powder form.
- Documenting the exposure in the employee's medical record.

The ASHP considers small spills to be those less than 5 ml. The 5 ml volume of material should be used to categorize spills as large or small. Spills of less than 5 ml or 5 gm outside a BSC should be cleaned up immediately by personnel wearing gowns, double latex gloves, and splash goggles. An appropriate NIOSH-approved respirator should be used for either powder or liquid spills where airborne powder or aerosol is or has been generated.

- Liquids should be wiped with absorbent gauze pads; solids should be wiped with wet absorbent gauze. The spill areas should then be cleaned three times using a detergent solution followed by clean water.
- Any broken glass fragments should be picked up using a small scoop (never the hands) and placed in a *"sharps"* container. The container should then go into an HD disposal bag, along with used absorbent pads and any other contaminated waste.
- Contaminated reusable items, for example, glassware and scoops, should be treated as outlined in institutional procedures.

When a large spill occurs, the area should be isolated and aerosol generation avoided. For spills larger than 5 ml, liquid spread is limited by gently covering with absorbent sheets or spill-control pads or pillows. If a powder is involved, damp cloths or towels should be used. Specific individuals should be trained to clean up large spills.

- Protective apparel, including respirators, should be used as with small spills when there is any suspicion of airborne powder or that an aerosol has been or will be generated. Most CDs are not volatile; however, this may not be true for all HDs. The volatility of the drug should be assessed in selecting the type of respiratory protection.
- All contaminated surfaces should be thoroughly cleaned three times with detergent and water. All contaminated absorbent sheets and other materials should be placed in the HD disposal bag.

Extensive spills within a BSC necessitate decontamination of all interior BSC surfaces after completion of the spill cleanup. The ASHP (1990) recommends this action for spills larger than 150 ml or the contents of one vial. If the HEPA filter of a BSC is contaminated, the unit should be labeled and sealed in plastic until the filter can be changed and disposed of properly by trained personnel wearing appropriate protective equipment.

Spill kits, clearly labeled, should be kept in or near preparation and administrative areas. Prior to cleanup, appropriate protective equipment should be donned. Absorbent sheets should be incinerable. Protective goggles and respirators should be cleaned with mild detergent and water after use.

### Storage and Transport

Access to areas where HDs are stored should be limited to authorized personnel with signs restricting entry (National Study Commission on Cytotoxic Exposure 1984). A list of drugs covered by HD policies and information on spill and emergency contact procedures should be posted or easily available to employees. Facilities used for storing HDs should not be used for other drugs, and should be designed to prevent containers from falling to the floor, e.g., bins with barrier fronts. Warning labels should be applied to all HD containers, as well as the shelves and bins where these containers are permanently stored.

Damaged shipping cartons should be opened in an isolated area or a BSC by a designated employee wearing double gloves, a gown, goggles, and appropriate respiratory protection. Individuals must be trained to process damaged packages as well.

The ASHP (1990) recommends that broken containers and contaminated packaging mats be placed in a *"sharps"* container and then into HD disposal bags. The bags should then be closed and placed in receptacles as described under Waste Disposal.

The appropriate protective equipment and waste disposal materials should be kept in the area where shipments are received, and employees should be trained in their use and the risks of exposure to HDs.

HDs should be securely capped or sealed, placed in sealed clear plastic bags, and transported in containers designed to avoid breakage.

Personnel involved in transporting HDs should be trained in spill procedures, including sealing off the contaminated area and calling for appropriate assistance.

## MEDICAL SURVEILLANCE

Workers who are potentially exposed to chemical hazards should be monitored in a systematic program of medical surveillance intended to prevent occupational injury and disease (ASHP 1990; National Study on Cytotoxic Exposure 1983; National Study Commission on Cytoxic Exposure 1984). The purpose of surveillance is to identify the earliest reversible biological effects so that exposure can be reduced or eliminated before the employee sustains irreversible damage. The occurrence of exposure-related disease or other adverse health effects should prompt immediate re-evaluation of primary preventive measures (e.g., engineering controls, personal protective equipment). In this manner, medical surveillance acts as a check on the appropriateness of controls already in use (McDiarmid and Jacobson-Kram 1989). For

detection and control of work-related health effects, job specific medical evaluations should be performed:

- before job placement
- periodically during employment
- following acute exposures
- at the time of job termination or transfer (exit examination)

This information should be collected and analyzed in a systematic fashion to allow early detection of disease patterns in individual workers and groups of workers.

## TRAINING AND INFORMATION DISSEMINATION

In compliance with the Hazard Communication Standard, all personnel involved in any aspect of the handling of covered HDs (physicians, nurses, pharmacists, housekeepers, employees involved in receiving, transport, or storage) must receive information and training to apprise them of the hazards of HDs present in the work area (National Study Commission on Cytotoxic Exposure 1983). Such information should be provided at the time of an employee's initial assignment to a work area where HDs are present and prior to assignments involving new hazards. The employer should provide annual refresher information and training.

The National Study Commission on Cytotoxic Exposure (1983) recommended that knowledge and competence of personnel be evaluated after the first orientation or training session, and then yearly, or more often if a need is perceived. Evaluation may involve direct observation of an individual's performance on the job. In addition, non-HD solutions should be used for evaluation of preparation technique; quinine, which will fluoresce under ultraviolet light, provides an easy mechanism for evaluation of technique.

It is essential that workers understand the carcinogenic potential and reproductive hazards of these drugs. Both females and males should understand the importance of avoiding exposure, especially early in pregnancy, so they can make informed decisions about the hazards involved. In addition, the facility's policy regarding reproductive toxicity of HDs should be explained to workers. Updated information should be provided to employees on a regular basis and whenever their jobs involve new hazards. Medical staff and other personnel who are not hospital employees should be informed of hospital policies and of the expectation that they will comply with these policies.

## RECORDKEEPING

Any workplace exposure record created in connection with HD handling shall be kept, transferred, and made available for at least thirty years and medical records shall be kept for the duration of employment plus thirty years in accordance with the Access to Employee Exposure and Medical Records Standard 29CFR 1910.20 (U.S. Department of Labor, OSHA 1989).

In addition, sound practice dictates that training records should include the following information:

- the dates of the training sessions
- the contents or a summary of the training sessions
- the names and qualifications of the persons conducting the training

- the names and job titles of all persons attending the training sessions

Training records should be maintained for three years from the date on which the training occurred.

## CONCLUSION

Safe handling guidelines were developed to reduce the risks of exposure to personnel who handle cytotoxic drugs and, although they are the basis for a major initiative to develop standard practice, there are still areas that require ongoing effort. These areas include but are not limited to nursing educational programs, home care, and nursing research.

With the expanding body of scientific knowledge regarding the potential hazards of handling cytotoxic drugs, oncology nurses are challenged to keep abreast of the latest information on the subject. Specifically, some studies show that oncology nurses do not always adhere to OSHA guidelines despite the knowledge about the potential hazards of working with cytotoxic drugs. Therefore, education and educational programs are necessary and should focus on the specific types of protective equipment recommended by the OSHA guidelines, their proper use, as well as the barriers to compliance. Ongoing, creative educational updates should be provided as new information becomes available.

Additionally, nurses have a professional responsibility to educate the public, specifically patients and caregivers, regarding safe practices when handling cancer chemotherapeutic agents or chemotherapy waste products. As patients are discharged early from the acute care setting to receive chemotherapy in their homes the clinical practice arena of home care will continue to expand. The OSHA guidelines must be reviewed regularly to ensure safe handling practices in the home remain up-to-date.

There is a need for more specific research related to utilization of OSHA guidelines. Including research to evaluate the longterm effects of working with cytotoxic agents especially research about reproductive risks (Valanis, Vollmer, and Steele 1999). Additionally, research and research topics should focus on compliance and knowledge of the OSHA guidelines for the members of multidisciplinary teams. This research needs to include various practice settings especially the home.

We have come far in setting the standard for safe handling of cytotoxic agents but we still have work to do. It is my hope that this chapter and ultimately this book will help improve nursing practice and patient care for the individual receiving cancer chemotherapy.

## BIBLIOGRAPHY

American National Standards Institute. (1968) Occupational and Educational Eye and Face Protection. *ANSI*, Z87.1.

American Society of Hospital Pharmacists. (1990). ASHP Technical Assistance Bulletin on Handling Cytotoxic and Hazardous Drugs. *American Journal of Hospital Pharmacy* 47(5): 1033–1049.

Anderson, R.W., Puckett, W.H., Dana, W.J., Nguyen, T.V., Theiss, J.C., and Matney, T.S. (1982). Risk of handling injectable antineoplastic agents. *American Journal of Hospital Pharmacy* 39(11): 1881–1887.

Avis, K.E., and Levchuck, J.W. (1984). Special considerations in the use of vertical laminar-flow workbenches. *American Journal of Hospital Pharmacy* 41(1): 81–87.

Barber, R.K. (1981) Fetal and neonatal effects of cytotoxic agents. *Obstetric Gynecology* 51: 41S–47S.

Benhamou, S., Pot-Deprun, J., Sancho-Garnier, H., and Chouroulinkov, I. (1988). Sister chromatid exchanges and chromosomal aberrations in lymphocytes of nurses handling cytostatic drugs. *International Journal of Cancer* 41(3): 350–353.

Bos, R.P., Leenars, A.O., Theuws, J.L., and Henderson, P.T. (1982). Mutagenicity of urine from nurses handling cytostatic drugs, influence of smoking. *International Archive of Occupational Environmental Health* 50: 359–369.

Burgaz, S., Ozdamar, Y.N., and Karakaya, A.E. (1988). A signal assay for the detection of genotoxic compounds: Application on the urines of cancer patients on chemotherapy and of nurses handling cytotoxic drugs. *Human Toxicology* 7(6): 557–560.

Chapman, R.M. (1984). Effect of cytotoxic therapy on sexuality and gonadal function. In M.C. Perry and J.W. Yarbro (eds.): *Toxicity of Chemotherapy*. Orlando: Grune and Stratton: 343–363.

Chen, C.H., Vazquez-Padua, M., and Cheng, Y.C. (1990). Effect of antihuman immunodeficiency virus nucleoside analogs on mDNA and its implications for delayed toxicity. *Molecular Pharmacology* 39: 625–628.

Christensen, C.J., Lemasters, G.K., and Wakeman, M.A. (1990). Work practices and policies of hospital pharmacists preparing antineoplastic agents. *Journal of Occupational Medicine* 32(6): 508–512.

Chrysostomou, A., Morley, A.A., and Seshadri, R. (1984). Mutation frequency in nurses and pharmacists working with cytotoxic drugs. *Australia New Zealand Journal of Medicine* 14: 831–834.

Connor, T.H., Laidlaw, J.L., Theiss, J.C., Anderson, R.W., and Matney, T.S. (1984). Permeability of latex and polyvinyl chloride gloves to carmustine. *American Journal of Hospital Pharmacy* 41(4): 676–679.

Crudi, C.B. (1980). A compounding dilemma: I've kept the drug sterile but have I contaminated myself? *NITA* 3: 77–80.

deWerk Neal, A., Wadden, R.A., and Chiou, W.L. (1983). Exposure of hospital workers to airborne antineoplastic agents. *American Journal of Hospital Pharmacy* 40(4): 597–601.

Doll, D.C. (1989). Aerosolised pentamidine. *Lancet* ii: 1284–1285.

Environmental Protection Agency. (1991) *Discarded Commercial Chemical Products, Off Specification*

*Species, Container Residues, and Spill Residues Thereof.* 40 CFR 261.33(f).

Everson, R.B., Ratcliffe, J.M., and Flack, P.M. (1985). Detection of low levels of urinary mutagen excretion by chemotherapy workers which was not related to occupational drug exposure. *Cancer Research* 45(12 Pt 1): 6487–6497.

Falck, K., Grohn, P., Sorsa, M., Vainio, H., Heinonen, E., and Holsti, L.R. (1979). Mutagenicity in urine of nurses handling cytostatic drugs. *Lancet* (8128): 1250–1251.

Falck, K., Sorsa, M., and Vainio, H. (1981). Use of the bacterial fluctuation test to detect mutagenicity in urine of nurses handling cytostatic drugs (abstract). *Mutation Research* 85: 236–237.

Ferguson, L.R., Everts, R., Robbie, M.A. et al. (1988). The use within New Zealand of cytogenetic approaches to monitoring of hospital pharmacists for exposure to cytotoxic drugs: Report of a pilot study in Auckland. *Australian Journal of Hospital Pharmacology* 18: 228–233.

Harrison, R., Bellows, J., and Rempel, D. (1988). Assessing exposures of health-care personnel to aerosols of ribavirin—California. *Morbidity and Mortality Weekly Report* 37: 560–563.

Hemminki, K., Kyyronen, P., and Lindbohm, M.L. (1985). Spontaneous abortions and malformations in the offspring of nurses exposed to anaesthetic gases, cytostatic drugs, and other potential hazards in hospitals, based on registered information of outcome. *Journal of Epidemiology Community Health* 39(2): 141–147.

Hirst, M., Tse, S., Mills, D.G., Levin, L., and White, D.F. (1984). Occupational exposure to cyclophosphamide. *Lancet* 1(8370): 186–188.

Hoy, R.H., and Stump, L.M. (1984). Effect of an air-venting filter device on aerosol production from vials. *American Journal of Hospital Pharmacy* 41(2): 324–326.

International Agency for Research on Cancer. (1975). *IARC Monographs on the Evaluation of the Carcinogenic Risk of Chemicals to Man: Some Aziridines, N-, S-, and O-mustards and Selenium* Vol. 9. Lyon, France: IARC.

———. (1982). *IARC Monographs on the Evaluation of the Carcinogenic Risk of Chemicals to Humans: Chemicals, Industrial Processes and Industries Associated with Cancer in Humans* Vol. 1–29(Suppl 4). Lyon, France: IARC.

———. (1987a). *IARC Monographs on the Evaluation of the Carcinogenic Risk of Chemicals to Humans; Genetic and Related Effects: An Updating of Selected IARC Monographs from Volumes 1–42* Vol 1–42(Suppl 6). Lyon, France: IARC

———. (1987b). *IARC Monographs on the Evaluation of the Carcinogenic Risk of Chemicals to Humans; Overall Evaluations of Carcinogenicity: An Updating of IARC Monographs Volumes 1 to 42* Vol 1–42(Suppl 7). Lyon, France: IARC.

———. (1990). *IARC Monographs on the Evaluation of the Carcinogenic Risk of Chemicals to Humans: Pharmaceutical Drugs* Vol 50. Lyon, France: IARC.

Jagun, O., Ryan, M., and Waldron, H.A. (1982). Urinary thioether excretion in nurses handling cytotoxic drugs. *Lancet* 2(8295): 443–444.

Juma, F.D., Rogers, H.J., Trounce, J.R., and Bradbrook, I.D. (1978). Pharmacokinetics of intravenous cycleophosphamide in man, estimated by gas-liquid chromatography. *Cancer Chemotherapy Pharmacology* 1:229–231.

Karakaya, A.E., Burgaz, S., and Bayhan, A. (1989). The significance of urinary thioethers as indicators of exposure to alkylating agents. *Archives of Toxicology* 13(Suppl): 117–119.

Kolmodin-Hedman, B., Hartvig, P., Sorsa, M., and Falck, K. (1983). Occupational handling of cytostatic drugs. *Archives of Toxicology* 54(1): 25–33.

Kyle, R.A. (1984). Second malignancies associated with chemotherapy. In M.C. Perry and J.W. Yarbro (eds.): *Toxicity of Chemotherapy*. Orlando, Fla.: Grune and Stratton, 479–506.

Laidlaw, J.L., Connor, T.H., Theiss, J.C., Anderson, R.W., and Matney, T.S. (1984). Permeability of latex and polyvinyl chloride gloves to 20 antineoplastic drugs. *American Journal of Hospital Pharmacy* 41(12): 2618–2623.

———. (1985). Permeability of four disposable protective-clothing materials to seven antineoplastic drugs. *American Journal of Hospital Pharmacy* 42(11): 2449–2454.

Matthews, T., and Boehme, R. (1988). Antiviral activity and mechanism of action of ganciclovir. *Reviews of Infectious Diseases* 10(Suppl 3): s490–s494.

McDevitt, J.J., Lees, P.S.J., and McDiarmid, M.A. (1993). Exposure of hospital pharmacists and nurses to antineoplastic agents. *Journal of Occupational Medicine* 35: 57–60.

McDiarmid, M.A., Egan, T., Furio, M., Bonacci, M., and Watts, S.R. (1988). Sampling for airborne fluorouracil in a hospital drug preparation area. *American Journal of Hospital Pharmacy* 43(8): 1942–1945.

McDiarmid, M.A., and Emmett, E.A. (1987). Biological monitoring and medical surveillance of workers exposed to antineoplastic agents. *Seminars in Occupational Medicine* 2: 109–117.

McDiarmid, M.A., Gurley, H.T., and Arrington, D. (1991). Pharmaceuticals as hospital hazards: Managing the risks. *Journal of Occupational Medicine* 33: 155–158.

McDiarmid, M.A, and Jacobson-Kram, D. (1989). Aerosolized pentamidine and public health. *Lancet* 2(8667): 863–864.

McDiarmid, M.A, Kolodner, K., Humphrey, F., Putman, D., and Jacobson-Kram, D. (1992). Baseline and phosphoramide mustard-induced sister- chromatid exchanges in pharmacists handling anticancer drugs. *Mutation Research* 279(3): 199–204.

McLendon, B.F., and Bron, A.F. (1978). Corneal toxicity from vinblastine solution. *British Journal of Ophthalmology* 62: 97–99.

National Sanitation Foundation. (1990). *Standard No. 49 for Class II (Laminar Flow) Biohazard Cabinetry.* Ann Arbor, MI: National Sanitation Foundation.

National Study Commission on Cytotoxic Exposure. (1983). *Recommendations for Handling Cytotoxic Agents.* Louis P. Jeffrey, Sc.D., Chairman, Rhode Island Hospital, Providence, Rhode Island.

———. (1984). *Consensus Responses to Unresolved Questions Concerning Cytotoxic Agents.* Louis P. Jeffrey, Sc.D., Chairman, Rhode Island Hospital, Providence, Rhode Island.

Nguyen, T.V., Theiss, J.C., and Matney, T.S. (1982). Exposure of pharmacy personnel to mutagenic antineoplastic drugs. *Cancer Research* 42(11): 4792–4796.

Nikula, E., Kiviniitty, K., Leisti, J., and Taskinen, P. (1984). Chromosome aberrations in lymphocytes of nurses handling cytostatic agents. *Scandinavian Journal of Work Environmental Health* 10: 71–74.

Norppa, H., Sorsa, M., Vainio, H., et al. (1980). Increased sister chromatid exchange frequencies in lymphocytes of nurses handling cytostatic drugs. *Scandinavian Journal of Work Environmental Health* 6: 229–301.

Oncology Nursing Society Clinical Practice Committee. (1997). *Cancer Chemotherapy Guidelines and Recommendations for Practice.* 2nd ed. Pittsburgh: Oncology Nursing Press.

Palmer, R.G., Dore, C.J., and Denman, A.M. (1984). Chlorambucil-induced chromosome damage to human lymphocytes is dose-dependent and cumulative. *Lancet* 1(8371): 246–249.

Physician's Desk Reference. (1991). *Physician's Desk Reference.* Oradell, N.J.: Medical Economics Data, 730.

Pohlova, H., Cerna, M., and Rossner, P. (1986). Chromosomal aberrations, SCE and urine mutagenicity in workers occupationally exposed to cytostatic drugs. *Mutation Research* 174(3): 213–217.

Pyy, L., Sorsa, M., and Hakala, E. (1988). Ambient monitoring of cyclophosphamide in manufacture and hospitals. *American Industrial Hygiene Association Journal* 49(6): 314–317.

Reich, S.D., and Bachur, N.R. (1975). Contact dermatitis associated with adriamycin (NSC-123127) and daunorubicin (NSC-82151). *Cancer Chemotherapy Reports* 59: 677–678.

Rogers, B., and Emmett, E.A. (1987). Handling antineoplastic agents: Urine mutagenicity in nurses. *IMAGE Journal of Nursing Scholarship* 19: 108–113.

Rosner, F. (1976). Acute leukemia as a delayed consequence of cancer chemotherapy. *Cancer* 37(2 Suppl): 1033–1036.

Sansivero, G., and Murray, S. (1989). Safe management of chemotherapy at home. *Oncology Nursing Forum* 16(5): 711–713.

Schafer, A.I. (1981). Teratogenic effects of antileukemic therapy. *Archives of Internal Medicine* 141(4): 514–515.

Selevan, S.G., Lindbolm, M.L., Hornung, R.W., and Hemminki, K. (1985). A study of occupational exposure to antineoplastic drugs and fetal loss in nurses. *New England Journal of Medicine* 313(19): 1173–1178.

Sieber, S.M., and Adamson, R.H. (1975). Toxicity of antineoplastic agents in man: Chromosomal aberrations, antifertility effects, congenital malformations, and carcinogenic potential. *Advanced Cancer Research* 22: 57–155.

Siebert, D., and Simon, U. (1973). Cyclophosphamide: pilot study of genetically active metabolites in the urine of a treated human patient. *Mutation Research* 19(1): 65–72.

Siever, S.M. (1975). Cancer chemotherapeutic agents and carcinogenesis. *Cancer Chemotherapy Reports* 59: 915–918.

Slevin, M.L., Ang, L.M., Johnston, A., and Turner, P. (1984). The efficiency of protective gloves used in the handling of cytotoxic drugs. *Cancer Chemotherapy Pharmacology* 12: 151–153.

Sorsa, M., Hemminki, K., and Vainio, H. (1985). Occupational exposure to anticancer drugs—potential and real hazards. *Mutation Research* 154(2): 135–149.

Sotaniemi, E.A., Sutinen, S., Arranto, A.J., et al. (1983). Liver damage in nurses handling cytostatic agents. *Acta Med. Scand.* 214: 181–189.

Stellman, J.M. (1987). The spread of chemotherapeutic agents at work: Assessment through stimulation. *Cancer Investigation* 5(2): 75–81.

Stephens, J.D., Golbus, M.S., Miller, T.R., Wilber, R.R., and Epstein, C.J. (1980). Multiple congenital abnormalities in a fetus exposed to 5-fluorouracil during the first trimester. *American Journal of Obstetrics and Gynecology* 137(6): 747–749.

Stiller, A., Obe, G., Bool, I., and Pribilla, W. (1983). No elevation of the frequencies of chromosomal aberrations as a consequence of handling cytostatic drugs. *Mutation Research* 121(3–4):253–259.

Stoikes, M.E., Carlson, J.D., Farris, F.F., and Walker, P.R. (1987). Permeability of latex and polyvinyl chloride gloves to fluorouracil and methotrexate. *American Journal of Hospital Pharmacy* 44: 1341–1346.

Stucker, I., Hirsch, A., and Doloy, T. (1986). Urine mutagenicity, chromosomal abnormalities and sister chromatid exchanges in lymphocytes of nurses handling cytostatic drugs. *International Archives of Occupational Environmental Health* 57: 195–205.

Stucker, I., Caillard, J.F., Collin, R. et al. (1990). Risk of spontaneous abortion among nurses handling antineoplastic drugs. *Scandinavian Journal of Work Environment Health* 16: 102–107.

U.S. Department of Health and Human Services. Public Health Service. National Institutes of Health. (1992). *Recommendations for the Safe Handling of Cytotoxic Drugs.* NIH Publication 92-2621.

U.S. Department of Health and Human Services. Public Health Service. Centers for Disease Control. National Institute for Occupational Safety and Health. (1988). *Guidelines for Protecting the Safety and Health of Health Care Workers.* DHHS (NIOSH) Publication 88-119.

U.S. Department of Labor, Occupational Safety and Health Administration. (1996). *Controlling occupational exposure to hazardous drugs.* OSHA Instruction CPL2-2.20B. Washington, D.C.: Author.

———. (1991). *Occupational Exposure To Bloodborne Pathogens Standard* 29 CFR 1910.1030

———. (1990). *Access to Employee and Medical Records Standard.* 29 CFR 1910.20.

———. (1984). *Respiratory Protection Standard* 29 CFR 1910.134.

Vaccari, F.L., Tonat, K., DeChristoforo, R., Gallelli, J.F., and Zimmerman, P.F. (1984). Disposal of antineoplastic wastes at the NIH. *American Journal of Hospital Pharmacy* 41(1): 87–92.

Valanis, B., Vollmer, W.M., and Steele, P. (1999). Occupational exposure to antineoplastic agents: Self-reported miscarriages and stillbirths among nurses and pharmacists. Journal of Occupational and Environmental Medicine 41(8): 632–638.

Venitt, S., Crofton-Sleigh, C., Hunt, J., Speechley, V., and Briggs, K. (1984). Monitoring exposure of nursing and pharmacy personnel to cytotoxic drugs: Urinary mutation assays and urinary platinum as markers of absorption. *Lancet* 1(8368): 74–76.

Waksvik, H., Klepp, O., and Brogger, A. (1981). Chromosome analyses of nurses handling cytostatic agents. *Cancer Treatment Reports* 65(7–8): 607–610.

Wall, R.L., and Clausen, K.P. (1975). Carcinoma of the urinary bladder in patients receiving cyclophosphamide. *New England Journal of Medicine* 293(6): 271–273.

Weisburger, J.H., Griswold, D.P., Prejean, J.D., et al. (1975). Tumor induction by cytostatics: The carcinogenic properties of some of the principal drugs used in clinical cancer chemotherapy. *Recent Results Cancer Research* 52: 1–17.

Zimmerman, P.F., Larsen, R.K., Barkley, E.W., and Gallelli, J.F. (1981). Recommendations for the safe handling of injectable antineoplastic drug products. *American Journal of Hospital Pharmacy* 38(11): 1693–1695.

# Appendices

# COMMON TOXICITY CRITERIA (CTC)

| Adverse Event | Grade | | | | |
|---|---|---|---|---|---|
| | **0** | **1** | **2** | **3** | **4** |
| **ALLERGY/IMMUNOLOGY** | | | | | |
| Allergic reaction/ hypersensitivity (including drug fever) | none | transient rash, drug fever <38°C (<100.4°F) | urticaria, drug fever ≥38°C (≥100.4°F), and/or asymptomatic bronchospasm | symptomatic bronchospasm, requiring parenteral medication(s), with or without urticaria; allergy-related edema/angioedema | anaphylaxis |
| Note: Isolated urticaria, in the absence of other manifestations of an allergic or hypersensitivity reaction, is graded in the DERMATOLOGY/SKIN category. | | | | | |
| Allergic rhinitis (including sneezing, nasal stuffiness, postnasal drip) | none | mild, not requiring treatment | moderate, requiring treatment | - | - |
| Autoimmune reaction | none | serologic or other evidence of autoimmune reaction but patient is asymptomatic (e.g., vitiligo), all organ function is normal and no treatment is required | evidence of autoimmune reaction involving a non-essential organ or function (e.g., hypothyroidism), requiring treatment other than immunosuppressive drugs | reversible autoimmune reaction involving function of a major organ or other adverse event (e.g., transient colitis or anemia), requiring short-term immunosuppressive treatment | autoimmune reaction causing major grade 4 organ dysfunction; progressive and irreversible reaction; long-term administration of high-dose immuno-suppressive therapy required |
| Also consider Hypothyroidism, Colitis, Hemoglobin, Hemolysis. | | | | | |
| Serum sickness | none | - | - | present | - |
| Urticaria is graded in the DERMATOLOGY/SKIN category if it occurs as an isolated symptom. If it occurs with other manifestations of allergic or hypersensitivity reaction, grade as Allergic reaction/hypersensitivity above. | | | | | |
| Vasculitis | none | mild, not requiring treatment | symptomatic, requiring medication | requiring steroids | ischemic changes or requiring amputation |
| Allergy/Immunology - Other (Specify, _____) | none | mild | moderate | severe | life-threatening or disabling |
| **AUDITORY/HEARING** | | | | | |
| Conductive hearing loss is graded as Middle ear/hearing in the AUDITORY/HEARING category. | | | | | |
| Earache is graded in the PAIN category. | | | | | |
| External auditory canal | normal | external otitis with erythema or dry desquamation | external otitis with moist desquamation | external otitis with discharge, mastoiditis | necrosis of the canal soft tissue or bone |
| Note: Changes associated with radiation to external ear (pinnae) are graded under Radiation dermatitis in the DERMATOLOGY/SKIN category. | | | | | |

| Adverse Event | Grade 0 | 1 | 2 | 3 | 4 |
|---|---|---|---|---|---|
| Inner ear/hearing | normal | hearing loss on audiometry only | tinnitus or hearing loss, not requiring hearing aid or treatment | tinnitus or hearing loss, correctable with hearing aid or treatment | severe unilateral or bilateral hearing loss (deafness), not correctable |
| Middle ear/hearing | normal | serous otitis without subjective decrease in hearing | serous otitis or infection requiring medical intervention; subjective decrease in hearing; rupture of tympanic membrane with discharge | otitis with discharge, mastoiditis or conductive hearing loss | necrosis of the canal soft tissue or bone |
| Auditory/Hearing - Other (Specify, _____) | normal | mild | moderate | severe | life-threatening or disabling |

## BLOOD/BONE MARROW

| Adverse Event | Grade 0 | 1 | 2 | 3 | 4 |
|---|---|---|---|---|---|
| Bone marrow cellularity | normal for age | mildly hypocellular or ≤25% reduction from normal cellularity for age | moderately hypocellular or >25 - ≤50% reduction from normal cellularity for age or >2 but <4 weeks to recovery of normal bone marrow cellularity | severely hypocellular or >50 - ≤75% reduction in cellularity for age or 4 - 6 weeks to recovery of normal bone marrow cellularity | aplasia or >6 weeks to recovery of normal bone marrow cellularity |
| Normal ranges: | | | | | |
| *children (≤18 years)* | *90% cellularity average* | | | | |
| younger adults (19-59) | 60 - 70% cellularity average | | | | |
| older adults (≥60 years) | 50% cellularity average | | | | |
| Note: Grade Bone marrow cellularity only for changes related to treatment not disease. | | | | | |
| CD4 count | WNL | <LLN - 500/mm$^3$ | 200 - <500/mm$^3$ | 50 - <200/mm$^3$ | <50/mm$^3$ |
| Haptoglobin | normal | decreased | - | absent | - |
| Hemoglobin (Hgb) | WNL | <LLN - 10.0 g/dL<br><LLN - 100 g/L<br><LLN - 6.2 mmol/L | 8.0 - <10.0 g/dL<br>80 - <100 g/L<br>4.9 - <6.2 mmol/L | 6.5 - <8.0 g/dL<br>65 - <80 g/L<br>4.0 - <4.9 mmol/L | <6.5 g/dL<br><65 g/L<br><4.0 mmol/L |
| For leukemia studies or bone marrow infiltrative/ myelophthisic processes, if specified in the protocol. | WNL | 10 - <25% decrease from pretreatment | 25 - <50% decrease from pretreatment | 50 - <75% decrease from pretreatment | ≥75% decrease from pretreatment |
| Hemolysis (e.g., immune hemolytic anemia, drug-related hemolysis, other)<br><br>Also consider Haptoglobin, Hemoglobin. | none | only laboratory evidence of hemolysis [e.g., direct antiglobulin test (DAT, Coombs') schistocytes] | evidence of red cell destruction and ≥2gm decrease in hemoglobin, no transfusion | requiring transfusion and/or medical intervention (e.g., steroids) | catastrophic consequences of hemolysis (e.g., renal failure, hypotension, bronchospasm, emergency splenectomy) |

| Adverse Event | Grade | | | | |
|---|---|---|---|---|---|
| | **0** | **1** | **2** | **3** | **4** |
| Leukocytes (total WBC) | WNL | <LLN - 3.0 x 10$^9$ /L <br> <LLN - 3000/mm$^3$ | ≥2.0 - <3.0 x 10$^9$ /L <br> ≥2000 - <3000/mm$^3$ | ≥1.0 - <2.0 x 10$^9$ /L <br> ≥1000 - <2000/mm$^3$ | <1.0 x 10$^9$ /L <br> <1000/mm$^3$ |
| For BMT studies, if specified in the protocol. | WNL | ≥2.0 - <3.0 X 10$^9$/L <br> ≥2000 - <3000/mm$^3$ | ≥1.0 - <2.0 x 10$^9$ /L <br> ≥1000 - <2000/mm$^3$ | ≥0.5 - <1.0 x 10$^9$ /L <br> ≥500 - <1000/mm$^3$ | <0.5 x 10$^9$ /L <br> <500/mm$^3$ |
| *For pediatric BMT studies (using age, race and sex normal values), if specified in the protocol.* | | *≥75 - <100% LLN* | *≥50 - <75% LLN* | *≥25 - 50% LLN* | *<25% LLN* |
| Lymphopenia | WNL | <LLN - 1.0 x 10$^9$ /L <br> <LLN - 1000/mm$^3$ | ≥0.5 - <1.0 x 10$^9$ /L <br> ≥500 - <1000/mm$^3$ | <0.5 x 10$^9$ /L <br> <500/mm$^3$ | - |
| *For pediatric BMT studies (using age, race and sex normal values), if specified in the protocol.* | | *≥75 - <100%LLN* | *≥50 - <75%LLN* | *≥25 - <50%LLN* | *<25%LLN* |
| Neutrophils/granulocytes (ANC/AGC) | WNL | ≥1.5 - <2.0 x 10$^9$ /L <br> ≥1500 - <2000/mm$^3$ | ≥1.0 - <1.5 x 10$^9$ /L <br> ≥1000 - <1500/mm$^3$ | ≥0.5 - <1.0 x 10$^9$ /L <br> ≥500 - <1000/mm$^3$ | <0.5 x 10$^9$ /L <br> <500/mm$^3$ |
| For BMT studies, if specified in the protocol. | WNL | ≥1.0 - <1.5 x 10$^9$ /L <br> ≥1000 - <1500/mm$^3$ | ≥0.5 - <1.0 x 10$^9$ /L <br> ≥500 - <1000/mm$^3$ | ≥0.1 - <0.5 x 10$^9$ /L <br> ≥100 - <500/mm$^3$ | <0.1 x 10$^9$ /L <br> <100/mm$^3$ |
| For leukemia studies or bone marrow infiltrative/ myelophthisic process, if specified in the protocol. | WNL | 10 - <25% decrease from baseline | 25 - <50% decrease from baseline | 50 - <75% decrease from baseline | ≥75% decrease from baseline |
| Platelets | WNL | <LLN - 75.0 x 10$^9$ /L <br> <LLN - 75,000/mm$^3$ | ≥50.0 - <75.0 x 10$^9$ /L <br> ≥50,000 - <75,000/mm$^3$ | ≥10.0 - <50.0 x 10$^9$ /L <br> ≥10,000 - <50,000/mm$^3$ | <10.0 x 10$^9$ /L <br> <10,000/mm$^3$ |
| For BMT studies, if specified in the protocol. | WNL | ≥50.0 - <75.0 x 10$^9$ /L <br> ≥50,000 - <75,000/mm$^3$ | ≥20.0 - <50.0 x 10$^9$ /L <br> ≥20,000 - <50,000/mm$^3$ | ≥10.0 - <20.0 x 10$^9$ /L <br> ≥10,000 - <20,000/mm$^3$ | <10.0 x 10$^9$ /L <br> <10,000/mm$^3$ |
| For leukemia studies or bone marrow infiltrative/ myelophthisic process, if specified in the protocol. | WNL | 10 - <25% decrease from baseline | 25 - <50% decrease from baseline | 50 - <75% decrease from baseline | ≥75% decrease from baseline |
| Transfusion: Platelets | none | - | - | yes | platelet transfusions and other measures required to improve platelet increment; platelet transfusion refractoriness associated with life-threatening bleeding. (e.g., HLA or cross matched platelet transfusions) |
| For BMT studies, if specified in the protocol. | none | 1 platelet transfusion in 24 hours | 2 platelet transfusions in 24 hours | ≥3 platelet transfusions in 24 hours | platelet transfusions and other measures required to improve platelet increment; platelet transfusion refractoriness associated with life-threatening bleeding. (e.g., HLA or cross matched platelet transfusions) |
| Also consider Platelets. | | | | | |

| Adverse Event | Grade 0 | 1 | 2 | 3 | 4 |
|---|---|---|---|---|---|
| Transfusion: pRBCs | none | - | - | yes | - |
| For BMT studies, if specified in the protocol. | none | ≤2 u pRBC in 24 hours elective or planned | 3 u pRBC in 24 hours elective or planned | ≥4 u pRBC in 24 hours | hemorrhage or hemolysis associated with life-threatening anemia; medical intervention required to improve hemoglobin |
| *For pediatric BMT studies, if specified in the protocol.* | *none* | *≤15mL/kg in 24 hours elective or planned* | *>15 - ≤30mL/kg in 24 hours elective or planned* | *>30mL/kg in 24 hours* | *hemorrhage or hemolysis associated with life-threatening anemia; medical intervention required to improve hemoglobin* |
| Also consider Hemoglobin. | | | | | |
| Blood/Bone Marrow - Other (Specify, _____ ) | none | mild | moderate | severe | life-threatening or disabling |

### CARDIOVASCULAR (ARRHYTHMIA)

| Adverse Event | 0 | 1 | 2 | 3 | 4 |
|---|---|---|---|---|---|
| Conduction abnormality/ Atrioventricular heart block | none | asymptomatic, not requiring treatment (e.g., Mobitz type I second-degree AV block, Wenckebach) | symptomatic, but not requiring treatment | symptomatic and requiring treatment (e.g., Mobitz type II second-degree AV block, third-degree AV block) | life-threatening (e.g., arrhythmia associated with CHF, hypotension, syncope, shock) |
| Nodal/junctional arrhythmia/dysrhythmia | none | asymptomatic, not requiring treatment | symptomatic, but not requiring treatment | symptomatic and requiring treatment | life-threatening (e.g., arrhythmia associated with CHF, hypotension, syncope, shock) |
| Palpitations | none | present | - | - | - |
| Note: Grade palpitations <u>only</u> in the absence of a documented arrhythmia. | | | | | |
| Prolonged QTc interval (QTc >0.48 seconds) | none | asymptomatic, not requiring treatment | symptomatic, but not requiring treatment | symptomatic and requiring treatment | life-threatening (e.g., arrhythmia associated with CHF, hypotension, syncope, shock) |
| Sinus bradycardia | none | asymptomatic, not requiring treatment | symptomatic, but not requiring treatment | symptomatic and requiring treatment | life-threatening (e.g., arrhythmia associated with CHF, hypotension, syncope, shock) |
| Sinus tachycardia | none | asymptomatic, not requiring treatment | symptomatic, but not requiring treatment | symptomatic and requiring treatment of underlying cause | - |
| Supraventricular arrhythmias (SVT/atrial fibrillation/ flutter) | none | asymptomatic, not requiring treatment | symptomatic, but not requiring treatment | symptomatic and requiring treatment | life-threatening (e.g., arrhythmia associated with CHF, hypotension, syncope, shock) |
| Syncope (fainting) is graded in the NEUROLOGY category. | | | | | |
| Vasovagal episode | none | - | present without loss of consciousness | present with loss of consciousness | - |

| | Grade | | | | |
|---|---|---|---|---|---|
| **Adverse Event** | **0** | **1** | **2** | **3** | **4** |
| Ventricular arrhythmia (PVCs/bigeminy/trigeminy/ ventricular tachycardia) | none | asymptomatic, not requiring treatment | symptomatic, but not requiring treatment | symptomatic and requiring treatment | life-threatening (e.g., arrhythmia associated with CHF, hypotension, syncope, shock) |
| Cardiovascular/ Arrhythmia - Other (Specify, _____) | none | asymptomatic, not requiring treatment | symptomatic, but not requiring treatment | symptomatic, and requiring treatment of underlying cause | life-threatening (e.g., arrhythmia associated with CHF, hypotension, syncope, shock) |

## CARDIOVASCULAR (GENERAL)

| | | | | | |
|---|---|---|---|---|---|
| Acute vascular leak syndrome | absent | - | symptomatic, but not requiring fluid support | respiratory compromise or requiring fluids | life-threatening; requiring pressor support and/or ventilatory support |
| Cardiac-ischemia/infarction | none | non-specific T - wave flattening or changes | asymptomatic, ST - and T - wave changes suggesting ischemia | angina without evidence of infarction | acute myocardial infarction |
| Cardiac left ventricular function | normal | asymptomatic decline of resting ejection fraction of ≥10% but <20% of baseline value; shortening fraction ≥24% but <30% | asymptomatic but resting ejection fraction below LLN for laboratory or decline of resting ejection fraction ≥20% of baseline value; <24% shortening fraction | CHF responsive to treatment | severe or refractory CHF or requiring intubation |

CNS cerebrovascular ischemia is graded in the NEUROLOGY category.

| | | | | | |
|---|---|---|---|---|---|
| Cardiac troponin I (cTnI) | normal | - | - | levels consistent with unstable angina as defined by the manufacturer | levels consistent with myocardial infarction as defined by the manufacturer |
| Cardiac troponin T (cTnT) | normal | ≥0.03 - <0.05 ng/mL | ≥0.05 - <0.1 ng/mL | ≥0.1 - <0.2 ng/mL | ≥0.2 ng/mL |
| Edema | none | asymptomatic, not requiring therapy | symptomatic, requiring therapy | symptomatic edema limiting function and unresponsive to therapy or requiring drug discontinuation | anasarca (severe generalized edema) |
| Hypertension | none | asymptomatic, transient increase by >20 mmHg (diastolic) or to >150/100* if previously WNL; not requiring treatment | recurrent or persistent or symptomatic increase by >20 mmHg (diastolic) or to >150/100* if previously WNL; not requiring treatment | requiring therapy or more intensive therapy than previously | hypertensive crisis |

*Note: For pediatric patients, use age and sex appropriate normal values >95th percentile ULN.

| Adverse Event | Grade | | | | |
|---|---|---|---|---|---|
| | 0 | 1 | 2 | 3 | 4 |
| Hypotension | none | changes, but not requiring therapy (including transient orthostatic hypotension) | requiring brief fluid replacement or other therapy but not hospitalization; no physiologic consequences | requiring therapy and sustained medical attention, but resolves without persisting physiologic consequences | shock (associated with acidemia and impairing vital organ function due to tissue hypoperfusion) |

Also consider Syncope (fainting).

Notes: Angina or MI is graded as Cardiac-ischemia/infarction in the CARDIOVASCULAR (GENERAL) category.

*For pediatric patients, systolic BP 65 mmHg or less in infants up to 1 year old and 70 mmHg or less in children older than 1 year of age, use two successive or three measurements in 24 hours.*

| Adverse Event | 0 | 1 | 2 | 3 | 4 |
|---|---|---|---|---|---|
| Myocarditis | none | - | - | CHF responsive to treatment | severe or refractory CHF |
| Operative injury of vein/artery | none | primary suture repair for injury, but not requiring transfusion | primary suture repair for injury, requiring transfusion | vascular occlusion requiring surgery or bypass for injury | myocardial infarction; resection of organ (e.g., bowel, limb) |
| Pericardial effusion/ pericarditis | none | asymptomatic effusion, not requiring treatment | pericarditis (rub, ECG changes, and/or chest pain) | with physiologic consequences | tamponade (drainage or pericardial window required) |
| Peripheral arterial ischemia | none | - | brief episode of ischemia managed non-surgically and without permanent deficit | requiring surgical intervention | life-threatening or with permanent functional deficit (e.g., amputation) |
| Phlebitis (superficial) | none | - | present | - | - |

Notes: Injection site reaction is graded in the DERMATOLOGY/SKIN category.

Thrombosis/embolism is graded in the CARDIOVASCULAR (GENERAL) category.

Syncope (fainting) is graded in the NEUROLOGY category.

| Adverse Event | 0 | 1 | 2 | 3 | 4 |
|---|---|---|---|---|---|
| Thrombosis/embolism | none | - | deep vein thrombosis, not requiring anticoagulant | deep vein thrombosis, requiring anticoagulant therapy | embolic event including pulmonary embolism |

Vein/artery operative injury is graded as Operative injury of vein/artery in the CARDIOVASCULAR (GENERAL) category.

| Adverse Event | 0 | 1 | 2 | 3 | 4 |
|---|---|---|---|---|---|
| Visceral arterial ischemia (non-myocardial) | none | - | brief episode of ischemia managed non-surgically and without permanent deficit | requiring surgical intervention | life-threatening or with permanent functional deficit (e.g., resection of ileum) |
| Cardiovascular/ General - Other (Specify, _____) | none | mild | moderate | severe | life-threatening or disabling |

| Adverse Event | Grade | | | | |
|---|---|---|---|---|---|
| | 0 | 1 | 2 | 3 | 4 |

## COAGULATION

Note: See the HEMORRHAGE category for grading the severity of bleeding events.

| DIC (disseminated intravascular coagulation) | absent | - | - | laboratory findings present with <u>no</u> bleeding | laboratory findings <u>and</u> bleeding |

Also consider Platelets.

Note: Must have increased fibrin split products or D-dimer in order to grade as DIC.

| Fibrinogen | WNL | ≥0.75 - <1.0 x LLN | ≥0.5 - <0.75 x LLN | ≥0.25 - <0.5 x LLN | <0.25 x LLN |
| For leukemia studies or bone marrow infiltrative/ myelophthisic process, if specified in the protocol. | WNL | <20% decrease from pretreatment value or LLN | ≥20 - <40% decrease from pretreatment value or LLN | ≥40 - <70% decrease from pretreatment value or LLN | <50 mg |
| Partial thromboplastin time (PTT) | WNL | >ULN - ≤1.5 x ULN | >1.5 - ≤2 x ULN | >2 x ULN | - |

Phlebitis is graded in the CARDIOVASCULAR (GENERAL) category.

| Prothrombin time (PT) | WNL | >ULN - ≤1.5 x ULN | >1.5 - ≤2 x ULN | >2 x ULN | - |

Thrombosis/embolism is graded in the CARDIOVASCULAR (GENERAL) category.

| Thrombotic microangiopathy (e.g., thrombotic thrombocytopenic purpura/TTP or hemolytic uremic syndrome/HUS) | absent | - | - | laboratory findings present without clinical consequences | laboratory findings and clinical consequences, (e.g., CNS hemorrhage/ bleeding or thrombosis/ embolism or renal failure) requiring therapeutic intervention |
| For BMT studies, if specified in the protocol. | - | evidence of RBC destruction (schistocytosis) without clinical consequences | evidence of RBC destruction with elevated creatinine (≤3 x ULN) | evidence of RBC destruction with creatinine (>3 x ULN) not requiring dialysis | evidence of RBC destruction with renal failure requiring dialysis and/or encephalopathy |

Also consider Hemoglobin, Platelets, Creatinine.

Note: Must have microangiopathic changes on blood smear (e.g., schistocytes, helmet cells, red cell fragments).

| Coagulation - Other (Specify, _____) | none | mild | moderate | severe | life-threatening or disabling |

## CONSTITUTIONAL SYMPTOMS

| Fatigue (lethargy, malaise, asthenia) | none | increased fatigue over baseline, but not altering normal activities | moderate (e.g., decrease in performance status by 1 ECOG level <u>or</u> 20% Karnofsky or *Lansky*) <u>or</u> causing difficulty performing some activities | severe (e.g., decrease in performance status by ≥2 ECOG levels <u>or</u> 40% Karnofsky or *Lansky*) <u>or</u> loss of ability to perform some activities | bedridden or disabling |

Note: See Appendix III for performance status scales.

| Adverse Event | Grade | | | | |
|---|---|---|---|---|---|
| | 0 | 1 | 2 | 3 | 4 |
| Fever (in the absence of neutropenia, where neutropenia is defined as AGC <1.0 x $10^9$/L) | none | 38.0 - 39.0°C (100.4 - 102.2°F) | 39.1 - 40.0°C (102.3 - 104.0°F) | >40.0°C (>104.0°F) for <24hrs | >40.0°C (>104.0°F) for >24hrs |
| Also consider Allergic reaction/hypersensitivity. | | | | | |
| Note: The temperature measurements listed above are oral or tympanic. | | | | | |
| Hot flashes/flushes are graded in the ENDOCRINE category. | | | | | |
| Rigors, chills | none | mild, requiring symptomatic treatment (e.g., blanket) or non-narcotic medication | severe and/or prolonged, requiring narcotic medication | not responsive to narcotic medication | - |
| Sweating (diaphoresis) | normal | mild and occasional | frequent or drenching | - | - |
| Weight gain | <5% | 5 - <10% | 10 - <20% | ≥20% | - |
| Also consider Ascites, Edema, Pleural effusion (non-malignant). | | | | | |
| Weight gain associated with Veno-Occlusive Disease (VOD) for BMT studies, if specified in the protocol. | <2% | ≥2 - <5% | ≥5 - <10% | ≥10% or as ascites | ≥10% or fluid retention resulting in pulmonary failure |
| Also consider Ascites, Edema, Pleural effusion (non-malignant). | | | | | |
| Weight loss | <5% | 5 - <10% | 10 - <20% | ≥20% | - |
| Also consider Vomiting, Dehydration, Diarrhea. | | | | | |
| Constitutional Symptoms - Other (Specify, _____) | none | mild | moderate | severe | life-threatening or disabling |

## DERMATOLOGY/SKIN

| Adverse Event | 0 | 1 | 2 | 3 | 4 |
|---|---|---|---|---|---|
| Alopecia | normal | mild hair loss | pronounced hair loss | - | - |
| Bruising (in absence of grade 3 or 4 thrombocytopenia) | none | localized or in dependent area | generalized | - | - |
| Note: Bruising resulting from grade 3 or 4 thrombocytopenia is graded as Petechiae/purpura and Hemorrhage/bleeding with grade 3 or 4 thrombocytopenia in the HEMORRHAGE category, not in the DERMATOLOGY/SKIN category. | | | | | |
| Dry skin | normal | controlled with emollients | not controlled with emollients | - | - |
| Erythema multiforme (e.g., Stevens-Johnson syndrome, toxic epidermal necrolysis) | absent | - | scattered, but not generalized eruption | severe or requiring IV fluids (e.g., generalized rash or painful stomatitis) | life-threatening (e.g., exfoliative or ulcerating dermatitis or requiring enteral or parenteral nutritional support) |
| Flushing | absent | present | - | - | - |
| Hand-foot skin reaction | none | skin changes or dermatitis without pain (e.g., erythema, peeling) | skin changes with pain, not interfering with function | skin changes with pain, interfering with function | - |
| Injection site reaction | none | pain or itching or erythema | pain or swelling, with inflammation or phlebitis | ulceration or necrosis that is severe or prolonged, or requiring surgery | - |

| Adverse Event | Grade | | | | |
|---|---|---|---|---|---|
| | 0 | 1 | 2 | 3 | 4 |
| Nail changes | normal | discoloration or ridging (koilonychia) or pitting | partial or complete loss of nail(s) or pain in nailbeds | - | - |
| Petechiae is graded in the HEMORRHAGE category. | | | | | |
| Photosensitivity | none | painless erythema | painful erythema | erythema with desquamation | - |
| Pigmentation changes (e.g., vitiligo) | none | localized pigmentation changes | generalized pigmentation changes | - | - |
| Pruritus | none | mild or localized, relieved spontaneously or by local measures | intense or widespread, relieved spontaneously or by systemic measures | intense or widespread and poorly controlled despite treatment | - |
| Purpura is graded in the HEMORRHAGE category. | | | | | |
| Radiation dermatitis | none | faint erythema or dry desquamation | moderate to brisk erythema or a patchy moist desquamation, mostly confined to skin folds and creases; moderate edema | confluent moist desquamation ≥1.5 cm diameter and not confined to skin folds; pitting edema | skin necrosis or ulceration of full thickness dermis; may include bleeding not induced by minor trauma or abrasion |
| Note: Pain associated with radiation dermatitis is graded separately in the PAIN category as Pain due to radiation. | | | | | |
| Radiation recall reaction (reaction following chemotherapy in the absence of additional radiation therapy that occurs in a previous radiation port) | none | faint erythema or dry desquamation | moderate to brisk erythema or a patchy moist desquamation, mostly confined to skin folds and creases; moderate edema | confluent moist desquamation ≥1.5 cm diameter and not confined to skin folds; pitting edema | skin necrosis or ulceration of full thickness dermis; may include bleeding not induced by minor trauma or abrasion |
| Rash/desquamation | none | macular or papular eruption or erythema without associated symptoms | macular or papular eruption or erythema with pruritus or other associated symptoms covering <50% of body surface or localized desquamation or other lesions covering <50% of body surface area | symptomatic generalized erythroderma or macular, papular or vesicular eruption or desquamation covering ≥50% of body surface area | generalized exfoliative dermatitis or ulcerative dermatitis |
| Also consider Allergic reaction/hypersensitivity. | | | | | |
| Note:  Stevens-Johnson syndrome is graded separately as Erythema multiforme in the DERMATOLOGY/SKIN category. | | | | | |
| Rash/dermatitis associated with high-dose chemotherapy or BMT studies. | none | faint erythema or dry desquamation | moderate to brisk erythema or a patchy moist desquamation, mostly confined to skin folds and creases; moderate edema | confluent moist desquamation ≥1.5 cm diameter and not confined to skin folds; pitting edema | skin necrosis or ulceration of full thickness dermis; may include spontaneous bleeding not induced by minor trauma or abrasion |
| Rash/desquamation associated with graft versus host disease (GVHD) for BMT studies, if specified in the protocol. | None | macular or papular eruption or erythema covering <25% of body surface area without associated symptoms | macular or papular eruption or erythema with pruritus or other associated symptoms covering ≥25 - <50% of body surface or localized desquamation or other lesions covering ≥25 - <50% of body surface area | symptomatic generalized erythroderma or symptomatic macular, papular or vesicular eruption, with bullous formation, or desquamation covering ≥50% of body surface area | generalized exfoliative dermatitis or ulcerative dermatitis or bullous formation |
| Also consider Allergic reaction/hypersensitivity. | | | | | |
| Note:  Stevens-Johnson syndrome is graded separately as Erythema multiforme in the DERMATOLOGY/SKIN category. | | | | | |

| | Grade | | | | |
|---|---|---|---|---|---|
| **Adverse Event** | **0** | **1** | **2** | **3** | **4** |
| Urticaria (hives, welts, wheals) | none | requiring no medication | requiring PO or topical treatment or IV medication or steroids for <24 hours | requiring IV medication or steroids for ≥24 hours | - |
| Wound-infectious | none | cellulitis | superficial infection | infection requiring IV antibiotics | necrotizing fasciitis |
| Wound-non-infectious | none | incisional separation | incisional hernia | fascial disruption without evisceration | fascial disruption with evisceration |
| Dermatology/Skin - Other (Specify, _____) | none | mild | moderate | severe | life-threatening or disabling |

## ENDOCRINE

| | | | | | |
|---|---|---|---|---|---|
| Cushingoid appearance (e.g., moon face, buffalo hump, centripetal obesity, cutaneous striae) | absent | - | present | - | - |

Also consider Hyperglycemia, Hypokalemia.

| | | | | | |
|---|---|---|---|---|---|
| Feminization of male | absent | - | - | present | - |
| Gynecomastia | none | mild | pronounced or painful | pronounced or painful and requiring surgery | - |
| Hot flashes/flushes | none | mild or no more than 1 per day | moderate and greater than 1 per day | - | - |
| Hypothyroidism | absent | asymptomatic, TSH elevated, no therapy given | symptomatic or thyroid replacement treatment given | patient hospitalized for manifestations of hypothyroidism | myxedema coma |
| Masculinization of female | absent | - | - | present | - |
| SIADH (syndrome of inappropriate antidiuretic hormone) | absent | - | - | present | - |
| Endocrine - Other (Specify, _____) | none | mild | moderate | severe | life-threatening or disabling |

## GASTROINTESTINAL

Amylase is graded in the METABOLIC/LABORATORY category.

| | | | | | |
|---|---|---|---|---|---|
| Anorexia | none | loss of appetite | oral intake significantly decreased | requiring IV fluids | requiring feeding tube or parenteral nutrition |
| Ascites (non-malignant) | none | asymptomatic | symptomatic, requiring diuretics | symptomatic, requiring therapeutic paracentesis | life-threatening physiologic consequences |
| Colitis | none | - | abdominal pain with mucus and/or blood in stool | abdominal pain, fever, change in bowel habits with ileus or peritoneal signs, and radiographic or biopsy documentation | perforation or requiring surgery or toxic megacolon |

Also consider Hemorrhage/bleeding with grade 3 or 4 thrombocytopenia, Hemorrhage/bleeding without grade 3 or 4 thrombocytopenia, Melena/GI bleeding, Rectal bleeding/hematochezia, Hypotension.

| | | | | | |
|---|---|---|---|---|---|
| Constipation | none | requiring stool softener or dietary modification | requiring laxatives | obstipation requiring manual evacuation or enema | obstruction or toxic megacolon |

| Adverse Event | Grade | | | | |
|---|---|---|---|---|---|
| | 0 | 1 | 2 | 3 | 4 |
| Dehydration | none | dry mucous membranes and/or diminished skin turgor | requiring IV fluid replacement (brief) | requiring IV fluid replacement (sustained) | physiologic consequences requiring intensive care; hemodynamic collapse |
| Also consider Diarrhea, Vomiting, Stomatitis/pharyngitis (oral/pharyngeal mucositis), Hypotension. | | | | | |
| Diarrhea patients without colostomy: | none | increase of <4 stools/day over pre-treatment | increase of 4-6 stools/day, or nocturnal stools | increase of ≥7 stools/day or incontinence; or need for parenteral support for dehydration | physiologic consequences requiring intensive care; or hemodynamic collapse |
| patients with a colostomy: | none | mild increase in loose, watery colostomy output compared with pretreatment | moderate increase in loose, watery colostomy output compared with pretreatment, but not interfering with normal activity | severe increase in loose, watery colostomy output compared with pretreatment, interfering with normal activity | physiologic consequences, requiring intensive care; or hemodynamic collapse |
| Diarrhea associated with graft versus host disease (GVHD) for BMT studies, if specified in the protocol. | None | >500 - ≤1000mL of diarrhea/day | >1000 - ≤1500mL of diarrhea/day | >1500mL of diarrhea/day | severe abdominal pain with or without ileus |
| *For pediatric BMT studies, if specified in the protocol.* | | *>5 - ≤10 mL/kg of diarrhea/day* | *>10 - ≤15 mL/kg of diarrhea/day* | *>15 mL/kg of diarrhea/day* | - |
| Also consider Hemorrhage/bleeding with grade 3 or 4 thrombocytopenia, Hemorrhage/bleeding without grade 3 or 4 thrombocytopenia, Pain, Dehydration, Hypotension. | | | | | |
| Duodenal ulcer (requires radiographic or endoscopic documentation) | none | - | requiring medical management or non-surgical treatment | uncontrolled by outpatient medical management; requiring hospitalization | perforation or bleeding, requiring emergency surgery |
| Dyspepsia/heartburn | none | mild | moderate | severe | - |
| Dysphagia, esophagitis, odynophagia (painful swallowing) | none | mild dysphagia, but can eat regular diet | dysphagia, requiring predominantly pureed, soft, or liquid diet | dysphagia, requiring IV hydration | complete obstruction (cannot swallow saliva) requiring enteral or parenteral nutritional support, or perforation |
| Note: If the adverse event is radiation-related, grade <u>either</u> under Dysphagia-esophageal related to radiation <u>or</u> Dysphagia-pharyngeal related to radiation. | | | | | |
| Dysphagia-<u>esophageal</u> related to radiation | none | mild dysphagia, but can eat regular diet | dysphagia, requiring predominantly pureed, soft, or liquid diet | Dysphagia, requiring feeding tube, IV hydration or hyperalimentation | complete obstruction (cannot swallow saliva); ulceration with bleeding not induced by minor trauma or abrasion or perforation |
| Also consider Pain due to radiation, Mucositis due to radiation. | | | | | |
| Note: Fistula is graded separately as Fistula-esophageal. | | | | | |
| Dysphagia-<u>pharyngeal</u> related to radiation | none | mild dysphagia, but can eat regular diet | dysphagia, requiring predominantly pureed, soft, or liquid diet | dysphagia, requiring feeding tube, IV hydration or hyperalimentation | complete obstruction (cannot swallow saliva); ulceration with bleeding not induced by minor trauma or abrasion or perforation |
| Also consider Pain due to radiation, Mucositis due to radiation. | | | | | |
| Note: Fistula is graded separately as Fistula-pharyngeal. | | | | | |
| Fistula-esophageal | none | - | - | present | requiring surgery |
| Fistula-intestinal | none | - | - | present | requiring surgery |

| Adverse Event | Grade | | | | |
|---|---|---|---|---|---|
| | 0 | 1 | 2 | 3 | 4 |
| Fistula-pharyngeal | none | - | - | present | requiring surgery |
| Fistula-rectal/anal | none | - | - | present | requiring surgery |
| Flatulence | none | mild | moderate | - | - |
| Gastric ulcer (requires radiographic or endoscopic documentation) | none | - | requiring medical management or non-surgical treatment | bleeding without perforation, uncontrolled by outpatient medical management; requiring hospitalization or surgery | perforation or bleeding, requiring emergency surgery |

Also consider Hemorrhage/bleeding with grade 3 or 4 thrombocytopenia, Hemorrhage/bleeding without grade 3 or 4 thrombocytopenia.

| Gastritis | none | - | requiring medical management or non-surgical treatment | uncontrolled by out-patient medical management; requiring hospitalization or surgery | life-threatening bleeding, requiring emergency surgery |
|---|---|---|---|---|---|

Also consider Hemorrhage/bleeding with grade 3 or 4 thrombocytopenia, Hemorrhage/bleeding without grade 3 or 4 thrombocytopenia.

Hematemesis is graded in the HEMORRHAGE category.

Hematochezia is graded in the HEMORRHAGE category as Rectal bleeding/hematochezia.

| Ileus (or neuroconstipation) | none | - | intermittent, not requiring intervention | requiring non-surgical intervention | requiring surgery |
|---|---|---|---|---|---|
| Mouth dryness | normal | mild | moderate | - | - |

Mucositis

Notes: Mucositis not due to radiation is graded in the GASTROINTESTINAL category for specific sites: Colitis, Esophagitis, Gastritis, Stomatitis/pharyngitis (oral/pharyngeal mucositis), and Typhlitis; or the RENAL/GENITOURINARY category for Vaginitis.

Radiation-related mucositis is graded as Mucositis due to radiation.

| Mucositis due to radiation | none | erythema of the mucosa | patchy pseudomembranous reaction (patches generally ≤1.5 cm in diameter and non-contiguous) | confluent pseudomembranous reaction (contiguous patches generally >1.5 cm in diameter) | necrosis or deep ulceration; may include bleeding not induced by minor trauma or abrasion |
|---|---|---|---|---|---|

Also consider Pain due to radiation.

Notes: Grade radiation mucositis of the larynx here.

Dysphagia related to radiation is also graded as either Dysphagia-esophageal related to radiation or Dysphagia-pharyngeal related to radiation, depending on the site of treatment.

| Nausea | none | able to eat | oral intake significantly decreased | no significant intake, requiring IV fluids | - |
|---|---|---|---|---|---|
| Pancreatitis | none | - | - | abdominal pain with pancreatic enzyme elevation | complicated by shock (acute circulatory failure) |

Also consider Hypotension.

Note: Amylase is graded in the METABOLIC/LABORATORY category.

Pharyngitis is graded in the GASTROINTESTINAL category as Stomatitis/pharyngitis (oral/pharyngeal mucositis).

| Adverse Event | Grade 0 | 1 | 2 | 3 | 4 |
|---|---|---|---|---|---|
| Proctitis | none | increased stool frequency, occasional blood-streaked stools or rectal discomfort (including hemorrhoids) not requiring medication | increased stool frequency, bleeding, mucus discharge, or rectal discomfort requiring medication; anal fissure | increased stool frequency/diarrhea requiring parenteral support; rectal bleeding requiring transfusion; or persistent mucus discharge, necessitating pads | perforation, bleeding or necrosis or other life-threatening complication requiring surgical intervention (e.g., colostomy) |

Also consider Hemorrhage/bleeding with grade 3 or 4 thrombocytopenia, Hemorrhage/bleeding without grade 3 or 4 thrombocytopenia, Pain due to radiation.

Notes: Fistula is graded separately as Fistula-rectal/anal.

Proctitis occurring more than 90 days after the start of radiation therapy is graded in the RTOG/EORTC Late Radiation Morbidity Scoring Scheme. (See Appendix IV)

| Adverse Event | 0 | 1 | 2 | 3 | 4 |
|---|---|---|---|---|---|
| Salivary gland changes | none | slightly thickened saliva; may have slightly altered taste (e.g., metallic); additional fluids may be required | thick, ropy, sticky saliva; markedly altered taste; alteration in diet required | - | acute salivary gland necrosis |
| Sense of smell | normal | slightly altered | markedly altered | - | - |
| Stomatitis/pharyngitis (oral/pharyngeal mucositis) | none | painless ulcers, erythema, or mild soreness in the absence of lesions | painful erythema, edema, or ulcers, but can eat or swallow | painful erythema, edema, or ulcers requiring IV hydration | severe ulceration or requires parenteral or enteral nutritional support or prophylactic intubation |
| For BMT studies, if specified in the protocol. | none | painless ulcers, erythema, or mild soreness in the absence of lesions | painful erythema, edema or ulcers but can swallow | painful erythema, edema, or ulcers preventing swallowing or requiring hydration or parenteral (or enteral) nutritional support | severe ulceration requiring prophylactic intubation or resulting in documented aspiration pneumonia |

Note: Radiation-related mucositis is graded as Mucositis due to radiation.

| Adverse Event | 0 | 1 | 2 | 3 | 4 |
|---|---|---|---|---|---|
| Taste disturbance (dysgeusia) | normal | slightly altered | markedly altered | - | - |
| Typhlitis (inflammation of the cecum) | none | - | - | abdominal pain, diarrhea, fever, and radiographic or biopsy documentation | perforation, bleeding or necrosis or other life-threatening complication requiring surgical intervention (e.g., colostomy) |

Also consider Hemorrhage/bleeding with grade 3 or 4 thrombocytopenia, Hemorrhage/bleeding without grade 3 or 4 thrombocytopenia, Hypotension, Febrile neutropenia.

| Adverse Event | 0 | 1 | 2 | 3 | 4 |
|---|---|---|---|---|---|
| Vomiting | none | 1 episode in 24 hours over pretreatment | 2-5 episodes in 24 hours over pretreatment | ≥6 episodes in 24 hours over pretreatment; or need for IV fluids | requiring parenteral nutrition; or physiologic consequences requiring intensive care; hemodynamic collapse |

Also consider Dehydration.

Weight gain is graded in the CONSTITUTIONAL SYMPTOMS category.

Weight loss is graded in the CONSTITUTIONAL SYMPTOMS category.

| Adverse Event | 0 | 1 | 2 | 3 | 4 |
|---|---|---|---|---|---|
| Gastrointestinal - Other (Specify, _____) | none | mild | moderate | severe | life-threatening or disabling |

| Adverse Event | Grade | | | | |
|---|---|---|---|---|---|
| | 0 | 1 | 2 | 3 | 4 |

## HEMORRHAGE

Notes: Transfusion in this section refers to pRBC infusion.

For any bleeding with grade 3 or 4 platelets (<50,000), always grade Hemorrhage/bleeding with grade 3 or 4 thrombocytopenia. Also consider Platelets, Transfusion: pRBCs, and Transfusion: platelets in addition to grading severity by grading the site or type of bleeding.

If the site or type of Hemorrhage/bleeding is listed, also use the grading that incorporates the site of bleeding: CNS Hemorrhage/bleeding, Hematuria, Hematemesis, Hemoptysis, Hemorrhage/bleeding with surgery, Melena/lower GI bleeding, Petechiae/purpura (Hemorrhage/bleeding into skin), Rectal bleeding/hematochezia, Vaginal bleeding.

If the platelet count is ≥50,000 and the site or type of bleeding is listed, grade the specific site. If the site or type is not listed and the platelet count is ≥50,000, grade Hemorrhage/bleeding without grade 3 or 4 thrombocytopenia and specify the site or type in the OTHER category.

| Adverse Event | 0 | 1 | 2 | 3 | 4 |
|---|---|---|---|---|---|
| Hemorrhage/bleeding with grade 3 or 4 thrombocytopenia | none | mild without transfusion | | requiring transfusion | catastrophic bleeding, requiring major non-elective intervention |

Also consider Platelets, Hemoglobin, Transfusion: platelets, Transfusion: pRBCs, site or type of bleeding. If the site is not listed, grade as Hemorrhage-Other (Specify site, _____).

Note: This adverse event must be graded for any bleeding with grade 3 or 4 thrombocytopenia.

| Adverse Event | 0 | 1 | 2 | 3 | 4 |
|---|---|---|---|---|---|
| Hemorrhage/bleeding without grade 3 or 4 thrombocytopenia | none | mild without transfusion | | requiring transfusion | catastrophic bleeding requiring major non-elective intervention |

Also consider Platelets, Hemoglobin, Transfusion: platelets, Transfusion: pRBCs, Hemorrhage - Other (Specify site, _____).

Note: Bleeding in the absence of grade 3 or 4 thrombocytopenia is graded here only if the specific site or type of bleeding is not listed elsewhere in the HEMORRHAGE category. Also grade as Other in the HEMORRHAGE category.

| Adverse Event | 0 | 1 | 2 | 3 | 4 |
|---|---|---|---|---|---|
| CNS hemorrhage/bleeding | none | - | - | bleeding noted on CT or other scan with no clinical consequences | hemorrhagic stroke or hemorrhagic vascular event (CVA) with neurologic signs and symptoms |
| Epistaxis | none | mild without transfusion | - | requiring transfusion | catastrophic bleeding, requiring major non-elective intervention |
| Hematemesis | none | mild without transfusion | - | requiring transfusion | catastrophic bleeding, requiring major non-elective intervention |
| Hematuria (in the absence of vaginal bleeding) | none | microscopic only | intermittent gross bleeding, no clots | persistent gross bleeding or clots; may require catheterization or instrumentation, or transfusion | open surgery or necrosis or deep bladder ulceration |
| Hemoptysis | none | mild without transfusion | - | requiring transfusion | catastrophic bleeding, requiring major non-elective intervention |
| Hemorrhage/bleeding associated with surgery | none | mild without transfusion | - | requiring transfusion | catastrophic bleeding, requiring major non-elective intervention |

Note: Expected blood loss at the time of surgery is not graded as an adverse event.

| Adverse Event | 0 | 1 | 2 | 3 | 4 |
|---|---|---|---|---|---|
| Melena/GI bleeding | none | mild without transfusion | - | requiring transfusion | catastrophic bleeding, requiring major non-elective intervention |

| Adverse Event | Grade | | | | |
|---|---|---|---|---|---|
| | 0 | 1 | 2 | 3 | 4 |
| Petechiae/purpura (hemorrhage/bleeding into skin or mucosa) | none | rare petechiae of skin | petechiae or purpura in dependent areas of skin | generalized petechiae or purpura of skin or petechiae of any mucosal site | - |
| Rectal bleeding/ hematochezia | none | mild without transfusion or medication | persistent, requiring medication (e.g., steroid suppositories) and/or break from radiation treatment | requiring transfusion | catastrophic bleeding, requiring major non-elective intervention |
| Vaginal bleeding | none | spotting, requiring <2 pads per day | requiring ≥2 pads per day, but not requiring transfusion | requiring transfusion | catastrophic bleeding, requiring major non-elective intervention |
| Hemorrhage - Other (Specify site, _____) | none | mild without transfusion | - | requiring transfusion | catastrophic bleeding, requiring major non-elective intervention |

## HEPATIC

| Adverse Event | 0 | 1 | 2 | 3 | 4 |
|---|---|---|---|---|---|
| Alkaline phosphatase | WNL | >ULN - 2.5 x ULN | >2.5 - 5.0 x ULN | >5.0 - 20.0 x ULN | >20.0 x ULN |
| Bilirubin | WNL | >ULN - 1.5 x ULN | >1.5 - 3.0 x ULN | >3.0 - 10.0 x ULN | >10.0 x ULN |
| Bilirubin associated with graft versus host disease (GVHD) for BMT studies, if specified in the protocol. | normal | ≥2 - <3 mg/100 mL | ≥3 - <6 mg/100 mL | ≥6 - <15 mg/100 mL | ≥15 mg/100 mL |
| GGT (γ - Glutamyl transpeptidase) | WNL | >ULN - 2.5 x ULN | >2.5 - 5.0 x ULN | >5.0 - 20.0 x ULN | >20.0 x ULN |
| Hepatic enlargement | absent | - | - | present | - |
| Note: Grade Hepatic enlargement only for treatment related adverse event including Veno-Occlusive Disease. | | | | | |
| Hypoalbuminemia | WNL | <LLN - 3 g/dL | ≥2 - <3 g/dL | <2 g/dL | - |
| Liver dysfunction/ failure (clinical) | normal | - | - | asterixis | encephalopathy or coma |
| Portal vein flow | normal | - | decreased portal vein flow | reversal/retrograde portal vein flow | - |
| SGOT (AST) (serum glutamic oxaloacetic transaminase) | WNL | >ULN - 2.5 x ULN | >2.5 - 5.0 x ULN | >5.0 - 20.0 x ULN | >20.0 x ULN |
| SGPT (ALT) (serum glutamic pyruvic transaminase) | WNL | >ULN - 2.5 x ULN | >2.5 - 5.0 x ULN | >5.0 - 20.0 x ULN | >20.0 x ULN |
| Hepatic - Other (Specify, _____) | none | mild | moderate | severe | life-threatening or disabling |

## INFECTION/FEBRILE NEUTROPENIA

| Adverse Event | 0 | 1 | 2 | 3 | 4 |
|---|---|---|---|---|---|
| Catheter-related infection | none | mild, no active treatment | moderate, localized infection, requiring local or oral treatment | severe, systemic infection, requiring IV antibiotic or antifungal treatment or hospitalization | life-threatening sepsis (e.g., septic shock) |

| | | | Grade | | |
|---|---|---|---|---|---|
| **Adverse Event** | **0** | **1** | **2** | **3** | **4** |
| Febrile neutropenia (fever of unknown origin without clinically or microbiologically documented infection)<br><br>(ANC <1.0 x $10^9$/L, fever ≥38.5°C)<br><br>Also consider Neutrophils.<br><br>Note: Hypothermia instead of fever may be associated with neutropenia and is graded here. | none | - | - | Present | Life-threatening sepsis (e.g., septic shock) |
| Infection (documented clinically or microbiologically) with grade 3 or 4 neutropenia<br><br>(ANC <1.0 x $10^9$/L)<br><br>Also consider Neutrophils.<br><br>Notes: Hypothermia instead of fever may be associated with neutropenia and is graded here.<br><br>In the absence of documented infection grade 3 or 4 neutropenia with fever is graded as Febrile neutropenia. | none | - | - | present | life-threatening sepsis (e.g., septic shock) |
| Infection with unknown ANC<br><br>Note: This adverse event criterion is used in the rare case when ANC is unknown. | none | - | - | present | life-threatening sepsis (e.g., septic shock) |
| Infection without neutropenia<br><br>Also consider Neutrophils. | none | mild, no active treatment | moderate, localized infection, requiring local or oral treatment | severe, systemic infection, requiring IV antibiotic or antifungal treatment, or hospitalization | life-threatening sepsis (e.g., septic shock) |
| Wound-infectious is graded in the DERMATOLOGY/SKIN category. | | | | | |
| Infection/Febrile Neutropenia - Other (Specify, _____) | none | mild | moderate | severe | life-threatening or disabling |

## LYMPHATICS

| | | | | | |
|---|---|---|---|---|---|
| Lymphatics | normal | mild lymphedema | moderate lymphedema requiring compression; lymphocyst | severe lymphedema limiting function; lymphocyst requiring surgery | severe lymphedema limiting function with ulceration |
| Lymphatics - Other (Specify, _____) | none | mild | moderate | severe | life-threatening or disabling |

## METABOLIC/LABORATORY

| | | | | | |
|---|---|---|---|---|---|
| Acidosis (metabolic or respiratory) | normal | pH <normal, but ≥7.3 | - | pH <7.3 | pH <7.3 with life-threatening physiologic consequences |
| Alkalosis (metabolic or respiratory) | normal | pH >normal, but ≤7.5 | - | pH >7.5 | pH >7.5 with life-threatening physiologic consequences |
| Amylase | WNL | >ULN - 1.5 x ULN | >1.5 - 2.0 x ULN | >2.0 - 5.0 x ULN | >5.0 x ULN |
| Bicarbonate | WNL | <LLN - 16 mEq/dL | 11 - 15 mEq/dL | 8 - 10 mEq/dL | <8 mEq/dL |

| Adverse Event | Grade | | | | |
|---|---|---|---|---|---|
| | 0 | 1 | 2 | 3 | 4 |
| CPK (creatine phosphokinase) | WNL | >ULN - 2.5 x ULN | >2.5 - 5 x ULN | >5 - 10 x ULN | >10 x ULN |
| Hypercalcemia | WNL | >ULN - 11.5 mg/dL<br>>ULN - 2.9 mmol/L | >11.5 - 12.5 mg/dL<br>>2.9 - 3.1 mmol/L | >12.5 - 13.5 mg/dL<br>>3.1 - 3.4 mmol/L | >13.5 mg/dL<br>>3.4 mmol/L |
| Hypercholesterolemia | WNL | >ULN - 300 mg/dL<br>>ULN - 7.75 mmol/L | >300 - 400 mg/dL<br>>7.75 - 10.34 mmol/L | >400 - 500 mg/dL<br>>10.34 - 12.92 mmol/L | >500 mg/dL<br>>12.92 mmol/L |
| Hyperglycemia | WNL | >ULN - 160 mg/dL<br>>ULN - 8.9 mmol/L | >160 - 250 mg/dL<br>>8.9 - 13.9 mmol/L | >250 - 500 mg/dL<br>>13.9 - 27.8 mmol/L | >500 mg/dL<br>>27.8 mmol/L or acidosis |
| Hyperkalemia | WNL | >ULN - 5.5 mmol/L | >5.5 - 6.0 mmol/L | >6.0 - 7.0 mmol/L | >7.0 mmol/L |
| Hypermagnesemia | WNL | >ULN - 3.0 mg/dL<br>>ULN - 1.23 mmol/L | - | >3.0 - 8.0 mg/dL<br>>1.23 - 3.30 mmol/L | >8.0 mg/dL<br>>3.30 mmol/L |
| Hypernatremia | WNL | >ULN - 150 mmol/L | >150 - 155 mmol/L | >155 - 160 mmol/L | >160 mmol/L |
| Hypertriglyceridemia | WNL | >ULN - 2.5 x ULN | >2.5 - 5.0 x ULN | >5.0 - 10 x ULN | >10 x ULN |
| Hyperuricemia | WNL | >ULN - ≤10 mg/dL<br>≤0.59 mmol/L without physiologic consequences | - | >ULN - ≤10 mg/dL<br>≤0.59 mmol/L with physiologic consequences | >10 mg/dL<br>>0.59 mmol/L |

Also consider Tumor lysis syndrome, Renal failure, Creatinine, Hyperkalemia.

| Adverse Event | 0 | 1 | 2 | 3 | 4 |
|---|---|---|---|---|---|
| Hypocalcemia | WNL | <LLN - 8.0 mg/dL<br><LLN - 2.0 mmol/L | 7.0 - <8.0 mg/dL<br>1.75 - <2.0 mmol/L | 6.0 - <7.0 mg/dL<br>1.5 - <1.75 mmol/L | <6.0 mg/dL<br><1.5 mmol/L |
| Hypoglycemia | WNL | <LLN - 55 mg/dL<br><LLN - 3.0 mmol/L | 40 - <55 mg/dL<br>2.2 - <3.0 mmol/L | 30 - <40 mg/dL<br>1.7 - <2.2 mmol/L | <30 mg/dL<br><1.7 mmol/L |
| Hypokalemia | WNL | <LLN - 3.0 mmol/L | - | 2.5 - <3.0 mmol/L | <2.5 mmol/L |
| Hypomagnesemia | WNL | <LLN - 1.2 mg/dL<br><LLN - 0.5 mmol/L | 0.9 - <1.2 mg/dL<br>0.4 - <0.5 mmol/L | 0.7 - <0.9 mg/dL<br>0.3 - <0.4 mmol/L | <0.7 mg/dL<br><0.3 mmol/L |
| Hyponatremia | WNL | <LLN - 130 mmol/L | - | 120 - <130 mmol/L | <120 mmol/L |
| Hypophosphatemia | WNL | <LLN -2.5 mg/dL<br><LLN - 0.8 mmol/L | ≥2.0 - <2.5 mg/dL<br>≥0.6 - <0.8 mmol/L | ≥1.0 - <2.0 mg/dL<br>≥0.3 - <0.6 mmol/L | <1.0 mg/dL<br><0.3 mmol/L |

Hypothyroidism is graded in the ENDOCRINE category.

| Adverse Event | 0 | 1 | 2 | 3 | 4 |
|---|---|---|---|---|---|
| Lipase | WNL | >ULN - 1.5 x ULN | >1.5 - 2.0 x ULN | >2.0 - 5.0 x ULN | >5.0 x ULN |
| Metabolic/Laboratory - Other (Specify, _____) | none | mild | moderate | severe | life-threatening or disabling |

## MUSCULOSKELETAL

Arthralgia is graded in the PAIN category.

| Adverse Event | 0 | 1 | 2 | 3 | 4 |
|---|---|---|---|---|---|
| Arthritis | none | mild pain with inflammation, erythema or joint swelling but not interfering with function | moderate pain with inflammation, erythema, or joint swelling interfering with function, but not interfering with activities of daily living | severe pain with inflammation, erythema, or joint swelling and interfering with activities of daily living | disabling |

| Adverse Event | Grade | | | | |
|---|---|---|---|---|---|
| | **0** | **1** | **2** | **3** | **4** |
| Muscle weakness (not due to neuropathy) | normal | asymptomatic with weakness on physical exam | symptomatic and interfering with function, but not interfering with activities of daily living | symptomatic and interfering with activities of daily living | bedridden or disabling |
| Myalgia [tenderness or pain in muscles] is graded in the PAIN category. | | | | | |
| Myositis (inflammation/damage of muscle) | none | mild pain, not interfering with function | pain interfering with function, but not interfering with activities of daily living | pain interfering with function and interfering with activities of daily living | bedridden or disabling |
| Also consider CPK. | | | | | |
| Note: Myositis implies muscle damage (i.e., elevated CPK). | | | | | |
| Osteonecrosis (avascular necrosis) | none | asymptomatic and detected by imaging only | symptomatic and interfering with function, but not interfering with activities of daily living | symptomatic and interfering with activities of daily living | symptomatic; or disabling |
| Musculoskeletal - Other (Specify, _____) | none | mild | moderate | severe | life-threatening or disabling |

## NEUROLOGY

| Adverse Event | Grade | | | | |
|---|---|---|---|---|---|
| | **0** | **1** | **2** | **3** | **4** |
| Aphasia, receptive and/or expressive, is graded under Speech impairment in the NEUROLOGY category. | | | | | |
| Arachnoiditis/meningismus/ radiculitis | absent | mild pain not interfering with function | moderate pain interfering with function, but not interfering with activities of daily living | severe pain interfering with activities of daily living | unable to function or perform activities of daily living; bedridden; paraplegia |
| Also consider Headache, Vomiting, Fever. | | | | | |
| Ataxia (incoordination) | normal | asymptomatic but abnormal on physical exam, and not interfering with function | mild symptoms interfering with function, but not interfering with activities of daily living | moderate symptoms interfering with activities of daily living | bedridden or disabling |
| CNS cerebrovascular ischemia | none | - | - | transient ischemic event or attack (TIA) | permanent event (e.g., cerebral vascular accident) |
| CNS hemorrhage/bleeding is graded in the HEMORRHAGE category. | | | | | |
| *Cognitive disturbance/ learning problems* | *none* | *cognitive disability; not interfering with work/school performance; preservation of intelligence* | *cognitive disability; interfering with work/school performance; decline of 1 SD (Standard Deviation) or loss of developmental milestones* | *cognitive disability; resulting in significant impairment of work/school performance; cognitive decline >2 SD* | *inability to work/frank mental retardation* |

| Adverse Event | Grade | | | | |
|---|---|---|---|---|---|
| | **0** | **1** | **2** | **3** | **4** |
| Confusion | normal | confusion or disorientation or attention deficit of brief duration; resolves spontaneously with no sequelae | confusion or disorientation or attention deficit interfering with function, but not interfering with activities of daily living | confusion or delirium interfering with activities of daily living | harmful to others or self; requiring hospitalization |
| Cranial neuropathy is graded in the NEUROLOGY category as Neuropathy-cranial. | | | | | |
| Delusions | normal | - | - | present | toxic psychosis |
| Depressed level of consciousness | normal | somnolence or sedation not interfering with function | somnolence or sedation interfering with function, but not interfering with activities of daily living | obtundation or stupor; difficult to arouse; interfering with activities of daily living | coma |
| Note: Syncope (fainting) is graded in the NEUROLOGY category. | | | | | |
| Dizziness/lightheadedness | none | not interfering with function | interfering with function, but not interfering with activities of daily living | interfering with activities of daily living | bedridden or disabling |
| Dysphasia, receptive and/or expressive, is graded under Speech impairment in the NEUROLOGY category. | | | | | |
| Extrapyramidal/ involuntary movement/ restlessness | none | mild involuntary movements not interfering with function | moderate involuntary movements interfering with function, but not interfering with activities of daily living | severe involuntary movements or torticollis interfering with activities of daily living | bedridden or disabling |
| Hallucinations | normal | - | - | present | toxic psychosis |
| Headache is graded in the PAIN category. | | | | | |
| Insomnia | normal | occasional difficulty sleeping not interfering with function | difficulty sleeping interfering with function, but not interfering with activities of daily living | frequent difficulty sleeping, interfering with activities of daily living | - |
| Note: This adverse event is graded when insomnia is related to treatment. If pain or other symptoms interfere with sleep do NOT grade as insomnia. | | | | | |
| *Irritability (children <3 years of age)* | *normal* | *mild; easily consolable* | *moderate; requiring increased attention* | *severe; inconsolable* | *-* |
| Leukoencephalopathy associated radiological findings | none | mild increase in SAS (subarachnoid space) and/or mild ventriculomegaly; and/or small (+/- multiple) focal T2 hyperintensities, involving periventricular white matter or <1/3 of susceptible areas of cerebrum | moderate increase in SAS; and/or moderate ventriculomegaly; and/or focal T2 hyperintensities extending into centrum ovale; or involving 1/3 to 2/3 of susceptible areas of cerebrum | severe increase in SAS; severe ventriculomegaly; near total white matter T2 hyperintensities or diffuse low attenuation (CT); focal white matter necrosis (cystic) | severe increase in SAS; severe ventriculomegaly; diffuse low attenuation with calcification (CT); diffuse white matter necrosis (MRI) |
| Memory loss | normal | memory loss not interfering with function | memory loss interfering with function, but not interfering with activities of daily living | memory loss interfering with activities of daily living | amnesia |

| Adverse Event | Grade | | | | |
|---|---|---|---|---|---|
| | 0 | 1 | 2 | 3 | 4 |
| Mood alteration-anxiety, agitation | normal | mild mood alteration not interfering with function | moderate mood alteration interfering with function, but not interfering with activities of daily living | severe mood alteration interfering with activities of daily living | suicidal ideation or danger to self |
| Mood alteration-depression | normal | mild mood alteration not interfering with function | moderate mood alteration interfering with function, but not interfering with activities of daily living | severe mood alteration interfering with activities of daily living | suicidal ideation or danger to self |
| Mood alteration-euphoria | normal | mild mood alteration not interfering with function | moderate mood alteration interfering with function, but not interfering with activities of daily living | severe mood alteration interfering with activities of daily living | danger to self |
| Neuropathic pain is graded in the PAIN category. | | | | | |
| Neuropathy-cranial | absent | - | present, not interfering with activities of daily living | present, interfering with activities of daily living | life-threatening, disabling |
| Neuropathy-motor | normal | subjective weakness but no objective findings | mild objective weakness interfering with function, but not interfering with activities of daily living | objective weakness interfering with activities of daily living | paralysis |
| Neuropathy-sensory | normal | loss of deep tendon reflexes or paresthesia (including tingling) but not interfering with function | objective sensory loss or paresthesia (including tingling), interfering with function, but not interfering with activities of daily living | sensory loss or paresthesia interfering with activities of daily living | permanent sensory loss that interferes with function |
| Nystagmus | absent | present | - | - | - |
| Also consider Vision-double vision. | | | | | |
| Personality/behavioral | normal | change, but not disruptive to patient or family | disruptive to patient or family | disruptive to patient and family; requiring mental health intervention | harmful to others or self; requiring hospitalization |
| Pyramidal tract dysfunction (e.g., ↑ tone, hyperreflexia, positive Babinski, ↓ fine motor coordination) | normal | asymptomatic with abnormality on physical examination | symptomatic or interfering with function but not interfering with activities of daily living | interfering with activities of daily living | bedridden or disabling; paralysis |
| Seizure(s) | none | - | seizure(s) self-limited and consciousness is preserved | seizure(s) in which consciousness is altered | seizures of any type which are prolonged, repetitive, or difficult to control (e.g., status epilepticus, intractable epilepsy) |
| Speech impairment (e.g., dysphasia or aphasia) | normal | - | awareness of receptive or expressive dysphasia, not impairing ability to communicate | receptive or expressive dysphasia, impairing ability to communicate | inability to communicate |
| Syncope (fainting) | absent | - | - | present | - |
| Also consider CARDIOVASCULAR (ARRHYTHMIA), Vasovagal episode, CNS cerebrovascular ischemia. | | | | | |

| Adverse Event | Grade | | | | |
|---|---|---|---|---|---|
| | **0** | **1** | **2** | **3** | **4** |
| Tremor | none | mild and brief or intermittent but not interfering with function | moderate tremor interfering with function, but not interfering with activities of daily living | severe tremor interfering with activities of daily living | - |
| Vertigo | none | not interfering with function | interfering with function, but not interfering with activities of daily living | interfering with activities of daily living | bedridden or disabling |
| Neurology - Other (Specify, _____) | none | mild | moderate | severe | life-threatening or disabling |

## OCULAR/VISUAL

| Adverse Event | 0 | 1 | 2 | 3 | 4 |
|---|---|---|---|---|---|
| Cataract | none | asymptomatic | symptomatic, partial visual loss | symptomatic, visual loss requiring treatment or interfering with function | - |
| Conjunctivitis | none | abnormal ophthalmologic changes, but asymptomatic or symptomatic without visual impairment (i.e., pain and irritation) | symptomatic and interfering with function, but not interfering with activities of daily living | symptomatic and interfering with activities of daily living | - |
| Dry eye | normal | mild, not requiring treatment | moderate or requiring artificial tears | - | - |
| Glaucoma | none | increase in intraocular pressure but no visual loss | increase in intraocular pressure with retinal changes | visual impairment | unilateral or bilateral loss of vision (blindness) |
| Keratitis (corneal inflammation/ corneal ulceration) | none | abnormal ophthalmologic changes but asymptomatic or symptomatic without visual impairment (i.e., pain and irritation) | symptomatic and interfering with function, but not interfering with activities of daily living | symptomatic and interfering with activities of daily living | unilateral or bilateral loss of vision (blindness) |
| Tearing (watery eyes) | none | mild: not interfering with function | moderate: interfering with function, but not interfering with activities of daily living | interfering with activities of daily living | - |
| Vision-blurred vision | normal | - | symptomatic and interfering with function, but not interfering with activities of daily living | symptomatic and interfering with activities of daily living | - |
| Vision-double vision (diplopia) | normal | - | symptomatic and interfering with function, but not interfering with activities of daily living | symptomatic and interfering with activities of daily living | - |
| Vision-flashing lights/floaters | normal | mild, not interfering with function | symptomatic and interfering with function, but not interfering with activities of daily living | symptomatic and interfering with activities of daily living | - |

| Adverse Event | Grade | | | | |
|---|---|---|---|---|---|
| | **0** | **1** | **2** | **3** | **4** |
| Vision-night blindness (nyctalopia) | normal | abnormal electro-retinography but asymptomatic | symptomatic and interfering with function, but not interfering with activities of daily living | symptomatic and interfering with activities of daily living | - |
| Vision-photophobia | normal | - | symptomatic and interfering with function, but not interfering with activities of daily living | symptomatic and interfering with activities of daily living | - |
| Ocular/Visual - Other (Specify, _____) | normal | mild | moderate | severe | unilateral or bilateral loss of vision (blindness) |

## PAIN

| Adverse Event | 0 | 1 | 2 | 3 | 4 |
|---|---|---|---|---|---|
| Abdominal pain or cramping | none | mild pain not interfering with function | moderate pain: pain or analgesics interfering with function, but not interfering with activities of daily living | severe pain: pain or analgesics severely interfering with activities of daily living | disabling |
| Arthralgia (joint pain) | none | mild pain not interfering with function | moderate pain: pain or analgesics interfering with function, but not interfering with activities of daily living | severe pain: pain or analgesics severely interfering with activities of daily living | disabling |
| Arthritis (joint pain with clinical signs of inflammation) is graded in the MUSCULOSKELETAL category. | | | | | |
| Bone pain | none | mild pain not interfering with function | moderate pain: pain or analgesics interfering with function, but not interfering with activities of daily living | severe pain: pain or analgesics severely interfering with activities of daily living | disabling |
| Chest pain (non-cardiac and non-pleuritic) | none | mild pain not interfering with function | moderate pain: pain or analgesics interfering with function, but not interfering with activities of daily living | severe pain: pain or analgesics severely interfering with activities of daily living | disabling |
| Dysmenorrhea | none | mild pain not interfering with function | moderate pain: pain or analgesics interfering with function, but not interfering with activities of daily living | severe pain: pain or analgesics severely interfering with activities of daily living | disabling |
| Dyspareunia | none | mild pain not interfering with function | moderate pain interfering with sexual activity | severe pain preventing sexual activity | - |
| Dysuria is graded in the RENAL/GENITOURINARY category. | | | | | |
| Earache (otalgia) | none | mild pain not interfering with function | moderate pain: pain or analgesics interfering with function, but not interfering with activities of daily living | severe pain: pain or analgesics severely interfering with activities of daily living | disabling |
| Headache | none | mild pain not interfering with function | moderate pain: pain or analgesics interfering with function, but not interfering with activities of daily living | severe pain: pain or analgesics severely interfering with activities of daily living | disabling |

| Adverse Event | Grade | | | | |
|---|---|---|---|---|---|
| | **0** | **1** | **2** | **3** | **4** |
| Hepatic pain | none | mild pain not interfering with function | moderate pain: pain or analgesics interfering with function, but not interfering with activities of daily living | severe pain: pain or analgesics severely interfering with activities of daily living | disabling |
| Myalgia (muscle pain) | none | mild pain not interfering with function | moderate pain: pain or analgesics interfering with function, but not interfering with activities of daily living | severe pain: pain or analgesics severely interfering with activities of daily living | disabling |
| Neuropathic pain (e.g., jaw pain, neurologic pain, phantom limb pain, post-infectious neuralgia, or painful neuropathies) | none | mild pain not interfering with function | moderate pain: pain or analgesics interfering with function, but not interfering with activities of daily living | severe pain: pain or analgesics severely interfering with activities of daily living | disabling |
| Pain due to radiation | none | mild pain not interfering with function | moderate pain: pain or analgesics interfering with function, but not interfering with activities of daily living | severe pain: pain or analgesics severely interfering with activities of daily living | disabling |
| Pelvic pain | none | mild pain not interfering with function | moderate pain: pain or analgesics interfering with function, but not interfering with activities of daily living | severe pain: pain or analgesics severely interfering with activities of daily living | disabling |
| Pleuritic pain | none | mild pain not interfering with function | moderate pain: pain or analgesics interfering with function, but not interfering with activities of daily living | severe pain: pain or analgesics severely interfering with activities of daily living | disabling |
| Rectal or perirectal pain (proctalgia) | none | mild pain not interfering with function | moderate pain: pain or analgesics interfering with function, but not interfering with activities of daily living | severe pain: pain or analgesics severely interfering with activities of daily living | disabling |
| Tumor pain (onset or exacerbation of tumor pain due to treatment) | none | mild pain not interfering with function | moderate pain: pain or analgesics interfering with function, but not interfering with activities of daily living | severe pain: pain or analgesics severely interfering with activities of daily living | disabling |
| Tumor flare is graded in the SYNDROME category. | | | | | |
| Pain - Other (Specify, _____) | none | mild | moderate | severe | disabling |

## PULMONARY

| Adverse Event | Grade | | | | |
|---|---|---|---|---|---|
| | **0** | **1** | **2** | **3** | **4** |
| Adult Respiratory Distress Syndrome (ARDS) | absent | - | - | - | present |
| Apnea | none | - | - | present | requiring intubation |

| Adverse Event | Grade | | | | |
|---|---|---|---|---|---|
| | 0 | 1 | 2 | 3 | 4 |
| Carbon monoxide diffusion capacity ($DL_{CO}$) | ≥90% of pretreatment or normal value | ≥75 - <90% of pretreatment or normal value | ≥50 - <75% of pretreatment or normal value | ≥25 - <50% of pretreatment or normal value | <25% of pretreatment or normal value |
| Cough | absent | mild, relieved by non-prescription medication | requiring narcotic antitussive | severe cough or coughing spasms, poorly controlled or unresponsive to treatment | - |
| Dyspnea (shortness of breath) | normal | - | dyspnea on exertion | dyspnea at normal level of activity | dyspnea at rest or requiring ventilator support |
| $FEV_1$ | ≥90% of pretreatment or normal value | ≥75 - <90% of pretreatment or normal value | ≥50 - <75% of pretreatment or normal value | ≥25 - <50% of pretreatment or normal value | <25% of pretreatment or normal value |
| Hiccoughs (hiccups, singultus) | none | mild, not requiring treatment | moderate, requiring treatment | severe, prolonged, and refractory to treatment | - |
| Hypoxia | normal | - | decreased $O_2$ saturation with exercise | decreased $O_2$ saturation at rest, requiring supplemental oxygen | decreased $O_2$ saturation, requiring pressure support (CPAP) or assisted ventilation |
| Pleural effusion (non-malignant) | none | asymptomatic and not requiring treatment | symptomatic, requiring diuretics | symptomatic, requiring $O_2$ or therapeutic thoracentesis | life-threatening (e.g., requiring intubation) |
| Pleuritic pain is graded in the PAIN category. | | | | | |
| Pneumonitis/pulmonary infiltrates | none | radiographic changes but asymptomatic or symptoms not requiring steroids | radiographic changes and requiring steroids or diuretics | radiographic changes and requiring oxygen | radiographic changes and requiring assisted ventilation |
| Pneumothorax | none | no intervention required | chest tube required | sclerosis or surgery required | life-threatening |
| Pulmonary embolism is graded as Thrombosis/embolism in the CARDIOVASCULAR (GENERAL) category. | | | | | |
| Pulmonary fibrosis | none | radiographic changes, but asymptomatic or symptoms not requiring steroids | requiring steroids or diuretics | requiring oxygen | requiring assisted ventilation |
| Note: Radiation-related pulmonary fibrosis is graded in the RTOG/EORTC Late Radiation Morbidity Scoring Scheme-Lung. (See Appendix IV) | | | | | |
| Voice changes/stridor/larynx (e.g., hoarseness, loss of voice, laryngitis) | normal | mild or intermittent hoarseness | persistent hoarseness, but able to vocalize; may have mild to moderate edema | whispered speech, not able to vocalize; may have marked edema | marked dyspnea/stridor requiring tracheostomy or intubation |
| Notes: Cough from radiation is graded as cough in the PULMONARY category. | | | | | |
| Radiation-related hemoptysis from larynx/pharynx is graded as Grade 4 Mucositis due to radiation in the GASTROINTESTINAL category. Radiation-related hemoptysis from the thoracic cavity is graded as Grade 4 Hemoptysis in the HEMORRHAGE category. | | | | | |
| Pulmonary - Other (Specify, _____) | none | mild | moderate | severe | life-threatening or disabling |

| Adverse Event | Grade | | | | |
|---|---|---|---|---|---|
| | 0 | 1 | 2 | 3 | 4 |
| **RENAL/GENITOURINARY** | | | | | |
| Bladder spasms | absent | mild symptoms, not requiring intervention | symptoms requiring antispasmodic | severe symptoms requiring narcotic | - |
| Creatinine | WNL | >ULN - 1.5 x ULN | >1.5 - 3.0 x ULN | >3.0 - 6.0 x ULN | >6.0 x ULN |
| Note: Adjust to age-appropriate levels for pediatric patients. | | | | | |
| Dysuria (painful urination) | none | mild symptoms requiring no intervention | symptoms relieved with therapy | symptoms not relieved despite therapy | - |
| Fistula or GU fistula (e.g., vaginal, vesicovaginal) | none | - | - | requiring intervention | requiring surgery |
| Hemoglobinuria | - | present | - | - | - |
| Hematuria (in the absence of vaginal bleeding) is graded in the HEMORRHAGE category. | | | | | |
| Incontinence | none | with coughing, sneezing, etc. | spontaneous, some control | no control (in the absence of fistula) | - |
| Operative injury to bladder and/or ureter | none | - | injury of bladder with primary repair | sepsis, fistula, or obstruction requiring secondary surgery; loss of one kidney; injury requiring anastomosis or re-implantation | septic obstruction of both kidneys or vesicovaginal fistula requiring diversion |
| Proteinuria | normal or <0.15 g/24 hours | 1+ or 0.15 - 1.0 g/24 hours | 2+ to 3+ or 1.0 - 3.5 g/24 hours | 4+ or >3.5 g/24 hours | nephrotic syndrome |
| Note: If there is an inconsistency between absolute value and dip stick reading, use the absolute value for grading. | | | | | |
| Renal failure | none | - | - | requiring dialysis, but reversible | requiring dialysis and irreversible |
| Ureteral obstruction | none | unilateral, not requiring surgery | - | bilateral, not requiring surgery | stent, nephrostomy tube, or surgery |
| Urinary electrolyte wasting (e.g., Fanconi's syndrome, renal tubular acidosis) | none | asymptomatic, not requiring treatment | mild, reversible and manageable with oral replacement | reversible but requiring IV replacement | irreversible, requiring continued replacement |
| Also consider Acidosis, Bicarbonate, Hypocalcemia, Hypophosphatemia. | | | | | |
| Urinary frequency/urgency | normal | increase in frequency or nocturia up to 2 x normal | increase >2 x normal but <hourly | hourly or more with urgency, or requiring catheter | - |
| Urinary retention | normal | hesitancy or dribbling, but no significant residual urine; retention occurring during the immediate postoperative period | hesitancy requiring medication or occasional in/out catheterization (<4 x per week), or operative bladder atony requiring indwelling catheter beyond immediate postoperative period but for <6 weeks | requiring frequent in/out catheterization (≥4 x per week) or urological intervention (e.g., TURP, suprapubic tube, urethrotomy) | bladder rupture |

| Adverse Event | Grade | | | | |
|---|---|---|---|---|---|
| | 0 | 1 | 2 | 3 | 4 |
| Urine color change (not related to other dietary or physiologic cause e.g., bilirubin, concentrated urine, hematuria) | normal | asymptomatic, change in urine color | - | - | - |
| Vaginal bleeding is graded in the HEMORRHAGE category. | | | | | |
| Vaginitis (not due to infection) | none | mild, not requiring treatment | moderate, relieved with treatment | severe, not relieved with treatment, or ulceration not requiring surgery | ulceration requiring surgery |
| Renal/Genitourinary - Other (Specify, _____) | none | mild | moderate | severe | life-threatening or disabling |

## SECONDARY MALIGNANCY

| Adverse Event | 0 | 1 | 2 | 3 | 4 |
|---|---|---|---|---|---|
| Secondary Malignancy - Other (Specify type, _____) excludes metastasis from initial primary | none | - | - | - | present |

## SEXUAL/REPRODUCTIVE FUNCTION

| Adverse Event | 0 | 1 | 2 | 3 | 4 |
|---|---|---|---|---|---|
| Dyspareunia is graded in the PAIN category. | | | | | |
| Dysmenorrhea is graded in the PAIN category. | | | | | |
| Erectile impotence | normal | mild (erections impaired but satisfactory) | moderate (erections impaired, unsatisfactory for intercourse) | no erections | - |
| Female sterility | normal | - | - | sterile | - |
| Feminization of male is graded in the ENDOCRINE category. | | | | | |
| Irregular menses (change from baseline) | normal | occasionally irregular or lengthened interval, but continuing menstrual cycles | very irregular, but continuing menstrual cycles | persistent amenorrhea | - |
| Libido | normal | decrease in interest | severe loss of interest | - | - |
| Male infertility | - | - | oligospermia (low sperm count) | azoospermia (no sperm) | - |
| Masculinization of female is graded in the ENDOCRINE category. | | | | | |
| Vaginal dryness | normal | mild | requiring treatment and/or interfering with sexual function, dyspareunia | - | - |
| Sexual/Reproductive Function - Other (Specify, _____) | none | mild | moderate | severe | disabling |

## SYNDROMES (not included in previous categories)

| | | | | | |
|---|---|---|---|---|---|
| Acute vascular leak syndrome is graded in the CARDIOVASCULAR (GENERAL) category. | | | | | |
| ARDS (Adult Respiratory Distress Syndrome) is graded in the PULMONARY category. | | | | | |

| Adverse Event | Grade | | | | |
|---|---|---|---|---|---|
| | **0** | **1** | **2** | **3** | **4** |
| Autoimmune reactions are graded in the ALLERGY/IMMUNOLOGY category. | | | | | |
| DIC (disseminated intravascular coagulation) is graded in the COAGULATION category. | | | | | |
| Fanconi's syndrome is graded as Urinary electrolyte wasting in the RENAL/GENITOURINARY category. | | | | | |
| Renal tubular acidosis is graded as Urinary electrolyte wasting in the RENAL/GENITOURINARY category. | | | | | |
| Stevens-Johnson syndrome (erythema multiforme) is graded in the DERMATOLOGY/SKIN category. | | | | | |
| SIADH (syndrome of inappropriate antidiuretic hormone) is graded in the ENDOCRINE category. | | | | | |
| Thrombotic microangiopathy (e.g., thrombotic thrombocytopenic purpura/TTP or hemolytic uremic syndrome/HUS) is graded in the COAGULATION category. | | | | | |
| Tumor flare | none | mild pain not interfering with function | moderate pain; pain or analgesics interfering with function, but not interfering with activities of daily living | severe pain; pain or analgesics interfering with function and interfering with activities of daily living | Disabling |
| Also consider Hypercalcemia. | | | | | |
| Note: Tumor flare is characterized by a constellation of symptoms and signs in direct relation to initiation of therapy (e.g., anti-estrogens/androgens or additional hormones). The symptoms/signs include tumor pain, inflammation of visible tumor, hypercalcemia, diffuse bone pain, and other electrolyte disturbances. | | | | | |
| Tumor lysis syndrome | absent | - | - | present | - |
| Also consider Hyperkalemia, Creatinine. | | | | | |
| Urinary electrolyte wasting (e.g., Fanconi's syndrome, renal tubular acidosis) is graded in the RENAL/GENITOURINARY category. | | | | | |
| Syndromes - Other (Specify, _____ ) | none | mild | moderate | severe | life-threatening or disabling |

## Appendix 2. Cancer Chemotherapy Agents Compatibility Chart

*Part A: Oncology Product with Oncology Products*

| Oncology Product A | Oncology Product B | Condition* | Diluting Solution | Concentration of Products | Stability and Compatibility Comments |
|---|---|---|---|---|---|
| *Bleomycin* | Cisplatin | Y | Not applicable | 3 units/mL & 1 mg/mL | No visible precipitate after sequential injection. |
| | Cisplatin & Cytarabine | A | Sodium Chloride 0.9% | 0.12 units/mL & 0.2 mg/mL & 1.05 mg/mL | Stable for 24 hours at 25°C. |
| | Cyclophosphamide | Y | Not applicable | 3 units/mL & 20 mg/mL | No visible precipitate after sequential injection. |
| | Cytarabine & Cisplatin | A | Sodium Chloride 0.9% | 0.12 units/mL & 1.05 mg/mL & 0.2 mg/mL | Stable for 24 hours at 25°C. |
| | Doxorubicin | Y | Not applicable | 3 units/mL & 2 mg/mL | No visible precipitate after sequential injection. |
| | Fludarabine | Y | Not applicable | 1 unit/mL & 1 mg/mL | Physically compatible for 4 hours at room temperature in fluorescent light. |
| | Fluorouracil | A | Sodium Chloride 0.9% | 0.02–0.03 units/mL & 1 mg/mL | Stable for 7 days at 4°C. May adsorb onto plastic. |
| | Fluorouracil | Y | Not applicable | 3 units/mL & 50 mg/mL | No visible precipitate after sequential injection. |
| | Methotrexate | A | Sodium Chloride 0.9% | 0.02–0.03 units/mL & 0.25–0.5 mg/mL | Unstable. Drug decomposes within 7 days at 4°C. |
| | Methotrexate | Y | Not applicable | 3 units/mL & 25 mg/mL | No visible precipitate after sequential injection. |
| | Mitomycin | A | Sodium Chloride 0.9% | 0.02–0.03 units/mL & 0.01–0.05 mg/mL | Unstable. Drug decomposes within 7 days at 4°C. |
| | Mitomycin | Y | Not applicable | 3 units/mL & 0.5 mg/mL | No visible precipitate after sequential injection. |
| | Vinblastine | A | Sodium Chloride 0.9% | 0.02–0.03 units/mL & 0.01–0.1 mg/mL | Stable for 7 days at 4°C. May adsorb onto plastic. |
| | Vinblastine | Y | Not applicable | 3 units/mL & 1 mg/mL | No visible precipitate after sequential injection. |
| | Vincristine | A | Sodium Chloride 0.9% | 0.02–0.03 units/mL & 0.05–0.1 mg/mL | Stable for 7 days at 4°C. May adsorb onto plastic. |
| | Vincristine | Y | Not applicable | 3 units/mL & 1 mg/mL | No visible precipitate after sequential injection. |
| *Carboplatin* | Fludarabine | Y | Dextrose 5% | 1 mg/mL & 5 mg/mL | Physically compatible for 4 hours at room temperature in fluorescent light. |
| | Fluorouracil | A | Sterile Water | 1 mg/mL & 10 mg/mL | Unstable. Greater than 20% loss of carboplatin within 24 hours at room temperature. |
| | Ifosfamide | A | Sterile Water | 1 mg/mL & 1 mg/mL | Both drugs stable for 5 days at room temperature. |
| | Ifosfamide & Etoposide | A | Sterile Water | 1 mg/mL & 2 mg/mL & 0.2 mg/mL | All drugs stable for 7 days at room temperature. |

*Condition: A = Admixture (drugs are used as an admixture in the IV bag).
Y = Y-site (drugs are combined at the Y-site in the IV line).

*Note:* Please consult complete prescribing information for any product mentioned.

| Drug | Combined with | A/Y | Diluent | Concentration | Stability |
|---|---|---|---|---|---|
| Mesna | | A | Sterile Water | 1 mg/mL & 1 mg/mL | Unstable. Greater than 10% loss of carboplatin within 24 hours at room temperature. |
| *Carmustine* | Cisplatin | A | See manufacturer's package inserts | 1.4 mg/mL & 0.86 mg/mL | Both drugs stable for 3 hours at 23°C. |
| | Fludarabine | Y | Dextrose 5% | 1.5 mg/mL & 1 mg/mL | Stable for 4 hours at room temperature in fluorescent light. |
| *Cisplatin* | Bleomycin & Cytarabine | A | Sodium Chloride 0.9% | 0.2 mg/mL & 0.12 units/mL & 1.05 mg/mL | Stable for 24 hours at 25°C. |
| | Carmustine | A | Dextrose 5% | 0.86 mg/mL & 1.4 mg/mL | Both drugs stable for 3 hours at 23°C. |
| | Carmustine | A | Sodium Chloride 0.9% | 0.86 mg/mL & 1.4 mg/mL | Both drugs stable for 3 hours at 23°C. |
| | Cyclophosphamide & Etoposide | A/Y | Sodium Chloride 0.9% | 0.2 mg/mL & 2 mg/mL & 0.2 mg/mL | Stable for 7 days at room temperature. |
| | Cytarabine & Bleomycin | A | Sodium Chloride 0.9% | 0.2 mg/mL & 1.05 mg/mL & 0.12 units/mL | Stable for 24 hours at 25°C. |
| | Etoposide | A | Dextrose 5% & Sodium Chloride 0.45% | 0.2 mg/mL & 0.2–0.4 mg/mL | Stable for 24 hours at 25°C. |
| | Etoposide | A | Sodium Chloride 0.9% | 0.2 mg/mL & 0.2 mg/mL | Stable for 15 days at room temperature when protected from light. |
| | Etoposide | A | Sodium Chloride 0.9% | 0.2 mg/mL & 0.2–0.4 mg/mL | Stable for 24 hours at 25°C. |
| | Etoposide | A | Sodium Chloride 0.9% | 10 mg/mL & 20 mg/mL | Both drugs stable for 7 days in PVC containers. |
| | Floxuridine | A | Sodium Chloride 0.9% | 0.5 mg/mL & 10 mg/mL | Physically compatible for 14 days when protected from light; however, a 13% loss and an 18% loss of floxuridine occur at 7 days and at 14 days, respectively. |
| | Floxuridine & Leucovorin | A | Sodium Chloride 0.9% | 0.2 mg/mL & 0.7 mg/mL & 0.14 mg/mL | All drugs stable for 7 days. |
| | Fluorouracil | A | Sodium Chloride 0.9% | 0.2 mg/mL & 1 mg/mL | Unstable. 10% loss of cisplatin in 1.5 hours and 25% loss in 4 hours at 25°C in fluorescent light. |
| | Fluorouracil | Y | Not applicable | 1 mg/mL & 50 mg/mL | No visible precipitate after sequential injection. |
| | Ifosfamide | A | Sodium Chloride 0.9% | 0.2 mg/mL & 20 mg/mL | Both drugs stable for 7 days at room temperature. |
| *Cyclophosphamide* | Bleomycin | Y | Not applicable | 20 mg/mL & 3 units/mL | No visible precipitate after sequential injection. |
| | Cisplatin | Y | Not applicable | 20 mg/mL & 1 mg/mL | No visible precipitate after sequential injection. |
| | Cisplatin & Etoposide | A | Sodium Chloride 0.9% | 2 mg/mL & 0.2 mg/mL & 0.2 mg/mL | All drugs stable for 7 days at room temperature |

*(continued)*

## Appendix 2. Cancer Chemotherapy Agents Compatibility Chart (continued)

*Part A: Oncology Product with Oncology Products*

| Oncology Product A | Oncology Product B | Condition* | Diluting Solution | Concentration of Products | Stability and Compatibility Comments |
|---|---|---|---|---|---|
| Cyclophosphamide (continued) | Doxorubicin | A | Sodium Chloride 0.9% | 0.67 mg & 11.7 mg/mL | Both drugs stable for 7 days at 25°C. |
| | Doxorubicin | Y | Not applicable | 20 mg/mL & 2 mg/mL | No visible precipitate after sequential injection. |
| | Fludarabine | Y | Dextrose 5% | 10 mg/mL & 1 mg/mL | Physically compatible for 4 hours at room temperature in fluorescent light. |
| | Fluorouracil | A | Sodium Chloride 0.9% | 1.67 mg/mL & 8.3 mg/mL | Both drugs stable for 15 days at room temperature. |
| | Fluorouracil | Y | Not applicable | 20 mg/mL & 50 mg/mL | No visible precipitate after sequential injection. |
| | Methotrexate | A | Sodium Chloride 0.9% | 1.67 mg/mL & 0.025 mg/mL | 9.3% loss of cyclophosphamide along with a degradation product at 7 days at room temperature. Also, a pH change occurs from 6.30 to 4.57. No loss of methotrexate within 14 days. |
| | Methotrexate | Y | Not applicable | 20 mg/mL & 25 mg/mL | No visible precipitate after sequential injection. |
| | Methotrexate & Fluorouracil | A | Sodium Chloride 0.9% | 1.67 mg/mL & 0.025 mg/mL & 8.3 mg/mL | 9.3% loss of cyclophosphamide within 7 days at room temperature; other drugs are stable. |
| | Mitomycin | Y | Not applicable | 20 mg/mL & 0.5 mg/mL | No visible precipitate after sequential injection. |
| | Vinblastine | Y | Not applicable | 20 mg/mL & 1 mg/mL | No visible precipitate after sequential injection. |
| | Vincristine | Y | Not applicable | 20 mg/mL & 1 mg/mL | No visible precipitate after sequential injection. |
| Cytarabine | Bleomycin & Cisplatin | A | Sodium Chloride 0.9% | 1.05 mg/mL & 0.12 units/mL & 0.2 mg/mL | Stable for 24 hours at 25°C. |
| | Cisplatin & Bleomycin | A | Sodium Chloride 0.9% | 1.05 mg/mL & 0.2 mg/mL & 0.12 units/mL | Stable for 24 hours at 25°C. |
| | Daunorubicin & Etoposide | A | Dextrose 5% | 200 mg & 25 mg & 300 mg | All drugs stable for 72 hours at 20°C. |
| | Daunorubicin & Etoposide | A | Sodium Chloride 0.45% | 200 mg & 25 mg & 300 mg | All drugs stable for 72 hours at 20°C. |
| | Etoposide & Daunorubicin | A | Dextrose 5% | 200 mg & 300 mg & 25 mg | All drugs stable for 72 hours at 20°C. |
| | Etoposide & Daunorubicin | A | Sodium Chloride 0.45% | 200 mg & 300 mg & 25 mg | All drugs stable for 72 hours at 20°C. |
| | Fludarabine | Y | Dextrose 5% | 50 mg/mL & 1 mg/mL | No visible precipitate at 4 hours at room temperature in fluorescent light. |
| | Fluorouracil | A | Dextrose 5% | 0.4 mg/mL & 0.25 mg/mL | Both drugs stable for 8 hours at 25°C. No significant UV spectrum changes. |
| | Methotrexate | A | Dextrose 5% | 0.4 mg/mL & 0.2 mg/mL | Both drugs stable for 8 hours at 25°C. No significant UV spectrum changes. |

| Drug | | Code | Solution | Concentration | Comments |
|---|---|---|---|---|---|
| | Methotrexate | A | Dextrose 5% | 30–50 mg/12 mL & 12 mg/12 mL | Hydrocortisone Sodium Succinate 15–25 mg/12 mL. All drugs stable for 24 hours at 25°C. |
| | Methotrexate | A | Elliot's B Solution | 30–50 mg/12 mL & 12 mg/12 mL | Hydrocortisone Sodium Succinate 12 mL. All drugs stable for 10 hours at 25°C. |
| | Methotrexate | A | Lactated Ringer's | 30–50 mg/12 mL & 12 mg/12 mL | Hydrocortisone Sodium Succinate 15–25 mg/12 mL. All drugs stable for 24 hours at 25°C. |
| | Methotrexate | A | Sodium Chloride 0.9% | 30–50 mg/12 mL & 12 mg/12 mL | Hydrocortisone Sodium Succinate 15–25 mg/12 mL. All drugs stable for 24 hours at 25°C. |
| | Vincristine | A | Dextrose 5% | 0.016 mg/mL & 0.004 mg/mL | Both drugs stable for 8 hours at 25°C. No significant UV spectrum changes. |
| *Daunorubicin* | Cytarabine & Etoposide | A | Dextrose 5% | 25 mg & 200 mg & 300 mg | All drugs stable for 72 hours at 20°C. |
| | Cytarabine & Etoposide | A | Sodium Chloride 0.45% | 25 mg & 200 mg & 300 mg | All drugs stable for 72 hours at 20°C. |
| | Etoposide & Cytarabine | A | Dextrose 5% | 25 mg & 300 mg & 200 mg | All drugs stable for 72 hours at 20°C. |
| | Etoposide & Cytarabine | A | Sodium Chloride 0.45% | 25 mg & 300 mg & 200 mg | All drugs stable for 72 hours at 20°C. |
| | Fludarabine | Y | Dextrose 5% | 2 mg/mL & 1 mg/mL | Incompatible. Slight haze forms at 4 hours at room temperature, visible in high-intensity light. |
| *Doxorubicin* | Bleomycin | Y | Not applicable | 2 mg/mL & 3 units/mL | No visible precipitate after sequential injection. |
| | Cisplatin | Y | Not applicable | 2 mg/mL & 1 mg/mL | No visible precipitate after sequential injection. |
| | Cyclophosphamide | Y | Not applicable | 2 mg/mL & 20 mg/mL | No visible precipitate after sequential injection. |
| | Cyclophosphamide | A | Sodium Chloride 0.9% | 11.7 mg/mL & 0.67 mg/mL | Both drugs stable for 7 days at 25°C. |
| | Fludarabine | Y | Dextrose 5% | 2 mg/mL & 1 mg/mL | Physically compatible for 4 hours at room temperature in fluorescent light. |
| | Fluorouracil | A | Dextrose 5% | 0.01 mg/mL & 0.25 mg/mL | Incompatible. Precipitates and color changes. |
| | Fluorouracil | Y | Not applicable | 2 mg/mL & 50 mg/mL | No visible precipitate after sequential injection. |
| | Methotrexate | Y | Not applicable | 2 mg/mL & 25 mg/mL | No visible precipitate after sequential injection. |
| | Mitomycin | Y | Not applicable | 2 mg/mL & 0.5 mg/mL | No visible precipitate after sequential injection. |
| | Vinblastine | A | Sodium Chloride 0.9% | 0.5–1.5 mg/mL & 0.075–0.15 mg/mL | May be stable for 10 days at 8° to 32°C; however, HPLC erratic. |
| | Vinblastine | Y | Not applicable | 2 mg/mL & 1 mg/mL | No visible precipitate after sequential injection. |
| | Vincristine | A | Dextrose 2.5% & Sodium Chloride 0.45% | 1.4 mg/mL & 0.033 mg/mL | Both drugs stable for 14 days at 25°C. |
| | Vincristine | A | Sodium Chloride 0.9% | 1.4 mg/mL & 0.033 mg/mL | Both drugs stable for 14 days at 25°C. |

## Appendix 2.  Cancer Chemotherapy Agents Compatibility Chart (continued)

### Part A: Oncology Product with Oncology Products

| Oncology Product A | Oncology Product B | Condition* | Diluting Solution | Concentration of Products | Stability and Compatibility Comments |
|---|---|---|---|---|---|
| *Doxorubicin (continued)* | Vincristine | A | Sodium Chloride 0.45% & Ringer's | 1.4 mg/mL & 0.033 mg/mL | Both drugs stable for 1 days and 7 days, respectively, at 25°C. |
| | Vincristine | Y | Not applicable | 2 mg/mL & 1 mg/mL | No visible precipitate after sequential injection. |
| *Etoposide* | Cisplatin | A | Dextrose 5% & Sodium Chloride 0.45% | 0.2 mg/mL & 0.2 mg/mL | Stable for 24 hours at 25°C. |
| | Cisplatin | A | Dextrose 5% & Sodium Chloride 0.45% | 0.4 mg/mL & 0.2 mg/mL | Mannitol 1.875% & Potassium Chloride 0.02 mEq/mL. Stable for 24 hours at 25°C. |
| | Cisplatin | A | Sodium Chloride 0.9% | 0.2 mg/mL & 0.2 mg/mL | Both drugs stable for 15 days at room temperature when protected from light. |
| | Cisplatin | A | Sodium Chloride 0.9% | 0.2–0.4 mg/mL & 0.2 mg/mL | Stable for 24 hours at 25°C. |
| | Cisplatin | A | Sodium Chloride 0.9% | 0.4 mg/mL & 0.2 mg/mL | Both drugs stable for 7 days in PVC containers. |
| | Cisplatin | A | Sodium Chloride 0.9% | 0.4 mg/mL & 0.2 mg/mL | Physically compatible for 48 hours at 22°C in fluorescent light or in the dark. |
| | Cisplatin & Cyclophosphamide | A | Sodium Chloride 0.9% | 0.2 mg/mL & 0.2 mg/mL & 2 mg/mL | All drugs stable for 7 days at room temperature. |
| | Cisplatin & Floxuridine | A | Sodium Chloride 0.9% | 0.3 mg/mL & 0.2 mg/mL & 0.7 mg/mL | All drugs stable for 7 days at room temperature. |
| | Cytarabine & Daunorubicin | A | Dextrose 5% | 300 mg & 200 mg & 25 mg | All drugs stable for 72 hours at 20°C. |
| | Cytarabine & Daunorubicin | A | Dextrose 5% & Sodium Chloride 0.45% | 0.4 mg/mL & 0.267 mg/mL & 0.033 mg/mL | Physically compatible and stable for 72 hours at 20°C. |
| | Cytarabine & Daunorubicin | A | Sodium Chloride 0.45% | 300 mg & 200 mg & 25 mg | All drugs stable for 72 hours at 20°C. |
| | Daunorubicin | A | Dextrose 5% & Sodium Chloride 0.45% | 0.4 mg/mL & 0.033 mg/mL | Physically compatible and stable for 72 hours at 20°C. |
| | Daunorubicin & Cytarabine | A | Dextrose 5% | 300 mg & 25 mg & 200 mg | All drugs stable for 72 hours at 20°C. |
| | Daunorubicin & Cytarabine | A | Sodium Chloride 0.45% | 300 mg & 25 mg & 200 mg | All drugs stable for 72 hours at 20°C. |
| | Fludarabine | Y | Dextrose 5% | 0.4 mg/mL & 1 mg/mL | Physically compatible for 4 hours at room temperature in fluorescent light. |

| Drug | Second Drug | | Concentration | Diluent | Notes |
|---|---|---|---|---|---|
| | Fluorouracil | A | 0.2 mg/mL & 10 mg/mL | Sodium Chloride 0.9% | Stable for 7 days at room temperature and for 1 day at 35°C. |
| | Ifosfamide | A | 0.2 mg/mL & 2 mg/mL | Sodium Chloride 0.9% | Stable for 7 days at room temperature. |
| | Ifosfamide & Carboplatin | A | 0.2 mg/mL & 2 mg/mL & 1 mg/mL | Sterile Water | Stable for 5 days at room temperature. |
| | Ifosfamide & Cisplatin | A | 0.2 mg/mL & 2 mg/mL & 0.2 mg/mL | Sodium Chloride 0.9% | Stable for 5 days at room temperature. |
| | Mitoxantrone | A | 0.5 mg/mL & 0.05 mg/mL | Sodium Chloride 0.9% | Stable for 22 hours at room temperature. |
| *Floxuridine* | Carboplatin | A | 10 mg/mL & 1 mg/mL | Sterile Water | Both drugs stable for 7 days at room temperature. |
| | Cisplatin | A | 10 mg/mL & 0.5 mg/mL | Sodium Chloride 0.9% | Physically compatible; however, a 13% loss of floxuridine occurs within 7 days. |
| | Cisplatin & Etoposide | A | 0.7 mg/mL & 0.2 mg/mL & 0.3 mg/mL | Sodium Chloride 0.9% | All drugs stable for 7 days at room temperature. |
| | Cisplatin & Leucovorin | A | 0.7 mg/mL & 0.2 mg/mL & 0.14 mg/mL | Sodium Chloride 0.9% | All drugs stable for 7 days at room temperature. |
| | Etoposide | A | 10 mg/mL & 0.2 mg/mL | Sodium Chloride 0.9% | Both drugs stable for 15 days at room temperature. |
| | Fludarabine | Y | 3 mg/mL & 1 mg/mL | Dextrose 5% | Physically compatible for 4 hours at room temperature in fluorescent light. |
| | Fluorouracil | A | 10 mg/mL & 10 mg/mL | Sodium Chloride 0.9% | Both drugs stable for 15 days at room temperature. |
| | Flurouracil & Leucovorin | A | 0.7 mg/mL & 5 mg/mL & 0.14 mg/mL | Sodium Chloride 0.9% | All drugs stable for 15 days at room temperature. |
| | Leucovorin | A | 1 mg/mL & 0.03 mg/mL | Sodium Chloride 0.9% | Physically compatible and stable for 48 hours at 4°C and at 20°C. No loss of floxuridine and 10% loss of leucovorin within 48 hours at 40°C. |
| *Fludarabine* | Bleomycin | Y | 1 mg/mL & 1 unit/mL | Dextrose 5% & Sodium Chloride 0.9% | Physically compatible for 4 hours at room temperature in fluorescent light. |
| | Carboplatin | Y | 1 mg/mL & 5 mg/mL | Dextrose 5% | Physically compatible for 4 hours at room temperature in fluorescent light. |
| | Carmustine | Y | 1 mg/mL & 1.5 mg/mL | Dextrose 5% | Physically compatible for 4 hours at room temperature in fluorescent light. |
| | Cisplatin | Y | 1 mg/mL & 1 mg/mL | Dextrose 5% | Physically compatible for 4 hours at room temperature in fluorescent light. |
| | Cyclophosphamide | Y | 1 mg/mL & 10 mg/mL | Dextrose 5% | Physically compatible for 4 hours at room temperature in fluorescent light. |

(continued)

**Appendix 2.  Cancer Chemotherapy Agents Compatibility Chart (continued)**

*Part A: Oncology Product with Oncology Products*

| Oncology Product A | Oncology Product B | Condition* | Diluting Solution | Concentration of Products | Stability and Compatibility Comments |
|---|---|---|---|---|---|
| *Fludarabine* (*continued*) | Cytarabine | Y | Dextrose 5% | 1 mg/mL & 50 mg/mL | Physically compatible for 4 hours at room temperature in fluorescent light. |
| | Dacarbazine | Y | Dextrose 5% | 1 mg/mL & 4 mg/mL | Physically compatible for 4 hours at room temperature in fluorescent light. |
| | Dactinomycin | Y | Dextrose 5% | 1 mg/mL & 0.01 mg/mL | Physically compatible for 4 hours at room temperature in fluorescent light. |
| | Daunorubicin | Y | Dextrose 5% | 1 mg/mL & 2 mg/mL | Incompatible for 4 hours at room temperature in fluorescent light. |
| | Doxorubicin | Y | Dextrose 5% | 1 mg/mL & 2 mg/mL | Physically compatible for 4 hours at room temperature in fluorescent light. |
| | Etoposide | Y | Dextrose 5% | 1 mg/mL & 0.4 mg/mL | Physically compatible for 4 hours at room temperature in fluorescent light. |
| | Floxuridine | Y | Dextrose 5% | 1 mg/mL & 3 mg/mL | Physically compatible for 4 hours at room temperature in fluorescent light. |
| | Fluorouracil | Y | Dextrose 5% | 1 mg/mL & 16 mg/mL | Physically compatible for 4 hours at room temperature in fluorescent light. |
| | Ifosfamide | Y | Dextrose 5% | 1 mg/mL & 25 mg/mL | Physically compatible for 4 hours at room temperature in fluorescent light. |
| | Mechlorethamine | Y | Dextrose 5% | 1 mg/mL & 1 mg/mL | Physically compatible for 4 hours at room temperature in fluorescent light. |
| | Mesna | Y | Dextrose 5% | 1 mg/mL & 10 mg/mL | Physically compatible for 4 hours at room temperature in fluorescent light. |
| | Methotrexate | Y | Dextrose 5% | 1 mg/mL & 15 mg/mL | Physically compatible for 4 hours at room temperature in fluorescent light. |
| | Mitoxantrone | Y | Dextrose 5% | 1 mg/mL & 0.5 mg/mL | Physically compatible for 4 hours at room temperature in fluorescent light. |
| | Pentostatin | Y | Dextrose 5% & Sodium Chloride 0.9% | 1 mg/mL & 0.4 mg/mL | Physically compatible for 4 hours at room temperature in fluorescent light. |
| | Vinblastine | Y | Dextrose 5% | 1 mg/mL & 1 mg/mL | Physically compatible for 4 hours at room temperature in fluorescent light. |
| | Vincristine | Y | Dextrose 5% | 1 mg/mL & 1 mg/mL | Physically compatible for 4 hours at room temperature in fluorescent light. |

**Fluorouracil**

| Drug | Code | Diluent | Concentration | Comments |
|---|---|---|---|---|
| Bleomycin | A | Sodium Chloride 0.9% | 1 mg/mL & 0.02–0.03 units/mL | Stable for 7 days at 4°C. May adsorb onto plastic. |
| Carboplatin | A | Sterile Water | 10 mg/mL & 1 mg/mL | Unstable. Greater than 20% loss of carboplatin within 24 hours at room temperature. |
| Cisplatin | A | Sodium Chloride 0.9% | 1 mg/mL & 0.2 mg/mL | Unstable. Greater than 10% loss of cisplatin within 1.5 hours and 25% loss within 4 hours at 25°C in light or dark. |
| Cisplatin | Y | Not applicable | 50 mg/mL & 1 mg/mL | No visible precipitate after sequential injection. |
| Cyclophosphamide | A | Sodium Chloride 0.9% | 8.3 mg/mL & 1.67 mg/mL | Both drugs stable for 15 days at room temperature. |
| Cyclophosphamide | Y | Not applicable | 50 mg/mL & 20 mg/mL | No visible precipitate after sequential injection. |
| Cyclophosphamide & Methotrexate | A | Sodium Chloride 0.9% | 8.3 mg/mL & 1.67 mg/mL & 0.025 mg/mL | 9.3% loss of cyclophosphamide within 7 days at room temperature. |
| Cytarabine | A | Dextrose 5% | 0.25 mg/mL & 0.4 mg/mL | Both drugs stable for 8 hours at 25°C. No significant UV spectrum changes. |
| Doxorubicin | A | Sodium Chloride 0.9% | 0.25 mg/mL & 0.01 mg/mL | Incompatible. Color changes to purple. |
| Doxorubicin | Y | Not applicable | 50 mg/mL & 2 mg/mL | No visible precipitate after sequential injection. |
| Etoposide | A | Sodium Chloride 0.9% | 10 mg/mL & 0.2 mg/mL | Both drugs stable for 7 days at room temperature and for 1 day at 35°C. |
| Floxuridine | A | Sodium Chloride 0.9% | 10 mg/mL & 10 mg/mL | Both drugs stable for 15 days at room temperature. |
| Floxurine & Leucovorin | A | Sodium Chloride 0.9% | 5 mg/mL & 0.7 mg/mL & 0.14 mg/mL | All drugs stable for 15 days at room temperature. |
| Ifosfamide | A | Sodium Chloride 0.9% | 10 mg/mL & 2 mg/mL | Both drugs stable for 5 days at room temperature. |
| Leucovorin | A | Sodium Chloride 0.9% | 10 mg/mL & 0.2 mg/mL | Both drugs stable for 15 days at room temperature when protected from light. |
| Leucovorin | Y | Not applicable | 50 mg/mL & 10 mg/mL | No visible precipitate after sequential injection. |
| Methotrexate | A | Dextrose 5% | 0.25 mg/mL & 0.2 mg/mL | Unstable. Both drugs decompose within 1 hour at 25°C. Altered UV spectrum. |
| Methotrexate | A | Fluorouracil (as diluent) | 500 mg/10 mL & 50 mg/10 mL | Both drugs stable for 24 hours at 25°C. |
| Methotrexate | A | Sodium Chloride 0.9% | 10 mg/mL & 0.03 mg/mL | Both drugs stable for 15 days at room temperature. |
| Methotrexate | Y | Not applicable | 50 mg/mL & 25 mg/mL | No visible precipitate after sequential injection. |
| Mitomycin | Y | Not applicable | 50 mg/mL & 0.5 mg/mL | No visible precipitate after sequential injection. |
| Vinblastine | Y | Not applicable | 50 mg/mL & 1 mg/mL | No visible precipitate after sequential injection. |
| Vincristine | A | Dextrose 5% | 0.01 mg/mL & 0.004 mg/mL | Both drugs stable for 8 hours at 25°C. No UV spectrum changes. |
| Vincristine | Y | Not applicable | 50 mg/mL & 1 mg/mL | No visible precipitate after sequential injection. |

*(continued)*

## Appendix 2. Cancer Chemotherapy Agents Compatibility Chart (*continued*)

*Part A: Oncology Product with Oncology Products*

| Oncology Product A | Oncology Product B | Condition* | Diluting Solution | Concentration of Products | Stability and Compatibility Comments |
|---|---|---|---|---|---|
| *Ifosfamide* | Carboplatin | A | Sterile Water | 1 mg/mL & 1 mg/mL | Both drugs stable for 5 days at room temperature. |
| | Carboplatin & Etoposide | A | Sterile Water | 2 mg/mL & 1 mg/mL & 0.2 mg/mL | All drugs stable for 7 days at room temperature. |
| | Cisplatin | A | Sodium Chloride 0.9% | 2 mg/mL & 0.2 mg/mL | Both drugs stable for 7 days at room temperature. |
| | Cisplatin & Etoposide | A | Sodium Chloride 0.9% | 2 mg/mL & 0.2 mg/mL & 0.2 mg/mL | All drugs stable for 5 days at room temperature. |
| | Etoposide | A | Sodium Chloride 0.9% | 2 mg/mL & 0.2 mg/mL | Both drugs stable for 5 days at room temperature. |
| | Fludarabine | Y | Dextrose 5% | 25 mg/mL & 1 mg/mL | Physically compatible for 4 hours at room temperature in fluorescent light. |
| | Fluorouracil | A | Sodium Chloride 0.9% | 2 mg/mL & 10 mg/mL | Both drugs stable for 5 days at room temperature. |
| | Mesna | A | Dextrose 5% | 0.6 mg/mL & 0.6 mg/mL | Both drugs stable for 24 hours at room temperature. |
| | Mesna | A | Dextrose 5% | 3.3 mg/mL & 3.3 mg/mL | Physically compatible and stable for 24 hours at 21°C in fluorescent light. |
| | Mesna | A | Dextrose 5% | 5 mg/mL & 5 mg/mL | Physically compatible and stable for 24 hours at 21°C in fluorescent light. |
| | Mesna | A | Dextrose 5% & Sodium Chloride 0.45% | 0.6 mg/mL & 0.6 mg/mL | Both drugs stable for 24 hours at room temperature. |
| | Mesna | A | Lactated Ringer's | 0.6 mg/mL & 0.6 mg/mL | Both drugs stable for 24 hours at room temperature. |
| | Mesna | A | Lactated Ringer's | 3.3 mg/mL & 3.3 mg/mL | Physically compatible and stable for 24 hours at 21°C in fluorescent light. |
| | Mesna | A | Lactated Ringer's | 5 mg/mL & 5 mg/mL | Physically compatible and stable for 24 hours at 21°C in fluorescent light. |
| | Mesna | A | Sodium Chloride 0.9% | 0.6 mg/mL & 0.6 mg/mL | Both drugs stable for 24 hours at room temperature. |
| | Mesna | A | Sodium Chloride 0.9% | 50 mg/mL & 40 mg/mL | Both drugs stable for 14 days at room temperature. |
| | Mesna | A | Sodium Chloride 0.9% | 83.3 mg/mL & 79 mg/mL | No loss of ifosfamide within 9 days at room temperature; however, a 7% loss occurs within 9 days at 37°C. Mesna not tested. |

| | | | | | |
|---|---|---|---|---|---|
| *Leucovorin* | Bleomycin | Y | Not applicable | 10 mg/mL & 3 units/mL | No visible precipitate after sequential injection. |
| | Cisplatin | A | Sodium Chloride 0.9% | 0.14 mg/mL & 0.2 mg/mL | Both drugs stable for 15 days at room temperature when protected from light. |
| | Cisplatin | Y | Not applicable | 10 mg/mL & 1 mg/mL | No visible precipitate after sequential injection. |
| | Cisplatin & Floxuridine | A | Sodium Chloride 0.9% | 0.14 mg/mL & 0.2 mg/mL & 0.7 mg/mL | All drugs stable for 7 days at room temperature. |
| | Cyclophosphamide | Y | Not applicable | 10 mg/mL & 20 mg/mL | No visible precipitate after sequential injection. |
| | Doxorubicin | Y | Not applicable | 10 mg/mL & 2 mg/mL | No visible precipitate after sequential injection. |
| | Floxuridine | A | Sodium Chloride 0.9% | 0.03 mg/mL & 1 mg/mL | Physically compatible and stable for 48 hours at 4°C and 20°C. No loss of floxuridine and 10% loss of leucovorin within 48 hours at 40°C. |
| | Floxuridine | A | Sodium Chloride 0.9% | 0.2 mg/mL & 10 mg/mL | Both drugs stable for 15 days at room temperature when protected from light. |
| | Floxuridine | A | Sodium Chloride 0.9% | 0.24 mg/mL & 2 mg/mL | Physically compatible and stable for 48 hours at 4°C and at 20°C. No loss of floxuridine and 7% loss of leucovorin within 48 hours at 40°C. |
| | Floxuridine | A | Sodium Chloride 0.9% | 0.96 mg/mL & 4 mg/mL | Physically compatible and stable for 48 hours at 4°C, 20°C, and 40°C. |
| | Floxuridine & Fluorouracil | A | Sodium Chloride 0.9% | 0.14 mg/mL & 0.7 mg/mL & 5 mg/mL | All drugs stable for 15 days at room temperature. |
| | Fluorouracil | A | Sodium Chloride 0.9% | 0.2 mg/mL & 10 mg/mL | Both drugs stable for 15 days at room temperature when protected from light. |
| | Fluorouracil | Y | Not applicable | 10 mg/mL & 50 mg/mL | No visible precipitate after sequential injection. |
| | Methotrexate | Y | Not applicable | 10 mg/mL & 25 mg/mL | No visible precipitate after sequential injection. |
| | Mitomycin | Y | Not applicable | 10 mg/mL & 0.5 mg/mL | No visible precipitate after sequential injection. |
| | Vinblastine | Y | Not applicable | 10 mg/mL & 1 mg/mL | No visible precipitate after sequential injection. |
| | Vincristine | Y | Not applicable | 10 mg/mL & 1 mg/mL | No visible precipitate after sequential injection. |
| *Mechlorethamine* | Fludarabine | Y | Dextrose 5% | 1 mg/mL & 1 mg/mL | Physically compatible for 4 hours at room temperature in fluorescent light. |
| *Mesna* | Carboplatin | A | Sterile Water | 1 mg/mL & 1 mg/mL | Unstable. Greater than 10% loss of carboplatin within 24 hours at room temperature. |
| | Cisplatin | A | Sodium Chloride 0.9% | 0.11 mg/mL & 0.067 mg/mL | Unstable. Weakly detectable cisplatin after 1 hour. |
| | Cisplatin | A | Sodium Chloride 0.9% | 3.3 mg/mL & 0.067 mg/mL | Unstable. No detectable cisplatin after 1 hour. |
| | Ifosfamide | A | Dextrose 5% | 0.6 mg/mL & 0.6 mg/mL | Stable for 24 hours at room temperature. |
| | Ifosfamide | A | Dextrose 5% Lactated Ringer's | 3.3 mg/mL & 5 mg/mL | Physically compatible for 24 hours at room temperature. |

(continued)

## Appendix 2. Cancer Chemotherapy Agents Compatibility Chart (continued)

*Part A: Oncology Product with Oncology Products*

| Oncology Product A | Oncology Product B | Condition* | Diluting Solution | Concentration of Products | Stability and Compatibility Comments |
|---|---|---|---|---|---|
| *Mesna* (continued) | Ifosfamide | A | Dextrose 5% & Sodium Chloride 0.9% | 0.6 mg/mL & 0.6 mg/mL | Stable for 24 hours at room temperature in polyethylene containers. |
| | Ifosfamide | A | Lactated Ringer's | 0.6 mg/mL 0.6 mg/mL | Stable for 24 hours at room temperature. |
| | Ifosfamide | A | Sodium Chloride 0.9% | 0.6 mg/mL & 0.6 mg/mL | Stable for 24 hours at room temperature. |
| | Ifosfamide | A | Sodium Chloride 0.9% | 40 mg/mL & 50 mg/mL | Stable for 14 days at room temperature. |
| | Ifosfamide | A | Sodium Chloride 0.9% | 79 mg/mL & 83.3 mg/mL | No loss of ifosfamide within 9 days at room temperature; however, a 7% loss occurs within 9 days at 37°C. Mesna not tested. |
| *Methotrexate* | Bleomycin | A | Sodium Chloride 0.9% | 0.25–0.5 mg/mL & 0.02–0.03 units/mL | Unstable. Drug decomposes within 7 days at 4°C. |
| | Bleomycin | Y | Not applicable | 25 mg/mL & 3 units/mL | No visible precipitate after sequential injection. |
| | Cisplatin | Y | Not applicable | 25 mg/mL & 1 mg/mL | No visible precipitate after sequential injection. |
| | Cyclophosphamide | A | Sodium Chloride 0.9% | 0.025 mg/mL & 1.67 mg/mL | Less than 7% loss of cyclophosphamide within 14 days at room temperature. |
| | Cyclophosphamide & Fluorouracil | A | Sodium Chloride 0.9% | 0.025 mg/mL & 1.67 mg/mL | 9.3% loss of cyclophosphamide within 7 days at room temperature. |
| | Cytarabine | A | Dextrose 5% | 0.2 mg/mL & 0.4 mg/mL | Both drugs stable for 8 hours at 25°C. No UV spectrum changes. |
| | Cytarabine | A | Dextrose 5% | 12 mg/12 mL & 30–50 mg/12 mL | Hydrocortisone Sodium Succinate 15–25 mg/ 12 mL. All drugs stable for 24 hours at 25°C. |
| | Cytarabine | A | Elliot's B Solution | 12 mg/12 mL & 30–50 mg/12 mL | Hydrocortisone Sodium Succinate 15–25 mg/ 12 mL. All drugs stable for 10 hours at 25°C. |
| | Cytarabine | A | Lactated Ringer's | 12 mg/12 mL & 30–50 mg/12 mL | Hydrocortisone Sodium succinate 15–25 mg/ 12 mL. All drugs stable for 24 hours at 25°C. |
| | Cytarabine | A | Sodium Chloride 0.9% | 12 mg/12 mL & 30–50 mg/12 mL | Hydrocortisone Sodium succinate 15–25 mg/ 12 mL. All drugs stable for 24 hours at 25°C. |
| | Doxorubicin | Y | Not applicable | 25 mg/mL & 2 mg/mL | No visible precipitate after sequential injection. |
| | Fludarabine | Y | Dextrose 5% | 0.2 mg/mL & 1 mg/mL | Physically compatible for 4 hours at room temperature in fluorescent light. |
| | Fluorouracil | A | Dextrose 5% | 0.2 mg/mL & 0.25 mg/mL | Unstable. Both drugs decompose within 1 hour at 25°C. Altered UV spectrum. |
| | Fluorouracil | A | Fluorouracil (as Diluent) | 50 mg/10 mL & 500 mg/10 mL | Both drugs stable for 24 hours at 25°C. |

| | | | | | |
|---|---|---|---|---|---|
| | Fluorouracil | A | Sodium Chloride 0.9% | 0.03 mg/mL & 10 mg/mL | Both drugs stable for 15 days at room temperature. |
| | Leucovorin | Y | Not applicable | 25 mg/mL & 10 mg/mL | No visible precipitate after sequential injection. |
| | Mitomycin | Y | Not applicable | 25 mg/mL & 0.5 mg/mL | No visible precipitate after sequential injection. |
| | Vinblastine | Y | Not applicable | 25 mg/mL & 1 mg/mL | No visible precipitate after sequential injection. |
| | Vincristine | A | Dextrose 5% | 0.008–0.1 mg/mL & 0.004–0.01 mg/mL | Both drugs stable for 8 hours at 25°C. No UV spectrum changes. |
| | Vincristine | Y | Not applicable | 25 mg/mL & 1 mg/mL | No visible precipitate after sequential injection. |
| *Mitomycin* | Bleomycin | A | Sodium Chloride 0.9% | 0.01 mg/mL & 0.02 units/mL | Unstable. 20% loss of bleomycin within 7 days at 4°C. |
| | Bleomycin | A | Sodium Chloride 0.9% | 0.01 mg/mL & 0.03 units/mL | Unstable. 20% loss of bleomycin within 7 days at 4°C. |
| | Bleomycin | A | Sodium Chloride 0.9% | 0.01–0.05 mg/mL & 0.02–0.03 units/mL | Unstable. Drug decomposes within 7 days at 4°C. |
| | Bleomycin | A | Sodium Chloride 0.9% | 0.05 mg/mL & 0.02 units/mL | Unstable. 52% loss of bleomycin within 7 days at 4°C. |
| | Bleomycin | A | Sodium Chloride 0.9% | 0.05 mg/mL & 0.03 units/mL | Unstable. 52% loss of bleomycin within 7 days at 4°C. |
| | Bleomycin | Y | Not applicable | 0.5 mg/mL & 3 units/mL | No visible precipitate after sequential injection. |
| | Cisplatin | Y | Not applicable | 0.5 mg/mL & 1 mg/mL | No visible precipitate after sequential injection. |
| | Cyclophosphamide | Y | Not applicable | 0.5 mg/mL & 20 mg/mL | No visible precipitate after sequential injection. |
| | Doxorubicin | Y | Not applicable | 0.5 mg/mL & 2 mg/mL | No visible precipitate after sequential injection. |
| | Fluorouracil | Y | Not applicable | 0.5 mg/mL & 50 mg/mL | No visible precipitate after sequential injection. |
| | Leucovorin | Y | Not applicable | 0.5 mg/mL & 10 mg/mL | No visible precipitate after sequential injection. |
| | Methotrexate | Y | Not applicable | 0.5 mg/mL & 25 mg/mL | No visible precipitate after sequential injection. |
| | Vinblastine | Y | Not applicable | 0.5 mg/mL & 1 mg/mL | No visible precipitate after sequential injection. |
| | Vincristine | Y | Not applicable | 0.5 mg/mL & 1 mg/mL | No visible precipitate after sequential injection. |
| *Mitoxantrone* | Fludarabine | Y | Dextrose 5% | 0.5 mg/mL & 1 mg/mL | Physically compatible for 4 hours at room temperature. |
| *Paclitaxel* | Bleomycin | Y | Dextrose 5% | 1.2 mg/mL & 1 unit/mL | No precipitate or change in color or turbidity within 4 hours. |
| | Carboplatin | Y | Dextrose 5% | 1.2 mg/mL & 5 mg/mL | No visible precipitate after sequential injection. |
| | Cisplatin | Y | Dextrose 5% | 1.2 mg/mL & 1 mg/mL | No visible precipitate after sequential injection. |
| | Cyclophosphamide | Y | Dextrose 5% | 1.2 mg/mL & 10 mg/mL | No visible precipitate after sequential injection. |
| | Cytarabine | Y | Dextrose 5% | 1.2 mg/mL & 50 mg/mL | No visible precipitate after sequential injection. |
| | Dacarbazine | Y | Dextrose 5% | 1.2 mg/mL & 4 mg/mL | No precipitate or change in color or turbidity within 4 hours. |
| | Doxorubicin | Y | Dextrose 5% | 1.2 mg/mL & 2 mg/mL | No visible precipitate after sequential injection. |

*(continued)*

## Appendix 2. Cancer Chemotherapy Agents Compatibility Chart (continued)

### Part A: Oncology Product with Oncology Products

| Oncology Product A | Oncology Product B | Condition* | Diluting Solution | Concentration of Products | Stability and Compatibility Comments |
|---|---|---|---|---|---|
| *Paclitaxel* (continued) | Etoposide | Y | Dextrose 5% | 1.2 mg/mL & 0.4 mg/mL | No visible precipitate after sequential injection. |
| | Floxuridine | Y | Dextrose 5% | 1.2 mg/mL & 3 mg/mL | No precipitate or change in color or turbidity within 4 hours. |
| | Fluorouracil | Y | Dextrose 5% | 1.2 mg/mL & 16 mg/mL | No visible precipitate after sequential injection. |
| | Ifosfamide | Y | Dextrose 5% | 1.2 mg/mL & 25 mg/mL | No precipitate or change in color or turbidity within 4 hours. |
| | Methotrexate | Y | Dextrose 5% | 1.2 mg/mL & 15 mg/mL | No visible precipitate after sequential injection. |
| | Mitoxantrone | Y | Dextrose 5% | 1.2 mg/mL & 0.5 mg/mL | Incompatible. Decreased turbidity, below normal range. |
| | Vinblastine | Y | Dextrose 5% | 1.2 mg/mL & 0.12 mg/mL | No precipitate or change in color or turbidity within 4 hours. |
| | Vincristine | Y | Dextrose 5% | 1.2 mg/mL & 0.05 mg/mL | No precipitate or change in color or turbidity within 4 hours. |
| *Sargramostim* (GM-CSF) | Bleomycin | Y | Sodium Chloride 0.9% | 10 µg/mL & 1 unit/mL | Physically compatible for 4 hours at 22°C in fluorescent light. |
| | Carmustine | Y | Sodium Chloride 0.9% | 10 µg/mL & 1.5 unit/mL | Physically compatible for 4 hours at 22°C in fluorescent light. |
| | Cisplatin | Y | Sodium Chloride 0.9% | 10 µg/mL & 1 mg/mL | Physically compatible for 4 hours at 22°C in fluorescent light. |
| | Etoposide | Y | Sodium Chloride 0.9% | 10 µg/mL & 0.4 mg/mL | Physically compatible for 4 hours at 22°C in fluorescent light. |
| | Fludarabine | Y | Sodium Chloride 0.9% | 10 µg/mL & 3 mg/mL | Physically compatible for 4 hours at 22°C in fluorescent light. |
| | Fluorouracil | Y | Sodium Chloride 0.9% | 10 µg/mL & 16 mg/mL | Physically compatible for 4 hours at 22°C in fluorescent light. |
| | Idarubicin | Y | Sodium Chloride 0.9% | 10 µg/mL & 0.5 mg/mL | Incompatible. Haze forms immediately. |
| | Ifosfamide | Y | Sodium Chloride 0.9% | 10 µg/mL & 25 mg/mL | Physically compatible for 4 hours at 22°C in fluorescent light. |
| | Mechlorethamine | Y | Sodium Chloride 0.9% | 10 µg/mL & 1 mg/mL | Physically compatible for 4 hours at 22°C in fluorescent light. |
| | Methotrexate | Y | Sodium Chloride 0.9% | 10 µg/mL & 15 mg/mL | Physically compatible for 4 hours at 22°C in fluorescent light. |
| | Mitomycin | Y | Sodium Chloride 0.9% | 10 µg/mL & 0.5 mg/mL | Incompatible. Haze forms within 30 minutes. |
| | Mitoxantrone | Y | Sodium Chloride 0.9% | 10 µg/mL & 0.5 mg/mL | Physically compatible for 4 hours at 22°C in fluorescent light. |

| | Drug | | Diluent | Concentration | Comments |
|---|---|---|---|---|---|
| | Pentostatin | Y | Sodium Chloride 0.9% | 10 µg/mL & 0.4 mg/mL | Physically compatible for 4 hours at 22°C in in fluorescent light. |
| | Vinblastine | Y | Sodium Chloride 0.9% | 10 µg/mL & 0.12 mg/mL | Physically compatible for 4 hours at 22°C in fluorescent light. |
| | Vincristine | Y | Sodium Chloride 0.9% | 10 µg/mL & 0.05 mg/mL | Physically compatible for 4 hours at 22°C in fluorescent light. |
| *Vinblastine* | Bleomycin | A | Sodium Chloride 0.9% | 0.01–0.1 mg/mL & 0.02–0.03 units/mL | Stable for 7 days at 4°C. May adsorb onto plastic. |
| | Bleomycin | Y | Not applicable | 1 mg/mL & 3 units/mL | No visible precipitate after sequential injection. |
| | Cisplatin | Y | Not applicable | 1 mg/mL & 1 mg/mL | No visible precipitate after sequential injection. |
| | Cyclophosphamide | Y | Not applicable | 1 mg/mL & 20 mg/mL | No visible precipitate after sequential injection. |
| | Doxorubicin | A | Sodium Chloride 0.9% | 0.075–0.15 mg/mL & 0.5–1.5 mg/mL | May be stable for 10 days at 8° to 32°C; however, HPLC erratic. |
| | Doxorubicin | Y | Not applicable | 1 mg/mL & 2 mg/mL | No visible precipitate after sequential injection. |
| | Fludarabine | Y | Dextrose 5% | 0.12 mg/mL & 1 mg/mL | Physically compatible for 4 hours at room temperature in fluorescent light. |
| | Leucovorin | Y | Not applicable | 1 mg/mL & 10 mg/mL | No visible precipitate after sequential injection. |
| | Methotrexate | Y | Not applicable | 1 mg/mL & 25 mg/mL | No visible precipitate after sequential injection. |
| | Mitomycin | Y | Not applicable | 1 mg/mL & 0.5 mg/mL | No visible precipitate after sequential injection. |
| | Vincristine | Y | Not applicable | 1 mg/mL & 1 mg/mL | No visible precipitate after sequential injection. |
| *Vincristine* | Bleomycin | A | Sodium Chloride 0.9% | 0.05–0.1 mg/mL & 0.02–0.03 units/mL | Stable for 7 days at 4°C. May adsorb onto plastic. |
| | Bleomycin | Y | Not Applicable | 1 mg/mL & 3 units/mL | No visible precipitate after sequential injection. |
| | Cisplatin | Y | Not Applicable | 1 mg/mL & 1 mg/mL | No visible precipitate after sequential injection. |
| | Cyclophosphamide | Y | Not Applicable | 1 mg/mL & 20 mg/mL | No visible precipitate after sequential injection. |
| | Cytarabine | A | Dextrose 5% | 0.004 mg/mL & 0.016 mg/mL | Both drugs stable for 8 hours at 25°C. No significant UV spectrum changes. |
| | Doxorubicin | A | Dextrose 2.5% & Sodium Chloride 0.45% | 0.033 mg/mL & 1.4 mg/mL | Both drugs stable for 14 days at 25°C. |
| | Doxorubicin | A | Sodium Chloride 0.9% | 0.033 mg/mL & 1.4 mg/mL | Both drugs stable for 14 days at 25°C. |
| | Doxorubicin | A | Sodium Chloride 0.45% & Ringer's | 0.033 mg/mL & 1.4 mg/mL | Both drugs stable for 7 days and 1 day, respectively, at 25°C. |
| | Doxorubicin | Y | Not applicable | 1 mg/mL & 2 mg/mL | No visible precipitate after sequential injection. |
| | Fludarabine | Y | Dextrose 5% | 1 mg/mL & 1 mg/mL | Physically compatible for 4 hours at room temperature in fluorescent light. |

*(continued)*

## Appendix 2. Cancer Chemotherapy Agents Compatibility Chart (continued)

### Part A: Oncology Product with Oncology Products

| Oncology Product A | Oncology Product B | Condition* | Diluting Solution | Concentration of Products | Stability and Compatibility Comments |
|---|---|---|---|---|---|
| *Vincristine* (continued) | Fluorouracil | A | Dextrose 5% | 0.004 mg/mL & 0.01 mg/mL | Both drugs stable for 8 hours at 25°C. No UV spectrum changes. |
| | Fluorouracil | Y | Not applicable | 1 mg/mL & 50 mg/mL | No visible precipitate after sequential injection. |
| | Leucovorin | Y | Not applicable | 1 mg/mL & 10 mg/mL | No visible precipitate after sequential injection. |
| | Methotrexate | A | Dextrose 5% | 0.004–0.01 mg/mL & 0.008–0.1 mg/mL | Both drugs stable for 8 hours at 25°C. No UV spectrum changes. |
| | Methotrexate | Y | Not applicable | 1 mg/mL & 25 mg/mL | No visible precipitate after sequential injection. |
| | Mitomycin | Y | Not applicable | 1 mg/mL & 0.5 mg/mL | No visible precipitate after sequential injection. |
| | Vinblastine | Y | Not applicable | 1 mg/mL & 1 mg/mL | No visible precipitate after sequential injection. |

### Part B: Oncology Product with Other Products

| Oncology Product | Other Product | Condition* | Diluting Solution | Concentration of Products | Stability and Compatibility Comments |
|---|---|---|---|---|---|
| *Bleomycin* | Amikacin Sulfate | A | Sodium Chloride 0.9% | 0.02–0.03 units/mL & 1.25 mg/mL | Stable for 7 days at 4°C. |
| | Aminophylline | A | Sodium Chloride 0.9% | 0.02–0.03 units/mL & 0.25 mg/mL | Unstable. Drug decomposes within 7 days at 4°C. |
| | Ascorbid Acid | A | Sodium Chloride 0.9% | 0.02–0.03 units/mL & 2.5–5 mg/mL | Unstable. Drug decomposes within 7 days at 4°C. |
| | Carbenicillin Disodium | A | Sodium Chloride 0.9% | 0.02–0.03 units/mL & 4–12 mg/mL | Unstable. Drug decomposes within 7 days at 4°C. |
| | Cefazolin Sodium | A | Sodium Chloride 0.9% | 0.02–0.03 units/mL & 1 mg/mL | Unstable. Drug decomposes within 7 days at 4°C. |
| | Cephalothin Sodium | A | Sodium Chloride 0.9% | 0.02–0.03 units/mL & 2.5–5 mg/mL | Unstable. Drug decomposes within 7 days at 4°C. |
| | Cephapirin Sodium | A | Sodium Chloride 0.9% | 0.02–0.03 units/mL & 3 mg/mL | Stable for 7 days at 4°C. May adsorb onto plastic. |
| | Dexamethasone Sodium Phosphate | A | Sodium Chloride 0.9% | 0.02–0.03 units/mL & 0.05 mg/mL | Stable for 7 days at 4°C. May adsorb onto plastic. |
| | Diazepam | A | Sodium Chloride 0.9% | 0.02–0.03 units/mL & 0.05–1 mg/mL | Incompatible. |
| | Diphenydramine Hydrochloride | A | Sodium Chloride 0.9% | 0.02–0.03 units/mL & 0.1mg/mL | Stable for 7 days at 4°C. May adsorb onto plastic. |
| | Droperidol | Y | Not applicable | 3 units/mL & 2.5 mg/mL | No visible precipitate after sequential injection. |
| | Gentamicin Sulfate | A | Sodium Chloride 0.9% | 0.02–0.03 units/mL & 0.1–0.6 mg/mL | Stable for 7 days at 4°C. May adsorb onto plastic. |

| Drug | Compatible Drug | | Solution | Concentration | Remarks |
|---|---|---|---|---|---|
| | Heparin Sodium | A | Dextrose 5% | 0.02–0.03 units/mL & 10–1,000 units/mL | Stable for 24 hours. May adsorb onto plastic. |
| | Heparin Sodium | A | Sodium Chloride 0.9% | 0.02–0.03 units/mL & 10–200 units/mL | Stable for 7 days at 4°C. May adsorb onto plastic. |
| | Heparin Sodium | Y | Not applicable | 3 units/mL & 1,000 units/mL | No visible precipitate after sequential injection. |
| | Hydrocortisone Sodium Phosphate | A | Sodium Chloride 0.9% | 0.02–0.03 units/mL & 0.1–2 mg/mL | Stable for 7 days at 4°C. May adsorb onto plastic. |
| | Hydrocortisone Sodium Succinate | A | Sodium Chloride 0.9% | 0.02–0.03 units/mL & 0.3–2.5 mg/mL | Unstable. Drug decomposes within 7 days at 4°C. |
| | Leucovorin Calcium | Y | Not applicable | 3 units/mL & 10 mg/mL | No visible precipitate after sequential injection. |
| | Methoclopramide Hydrochloride | Y | Not applicable | 3 units/mL & 5 mg/mL | No visible precipitate after sequential injection. |
| | Nafcillin Sodium | A | Sodium Chloride 0.9% | 0.02–0.03 units/mL & 2.5 mg/mL | Unstable. Drug decomposes within 7 days at 4°C. |
| | Ondansetron Hydrochloride | Y | Sodium Chloride 0.9% | 1 unit/mL & 1 mg/mL | Physically compatible for 4 hours at 22°C in fluorescent light. |
| | Penicillin G Sodium | A | Sodium Chloride 0.9% | 0.02–0.03 units/mL & 0.5 mg/mL | Unstable. Drug decomposes within 7 days at 4°C. |
| | Phenytoin Sodium | A | Sodium Chloride 0.9% | 0.02–0.03 units/mL & 0.5 mg/mL | Stable for 7 days at 4°C. May adsorb onto plastic. |
| | Sargramostim | Y | Sodium Chloride 0.9% | 1 unit/mL & 10 µg/mL | Physically compatible for 4 hours at 22°C in fluorescent light. |
| | Streptomycin Sulfate | A | Sodium Chloride 0.9% | 0.02–0.03 units/mL & 4 mg/mL | Stable for 7 days at 4°C. May adsorb onto plastic. |
| | Sulfate Terbutaline | A | Sodium Chloride 0.9% | 0.02–0.03 units/mL & 0.0075 mg/mL | Unstable. Drug decomposes within 7 days at 4°C. |
| | Tobramycin Sulfate | A | Sodium Chloride 0.9% | 0.02–0.03 units/mL & 0.5 mg/mL | Stable for 7 days at 4°C. May adsorb onto plastic. |
| *Carboplatin* | Ondansetron Hydrochloride | Y | Sodium Chloride 0.9% | 0.18–9.9 µg/mL & 16–160 µg/mL | Physically compatible when carboplatin is administered over 10 to 60 minutes. |
| | Ondansetron Hydrochloride | Y | Dextrose 5% | 5 mg/mL & 1 mg/mL | Physically compatible for 4 hours at 22°C in fluorescent light. |
| | Sargramostim | Y | Sodium Chloride 0.9% | 5 mg/mL & 10 µg/mL | Physically compatible for 4 hours in 22°C in fluorescent light. |
| *Carmustine* | Ondansetron Hydrochloride | Y | Dextrose 5% & Sodium Chloride 0.9% | 1.5 mg/mL & 1 mg/mL | Physically compatible for 4 hours at 22°C in fluorescent light. |
| | Sargramostim | Y | Sodium Chloride 0.9% | 5 mg/mL & 10 µg/mL | Physically compatible for 4 hours at 22°C in fluorescent light. |

*(continued)*

## Appendix 2. Cancer Chemotherapy Agents Compatibility Chart (continued)

*Part B: Oncology Product with Other Products*

| Oncology Product | Other Product | Condition* | Diluting Solution | Concentration of Products | Stability and Compatibility Comments |
|---|---|---|---|---|---|
| *Carmustine (continued)* | Sodium Bicarbonate | A | Dextrose 5% | 0.1 mg/mL & 0.1 mEq/mL | Unstable. Drug decomposes within 1 hour at 25°C. |
| | Sodium Bicarbonate | A | Sodium Chloride 0.9% | 0.1 mg/mL & 0.1 mEq/mL | Unstable. Drug decomposes within 1 hour at 25°C. |
| *Cisplatin* | Droperidol | Y | Not applicable | 2.5 mg/mL & 1 mg/mL | No visible precipitate after sequential injection. |
| | Furosemide | Y | Not applicable | 1 mg/mL & 10 mg/mL | No visible precipitate after sequential injection. |
| | Heparin Sodium | Y | Not applicable | 1 mg/mL & 1,000 units/mL | No visible precipitate after sequential injection. |
| | Hydroxyzine Hydrochloride | A | Sodium Chloride 0.9% | 0.2 mg/mL & 0.5 mg/mL | Physically compatible for 48 hours at room temperature in glass containers. |
| | Leucovorin Calcium | A | Sodium Chloride 0.9% | 0.2 mg/mL & 0.14 mg/mL | Both drugs stable for 15 days at room temperature when protected from light. |
| | Leucovorin Calcium | Y | Not applicable | 1 mg/mL & 10 mg/mL | No visible precipitate after sequential injection. |
| | Magnesium Sulfate | A | Dextrose 5% & Sodium Chloride 0.45% | 0.05 mg/mL & 1 mg/mL | Physically compatible for 48 hours at 25°C and for 96 hours at 4°C in PVC containers. |
| | Magnesium Sulfate | A | Dextrose 5% & Sodium Chloride 0.45% | 0.2 mg/mL & 2 mg/mL | Physically compatible for 48 hours at 25°C and for 96 hours at 4°C in PVC containers. |
| | Mannitol | A | Dextrose 5% & Sodium Chloride 0.45% | 0.05 mg/mL & 18.75 mg/mL | Physically compatible for 48 hours at 25°C and for 96 hours at 4°C in PVC containers. |
| | Mesna | A | Sodium Chloride 0.9% | 0.067 mg/mL & 0.11 mg/mL | Unstable. Weakly detectable cisplatin after 1 hour. |
| | Mesna | A | Sodium Chloride 0.9% | 0.067 mg/mL & 3.3 mg/mL | Unstable. No detectable cisplatin after 1 hour. |
| | Metoclopramide Hydrochloride | Y | Not applicable | 1 mg/mL & 5 mg/mL | No visible precipitate after sequential injection. |
| | Metoclopramide Hydrochloride | A | See manufacturer's package insert | 173 mg & 10–160 mg | Use immediately. |
| | Ondansetron Hydrochloride | Y | Sodium Chloride 0.9% | 0.48 mg/mL & 16–160 µg/mL | Physically compatible when cisplatin is administered over 1 to 8 hours. |
| | Ondansetron Hydrochloride | Y | Sodium Chloride 0.9% | 1 mg/mL & 1 mg/mL | Physically compatible for 4 hours at 22°C in fluorescent light. |
| | Sargramostim | Y | Sodium Chloride 0.9% | 1 mg/mL & 10 µg/mL | Physically compatible for 4 hours at 22°C in fluorescent light. |

| | | | | | |
|---|---|---|---|---|---|
| *Cyclophosphamide* | Amikacin Sulfate | Y | Dextrose 5% | 20 mg/mL & 5 mg/mL | Physically compatible for 4 hours at 25°C in fluorescent light. |
| | Ampicillin Sodium | Y | Dextrose 5% | 20 mg/mL & 20 mg/mL | Physically compatible for 4 hours at 25°C in fluorescent light. |
| | Ampicillin Sodium | Y | Sodium Chloride 0.9% | 20 mg/mL & 20 mg/mL | Physically compatible for 4 hours at 25°C in fluorescent light. |
| | Azlocillin Sodium | Y | Dextrose 5% | 20 mg/mL & 20 mg/mL | Physically compatible for 4 hours at 25°C in fluorescent light. |
| | Cefamandole Nafate | Y | Dextrose 5% | 20 mg/mL & 20 mg/mL | Physically compatible for 4 hours at 25°C in fluorescent light. |
| | Cefazolin Sodium | Y | Dextrose 5% | 20 mg/mL & 20 mg/mL | Physically compatible for 4 hours at 25°C in fluorescent light. |
| | Cefoperazone Sodium | Y | Dextrose 5% | 20 mg/mL & 20 mg/mL | Physically compatible for 4 hours at 25°C in fluorescent light. |
| | Ceforanide | Y | Dextrose 5% | 20 mg/mL & 20 mg/mL | Physically compatible for 4 hours at 25°C in fluorescent light. |
| | Cefotaxime Sodium | Y | Dextrose 5% | 20 mg/mL & 20 mg/mL | Physically compatible for 4 hours at 25°C in fluorescent light. |
| | Cefoxitin Sodium | Y | Dextrose 5% | 20 mg/mL & 20 mg/mL | Physically compatible for 4 hours at 25°C in fluorescent light. |
| | Cefuroxime Sodium | Y | Dextrose 5% | 20 mg/mL & 30 mg/mL | Physically compatible for 4 hours at 25°C in fluorescent light. |
| | Cephalothin Sodium | Y | Dextrose 5% | 20 mg/mL & 20 mg/mL | Physically compatible for 4 hours at 25°C in fluorescent light. |
| | Cephapirin Sodium | Y | Dextrose 5% | 20 mg/mL & 20 mg/mL | Physically compatible for 4 hours at 25°C in fluorescent light. |
| | Chloramphenicol Sodium Succinate | Y | Dextrose 5% | 20 mg/mL & 20 mg/mL | Physically compatible for 4 hours at 25°C in fluorescent light. |
| | Clindamycin Phosphate | Y | Dextrose 5% | 20 mg/mL & 12 mg/mL | Physically compatible for 4 hours at 25°C in fluorescent light. |
| | Doxycycline Hyclate | Y | Dextrose 5% | 20 mg/mL & 1 mg/mL | Physically compatible for 4 hours at 25°C in fluorescent light. |
| | Droperidol | Y | Not applicable | 20 mg/mL & 2.5 mg/mL | No visible precipitate after sequential injection. |
| | Erythromycin Lactobionate | Y | Dextrose 5% | 20 mg/mL & 5 mg/mL | Physically compatible for 4 hours at 25°C in fluorescent light. |
| | Furosemide | Y | Not applicable | 20 mg/mL & 10 mg/mL | No visible precipitate after sequential injection. |
| | Gentamicin Sulfate | Y | Dextrose 5% | 20 mg/mL & 1.6 mg/mL | Physically compatible for 4 hours at 25°C in fluorescent light. |
| | Heparin Sodium | Y | Not applicable | 20 mg/mL & 1,000 units/mL | No visible precipitate after sequential injection. |
| | Hydroxyzine Hydrocloride | A | Dextrose 5% | 1 mg/mL & 0.5 mg/mL | Physically compatible for 48 hours. |

*(continued)*

**Appendix 2. Cancer Chemotherapy Agents Compatibility Chart (continued)**

*Part B: Oncology Product with Other Products*

| Oncology Product | Other Product | Condition* | Diluting Solution | Concentration of Products | Stability and Compatibility Comments |
|---|---|---|---|---|---|
| *Cyclophosphamide* (continued) | Kanamycin Sulfate | Y | Dextrose 5% | 20 mg/mL & 2.5 mg/mL | Physically compatible for 4 hours at 25°C in fluorescent light. |
| | Leucovorin Sodium | Y | Not applicable | 20 mg/mL & 10 mg/mL | No visible precipitate after sequential injection. |
| | Metoclopramide Hydrochloride | Y | Not applicable | 20 mg/mL & 5 mg/mL | No visible precipitate after sequential injection. |
| | Metoclopramide Hydrochloride | A | See manufacturer's package insert | 560 mg & 10–160 mg | Physically compatible for 24 hours at 25°C. |
| | Metronidazole | Y | Dextrose 5% | 20 mg/mL & 5 mg/mL | Physically compatible for 4 hours at 25°C in fluorescent light. |
| | Mezlocillin Sodium | Y | Dextrose 5% | 20 mg/mL & 80 mg/mL | Physically compatible for 4 hours at 25°C in fluorescent light. |
| | Minocycline Hydrochloride | Y | Dextrose 5% | 20 mg/mL & 0.2 mg/mL | Physically compatible for 4 hours at 25°C in fluorescent light. |
| | Moxalactam | Y | Dextrose 5% | 20 mg/mL & 20 mg/mL | Physically compatible for 4 hours at 25°C in fluorescent light. |
| | Nafcillin Sodium | Y | Dextrose 5% | 20 mg/mL & 20 mg/mL | Physically compatible for 4 hours at 25°C in fluorescent light. |
| | Ondansetron Hydrochloride | Y | Dextrose 5% & Sodium Chloride 0.9% | 10 mg/mL & 1 mg/mL | Physically compatible for 4 hours at 22°C in fluorescent light. |
| | Ondansetron Hydrochloride | Y | Not applicable | 20 mg/mL & 16–160 µg/mL | Physically compatible with cyclophosphamide as a 5-minute bolus. |
| | Oxacillin Sodium | Y | Dextrose 5% | 20 mg/mL & 20 mg/mL | Physically compatible for 4 hours at 25°C in fluorescent light. |
| | Penicillin G Potassium | Y | Dextrose 5% | 20 mg/mL & 100,000 units/mL | Physically compatible for 4 hours at 25°C in fluorescent light. |
| | Piperacillin Sodium | Y | Dextrose 5% | 20 mg/mL & 60 mg/mL | Physically compatible for 4 hours at 25°C in fluorescent light. |
| | Sargramostim | Y | Sodium Chloride 0.9% | 10 mg/mL & 10 µg/mL | Physically compatible for 4 hours at 22°C in fluorescent light. |
| | Tetracycline Hydrochloride | Y | Dextrose 5% | 20 mg/mL & 2.5 mg/mL | Physically compatible for 4 hours at 25°C in fluorescent light. |
| | Ticarcillin Disodium | Y | Dextrose 5% | 20 mg/mL & 30 mg/mL | Physically compatible for 4 hours at 25°C in fluorescent light. |
| | Tobramycin Sulfate | Y | Dextrose 5% | 20 mg/mL & 0.8 mg/mL | Physically compatible for 4 hours at 25°C in fluorescent light. |

| | Drug | Code | Solution | Concentration | Remarks |
|---|---|---|---|---|---|
| | Trimethoprim/Sulfamethoxazole | Y | Dextrose 5% | 20 mg/mL & 0.8/4 mg/mL | Physically compatible for 4 hours at 25°C in fluorescent light. |
| | Vancomycin Hydrochloride | Y | Dextrose 5% | 20 mg/mL & 5 mg/mL | Physically compatible for 4 hours at 25°C in fluorescent light. |
| *Cytarabine* | Carbenicillin Disodium | A | Dextrose 5% | 0.1 mg/mL & 0.6 mg/mL | Incompatible. Outside the pH range for carbenicillin. |
| | Cephalothin Sodium | A | Dextrose 5% | 0.8 mg/mL & 1 mg/mL | Both drugs stable for 8 hours at 25°C. |
| | Gentamicin Sulfate | A | Dextrose 5% | 0.1 mg/mL & 0.08 mg/mL | Physically compatible for 24 hours. |
| | Gentamicin Sulfate | A | Dextrose 5% | 0.3 mg/mL & 0.24 mg/mL | Incompatible. |
| | Heparin Sodium | A | Dextrose 5% & Sodium Chloride 0.9% | 0.5 mg/mL & 10–20 units/mL | Incompatible. Haze forms. |
| | Hydrocortisone Sodium Succinate | A | Dextrose 5% & Sodium Chloride 0.9% | 0.36 mg/mL & 0.5 mg/mL | Physically compatible for 40 hours. |
| | Hydrocortisone Sodium Succinate | A | Ringer's | 0.36 mg/mL & 0.5 mg/mL | Incompatible. |
| | Hydroxyzine Hydrochloride | A | Dextrose 5% | 1 mg/mL & 0.5 mg/mL | Physically compatible for 48 hours in glass containers. |
| | Insulin, Regular | A | Dextrose 5% | 0.1 mg/mL & 40 units/L | Incompatible. Fine precipitate. |
| | Insulin, Regular | A | Dextrose 5% | 0.5 mg/mL & 40 units/mL | Incompatible. Fine precipitate. |
| | Methylprednisolone Sodium Succinate | A | Dextrose 5% & Sodium Chloride 0.9% | 0.36 mg/mL & 0.25 mg/mL | Physically compatible for 24 hours. |
| | Methylprednisolone Sodium Succinate | A | Dextrose 10% & Sodium Chloride 0.9% | 0.36 mg/mL & 0.25 mg/mL | Physically compatible for 24 hours. |
| | Methylprednisolone Sodium Succinate | A | Sodium Lactate 1/6 molar | 0.36 mg/mL & 0.25 mg/mL | Incompatible. |
| | Methylprednisolone Sodium Succinate | A | Ringer's | 0.36 mg/mL & 0.25 mg/mL | Incompatible. |
| | Metoclopramide Hydrochloride | A | See manufacturer's package inserts | 50–500 mg & 10–160 mg | Physically compatible for 48 hours at 25°C. |
| | Nafcillin Sodium | A | Dextrose 5% | 0.1 mg/mL & 4 mg/mL | Incompatible. Precipitates. |
| | Ondansetron Hydrochloride | Y | Sodium Chloride 0.9% | 50 mg/mL & 1 mg/mL | Physically compatible for 4 hours at 22°C in fluorescent light. |
| | Oxacillin Sodium | A | Dextrose 5% | 0.1 mg/mL & 2 mg/mL | Incompatible. Outside the pH range for oxacillin. |
| | Penicillin G Sodium | A | Dextrose 5% | 0.2 mg/mL & 2 MU/L | Incompatible. Outside the pH range for penicillin G sodium. |

*(continued)*

## Appendix 2. Cancer Chemotherapy Agents Compatibility Chart (continued)

### Part B: Oncology Product with Other Products

| Oncology Product | Other Product | Condition* | Diluting Solution | Concentration of Products | Stability and Compatibility Comments |
|---|---|---|---|---|---|
| *Cytarabine* (continued) | Potassium Chloride | A | Dextrose 5% & Sodium Chloride 0.9% | 0.17 mg/mL & 80 mEq/L | Physically compatible for 24 hours. |
| | Potassium Chloride | A | Dextrose 5% & Sodium Chloride 0.9% | 2 mg/mL & 100 mEq/L | Physically compatible and stable for 8 days. |
| | Prednisolone Sodium Phosphate | A | Dextrose 5% | 0.4 mg/mL & 0.2 mg/mL | Both drugs stable for 8 hours at 25°C. |
| | Sargramostim | Y | Sodium Chloride 0.9% | 50 mg/mL & 10 µg/mL | Physically compatible for 4 hours at 22°C in fluorescent light. |
| | Sodium Bicarbonate | A | Dextrose 5% | 0.2–1 mg/mL & 0.05 mEq/mL | Stable for 7 days at 8°C and at 22°C inglass or PVC containers. |
| | Sodium Bicarbonate | A | Dextrose 5% & Sodium Chloride 0.225% | 0.2–1 mg/mL & 0.05 mEq/mL | Stable for 7 days at 8°C and at 22°C inglass or PVC containers. |
| *Dacarbazine* | Heparin Sodium | A | Sodium Chloride 0.9% | 10 mg/mL & 100 units/mL | Incompatible. Precipitates in IV line. |
| | Hydrocortisone Sodium Phosphate | A | Not stated | Not stated | Physically compatible. |
| | Hydrocortisone Sodium Succinate | A | Not stated | Not stated | Incompatible. Precipitates. |
| | Lidocaine Hydrochloride | A | Not stated | Not stated & 1% or 2% | Physically compatible. |
| | Metoclopramide Hydrochloride | A | See manufacturer's package inserts | 140 mg & 10–160 mg | Physically compatible for 8 hours at 25°C. |
| | Ondansetron Hydrochloride | Y | Dextrose 5% & Sodium Chloride 0.9% | 4 mg/mL & 1 mg/mL | Physically compatible for 4 hours at 22°C in fluorescent light. |
| | Sargramostim | Y | Sodium Chloride 0.9% | 4 mg/mL & 10 µg/mL | Physically compatible for 4 hours at 22°C in fluorescent light. |
| *Dactinomycin* | Ondansetron Hydrochloride | Y | Dextrose 5% & Sodium Chloride 0.9% | 0.01 mg/mL & 1 mg/mL | Physically compatible for 4 hours at 22°C in fluorescent light. |
| | Sargramostim | Y | Sodium Chloride 0.9% | 0.01 mg/mL & 10 µg/mL | Physically compatible for 4 hours at 22°C in fluorescent light. |

| Drug | Second Drug | A/Y | Solution | Concentration | Remarks |
|---|---|---|---|---|---|
| *Daunorubicin* | Dexamethasone Sodium Phosphate | A | Not stated | Not stated | Incompatible. Precipitates. |
| | Heparin Sodium | A | Dextrose 5% | 0.2 mg/mL & 4 units/mL | Incompatible. |
| | Hydrocortisone Sodium Succinate | A | Dextrose 5% | 0.2 mg/mL & 0.5 mg/mL | Physically compatible. |
| | Ondansetron Hydrochloride | Y | Dextrose 5% & Sodium Chloride 0.9% | 2 mg/mL & 1 mg/mL | Physically compatible for 4 hours at 22°C in fluorescent light. |
| *Doxorubicin* | Aminophylline | A | Not stated | Not stated | Incompatible. Color change. |
| | Cephalothin Sodium | A | Not stated | Not stated | Incompatible. Precipitates. |
| | Dexamethasone Sodium Phosphate | A | Not stated | Not stated | Incompatible. Precipitates. |
| | Diazepam | A | Not stated | Not stated | Incompatible. Precipitates. |
| | Droperidol | Y | Not applicable | 2 mg/mL & 2.5 mg/mL | No visible precipitate after sequential injection. |
| | Furosemide | A | See manufacturer's package inserts | 2 mg/mL & 10 mg/mL | Incompatible. Precipitates. |
| | Heparin Sodium | A | See manufacturer's package inserts | 2 mg/mL & 1,000 units/mL | Incompatible. Precipitates. |
| | Hydrocortisone Sodium Succinate | A | Not stated | Not stated | Incompatible. Precipitates. |
| | Leucovorin Calcium | Y | Not applicable | 2 mg/mL & 10 mg/mL | Not visible precipitate after sequential injection. |
| | Metoclopramide Hydrochloride | A | See manufacturer's package inserts | 103.8 mg & 10–160 mg | Physically compatible for 24 hours at 25°C. |
| | Ondansetron Hydrochloride | Y | Sodium Chloride 0.9% | 2 mg/mL & 1 mg/mL | Physically compatible for 4 hours at 22°C in fluorescent light. |
| | Sargramostim | Y | Sodium Chloride 0.9% | 2 mg/mL & 10 μg/mL | Physically compatible for 4 hours at 22°C in flourescent light. |
| *Etoposide* | Hydroxyzine Hydrochloride | A | Dextrose 5% | 1 mg/mL & 0.5 mg/mL | Physically compatible for 48 hours. |
| | Metoclopramide Hydrochloride | A | See manufacturer's package inserts | 86.5 mg & 10–160 mg | Physically compatible for 48 hours at 25°C. |
| | Morphine Sulfate | A | Not stated | Not stated & 50 mg/mL | Stable for 24 hours. |
| | Ondansetron Hydrochloride | Y | Dextrose 5% & Sodium Chloride 0.9% | 0.4 mg/mL & 1 mg/mL | Physically compatible for 4 hours at 22°C in fluorescent light. |
| | Potassium Chloride | A | Sodium Chloride 0.9% | 0.2–0.4 mg/mL & 0.04 mEq/mL | Physically compatible for 8 hours. |

*(continued)*

**Appendix 2. Cancer Chemotherapy Agents Compatibility Chart** (*continued*)

*Part B: Oncology Product with Other Products*

| Oncology Product | Other Product | Condition* | Diluting Solution | Concentration of Products | Stability and Compatibility Comments |
|---|---|---|---|---|---|
| *Etoposide* (*continued*) | Potassium Chloride | A | Dextrose 5% | 0.2–0.4 mg/mL & 0.04 mEq/mL | Physically compatible for 8 hours. |
| | Potassium Chloride | A | Lactated Ringer's | 0.2–0.4 mg/mL & 0.04 mEq/mL | Physically compatible for 8 hours. |
| | Potassium Chloride | A | Mannitol 10% | 0.2–0.4 mg/mL & 0.04 mEq/mL | Physically compatible for 8 hours. |
| | Sargramostim | Y | Sodium Chloride 0.9% | 0.4 mg/mL & 10 µg/mL | Physically compatible for 4 hours at room temperature in fluorescent light. |
| *Floxuridine* | Heparin Sodium | A | Sodium Chloride 0.9% | 2.5–12 mg/mL & 200 units/mL | Stable for 4 days at 37°C. |
| | Ondansetron Hydrochloride | Y | Dextrose 5% & Sodium Chloride 0.9% | 3 mg/mL & 1 mg/mL | Physically compatible for 4 hours at 22°C in fluorescent light. |
| *Fludarabine* | Acyclovir Sodium | Y | Dextrose 5% | 1 mg/mL & 7 mg/mL | Physically incompatible at 4 hours. Darker color visible. |
| | Amikacin Sulfate | Y | Dextrose 5% | 1 mg/mL & 5 mg/mL | Physically compatible for 4 hours at room temperature in fluorescent light. |
| | Aminophylline | Y | Dextrose 5% | 1 mg/mL & 2.5 mg/mL | Physically compatible for 4 hours at room temperature in fluorescent light. |
| | Amphotericin B | Y | Dextrose 5% | 1 mg/mL & 0.6 mg/mL | Incompatible. Small amount of precipitate forms within 4 hours at room temperature in fluorescent light. |
| | Ampicillin Sodium | Y | Dextrose 5% & Sodium Chloride 0.9% | 1 mg/mL & 20 mg/mL | Physically compatible for 4 hours at room temperature in fluorescent light. |
| | Ampicillin Sodium/ Sulbactam Sodium | Y | Dextrose 5% & Sodium Chloride 0.9% | 1 mg/mL & 20/10 mg/mL | Physically compatible for 4 hours at room temperature in fluorescent light. |
| | Aztreonam | Y | Dextrose 5% | 1 mg/mL & 40 mg/mL | Physically compatible for 4 hours at room temperature in fluorescent light. |
| | Butorphanol Tartrate | Y | Dextrose 5% | 1 mg/mL & 0.04 mg/mL | Physically compatible for 4 hours at room temperature in fluorescent light. |
| | Cefazolin Sodium | Y | Dextrose 5% | 1 mg/mL & 20 mg/mL | Physically compatible for 4 hours at room temperature in fluorescent light. |
| | Cefoperazone Sodium | Y | Dextrose 5% | 1 mg/mL & 40 mg/mL | Physically compatible for 4 hours at room temperature in fluorescent light. |

| Drug | | Solution | Concentration | Remarks |
|---|---|---|---|---|
| Cefonicid | Y | Dextrose 5% | 1 mg/mL & 20 mg/mL | Physically compatible for 4 hours at room temperature in fluorescent light. |
| Cefotaxime Sodium | Y | Dextrose 5% | 1 mg/mL & 20 mg/mL | Physically compatible for 4 hours at room temperature in fluorescent light. |
| Cefotetan Disodium | Y | Dextrose 5% | 1 mg/mL & 20 mg/mL | Physically compatible for 4 hours at room temperature in fluorescent light. |
| Ceftazidime | Y | Dextrose 5% | 1 mg/mL & 40 mg/mL | Physically compatible for 4 hours at room temperature in fluorescent light. |
| Ceftizoxime Sodium | Y | Dextrose 5% | 1 mg/mL & 20 mg/mL | Physically compatible for 4 hours at room temperature in fluorescent light. |
| Ceftriaxone Sodium | Y | Dextrose 5% | 1 mg/mL & 20 mg/mL | Physically compatible for 4 hours at room temperature in fluorescent light. |
| Cefuroxime Sodium | Y | Dextrose 5% | 1 mg/mL & 30 mg/mL | Physically compatible for 4 hours at room temperature in fluorescent light. |
| Chlorpromazine Hydrochloride | | Dextrose 5% | 1 mg/mL & 2 mg/mL | Incompatible. Haze forms within 30 minutes at room temperature in fluorescent light. |
| Cimetidine Hydrochloride | Y | Dextrose 5% | 1 mg/mL & 12 mg/mL | Physically compatible for 4 hours at room temperature in fluorescent light. |
| Clindamycin | Y | Dextrose 5% | 1 mg/mL & 10 mg/mL | Physically compatible for 4 hours at room temperature in fluorescent light. |
| Dexamethasone Sodium Phosphate | Y | Dextrose 5% | 1 mg/mL & 1 mg/mL | Physically compatible for 4 hours at room temperature in fluorescent light. |
| Diphenhydramine Hydrochloride | Y | Dextrose 5% | 1 mg/mL & 2 mg/mL | Physically compatible for 4 hours at room temperature in fluorescent light. |
| Doxycycline Hyclate | Y | Dextrose 5% | 1 mg/mL & 1 mg/mL | Physically compatible for 4 hours at room temperature in fluorescent light. |
| Droperidol | Y | Dextrose 5% | 1 mg/mL & 0.4 mg/mL | Physically compatible for 4 hours at room temperature in fluorescent light. |
| Famotidine | Y | Dextrose 5% | 1 mg/mL & 2 mg/mL | Physically compatible for 4 hours at room temperature in fluorescent light. |
| Fluconazole | Y | Dextrose 5% | 1 mg/mL & 2 mg/mL | Physically compatible for 4 hours at room temperature in fluorescent light. |
| Furosemide | Y | Dextrose 5% | 1 mg/mL & 3 mg/mL | Physically compatible for 4 hours at room temperature in fluorescent light. |
| Ganciclovir Sodium | Y | Dextrose 5% | 1 mg/mL & 20 mg/mL | Incompatible. Dark color forms within 4 hours at room temperature in fluorescent light. |
| Haloperidol Lactate | Y | Dextrose 5% | 1 mg/mL & 0.2 mg/mL | Physically compatible for 4 hours at room temperature in fluorescent light. |
| Heparin Sodium | Y | Dextrose 5% | 1 mg/mL & 40 units/mL | Physically compatible for 4 hours at room temperature in fluorescent light. |

(continued)

## Appendix 2. Cancer Chemotherapy Agents Compatibility Chart (continued)

*Part B: Oncology Product with Other Products*

| Oncology Product | Other Product | Condition* | Diluting Solution | Concentration of Products | Stability and Compatibility Comments |
|---|---|---|---|---|---|
| *Fludarabine* (continued) | Heparin Sodium | Y | Dextrose 5% | 1 mg/mL & 100 units/mL | Physically compatible for 4 hours at room temperature in fluorescent light. |
| | Heparin Sodium | Y | Dextrose 5% | 1 mg/mL & 1,000 units/mL | Physically compatible for 4 hours at room temperature in fluorescent light. |
| | Sargramostim | Y | Sodium Chloride 0.9% | 3 mg/mL & μg/mL | Physically compatible for 4 hours at 22°C in fluorescent light. |
| | Zidovudine | Y | Dextrose 5% | 1 mg/mL & 4 mg/mL | Physically compatible for 4 hours at room temperature in fluorescent light. |
| *Fluorouracil* | Cephalothin Sodium | A | Dextrose 5% | 0.5 mg/mL & 1 mg/mL | Both drugs stable for 8 hours at 25°C. No UV spectrum changes. |
| | Diazepam | A | Not stated | Not stated | Incompatible. Precipitates. |
| | Droperidol | A | See manufacturer's package inserts | 50 mg/mL & 2.5 mg/mL | Incompatible. Precipitates. |
| | Droperidol | Y | Not applicable | 50 mg/mL & 25 mg/mL | Incompatible. Precipitates immediately. |
| | Furosemide | Y | Not applicable | 50 mg/mL & 10 mg/mL | No visible precipitate after sequential injection. |
| | Heparin Sodium | Y | Not applicable | 50 mg/mL & 1,000 units/mL | No visible precipitate after sequential injection. |
| | Hydrocortisone Sodium Succinate | Y | Lactated Ringer's | 50 mg/mL & 10 mg/mL | Physically compatible for 4 hours at room temperature. |
| | Leucovorin Calcium | A | Sodium Chloride 0.9% | 10 mg/mL & 0.2 mg/mL | Stable for 15 days at room temperature when protected from light. |
| | Mannitol | Y | Dextrose 5% & Sodium Chloride 0.45% | 1 mg/mL & 200 mg/mL | No precipitate or color change after 24 hours. |
| | Mannitol | Y | Dextrose 5% & Sodium Chloride 0.9% | 1 mg/mL & 200 mg/mL | No precipitate or color change after 24 hours. |
| | Mannitol | Y | Dextrose 5% & Sodium Chloride 0.45% | 2 mg/mL & 200 mg/mL | No precipitate or color change after 24 hours. |
| | Mannitol | Y | Dextrose 5% & Sodium Chloride 0.9% | 2 mg/mL & 200 mg/mL | No precipitate or color change after 24 hours. |
| | Metoclopramide Hydrochloride | Y | Not applicable | 50 mg/mL & 5 mg/mL | No visible precipitate after sequential injection. |
| | Metoclopramide Hydrochloride | A | See manufacturer's package inserts | 840 mg & 10–160 mg | Incompatible. |

| Drug | | Agent | Concentration | Solution | Remarks |
|---|---|---|---|---|---|
| | Y | Ondansetron Hydrochloride | Not applicable | <0.8 mg/mL & 16–160 µg/mL | Physically compatible when fluorouracil is administered at 20 mL/hour. |
| | Y | Ondansetron Hydrochloride | Dextrose 5% & Sodium Chloride 0.9% | 16 mg/mL & 1 mg/mL | Incompatible. Precipitates immediately. |
| | Y | Potassium Chloride | Sodium Chloride 0.9% | 50 mg/mL & 40 mEq/L | Physically compatible for 4 hours at room temperature. |
| | A | Prednisolone Sodium Phosphate | Dextrose 5% | 0.25 mg/mL & 0.2 mg/mL | Both drugs stable for 8 hours at 25°C. No UV spectrum changes. |
| | Y | Sargramostim | Sodium Chloride 0.9% | 16 mg/mL & 10 µg/mL | Physically compatible for 4 hours at 22°C in fluorescent light. |
| | Y | Vitamin B Complex with Vitamin C | Sodium Chloride 0.9% | 50 mg/mL & 2 mg/mL | Physically compatible for 4 hours at room temperature. |
| *Idarubicin* | A | Heparin Sodium | Not stated | Not stated | Incompatible. Precipitates immediately. |
| | Y | Sargramostim | Sodium Chloride 0.9% | 0.5 mg/mL & 10 µg/mL | Incompatible. Haze forms immediately. |
| *Ifosfamide* | Y | Ondansetron Hydrochloride | Dextrose 5% & Sodium Chloride 0.9% | 25 mg/mL & 1 mg/mL | Physically compatible for 4 hours at 22°C in fluorescent light. |
| | Y | Sargramostim | Sodium Chloride 0.9% | 25 mg/ml & 10 µg/mL | Physically compatible for 4 hours at 22°C in fluorescent light. |
| *Leucovorin* | Y | Droperidol | Not applicable | 10 mg/mL & 2.5 mg/mL | Incompatible. Precipitates immediately. |
| | Y | Fluconazole | Not applicable | 10 mg/mL & 2 mg/mL | Physically compatible for 24 hours at room temperature in fluorescent light. |
| | Y | Foscarnet Sodium | Not applicable | 10 mg/mL & 24 mg/mL | Incompatible. Cloudy yellow solution. |
| | Y | Furosemide | Not applicable | 10 mg/mL & 10 mg/mL | No visible precipitate after sequential injection. |
| | Y | Heparin Sodium | Not applicable | 10 mg/mL & 1,000 units/mL | No visible precipitate after sequential injection. |
| | Y | Metoclopramide Hydrochloride | Not applicable | 10 mg/mL & 5 mg/mL | No visible precipitate after sequential injection. |
| *Mechlorethamine* | A | Methohexital Sodium | Dextrose 5% | 0.04 mg/mL & 2 mg/mL | Unstable. Drug decomposes within 3 hours. |
| | A | Methohexital Sodium | Sodium Chloride 0.9% | 0.04 mg/mL & 2 mg/mL | Unstable. Drug decomposes within 3 hours. |
| | Y | Ondansetron Hydrochloride | Sodium Chloride 0.9% | 1 mg/mL & 1 mg/mL | Physically compatible for 4 hours at 22°C in fluorescent light. |
| | Y | Sargramostim | Sodium Chloride 0.9% | 1 mg/mL & 10 µg/mL | Physically compatible for 4 hours at 22°C in fluorescent light. |

*(continued)*

## Appendix 2. Cancer Chemotherapy Agents Compatibility Chart (continued)

### Part B: Oncology Product with Other Products

| Oncology Product | Other Product | Condition* | Diluting Solution | Concentration of Products | Stability and Compatibility Comments |
|---|---|---|---|---|---|
| *Mesna* | Hydroxyzine Hydrochloride | A | Dextrose 5% | 3 mg/mL & 0.5 mg/mL | Physically compatible for 48 hours. |
| | Ondansetron Hydrochloride | Y | Dextrose 5% & Sodium Chloride 0.9% | 10 mg/mL & 1 mg/mL | Physically compatible for 4 hours at 22°C in fluorescent light. |
| | Sargramostim | Y | Sodium Chloride 0.9% | 10 mg/mL & 10 µg/mL | Physically compatible for 4 hours at 22°C in fluorescent light. |
| *Methotrexate* | Cephalothin Sodium | A | Dextrose 5% | 0.4 mg/mL & 1 mg/mL | Both drugs stable for 8 hours at 25°C. No UV spectrum changes. |
| | Droperidol | A | See manufacturer's package inserts | 25 mg/mL & 2.5 mg/mL | Incompatible. Precipitates. |
| | Furosemide | Y | Not applicable | 25 mg/mL & 10 mg/mL | No visible precipitate after sequential injection. |
| | Heparin Sodium | Y | Not applicable | 25 mg/mL & 1,000 units/mL | No visible precipitate after sequential injection. |
| | Hydroxyzine Hydrochloride | A | Dextrose 5% | 1 mg/mL & 0.5 mg/mL | Physically compatible at 48 hours. |
| | Hydroxyzine Hydrochloride | A | Dextrose 5% | 3 mg/mL & 0.5 mg/mL | Physically compatible at 48 hours. |
| | Leucovorin Calcium | Y | Not applicable | 25 mg/mL & 10 mg/mL | No visible precipitate after sequential injection. |
| | Metoclopramide Hydrochloride | Y | Not applicable | 25 mg/mL & 5 mg/mL | No visible precipitate after sequential injection. |
| | Metoclopramide Hydrochloride | A | See manufacturer's package inserts | 50–200 mg & 10–160 mg | Use immediately. |
| | Ondansetron Hydrochloride | Y | Dextrose 5% & Sodium Chloride 0.9% | 15 mg/mL & 1 mg/mL | Physically compatible for 4 hours at 22°C in fluorescent light. |
| | Prednisolone Sodium Phosphate | A | Dextrose 5% | 0.2 mg/mL & 0.2 mg/mL | Unstable. Both drugs decompose within 1 hour at 25°C. UV spectrum changes. |
| | Sargramostim | Y | Sodium Chloride 0.9% | 15 mg/mL & 10 µg/mL | Physically compatible for 4 hours at 22°C in fluorescent light. |
| | Sodium Bicarbonate | A | Dextrose 5% | 0.75 mg/mL & 0.05 mEq/mL | Stable for 7 days at 5°C and for 72 hours at 25°C when exposed to light. |
| | Vancomycin Hydrochloride | Y | Not applicable | Not stated & 0.51 mg/mL | Physically compatible for 1 hour during simultaneous fusion. |

| Drug | Agent | | Solution | Concentration | Remarks |
|---|---|---|---|---|---|
| *Mitomycin* | Droperidol | Y | Not applicable | 0.5 mg/mL & 2.5 mg/mL | No visible precipitate after sequential injection. |
| | Furosemide | Y | Not applicable | 0.5 mg/mL & 10 mg/mL | No visible precipitate after sequential injection. |
| | Heparin Sodium | Y | Not applicable | 0.5 mg/mL & 1,000 units/mL | No visible precipitate after sequential injection. |
| | Heparin Sodium | A | Sodium Chloride 0.9% | 5–15 mg/30 mL & 1,000–10,000 units/30 mL | Stable for 48 hours at 25°C. |
| | Leucovorin Calcium | Y | Not applicable | 0.5 mg/mL & 10 mg/mL | No visible precipitate after sequential injection. |
| | Ondansetron Hydrochloride | Y | Sodium Chloride 0.9% | 0.5 mg/mL & 1 mg/mL | Physically compatible for 4 hours at 22°C in fluorescent light. |
| | Sargramostim | Y | Sodium Chloride 0.9% | 0.5 mg/mL & 10 µg/mL | Incompatible. Slight haze forms in 30 minutes. |
| *Mitoxantrone* | Hydrocortisone Sodium Phosphate | A | Dextrose 5% | 0.05–0.2 mg/mL & 0.1–2 mg/mL | Incompatible. Blue precipitate forms in PVC containers. |
| | Hydrocortisone Sodium Phosphate | A | Dextrose 5% | 0.05–0.2 mg/mL & 0.1–2 mg/mL | Physically compatible in glass containers. |
| | Hydrocortisone Sodium Phosphate | A | Sodium Chloride 0.9% | 0.05–0.2 mg/mL & 0.1–2 mg/mL | Physically compatible and stable for 24 hours at room temperature. |
| | Ondansetron Hydrochloride | Y | Dextrose 5% & Sodium Chloride 0.9% | 0.5 mg/mL & 1 mg/mL | Physically compatible for 4 hours at 22°C in fluorescent light. |
| | Sargramostim | Y | Sodium Chloride 0.9% | 0.5 mg/mL & 10 µg/mL | Physically compatible for 4 hours at 22°C in fluorescent light. |
| *Paclitaxel* | Acyclovir Sodium | Y | Dextrose 5% | 1.2 mg/mL & 7 mg/mL | No precipitate or change in color or turbidity within 4 hours. |
| | Amikacin Sulfate | Y | Dextrose 5% | 1.2 mg/mL & 5 mg/mL | No precipitate or change in color or turbidity within 4 hours. |
| | Aminophylline | Y | Dextrose 5% | 1.2 mg/mL & 2.5 mg/mL | No precipitate or change in color or turbidity within 4 hours. |
| | Amphotericin B | Y | Dextrose 5% | 1.2 mg/mL & 0.6 mg/mL | Incompatible. Increased turbidity immediately. |
| | Ampicillin Sodium/ Sulbactam Sodium | Y | Dextrose 5% & Sodium Chloride 0.9% | 1.2 mg/mL & 20/10 mg/mL | No precipitate or change in color or turbidity within 4 hours. |
| | Butorphanol Tartrate | Y | Dextrose 5% | 1.2 mg/mL & 0.04 mg/mL | No precipitate or change in color or turbidity within 4 hours. |
| | Calcium Chloride | Y | Dextrose 5% | 1.2 mg/mL & 20 mg/mL | No precipitate or change in color or turbidity within 4 hours. |
| | Ceforanide | Y | Dextrose 5% | 1.2 mg/mL & 20 mg/mL | No precipitate or change in color or turbidity within 4 hours. |
| | Cefotetan Disodium | Y | Dextrose 5% | 1.2 mg/mL & 20 mg/mL | No precipitate or change in color or turbidity within 4 hours. |

(continued)

## Appendix 2. Cancer Chemotherapy Agents Compatibility Chart (continued)

*Part B: Oncology Product with Other Products*

| Oncology Product | Other Product | Condition* | Diluting Solution | Concentration of Products | Stability and Compatibility Comments |
|---|---|---|---|---|---|
| *Paclitaxel (continued)* | Ceftazidime | Y | Dextrose 5% | 1.2 mg/mL & 40 mg/mL | No precipitate or change in color or turbidity within 4 hours. |
| | Ceftriaxone Sodium | Y | Dextrose 5% | 1.2 mg/mL & 20 mg/mL | No precipitate or change in color or turbidity within 4 hours. |
| | Chlorpromazine Hydrochloride | Y | Dextrose 5% | 1.2 mg/mL & 2 mg/mL | Incompatible. Decreased turbidity, below normal range. |
| | Cimetidine Hydrochloride | Y | Dextrose 5% | 1.2 mg/mL & 12 mg/mL | No precipitate, color change, or gas production within 4 hours. |
| | Dexamethasone Sodium Phosphate | Y | Dextrose 5% | 1.2 mg/mL & 1 mg/mL | No precipitate, color change, or gas production within 4 hours. |
| | Diphenhydramine Hydrochloride | Y | Dextrose 5% | 1.2 mg/mL & 2 mg/mL | No precipitate, color change, or gas production within 4 hours. |
| | Droperidol | Y | Dextrose 5% | 1.2 mg/mL & 0.4 mg/mL | No precipitate or change in color or turbidity within 4 hours. |
| | Famotidine | Y | Dextrose 5% | 1.2 mg/mL & 2 mg/mL | No precipitate or change in color or turbidity within 4 hours. |
| | Fluconazole | Y | Dextrose 5% | 1.2 mg/mL & 2 mg/mL | No precipitate or change in color or turbidity within 4 hours. |
| | Furosemide | Y | Dextrose 5% | 1.2 mg/mL & 3 mg/mL | No precipitate or change in color or turbidity within 4 hours. |
| | Ganciclovir Sodium | Y | Dextrose 5% | 1.2 mg/mL & 20 mg/mL | No precipitate or change in color or turbidity within 4 hours. |
| | Gentamicin Sulfate | Y | Dextrose 5% | 1.2 mg/mL & 5 mg/mL | No precipitate or change in color or turbidity within 4 hours. |
| | Haloperidol Lactate | Y | Dextrose 5% | 1.2 mg/mL & 0.2 mg/mL | No precipitate, color change, or gas production within 4 hours. |
| | Heparin Sodium | Y | Dextrose 5% | 1.2 mg/mL & 100 units/mL | No precipitate or change in color or turbidity within 4 hours. |
| | Hydrocortisone Sodium Phosphate | Y | Dextrose 5% | 1.2 mg/mL & 1 mg/mL | No precipitate or change in color or turbidity within 4 hours. |
| | Hydrocortisone Sodium Succinate | Y | Dextrose 5% | 1.2 mg/mL & 1 mg/mL | Incompatible. Decreased turbidity, below normal range. |
| | Hydromorphone Hydrochloride | Y | Dextrose 5% | 1.2 mg/mL & 0.5 mg/mL | No precipitate or change in color or turbidity within 4 hours. |
| | Hydroxyzine Hydrochloride | Y | Dextrose 5% | 1.2 mg/mL & 4 mg/mL | Incompatible. Decreased turbidity, below normal range. |

| Drug | | Solution | Concentration | Remarks |
|---|---|---|---|---|
| Lorazepam | Y | Dextrose 5% | 1.2 mg/mL & 0.1 mg/mL | No precipitate or change in color or turbidity within 4 hours. |
| Magnesium Sulfate | Y | Dextrose 5% | 1.2 mg/mL & 100 mg/mL | No precipitate or change in color or turbidity within 4 hours. |
| Mannitol | Y | Dextrose 5% | 1.2 mg/mL & 150 mg/mL | No precipitate or change in color or turbidity within 4 hours. |
| Meperidine Hydrochloride | Y | Dextrose 5% | 1.2 mg/mL & 4 mg/mL | No precipitate or change in color or turbidity within 4 hours. |
| Mesna | Y | Dextrose 5% | 1.2 mg/mL & 10 mg/mL | No precipitate or change in color or turbidity within 4 hours. |
| Methylprednisolone Sodium Succinate | Y | Dextrose 5% | 1.2 mg/mL & 5 mg/mL | Incompatible. Decreased turbidity, below normal range. |
| Metoclopramide Hydrochloride | Y | Dextrose 5% | 1.2 mg/mL & 5 mg/mL | No precipitate or change in color or turbidity within 4 hours. |
| Morphine Sulfate | Y | Dextrose 5% | 1.2 mg/mL & 1 mg/mL | No precipitate or change in color or turbidity within 4 hours. |
| Nalbuphine Hydrochloride | Y | Dextrose 5% | 1.2 mg/mL & 10 mg/mL | No precipitate or change in color or turbidity within 4 hours. |
| Ondansetron Hydrochloride | Y | Dextrose 5% | 1.2 mg/mL & 0.5 mg/mL | No precipitate or change in color or turbidity within 4 hours. |
| Pentostatin | Y | Dextrose 5% & Sodium Chloride 0.9% | 1.2 mg/mL & 0.4 mg/mL | No precipitate or change in color or turbidity within 4 hours. |
| Potassium Chloride | Y | Dextrose 5% | 1.2 mg/mL & 0.1 mEq/L | No precipitate or change in color or turbidity within 4 hours. |
| Prochlorperazine Edisylate | Y | Dextrose 5% | 1.2 mg/mL & 0.5 mg/mL | No precipitate, color change, or gas production within 4 hours. |
| Ranitidine Hydrochloride | Y | Dextrose 5% | 1.2 mg/mL & 2 mg/mL | No precipitate, color change, or gas production within 4 hours. |
| Sodium Bicarbonate | Y | Dextrose 5% | 1.2 mg/mL & 1 mg/mL | No precipitate or change in color or turbidity within 4 hours. |
| Vancomycin Hydrochloride | Y | Dextrose 5% | 1.2 mg/mL & 10 mg/mL | No precipitate, color change, or gas production within 4 hours. |
| Zidovudine | Y | Dextrose 5% | 1.2 mg/mL & 4 mg/mL | No precipitate or change in color or turbidity within 4 hours. |
| *Pentostatin* Ondansetron Hydrochloride | Y | Sodium Chloride 0.9% | 0.4 mg/mL & 1 mg/mL | Physically compatible for 4 hours at 22°C in fluorescent light. |
| Sargramostim | Y | Sodium Chloride 0.9% | 0.4 mg/mL & 10 µg/mL | Physically compatible for 4 hours at 22°C in fluorescent light. |

*(continued)*

## Appendix 2. Cancer Chemotherapy Agents Compatibility Chart (continued)

*Part B: Oncology Product with Other Products*

| Oncology Product | Other Product | Condition* | Diluting Solution | Concentration of Products | Stability and Compatibility Comments |
|---|---|---|---|---|---|
| *Sargramostin (GM-CSF)* | Acyclovir Sodium | Y | Sodium Chloride 0.9% | 10 µg/mL & 7 mg/mL | Incompatible. White precipitate at 4 hours at room temperature in fluorescent light. |
| | Amikacin Sulfate | Y | Sodium Chloride 0.9% | 10 µg/mL & 5 mg/mL | No visible precipitate at 4 hours at room temperature in fluorescent light. |
| | Aminophylline | Y | Sodium Chloride 0.9% | 10 µg/mL & 2.5 mg/mL | No visible precipitate at 4 hours at room temperature in fluorescent light. |
| | Amphotericin B | Y | Dextrose 5% | 10 µg/mL & 0.6 mg/mL | No visible precipitate at 4 hours at room temperature in fluorescent light. |
| | Amphotericin B | Y | Sodium Chloride 0.9% | 10 µg/mL & 0.6 mg/mL | Incompatible. Immediate yellow precipitate. |
| | Ampicillin Sodium | Y | Sodium Chloride 0.9% | 10 µg/mL & 20 mg/mL | Incompatible. Precipitates at 4 hours at room temperature in fluorescent light. |
| | Ampicillin Sodium/ Sulbactam Sodium | Y | Sodium Chloride 0.9% | 10 µg/mL & 20/10 mg/mL | Incompatible. Precipitates at 4 hours at room temperature in fluorescent light. |
| | Aztreonam | Y | Sodium Chloride 0.9% | 10 µg/mL & 40 mg/mL | No visible precipitate at 4 hours at room temperature in fluorescent light. |
| | Calcium Gluconate | Y | Sodium Chloride 0.9% | 10 µg/mL & 40 mg/mL | No visible precipitate at 4 hours at room temperature in fluorescent light. |
| | Cefazolin Sodium | Y | Sodium Chloride 0.9% | 10 µg/mL & 20 mg/mL | No visible precipitate at 4 hours at room temperature in fluorescent light. |
| | Cefonicid Sodium | Y | Sodium Chloride 0.9% | 10 µg/mL & 20 mg/mL | Incompatible. Visible precipitate at 4 hours at room temperature in fluorescent light. |
| | Cefoperazone Sodium | Y | Sodium Chloride 0.9% | 10 µg/mL & 40 mg/mL | Incompatible. Slight haze forms immediately at room temperature in fluorescent light. |
| | Ceforanide | Y | Sodium Chloride 0.9% | 10 µg/mL & 20 mg/mL | No visible precipitate at 4 hours at room temperature in fluorescent light. |
| | Cefotaxime Sodium | Y | Sodium Chloride 0.9% | 10 µg/mL & 20 mg/mL | No visible precipitate at 4 hours at room temperature in fluorescent light. |
| | Cefotetan Disodium | Y | Sodium Chloride 0.9% | 10 µg/mL & 20 mg/mL | No visible precipitate at 4 hours at room temperature in fluorescent light. |
| | Ceftazidime | Y | Sodium Chloride 0.9% | 10 µg/mL & 40 mg/mL | Incompatible. Large visible particle at 4 hours at room temperature in fluorescent light. |
| | Ceftriaxone Sodium | Y | Sodium Chloride 0.9% | 10 µg/mL & 20 mg/mL | No visible precipitate at 4 hours at room temperature in fluorescent light. |
| | Cefuroxime Sodium | Y | Sodium Chloride 0.9% | 10 µg/mL & 30 mg/mL | No visible precipitate at 4 hours at room temperature in fluorescent light. |

| Chlorpromazine Hydrochloride | Y | Sodium Chloride 0.9% | 10 µg/mL & 2 mg/mL | Incompatible. Slight haze forms immediately at room temperature in fluorescent light. |
|---|---|---|---|---|
| Clindamycin Phosphate | Y | Sodium Chloride 0.9% | 10 µg/mL & 10 mg/mL | No visible precipitate at 4 hours at room temperature in fluorescent light. |
| Dexamethasone Sodium Phosphate | Y | Sodium Chloride 0.9% | 10 µg/mL & 1 mg/mL | No visible precipitate at 4 hours at room temperature in fluorescent light. |
| Diphenhydramine Hydrochloride | Y | Sodium Chloride 0.9% | 10 µg/mL & 1 mg/mL | No visible precipitate at 4 hours at room temperature in fluorescent light. |
| Doxycycline Hyclate | Y | Sodium Chloride 0.9% | 10 µg/mL & 1 mg/mL | No visible precipitate at 4 hours at room temperature in fluorescent light. |
| Droperidol | Y | Sodium Chloride 0.9% | 10 µg/mL & 0.4 mg/mL | No visible precipitate at 4 hours at room temperature in fluorescent light. |
| Famotidine | Y | Sodium Chloride 0.9% | 10 µg/mL & 2 mg/mL | No visible precipitate at 4 hours at room temperature in fluorescent light. |
| Fluconazole | Y | Sodium Chloride 0.9% | 10 µg/mL & 2 mg/mL | No visible precipitate at 4 hours at room temperature in fluorescent light. |
| Furosemide | Y | Sodium Chloride 0.9% | 10 µg/mL & 3 mg/mL | No visible precipitate at 4 hours at room temperature in fluorescent light. |
| Ganciclovir Sodium | Y | Sodium Chloride 0.9% | 10 µg/mL & 20 mg/mL | Incompatible. Fine precipitate at 4 hours at room temperature in fluorescent light. |
| Gentamicin Sulfate | Y | Sodium Chloride 0.9% | 10 µg/mL & 5 mg/mL | No visible precipitate at 4 hours at room temperature in fluorescent light. |
| Haloperidol Lactate | Y | Sodium Chloride 0.9% | 10 µg/mL & 0.2 mg/mL | Incompatible. Fine precipitate at 4 hours at room temperature in fluorescent light. |
| Heparin Sodium | Y | Sodium Chloride 0.9% | 10 µg/mL & 100 units/mL | No visible precipitate at 4 hours at room temperature in fluorescent light. |
| Hydrocortisone Sodium Phosphate | Y | Sodium Chloride 0.9% | 10 µg/mL & 1 mg/mL | Incompatible. Visible filamentous particle at 4 hours at room temperature in fluorescent light. |
| Hydrocortisone Sodium Succinate | Y | Sodium Chloride 0.9% | 10 µg/mL & 1 mg/mL | Incompatible. Visible particles within 1 hour at room temperature in fluorescent light. |
| Hydromorphone Hydrochloride | Y | Sodium Chloride 0.9% | 10 µg/mL & 0.5 mg/mL | Incompatible. Visible particles within 30 minutes at room temperature in fluorescent light. |
| Hydroxyzine Hydrochloride | Y | Sodium Chloride 0.9% | 10 µg/mL & 4 mg/mL | Incompatible. Haze and particles within 4 hours at room temperature in fluorescent light. |
| Imipenem-Cilastatin Sodium | Y | Sodium Chloride 0.9% | 10 µg/mL & 5 mg/mL | Incompatible. Visible precipitate within 4 hours at room temperature in fluorescent light. |
| Lorazepam | Y | Sodium Chloride 0.9% | 10 µg/mL & 0.1 mg/mL | Incompatible. Bluish haze forms within 1 hour at room temperature in fluorescent light. |
| Magnesium Sulfate | Y | Sodium Chloride 0.9% | 10 µg/mL & 100 mg/mL | No visible precipitate at 4 hours at room temperature in fluorescent light. |

(continued)

## Appendix 2. Cancer Chemotherapy Agents Compatibility Chart *(continued)*

*Part B: Oncology Product with Other Products*

| Oncology Product | Other Product | Condition* | Diluting Solution | Concentration of Products | Stability and Compatibility Comments |
|---|---|---|---|---|---|
| *Sargramostim (GM-CSF) (continued)* | Mannitol | Y | Sodium Chloride 0.9% | 10 µg/mL & 150 mg/mL | No visible precipitate at 4 hours at room temperature in fluorescent light. |
| | Meperidine Hydrochloride | Y | Sodium Chloride 0.9% | 10 µg/mL & 4 mg/mL | No visible precipitate at 4 hours at room temperature in fluorescent light. |
| | Mesna | Y | Sodium Chloride 0.9% | 10 µg/mL & 10 mg/mL | No visible precipitate at 4 hours at room temperature in fluorescent light. |
| | Methylprednisolone Sodium Succinate | Y | Sodium Chloride 0.9% | 10 µg/mL & 5 mg/mL | Incompatible. Visible particles within 4 hours at room temperature in fluorescent light. |
| | Metoclopramide Hydrochloride | Y | Sodium Chloride 0.9% | 10 µg/mL & 5 mg/mL | No visible precipitate at 4 hours at room temperature in fluorescent light. |
| | Metronidazole | Y | Sodium Chloride 0.9% | 10 µg/mL & 5 mg/mL | No visible precipitate at 4 hours at room temperature in fluorescent light. |
| | Mezlocillin Sodium | Y | Sodium Chloride 0.9% | 10 µg/mL & 40 mg/mL | No visible precipitate at 4 hours at room temperature in fluorescent light. |
| | Miconazole | Y | Sodium Chloride 0.9% | 10 µg/mL & 3.5 mg/mL | No visible precipitate at 4 hours at room temperature in fluorescent light. |
| | Minocycline Hydrochloride | Y | Sodium Chloride 0.9% | 10 µg/mL & 0.2 mg/mL | No visible precipitate at 4 hours at room temperature in fluorescent light. |
| | Mitomycin | Y | Sodium Chloride 0.9% | 10 µg/mL & 0.5 mg/mL | Incompatible. Haze forms within 30 minutes at room temperature in fluorescent light. |
| | Morphine Sulfate | Y | Sodium Chloride 0.9% | 10 µg/mL & 1 mg/mL | Incompatible. Haze and precipitate form within 1 hour at room temperature in fluorescent light. |
| | Nalbuphine Hydrochloride | Y | Sodium Chloride 0.9% | 10 µg/mL & 40 mg/mL | Incompatible. Haze forms within 30 minutes and filaments form within 4 hours at room temperature in fluorescent light. |
| | Netilmicin Sulfate | Y | Sodium Chloride 0.9% | 10 µg/mL & 5 mg/mL | No visible precipitate at 4 hours at room temperature in fluorescent light. |
| | Ondansetron Hydrochloride | Y | Sodium Chloride 0.9% | 10 µg/mL & 0.5 mg/mL | Incompatible. Filamentous particles within 30 minutes at room temperature in fluorescent light. |
| | Piperacillin Sodium | Y | Sodium Chloride 0.9% | 10 µg/mL & 40 mg/mL | Incompatible. Precipiates at 4 hours at room temperature in fluorescent light. |
| | Potassium Chloride | Y | Sodium Chloride 0.9% | 10 µg/mL & 0.1 mEq/mL | No visible precipitate at 4 hours at room temperature in fluorescent light. |
| | Prochlorperazine | Y | Sodium Chloride 0.9% | 10 µg/mL & 0.5 mg/mL | No visible precipitate at 4 hours at room temperature in fluorescent light. |
| | Promethazine Hydrochloride | Y | Sodium Chloride 0.9% | 10 µg/mL & 2 mg/mL | No visible precipitate at 4 hours at room temperature in fluorescent light. |

| Drug | | Solution | Concentration | Comments |
|---|---|---|---|---|
| Ranitidine Hydrochloride | Y | Sodium Chloride 0.9% | 10 µg/mL & 2 mg/mL | No visible precipitate at 4 hours at room temperature in fluorescent light. |
| Sodium Bicarbonate | Y | Sodium Chloride 0.9% | 10 µg/mL & 1 mEq/mL | Incompatible. Precipitates at 4 hours at room temperature in fluorescent light. |
| Tetracycline Hydrochloride | Y | Sodium Chloride 0.9% | 10 µg/mL & 2.5 mg/mL | No visible precipitate at 4 hours at room temperature in fluorescent light. |
| Ticarcillin Disodium | Y | Sodium Chloride 0.9% | 10 µg/mL & 30 mg/mL | No visible precipitate at 4 hours at room temperature in fluorescent light. |
| Ticarcillin Disodium/ Clavulanate Potassium | Y | Sodium Chloride 0.9% | 10 µg/mL & 31 mg/mL | No visible precipitate at 4 hours at room temperature in fluorescent light. |
| Tobramycin Sulfate | Y | Sodium Chloride 0.9% | 10 µg/mL & 5 mg/mL | Incompatible. Precipitate and filaments form at 4 hours at room temperature in fluorescent light. |
| Trimethoprim/ Sulfamethoxazole | Y | Sodium Chloride 0.9% | 10 µg/mL & 0.8/4 mg/mL | No visible precipitate at 4 hours at room temperature in fluorescent light. |
| Vancomycin Hydrochloride | Y | Sodium Chloride 0.9% | 10 µg/mL & 10 mg/mL | No visible precipitate at 4 hours at room temperature in fluorescent light. |
| Zidovudine | Y | Sodium Chloride 0.9% | 10 µg/mL & 4 mg/mL | No visible precipitate at 4 hours at room temperature in fluorescent light. |
| *Vinblastine* | | | | |
| Droperidol | Y | Not applicable | 1 mg/mL & 2.5 mg/mL | No visible precipitate after sequential injection. |
| Furosemide | A | See manufacturer's package inserts | 1 mg/mL & 10 mg/mL | Incompatible. Precipitates. |
| Furosemide | Y | Not applicable | 1 mg/mL & 10 mg/mL | Incompatible. Precipitates immediately. |
| Heparin Sodium | A | Sodium Chloride 0.9% | 1 mg/mL & 200 units/mL | Unstable. Drug decomposes within 24 hours at 37°C. |
| Heparin Sodium | Y | Not applicable | 1 mg/mL & 1,000 units/mL | No visible precipitate after sequential injection. |
| Leucovorin Calcium | Y | Not applicable | 1 mg/mL & 10 mg/mL | No visible precipitate after sequential injection. |
| Metoclopramide Hydrochloride | Y | Not applicable | 1 mg/mL & 5 mg/mL | No visible precipitate after sequential injection. |
| Metoclopramide Hydrocloride | A | See manufacturer's package inserts | 9.5 mg & 10–160 mg | Physically compatible for 48 hours at 25°C. |
| Ondansetron Hydrochloride | Y | Dextrose 5% & Sodium Chloride 0.9% | 0.12 mg/mL & 1 mg/mL | Physically compatible for 4 hours at 22°C in fluorescent light. |
| Sargramostim | Y | Sodium Chloride 0.9% | 0.12 mg/mL & 10 µg/mL | Physically compatible for 4 hours at 22°C in fluorescent light. |

*(continued)*

## Appendix 2. Cancer Chemotherapy Agents Compatibility Chart *(continued)*

*Part B: Oncology Product with Other Products*

| Oncology Product | Other Product | Condition* | Diluting Solution | Concentration of Products | Stability and Compatibility Comments |
|---|---|---|---|---|---|
| *Vincristine* | Droperidol | Y | Not applicable | 1 mg/mL & 2.5 mg/mL | No visible precipitate after sequential injection. |
| | Furosemide | A | See manufacturer's package inserts | 1 mg/mL & 10 mg/mL | Incompatible. Precipitates. |
| | Furosemide | Y | Not applicable | 1 mg/mL & 10 mg/mL | Incompatible. Precipitates immediately. |
| | Heparin Sodium | Y | Not applicable | 1 mg/mL & 1,000 units/mL | No visible precipitate after sequential injection. |
| | Leucovorin Calcium | Y | Not applicable | 1 mg/mL & 10 mg/mL | No visible precipitate after sequential injection. |
| | Metoclopramide Hydrochloride | A | See manufacturer's package inserts | 2.4 mg & 10–160 mg | Physically compatible for 48 hours at 25°C. |
| | Metoclopramide Hydrochloride | Y | Not applicable | 5 mg/mL & 1 mg/mL | No visible precipitate after sequential injection. |
| | Ondansetron Hydrochloride | Y | Dextrose 5% & Sodium Chloride 0.9% | 0.05 mg/mL & 1 mg/mL | Physically compatible for 4 hours at 22°C in fluorescent light. |
| | Sargramostim | Y | Sodium Chloride 0.9% | 0.05 mg/mL & 10 µg/mL | Physically compatible for 4 hours at 22°C in fluorescent light. |

*Source:* Chiron Therapeutics. Reprinted with permission.

## Appendix 3.   Nomograms for Determination of BSA from Height and Weight (Adults)*

| Height | Body surface area | Weight |
|---|---|---|
| cm 200 — 79 in | 2.80 m² | kg 150 — 330 lb |
| 78 | | 145 — 320 |
| 195 — 77 | 2.70 | 140 — 310 |
| 76 | | 135 — 300 |
| 190 — 75 | 2.60 | 130 — 290 |
| 74 | | |
| 185 — 73 | 2.50 | 125 — 280 |
| 72 | 2.40 | 120 — 270 |
| 180 — 71 | | — 260 |
| 70 | 2.30 | 115 — 250 |
| 175 — 69 | 2.20 | 110 — 240 |
| 68 | | 105 — 230 |
| 170 — 67 | 2.10 | 100 — 220 |
| 66 | | |
| 165 — 65 | 2.00 | 95 — 210 |
| 64 | 1.95 | 90 — 200 |
| 160 — 63 | 1.90 | |
| 62 | 1.85 | 85 — 190 |
| 155 — 61 | 1.80 | 80 — 180 |
| 60 | 1.75 | |
| 150 — 59 | 1.70 | 75 — 170 |
| 58 | 1.65 | — 160 |
| 145 — 57 | 1.60 | 70 — 150 |
| 56 | 1.55 | |
| 140 — 55 | 1.50 | 65 — 140 |
| 54 | 1.45 | 60 — 130 |
| 135 — 53 | 1.40 | |
| 52 | 1.35 | 55 — 120 |
| 130 — 51 | 1.30 | |
| 50 | | 50 — 110 |
| 125 — 49 | 1.25 | — 105 |
| 48 | 1.20 | 45 — 100 |
| 120 — 47 | 1.15 | — 95 |
| 46 | 1.10 | — 90 |
| 115 — 45 | 1.05 | 40 — 85 |
| 44 | 1.00 | — 80 |
| 110 — 43 | | 35 — 75 |
| 42 | 0.95 | — 70 |
| 105 — 41 | 0.90 | |
| 40 | | |
| cm 100 — 39 in | 0.86 m² | kg 30 — 66 lb |

*From the formula of DuBois and DuBois. *Arch. micrn. Med.* 17.863 (1916): $S = W^{0.696} \times H^{0.726} \times 71.84$, or log $S = $ log $W \times 0.425 + $ log $H \times 0.725 + 1.8564$ ($S = $ body surface in square centimeters; $W = $ weight in kilograms; $H = $ height in centimeters).

The body surface area is the point of intersection on the middle scale when a straight line joins the height and weight scales (e.g., Patient A weighs 109 kg and is 171 cm tall; the patient's BSA [m²] is 2.2).

*Source:* Hubbard, S.M., and Seipp, C.A. (1982). Administration of cancer treatments: Practical guide for physicians and oncology nurses. In V.J. DeVita, Jr., S. Hellman, S.A. Rosenberg (eds.): *Cancer Principles and Practices of Oncology*. Philadelphia: Lippincott, 1985.

# Appendix 4. Table of Standard Body Weights (Pounds & Kilograms)

*Men*

| Height | | Age | | | | | | | | | | | | |
| Feet | Inches | 25-29 | | 30-34 | | 35-39 | | 40-44 | | 45-49 | | 50-54 | | 55 up | |
| | | Lbs. | Kgs. | Lbs. | Kgs. | Lbs. | Kgs. | Lbs. | Kgs. | Lbs. | Kgs. | Lbs. | Kgs. | Lbs. | Kgs. |
| 4 | 11 | 122 | 55.5 | 125 | 56.8 | 127 | 57.7 | 130 | 59.1 | 132 | 60.0 | 133 | 60.5 | 134 | 60.9 |
| 5 | 0 | 124 | 56.4 | 127 | 57.7 | 129 | 58.6 | 132 | 60.0 | 134 | 60.9 | 135 | 61.4 | 136 | 61.8 |
| | 1 | 126 | 57.3 | 129 | 58.6 | 131 | 59.5 | 134 | 60.9 | 136 | 61.8 | 137 | 62.3 | 138 | 62.7 |
| | 2 | 128 | 58.2 | 131 | 59.5 | 133 | 60.5 | 136 | 61.8 | 138 | 62.7 | 139 | 63.2 | 140 | 63.6 |
| | 3 | 131 | 59.6 | 134 | 60.9 | 136 | 61.8 | 139 | 63.2 | 141 | 64.1 | 142 | 64.5 | 143 | 65.0 |
| | 4 | 134 | 60.9 | 137 | 62.3 | 140 | 63.6 | 142 | 64.6 | 144 | 65.5 | 145 | 65.9 | 146 | 66.4 |
| | 5 | 138 | 62.7 | 141 | 64.1 | 144 | 65.5 | 146 | 66.4 | 148 | 67.3 | 149 | 67.7 | 150 | 68.2 |
| | 6 | 142 | 64.5 | 145 | 65.9 | 148 | 67.3 | 150 | 68.2 | 152 | 69.1 | 153 | 69.5 | 154 | 70.0 |
| | 7 | 146 | 66.4 | 149 | 67.7 | 152 | 69.1 | 154 | 70.0 | 156 | 70.9 | 157 | 71.4 | 158 | 71.8 |
| | 8 | 150 | 68.2 | 154 | 70.0 | 157 | 71.4 | 159 | 72.3 | 161 | 73.2 | 162 | 73.6 | 163 | 74.1 |
| | 9 | 154 | 70.0 | 158 | 71.8 | 162 | 73.6 | 164 | 74.6 | 166 | 75.5 | 167 | 75.9 | 168 | 76.4 |
| | 10 | 158 | 71.8 | 163 | 74.1 | 167 | 75.9 | 169 | 76.8 | 171 | 77.7 | 172 | 78.2 | 173 | 78.6 |
| | 11 | 163 | 74.1 | 168 | 76.4 | 172 | 78.2 | 175 | 79.5 | 177 | 80.5 | 178 | 80.9 | 179 | 81.4 |
| 6 | 0 | 169 | 76.8 | 174 | 79.1 | 178 | 80.9 | 181 | 82.3 | 183 | 83.2 | 184 | 83.6 | 185 | 84.1 |
| | 1 | 175 | 79.5 | 180 | 81.8 | 184 | 83.6 | 187 | 85.0 | 190 | 86.4 | 191 | 86.8 | 192 | 87.3 |
| | 2 | 181 | 82.3 | 186 | 84.5 | 191 | 86.8 | 194 | 88.2 | 197 | 89.5 | 198 | 90.0 | 199 | 90.5 |
| | 3 | 187 | 85.0 | 192 | 87.3 | 197 | 89.5 | 201 | 91.4 | 204 | 92.7 | 205 | 93.2 | 206 | 93.6 |

*Women*

| Height | | Age | | | | | | | | | | | | |
| Feet | Inches | 25-29 | | 30-34 | | 35-39 | | 40-44 | | 45-49 | | 50-54 | | 55 up | |
| | | Lbs. | Kgs. | Lbs. | Kgs. | Lbs. | Kgs. | Lbs. | Kgs. | Lbs. | Kgs. | Lbs. | Kgs. | Lbs. | Kgs. |
| 4 | 11 | 116 | 52.7 | 119 | 54.1 | 122 | 55.5 | 126 | 57.3 | 129 | 58.6 | 131 | 59.6 | 132 | 60.0 |
| 5 | 0 | 118 | 53.6 | 121 | 55.0 | 124 | 56.4 | 128 | 58.2 | 131 | 59.5 | 133 | 60.5 | 134 | 60.9 |
| | 1 | 120 | 54.5 | 123 | 55.9 | 126 | 57.3 | 130 | 59.1 | 133 | 60.5 | 135 | 61.4 | 137 | 62.3 |
| | 2 | 122 | 55.5 | 125 | 56.8 | 129 | 58.6 | 133 | 60.5 | 136 | 61.8 | 138 | 62.7 | 140 | 63.6 |
| | 3 | 125 | 56.8 | 128 | 58.2 | 132 | 60.0 | 136 | 61.8 | 139 | 63.2 | 141 | 64.1 | 143 | 65.0 |
| | 4 | 129 | 58.6 | 132 | 60.0 | 136 | 61.7 | 139 | 63.2 | 142 | 64.5 | 144 | 65.5 | 146 | 66.4 |
| | 5 | 132 | 60.0 | 136 | 61.8 | 140 | 63.6 | 143 | 65.0 | 146 | 66.4 | 148 | 67.3 | 150 | 68.2 |
| | 6 | 136 | 61.8 | 140 | 63.8 | 144 | 65.5 | 147 | 66.8 | 151 | 68.6 | 152 | 69.1 | 153 | 69.6 |
| | 7 | 140 | 63.6 | 144 | 65.5 | 148 | 67.3 | 151 | 68.6 | 155 | 70.5 | 157 | 71.4 | 158 | 71.8 |
| | 8 | 144 | 65.5 | 148 | 67.3 | 152 | 69.1 | 155 | 70.5 | 159 | 72.3 | 162 | 73.6 | 163 | 74.1 |
| | 9 | 148 | 67.3 | 152 | 69.1 | 156 | 70.9 | 159 | 72.3 | 163 | 74.1 | 166 | 75.5 | 167 | 75.9 |
| | 10 | 152 | 69.1 | 155 | 70.5 | 159 | 72.3 | 162 | 73.6 | 166 | 75.5 | 170 | 77.3 | 173 | 78.6 |
| | 11 | 155 | 70.5 | 158 | 71.8 | 162 | 73.6 | 166 | 75.5 | 170 | 77.3 | 174 | 79.1 | 177 | 80.5 |
| 6 | 0 | 159 | 72.3 | 162 | 73.6 | 165 | 75.0 | 169 | 76.8 | 173 | 78.6 | 177 | 80.5 | 182 | 82.7 |

Occasionally drug doses are calculated on the basis of a person's standard or ideal body weight. Determine the patient's standard weight from above, and compare this with the patient's actual weight. Whichever of these two numbers is lower should be used to determine the patient's dosage.

*Source:* Barton-Burke, M., Wilkes, G., and Ingwersen, K. (1996). *Cancer Chemotherapy: A Nursing Process Approach.* 2nd ed. Sudbury, Mass.: Jones & Bartlett Publishers, 678.

# Appendix 5.  Nomograms for Determination of BSA from Height and Weight (Children)

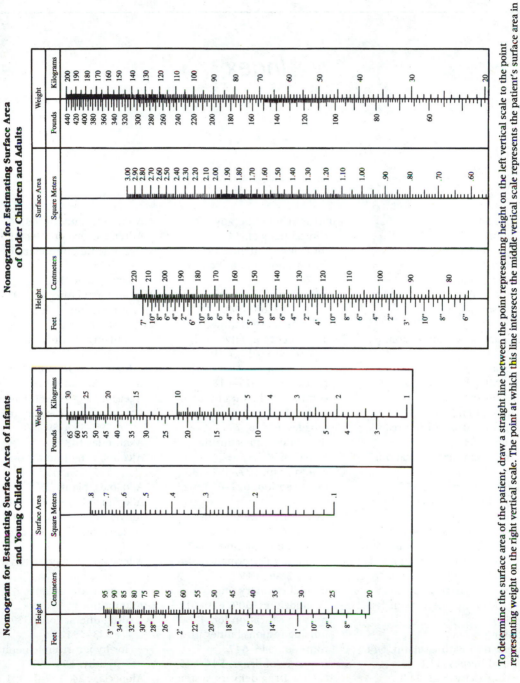

**Nomogram for Estimating Surface Area of Infants and Young Children**

**Nomogram for Estimating Surface Area of Older Children and Adults**

To determine the surface area of the patient, draw a straight line between the point representing height on the left vertical scale to the point representing weight on the right vertical scale. The point at which this line intersects the middle vertical scale represents the patient's surface area in square meters.

*Source:* Barton-Burke, M., Wilkes, G., and Ingwersen, K. (1996). *Cancer Chemotherapy: A Nursing Process Approach.* 2nd ed. Sudbury, Mass.: Jones & Bartlett Publishers, 679.

# Index